Brain Aging: Neurodegeneration and Therapeutic Interventions

Brain Aging: Neurodegeneration and Therapeutic Interventions

Edited by Isla Pearson

STATES
ACADEMIC PRESS
www.statesacademicpress.com

States Academic Press,
109 South 5th Street,
Brooklyn, NY 11249, USA

Visit us on the World Wide Web at:
www.statesacademicpress.com

ISBN: 978-1-63989-085-9

Cataloging-in-Publication Data

Brain aging : neurodegeneration and therapeutic interventions / edited by Isla Pearson.
p. cm.
Includes bibliographical references and index.
ISBN 978-1-63989-085-9
1. Brain--Aging. 2. Brain--Diseases--Age factors. 3. Nervous system--Degeneration.
4. Brain--Aging--Treatment. I. Pearson, Isla.

RC451.4.A5 B73 2022
618.976 89--dc23

Table of Contents

Preface

In my initial years as a student, I used to run to the library at every possible instance to grab a book and learn something new. Books were my primary source of knowledge and I would not have come such a long way without all that I learnt from them. Thus, when I was approached to edit this book; I became understandably nostalgic. It was an absolute honor to be considered worthy of guiding the current generation as well as those to come. I put all my knowledge and hard work into making this book most beneficial for its readers.

Aging causes changes in all the parts of the body including the brain. The size, vasculature and cognition of brain change with age. It causes changes at all levels, from molecules to morphology. Brain shrinks and incidence of stroke, dementia and white matter lesions increase with advancing age. There are changes in the levels of hormones and neurotransmitters. Regular exercise, low alcohol intake and a healthy diet are a few protective measures that reduce cardiovascular risk as well as aid the aging brain. The changes in the brain are not uniform in all regions. Another factor that affects the aging of brain and its cognitive performance is hormonal influence. Aging is one of the most important risk factors for neurodegenerative diseases such as Alzheimer's and Parkinson's disease. This book provides significant information of this discipline to help develop a good understanding of brain aging. The topics covered herein deal with the therapeutic interventions in brain aging. This book will prove to be immensely beneficial to students and researchers in this field.

I wish to thank my publisher for supporting me at every step. I would also like to thank all the authors who have contributed their researches in this book. I hope this book will be a valuable contribution to the progress of the field.

Editor

1

Implications of Mitochondrial Dynamics on Neurodegeneration and on Hypothalamic Dysfunction

Antonio Zorzano [1,2,3*] *and Marc Claret* [3,4*]

[1] *Molecular Medicine Program, Institute of Research in Biomedicine (IRB Barcelona), Barcelona, Spain,* [2] *Departament de Bioquímica i Biologia Molecular, Facultat de Biologia, Universitat de Barcelona, Barcelona, Spain,* [3] *CIBER de Diabetes y Enfermedades Metabólicas Asociadas, Instituto de Salud Carlos III, Barcelona, Spain,* [4] *Diabetes and Obesity Research Laboratory, Institut d'Investigacions Biomèdiques August Pi i Sunyer, Barcelona, Spain*

Edited by:
Enrique Cadenas,
University of Southern California, USA

Reviewed by:
Juan P. Bolanos,
University of Salamanca-CSIC, Spain
Catarina Oliveira,
University of Coimbra, Portugal

***Correspondence:**
Antonio Zorzano,
Molecular Medicine Program, Institute of Research in Biomedicine (IRB Barcelona), C/Baldiri Reixac 10, 08028 Barcelona, Spain
antonio.zorzano@irbbarcelona.org;
Marc Claret,
Diabetes and Obesity Research Laboratory, Institut d'Investigacions Biomèdiques August Pi i Sunyer, Centre Esther Koplowitz, C/Rosselló 149-153, 5th floor, 08036 Barcelona, Spain
mclaret@clinic.ub.es

Mitochondrial dynamics is a term that encompasses the movement of mitochondria along the cytoskeleton, regulation of their architecture, and connectivity mediated by tethering and fusion/fission. The importance of these events in cell physiology and pathology has been partially unraveled with the identification of the genes responsible for the catalysis of mitochondrial fusion and fission. Mutations in two mitochondrial fusion genes (*MFN2* and *OPA1*) cause neurodegenerative diseases, namely Charcot-Marie Tooth type 2A and autosomal dominant optic atrophy (ADOA). Alterations in mitochondrial dynamics may be involved in the pathophysiology of prevalent neurodegenerative conditions. Moreover, impairment of the activity of mitochondrial fusion proteins dysregulates the function of hypothalamic neurons, leading to alterations in food intake and in energy homeostasis. Here we review selected findings in the field of mitochondrial dynamics and their relevance for neurodegeneration and hypothalamic dysfunction.

Keywords: mitochondrial fission, mitochondrial fusion, mitofusin 2, obesity, food intake, neurodegenerative diseases

Introduction

Mitochondrial filaments were first reported in the mid-1800s upon the discovery of mitochondria. However, it was not until the 1990s that the improvement of mitochondrial dyes permitted the visualization of mitochondrial motion in different cellular models (Bereiter-Hahn and Voth, 1994; Nunnari et al., 1997; Cortese et al., 1998). Mitochondrial dynamics alludes to the movement of mitochondria along the cytoskeleton and also to changes in mitochondrial morphology, both parameters being controlled by fusion and fission events, which in turn lead to these organelles forming tubular or branched reticular networks.

The discovery of the first gene that participates in mitochondria fusion in *Drosophila melanogaster* came about in 1997 (Hales and Fuller, 1997). In the last years, genes that participate in mitochondrial fusion or fission have been identified (Yaffe, 1999). Although considerable advances have been made in the field of mitochondrial dynamics in recent years, the molecular elements that regulate fusion and fission remain unclear. In this regard, the physiological relevance of mitochondrial dynamics in mammals is not precisely understood, and the proteins that determine differences in mitochondrial morphology among distinct cell types need to be clarified.

Mitochondrial dynamics is required to facilitate inter-mitochondrial complementation, and it also participates in ensuring that mitochondria undergo maximal hyperfusion under conditions of cellular stress (Chen and Chan, 2005; Tondera et al., 2009). The fragmentation of mitochondria is also crucial in order for these organelles to undergo mitophagy (Twig et al., 2008), and balanced mitochondrial dynamics is key to the maintenance of an appropriate cell metabolism (Bach et al., 2003; Sebastian et al., 2012).

Major Processes and Proteins Involved in Mitochondrial Dynamics

Here we will review the proteins that participate in mitochondrial fusion and mitochondrial fission.

The Mitochondrial Fusion Machinery

Mitochondrial compartmentalization is ensured by fusion of the inner and outer mitochondrial membranes (Meeusen et al., 2004). The main proteins involved in this process are the outer membrane GTPases Mitofusins (Mfn1 and Mfn2) (Chen et al., 2003; Ishihara et al., 2004) and the inner membrane GTPase Optic atrophy 1 (OPA1) (Cipolat et al., 2004; Ishihara et al., 2006).

Mfn1 and Mfn2 are integral outer mitochondrial membrane proteins and modulate mitochondrial morphology by promoting mitochondria tethering and fusion (Koshiba et al., 2004). The functions of Mfn1 and Mfn2 seems to overlap, since Mfn1 partially rescues the defects caused by Mfn2 mutation (Detmer and Chan, 2007). *Mfn1* and *Mfn2* genes are widely expressed. Mfn1 gene expression is high in heart and is expressed at lower level in other human tissues. Mfn2 transcripts are abundant in heart and skeletal muscle and present at lower levels in other tissues (Santel et al., 2003).

Mfn1 shows two transmembrane domains at the C-terminus of the protein, near a heptad-repeat (HR) domain (Santel et al., 2003). The N-terminal region of Mfn1 contains a GTP-binding domain followed by a heptad-repeat domain (HR1) (Santel et al., 2003; Koshiba et al., 2004). The C-terminal HR domain is considered to mediate the first step of mitochondrial fusion, which consists of the tethering of two adjacent mitochondria through the formation of a dimeric antiparallel coiled-coil structure (Koshiba et al., 2004). These dimeric structures can be homotypic (Mfn1-Mfn1 or Mfn2-Mfn2) or heterotypic (Mfn1-Mfn2) (Chen et al., 2003; Koshiba et al., 2004). In addition, Mfn1 shows higher GTPase activity than Mfn2 (Ishihara et al., 2004). In this respect, mitochondria containing Mfn1 show greater tethering efficiency than mitochondria with Mfn2 (Ishihara et al., 2004).

Mfn1 shows both transcriptional and post-transcriptional or post-translational regulation (Santel et al., 2003). In this regard, Mfn1 is regulated by PGC-1α during postnatal cardiac growth (Martin et al., 2014). In contrast, Mfn1 is repressed by dexamethasome in liver and in hepatoma cells (Hernandez-Alvarez et al., 2013) and by microRNA 140 in cardiomyocytes (Li et al., 2014). Regarding post-translational regulation, Mfn1 undergoes ubiquitination mediated by MARCH-V (also named MITOL) or Parkin (Gegg et al., 2010; Park et al., 2010; Tanaka et al., 2010; Park and Cho, 2012), and deacetylation and activation mediated by HDAC6 (Lee et al., 2014). Mfn1 may be regulated through binding to MIB, a member of the quinone oxidoreductase subfamily of zinc-containing alcohol dehydrogenase proteins (Eura et al., 2006), and overexpression of MIB induces mitochondrial fragmentation, whereas MIB knockdown causes enhanced mitochondrial network structures (Eura et al., 2006).

As mentioned, Mfn2 is an integral outer mitochondrial membrane protein, which exposes both terminal ends to the cytosol (Rojo et al., 2002). The N-terminal GTPase activity of Mfn2 is key for its function in mitochondrial fusion (Chen et al., 2003; Eura et al., 2003). Mfn2 is essential for embryonic development, and ablation of Mfn2 causes placental dysfunction (Chen et al., 2003). Mfn2 exerts a key role in brain, and protects against neurodegeneration in the cerebellum (Chen et al., 2007) as well as in dopaminergic neurons (Lee et al., 2012; Pham et al., 2012). In addition, Mfn2 repression in neurons leads to a delayed cell death upon excitotoxicity (Martorell-Riera et al., 2014). Mfn2 has been proposed to regulate cell proliferation and mitochondrial metabolism (Bach et al., 2003; Chen et al., 2004a, 2014; Pich et al., 2005). In addition, this protein promotes insulin signaling, and deficiency in muscle or liver causes impaired insulin signaling caused by excessive JNK activity and phosphorylation of IRS proteins at serine residues—the latter inhibiting the capacity to activate PI-3 kinase and downstream elements of the pathway (Sebastian et al., 2012). Whether Mfn2 modulates insulin signaling in other tissues such as brain, remains unknown.

The transcription factor Sp1 binds to and drives Mfn2 gene transcription both in skeletal muscle and in smooth muscle cells (Sorianello et al., 2012). The transcription factor Estrogen-Related Receptor-alpha (ERRα) also binds to the human Mfn2 promoter and stimulates transcription (Soriano et al., 2006). The transcription of Mfn2 is stimulated by the coactivators PGC-1α and PGC-1β—key factors in mitochondrial biogenesis (Scarpulla et al., 2012)— through physical/functional interaction with ERRα (Soriano et al., 2006; Liesa et al., 2008). Thus, PGC-1α or PGC1β overexpression induces Mfn2 in cells (Soriano et al., 2006; Liesa et al., 2008). PGC-1β is also necessary for the maintenance of Mfn2 in tissues, and PGC-1β KO mice show reduced Mfn2 in metabolically-relevant tissues (Liesa et al., 2008). In keeping with this, PGC-1β influences mitochondrial morphology through the promotion of mitochondrial elongation, and enhanced mitochondrial fusion (Liesa et al., 2008). Interestingly. overexpression of PGC-1β causes mitochondrial elongation in wild-type, and in Mfn1 KO MEF cells. However, such overexpression does not cause mitochondrial elongation in Mfn2 KO MEF cells (Liesa et al., 2008), which suggests that Mfn2 is required for the effects of PGC-1βon mitochondrial morphology. These data are also consistent with the reduced mitochondrial volume, independent of changes in mitochondrial number, detected in muscle from PGC-1β KO mice (Lelliott et al., 2006; Liesa et al., 2008). Based on all those evidences, Mfn2 undergoes transcriptional regulation.

In addition to this mechanism of control, Mfn2 is regulateded by proteasomal degradation. In this respect, Mfn2 undergoes ubiquitination catalyzed by Parkin (Gegg et al., 2010; Poole et al., 2010; Tanaka et al., 2010; Ziviani et al., 2010). Mfn2 is also ubiquitinated by the E3 ubiquitin ligases HUWE1, regulated by phosphorylation of JNK, and by the ubiquitin ligase Mul1 (Leboucher et al., 2012; Lokireddy et al., 2012). The processes of Mfn2 ubiquitination lead to Mfn2 degradation. The ubiquitin ligase MARCH-V (or MITOL) catalyzes lysine-63-linked polyubiquitination of Mfn2 but does not drive its proteasomal degradation (Sugiura et al., 2013). Mfn2 levels are also regulated by activation of the deubiquitinase USP30 (Yue et al., 2014).

Optic atrophy gene 1 (OPA1) is also a dynamin-related protein with GTPase activity. This protein is located in the intermembrane space, in the inner mitochondrial membrane and in the cristae volume (Misaka et al., 2002; Olichon et al., 2002; Satoh et al., 2003). OPA1 is essential for mitochondrial fusion (Cipolat et al., 2004; Chen et al., 2005). OPA1 shows high expression in brain, retina, liver, heart, skeletal muscle, and testis (Delettre et al., 2001; Cipolat et al., 2004). OPA1 maintains the normal structure of the optic nerve (Davies et al., 2007), and its deficiency causes alterations in the dendritic morphology of retinal ganglion cells (Williams et al., 2010). In addition, OPA1 promotes neuronal survival following excitotoxicity (Jahani-Asl et al., 2011).

Various OPA1 isoforms have been identified (Olichon et al., 2003; Cipolat et al., 2004; Griparic et al., 2004; Ishihara et al., 2006). The existence of multiple OPA1 isoforms and cleavage mechanisms may explain the role of this protein beyond mitochondrial inner membrane fusion, such as in cristae remodeling, supercomplex formation, and in the regulation of the selective fusion that determines mitochondrial autophagy (Frezza et al., 2006; Twig et al., 2008; Cogliati et al., 2013). OPA1 isoforms are generated from a single gene through alternative splicing and proteolysis. OPA1 isoforms are named as long and short on the basis of their electrophoretic mobility (Delettre et al., 2001; Olichon et al., 2007; Akepati et al., 2008). Both short and long forms are required for mitochondrial fusion, and thus constitutive OPA1 cleavage is required for efficient mitochondrial fusion (Song et al., 2007; DeVay et al., 2009). Some long OPA1 isoforms are constitutively cleaved by the intermembrane space AAA protease YME1L (Griparic et al., 2007; Song et al., 2007). The cleavage of OPA1 is also induced by mitochondrial depolarization, which reduces the abundance of long isoforms, increases the short OPA1 isoforms, and reduces mitochondrial fusion. This inducible OPA1 cleavage is also activated by ATP deficiency and by apoptosis (Baricault et al., 2007; Griparic et al., 2007) and it is catalyzed by the zinc metalloprotease OMA1 (Ehses et al., 2009; Head et al., 2009; Quiros et al., 2012). In this respect, OMA1 ablation causes a deficient mitochondrial activity and function in brown adipose tissue, and obesity (Quiros et al., 2012).

The Mitochondrial Fission Machinery

Mitochondrial fission describes the fragmentation of a mitochondrion into two. This process is necessary to drive damaged mitochondria through mitophagy (Kim et al., 2007), to pass mitochondria to daughter cells during mitosis, and to regulate apoptosis (Lee et al., 2004). Alterations in fission machinery increase the generation of reactive oxygen species (ROS) and lead to a heterogeneous population of mitochondria with non-uniform mitochondrial DNA distribution (Parone et al., 2008).

Dynamin-related protein 1 (Drp1) plays a key role in the catalysis of mitochondrial fission. Drp1 is a cytosolic protein that is recruited to the outer mitochondrial membrane, where it catalyzes mitochondrial division. Drp1 interacts with the mitochondrial proteins fission protein 1 homolog (Fis1), the mitochondrial fission factor (Mff), MiD49, and MiD51.

Drp1 is found mainly in the cytosol and, as a member of the dynamin protein family, it contains a GTPase domain and a GTPase effector domain. Drp1 assembles into multimeric ring complexes at mitochondrial fission sites, which leads to constriction following GTP hydrolysis to promote division (Bleazard et al., 1999; Van Der Bliek, 1999; Legesse-Miller et al., 2003; Ingerman et al., 2005; Lackner et al., 2009; Mears et al., 2011). Given that Drp 1 lacks domains involved in membrane binding, the recruitment of this molecule at the mitochondrial outer membrane requires the involvement of membrane proteins that act as receptors (Parone et al., 2008).

Drp1 is regulated by post-translational modifications such as S-nitrosylation, sumoylation, ubiquitination, and phosphorylation of serine residues, and they may regulate its recruitment to the mitochondria. S-nitrosylation enhances the pro-fission activity of Drp1 by inducing dimerization and enhancing GTPase activity (Cho et al., 2009). Drp1 S-nitrosylation and mitochondrial fragmentation have been detected by the ß-amyloid protein (Aβ), a mediator of Alzheimer's disease (AD) (Head et al., 2009). Drp1 can be also activated by sumoylation (Wasiak et al., 2007). Thus, SUMO-1 and its conjugating enzyme Ubc9 induce mitochondrial fission by stabilizing Drp1 (Harder et al., 2004). In contrast, the sentrin/SUMO-specific protease SENP5 reduces Drp1 levels, which reduces mitochondrial fission (Zunino et al., 2009). In addition, it has been proposed that MARCH V, a mitochondrial E3 ubiquitin ligase, participates in the translocation of Drp1 to mitochondria independently of changes in stability (Karbowski et al., 2007). Phosphorylation occurs on Ser616 and Ser637 (in reference to the human Drp1 sequence). Phosphorylation of Ser616 by cyclin-dependent kinase 1 (Cdk1/cyclin B) causes Drp1 recruitment to the mitochondria (Taguchi et al., 2007). Phosphorylation of Ser637 is catalyzed by protein kinase A (PKA), Calmodulin-dependent kinase, and Pim1 (Chang and Blackstone, 2007; Cribbs and Strack, 2007), and it inhibits Drp1 function. Dephosphorylation of the Ser637 residue by the protein phosphatase calcineurin recruits Drp1 to the mitochondria and promotes fission (Cribbs and Strack, 2007; Cereghetti et al., 2008).

Drp1 ablation in mice causes embryonic lethality. Drp1 knockout embryos present alterations in liver and heart development, increased apoptosis within the deep neural cortex, and deficient synapse formation (Ishihara et al., 2009). In addition, Drp1 loss-of-function delays cytochrome c release during apoptosis, thereby suggesting that this release is linked to mitochondrial fission (Ishihara et al., 2009).

The recruitment of the Drp1 ortholog in yeast (Dnm1) from the cytosol to the outer mitochondrial membrane occurs through association with the protein Fis1, resulting in the formation of a fission complex (Mozdy et al., 2000; Legesse-Miller et al., 2003; Yoon et al., 2003; Karren et al., 2005). Mammalian Fis1 is a small ubiquitous 17.2-kDa protein found throughout the mitochondrial network. Fis1 is anchored into the outer mitochondrial membrane via its COOH terminal part, which contains an alpha-helix, a transmembrane domain, and a COOH-terminal tail exposed to the inter-membrane space. The NH2-terminal part of the protein contains four distinct regions with five alpha-helices (Suzuki et al., 2003; Dohm et al., 2004); the first alpha-helix of Fis1 has been reported to be critical for its oligomerization and fission activity (Jofuku et al., 2005). The subsequent four alpha-helices make up two tetratrico-peptide repeat peptides, which are not required for Fis1 oligomerization but they participate in the protein-protein interactions required for fission (Jofuku et al., 2005). Overexpression of Fis1 causes mitochondrial fragmentation, whereas knockdown of this protein results in the formation of a highly fused mitochondrial network, thereby indicating that Fis1 activates mitochondrial fission (Mozdy et al., 2000; Yoon et al., 2003; Stojanovski et al., 2004; Karren et al., 2005). However, the observations that Drp1 can still be recruited to the mitochondrial outer membrane following knockdown of Fis1 (Lee et al., 2004; Wasiak et al., 2007) suggest that other proteins also participate in mammalian mitochondrial fission.

Mff (Gandre-Babbe and van der Bliek, 2008; Otera et al., 2010) is anchored to the outer mitochondrial membrane and it can recruit Drp1 independently of Fis1 (Otera et al., 2010). Absent in yeast, Mff represents a more recent acquisition of the mitochondrial fission machinery that is active in mammalian cells. Mff localizes in discrete sites on mitochondria, and its overexpression causes recruitment of Drp1 to mitochondria and mitochondrial fragmentation. Conversely, Mff deficiency leads to reduced Drp1 at the mitochondrial and to mitochondrial elongation (Otera et al., 2010).

MiD49 and MiD51 proteins share 65% identity and are anchored to the mitochondrial outer membrane through their N-terminal end (Simpson et al., 2000; Palmer et al., 2011). Like Drp1, MiD49/51 form puncta and rings around mitochondria. MiD49/51 recruit Drp1 to the mitochondria, whereas their loss-of-function reduces mitochondrial Drp1 association. Co-immunoprecipitation experiments have established that MiD49 interacts with Drp1. MiD49 and MiD51 can act independently of both Mff and Fis 1 (Loson et al., 2013).

Located in the outer mitochondrial membrane, ganglioside-induced differentiation-associated protein 1 (GDAP1) has been proposed to participate in mitochondrial fission (Cassereau et al., 2011). GDAP1 gain-of-function causes mitochondrial fragmentation, while its deficiency results in mitochondrial elongation (Niemann et al., 2005). Genetic manipulation of the *Drosophila* ortholog Gdap1 also leads to changes in the size, morphology and distribution of mitochondria and in neuronal and muscular degeneration (Lopez Del Amo et al., 2015).

Interaction of the Endoplasmic Reticulum and Mitochondria: Role of Proteins Involved in Mitochondrial Dynamics

Close appositions between the endoplasmic reticulum (ER) and mitochondria or mitochondria-ER contact sites have been observed by electron microscopy in fixed samples of several cell types and are unexplainable by fixation artifacts. These regions represent the sites of phospholipid exchange between the two organelles. The close contacts through which the ER communicates with mitochondria have been biochemically purified and are referred to as the mitochondria-associated ER membrane (MAM) (Vance, 1990). The interaction between mitochondria and the ER is crucial in mediating organelle-organelle signals, such as metabolic stress or cell death cues (**Figure 1**).

Mitochondria tethering to the ER via the MAM is a dynamic process. These ER-contiguous membranes contain multiple phospholipid- and glycosphingolipid-synthesizing enzymes, including long-chain fatty acid-CoA ligase type 4 (FACL4) and phosphatidylserine synthase-1, and they support the direct transfer of lipids between the ER and mitochondria (Stone and Vance, 2000; Cardenas et al., 2010). In addition to supporting lipid transfer, MAMs also exchange Ca^{2+} ions, which regulate processes such as ER chaperone-assisted folding of newly synthesized proteins and enzymes with dehydrogenase activity (Berridge, 2002). In this regard, the truncated variant of the sarcoendoplasmic reticulum Ca^{2+}-ATPase 1 (SERCA1T) is induced during ER stress, promotes the transfer of calcium from the ER to mitochondria, and induces apoptosis (Chami et al., 2008). Nearly 30 proteins that play relevant roles in organelle homeostasis are found in this compartment. Furthermore, proteomic studies of mouse brain MAM fractions have identified about 1000 proteins localized in MAMs (Poston et al., 2013). Chaperones, ion channels, proteins of mitochondrial dynamics, and metabolic enzymes are among the molecules detected in MAMs. Thus, the chaperone GRP-75 links the outer mitochondrial membrane protein VDAC with the N-terminus of the inositol 1,4,5-trisphosphate receptor (IP3R), and GRP-75 deficiency reduces calcium transfer from the ER to mitochondria (Szabadkai et al., 2006) (**Figure 2**). Another MAM-localized protein is the Sigma-1 receptor chaperone. Sigma-1 binds GRP-78 and its overexpression counteracts the ER stress response and prevents apoptosis mediated by the release of ER calcium (Hayashi and Su, 2007). PACS2, another protein localized in MAMs, is involved in the ER-mitochondria interaction. PACS2 silencing causes mitochondria and ER fragmentation and also ER stress characterized by enhanced GRP-78 expression and reduced apoptosis (Simmen et al., 2005). The ER protein Nogo also alters the ER-mitochondria unit (Sutendra et al., 2011).

Mfn2 was initially identified as a mitochondria fusion protein. However, it also plays a critical role in maintaining ER morphology by tethering mitochondria and the ER (de Brito and Scorrano, 2008) (**Figure 3**). *Mfn2* null mouse embryonic fibroblasts (MEFs) show a fragmented ER network, and

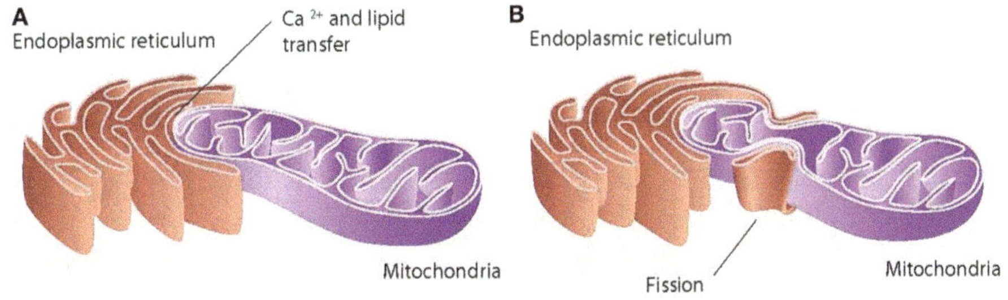

FIGURE 1 | ER–mitochondria contact sites. The ER interacts with mitochondria through close contacts that permit the transfer of calcium from the ER to mitochondria and that permit the exchange of lipids between those two organelles **(A)**. The ER also interacts with mitochondria through mitochondrial fission sites **(B)**.

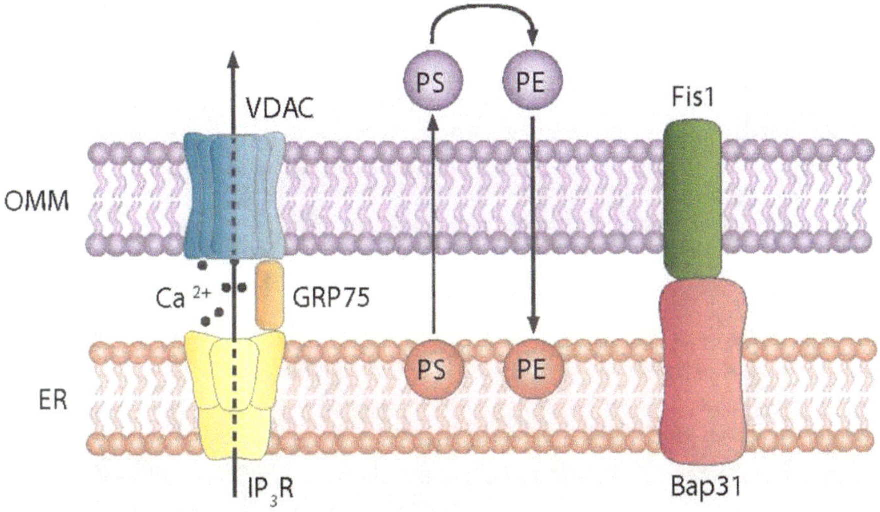

FIGURE 2 | Proteins and processes involved in the ER-mitochondria contact sites. Contact sites involve, among others, the exchange of phosphatidylserine (PS) and phosphatidylethanolamine (PE) between the ER and mitochondria and the formation of complexes between the ER and mitochondrial proteins, as shown.

the contact regions between mitochondria and the ER are significantly reduced (de Brito and Scorrano, 2008). In keeping with this view, Mfn2 loss-of-function in cells or in tissues such as muscle, liver or hypothalamus causes ER stress (Sebastian et al., 2012; Munoz et al., 2013; Schneeberger et al., 2013). Moreover, Mfn2 deficiency causes chronic activation of PERK, a process that plays a relevant role in the alterations detected under these conditions (**Figure 3**). Thus, PERK deficiency in Mfn2 null MEFs reduces ROS production, normalizes mitochondrial calcium, and improves mitochondrial morphology (Munoz et al., 2013).

Other proteins involved in mitochondrial dynamics, such as Drp1 and Fis1, are also associated with ER-mitochondria contact sites (Pitts et al., 1999; Iwasawa et al., 2011). In mammalian cells, the ER tubules contact the mitochondrial membrane at constriction sites marked by Drp1 and its receptor the Mff protein (Friedman et al., 2011). In fact, Drp1 and Mff are markers for ER-mitochondria contact sites. The ER-mitochondria contact is not disrupted by Drp1 or Mff depletion, thereby suggesting that such interactions are independent of division machinery recruitment (Friedman et al., 2011). Contact with the ER is therefore a feature of mitochondrial fission sites (**Figure 1**). This contact is also maintained after mitochondrial fission.

In all, alterations in the expression of Mfn2 lead to the disruption of ER-mitochondria communications and the ER plays a key role in the localization of mitochondrial fission sites.

Mutations in Genes Involved in Mitochondrial Dynamics Cause Neurodegenerative Disorders

In the nervous system, mitochondria are essential for energy production, calcium regulation, maintenance of plasma membrane potential, protein folding by chaperones, axonal and dendritic transport, and release and re-uptake of neurotransmitters at synapses. In the last years, mitochondrial dynamics has been reported to participate in the pathophysiology of neuronal disorders. In this respect, mutations in genes involved in mitochondrial dynamics have been shown to cause neuronal disorders.

Autosomal Dominant Optic Atrophy

Autosomal dominant optic atrophy (ADOA) has an estimated prevalence ranging from 1:12,000 to 1:50,000 and it is the most

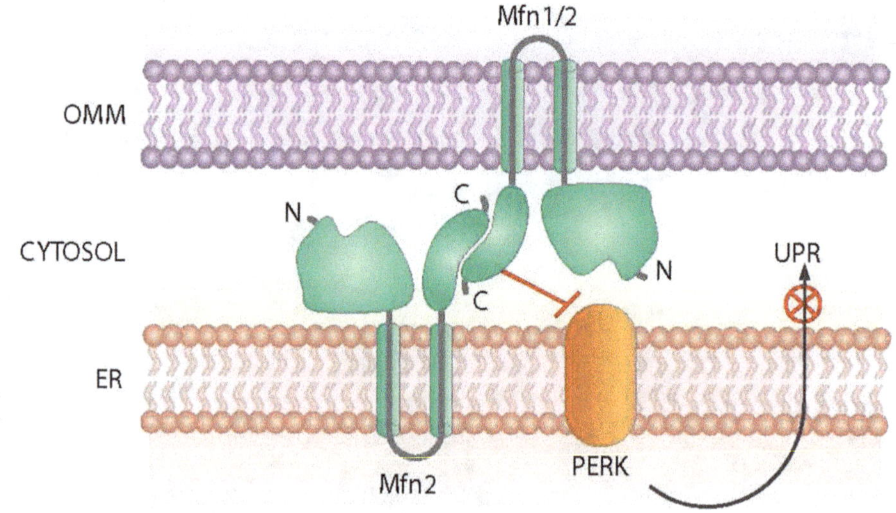

FIGURE 3 | Roles of Mfn2 on ER-mitochondria contact sites. Mfn2 participates in the tethering of mitochondria and the ER at contact sites. In addition, Mfn2 negatively regulates PERK, a protein kinase involved in the Unfolded Protein Response (UPR) and activated upon ER stress.

common form of inherited optic neuropathy. This disease is characterized by visual impairment in early childhood with moderate to severe loss of visual acuity, temporal optic disc pallor, abnormalities of color vision, and caecocentral visual field scotoma (Hoyt, 1980; Votruba et al., 1998; Johnston et al., 1999). Histopathological analysis suggests that the fundamental pathology of ADOA is a primary degeneration of retinal ganglion cells, followed by increasing atrophy of the optic nerve (Johnston et al., 1979; Kjer et al., 1983).

Most families with ADOA show pathogenic mutations in the *OPA1* gene (Olichon et al., 2006). More than 200 OPA1 gene mutations have been identified—these basically family-specific (Ferré et al., 2005). OPA1 mutations involve mainly substitutions, but also deletions and insertions (Delettre et al., 2001; Olichon et al., 2006). Near 50% of the mutations cause truncation of the OPA1 protein, and most of the mutations are detected in the GTPase domain and are thus likely to eliminate mitochondrial fusion. The pathogenesis of ADOA occurs, in most cases, as a result of haploinsufficiency (loss-of-function, Delettre et al., 2000). In this regard, OPA1 deficiency in mice induced by in-frame deletion of 27 amino acid residues in the GTPase domain or non-sense mutations causes the degeneration of retinal ganglion cells and disorganized mitochondrial cristae of optic nerve axons (Alavi et al., 2007; Davies et al., 2007). In addition to haploinsufficiency, ADOA can also develop as a result of a dominant negative mechanism (Delettre et al., 2000; Pesch et al., 2001; Baris et al., 2003; Kim et al., 2005).

Some human OPA1 mutations cause a specific form of disease, characterized by myopathy and progressive external ophtalmoplegia (Hudson et al., 2008), and has been named "OPA1 plus syndrome." This syndrome is also characterized by reduced mitochondrial DNA copy number. In keeping with this, patients with certain OPA1 mutations show multiple deletions in mitochondrial DNA in skeletal muscle (Amati-Bonneau et al., 2008; Hudson et al., 2008), and mice carrying the Opa1(delTTAG) mutation (found in 30% of all human patients with ADOA) show a multi-systemic phenotype (Sarzi et al., 2012).

Mfn2 Mutations: Charcot-Marie-Tooth Type 2A

Charcot-Marie-Tooth (CMT) disease is clinically characterized by weakness and distal muscle atrophy, predominantly of the lower extremities, and by sensory loss. CMT affects approximately 1 in 2500 individuals, thus making this condition one of the most common hereditary diseases and the most common hereditary neuropathy (Skre, 1974).

CMT2 is characterized by chronic axonal degeneration and regeneration, leading to steady loss of nerve fibers with normal or slightly reduced motor nerve conduction velocities ($\geq$38 m/s) (Dyck and Lambert, 1968). Mutations in MFN2 cause 20% of CMT2 cases (Lawson et al., 2005), and this the most prevalent axonal form of CMT. CMT2 cases show high variability in clinical symptoms. Furthermore, MFN2 mutations have been detected in CMT2 families and are associated with additional features such as spasticity (Zhu et al., 2005) and atrophy (Verhoeven et al., 2006).

Most of the MFN2 mutations found in CMT2A patients are missense (Zuchner et al., 2004; Kijima et al., 2005; Lawson et al., 2005; Zhu et al., 2005; Chung et al., 2006; Engelfried et al., 2006; Verhoeven et al., 2006). More than 50% are detected in the GTPase domain but they do not affect GTP binding (Baloh et al., 2007). In addition, MFN2 mutations have been detected in the following sites: in the NH2-terminal region; near or at the Ras-binding domain; in the vicinity of or at the HR1 region; and in the COOH terminus, specifically in the HR2 region, facing the cytoplasmic site.

The mutations of MFN2 responsible for CMT2A show autosomal dominant inheritance; consequently, they may show haploinsufficiency or a dominant gain-of-function. In keeping with this view, the overexpression of some mutant forms of MFN2 induces the aggregation of mitochondria in cultured rat dorsal root ganglion neurons and in MEFs, indicating the promotion of gain-of-function (Baloh et al., 2007; Detmer and Chan, 2007). The defective mitochondrial fusion activity of some Mfn2 mutants is rescued by Mfn1 gain-of-function, which is in keeping with the observation that Mfn1 physically associates with wild-type Mfn2 and mutant forms of CMT2A (Loiseau et al., 2007; Amiott et al., 2008).

Transgenic mice have been generated to express a mutant form of MFN2 with a presumed gain-of-function (T105M) specifically in motor neurons. These mice show a phenotype consistent with the clinical symptoms detected in CMT2A, and provide a system to determine the function of mitochondria in the axons of motor neurons (Detmer et al., 2008).

GDAP1 mutations are associated with type 4A CMT (CMT4A), the most frequently detected recessive form of CMT (Baxter et al., 2002; Cuesta et al., 2002). CMT4 is classically defined as a demyelinating form of the disease and it is associated with segmental de- and re-myelination, in contrast to CMT2, which shows axonal degeneration without demyelination (Berger et al., 2002; Suter and Scherer, 2003). However, analysis of the nerve conduction rates of subjects with GDAP1 mutations indicates that while some mutations show low nerve conduction rates (Baxter et al., 2002; Ammar et al., 2003; Senderek et al., 2003), others are characterized by normal rates (Nelis et al., 2002; Ammar et al., 2003; Boerkoel et al., 2003; De Sandre-Giovannoli et al., 2003; Sevilla et al., 2003). These data demonstrate that some of the GDAP1 mutations cause axonal loss rather than demyelinization.

Mitochondrial Dynamics and Prevalent Neurodegenerative Diseases

Both fusion and fission mechanisms participate in the mitochondrial life cycle and any disruption of their balance can alter the steady-state distribution of mitochondria. Specifically in neurons, the mitochondrial fusion/fission machinery is intimately and critically involved in the formation of synapses and dendritic spines. Thus, alterations in mitochondrial dynamics prevent these organelles from distributing to synapses, thus leading to a loss of mitochondria from dendritic spines and, consequently, to a reduction of synapse formation (Li et al., 2004). The mitochondrial dynamics proteins that control the distribution of mitochondria in dendrites also regulate the density and plasticity of synapses (Li et al., 2004). Thus, dominant-negative Drp1 or OPA1 overexpression (both of which reduce dendritic mitochondria) causes a decreased density of spines and synapses (Li et al., 2004). Consistent with this view, Drp1 ablation in mice shows developmental abnormalities, particularly in the forebrain (Ishihara et al., 2009). Given these considerations, a strong association between the expression/activity of proteins involved in mitochondrial dynamics and neurodegenerative diseases can be expected.

In this regard, brains from AD patients show fragmented and perinuclear mitochondria (Cho et al., 2009; Wang et al., 2009a), paralleled by increased expression of Fis1 and decreased expression of the fusion proteins Mfn1, Mfn2, and OPA1 (Wang et al., 2009a; Reddy et al., 2011). These data suggest that abnormal mitochondrial dynamics in neurons of AD patients may participate in the pathogenesis of the disease. In line with these observations, brains from AD patients show altered lipid metabolism (Schon and Area-Gomez, 2010), aberrant calcium homeostasis (Supnet and Bezprozvanny, 2010), enhanced unfolded protein response (UPR) (Hoozemans et al., 2005), and defects in energy metabolism (Ferreira et al., 2010). As to the factors responsible for mitochondrial dysfunction, overexpression of amyloid precursor protein (APP) or exposure to amyloid beta peptide (Abeta) induces mitochondrial fragmentation and abnormal distribution (Rui et al., 2006; Wang et al., 2008). Furthermore, exposure of neurons to oligomerized Abeta leads to S-nitrosylation of Drp1, causing mitochondrial fragmentation (Cho et al., 2009). Upregulated MAM function at the ER-mitochondrial interface and increased cross-talk between these two organelles has been reported in presenilin-mutant cells, and it may participate in the pathogenesis of AD (Area-Gomez et al., 2012).

Complex I activity is reduced in the substantia nigra of subjects with Parkinson's disease (PD), and various complex inhibitors (MPP^+, rotenone, and other pesticides) cause neuropathological changes similar to those observed in PD (Schapira et al., 2006). In this regard, rotenone and 6-hydroxydopamine have been shown to induce Drp1-dependent mitochondrial fragmentation in neuronal cells (Barsoum et al., 2006; Gomez-Lazaro et al., 2008). Mutations in Parkin and outer membrane kinase PTEN-induced putative kinase-1 (PINK1) have been reported in familial PD, and these proteins participate in a major mitochondrial quality control pathway (Pickrell and Youle, 2015). When the mitochondrial membrane potential decreases, PINK1 recruits Parkin to the mitochondria (Narendra et al., 2010). Parkin next ubiquitinates PINK1, thus trigering mitophagy. Parkin also ubiquitinates other targets such as Mfn1, Mfn2, Fis1, and Drp1, causing their proteasomal degradation (Tanaka et al., 2010; Ziviani et al., 2010; Chan et al., 2011; Wang et al., 2011). In agreement, loss of function of PINK1 or Parkin causes mitochondrial fragmentation (Exner et al., 2007; Lutz et al., 2009; Sandebring et al., 2009), and mammalian fibroblasts carrying PINK1 mutations from PD patients also exhibit mitochondrial fragmentation (Grunewald et al., 2009).

Huntington's disease (HD) is caused by an expansion of a CAG trinucleotide sequence that encodes a polyglutamine tract in the huntingtin protein. Mitochondrial dysfunction is also associated with the pathogenesis of HD (Brouillet et al., 1995; Tabrizi et al., 1999; Panov et al., 2002; Schapira et al., 2014). Thus, the striatum and frontal cortex of HD patients show an increased abundance of Fis1 and Drp1 (Costa et al., 2010) and decreased levels of Mfn1, Mfn2, and OPA1 (Shirendeb et al., 2011). This pattern of changes may lead to mitochondrial fragmentation in these subjects. As to the mechanisms responsible for mitochondrial fragmentation, overexpression of mutant huntingtin causes mitochondrial fragmentation and blockade of fragmentation prevents the cytotoxic effects of mutant huntingtin (Wang et al., 2009b). Furthermore, mutant huntingtin binds to Drp1 and enhances its GTPase activity (Song et al., 2011). In all, these studies support the notion that alterations in mitochondrial dynamics are involved in the pathogenesis of HD.

Hypothalamic Neuronal Circuits and Mitochondrial Function

The maintenance of energy homeostasis is fundamental to sustain life. In mammals, the central nervous system (CNS) plays a critical role in the regulation of appetite, energy expenditure, and metabolism through multiple and distributed neuronal circuits. The hypothalamus, which is made up of distinct nuclei, including the arcuate nucleus (ARC), the paraventricular nucleus, the lateral area, the dorsomedial nucleus and the ventromedial nucleus, is arguably the most important CNS region in metabolic control (Schneeberger et al., 2014). Extensive experimental evidence indicates that ARC is a key area in the neural hierarchy that regulates this biological process. The ARC holds at least two subsets of neurons—with opposite functions and reciprocally regulated—involved in systemic energy balance control. One set co-expresses orexigenic neuropeptides Agouti-related protein (AgRP) and Neuropeptide Y (NPY), while the other co-expresses anorexigenic neuropeptides cocaine- and amphetamine-regulated transcript (CART) and α-melanocyte-stimulating hormone (α-MSH, a product of proopiomelanocortin (POMC) processing) (Schneeberger et al., 2014).

The Melanocortin System

POMC and AgRP neurons, together with downstream neurons expressing melanocortin receptors (MCR) 3 and 4, form the melanocortin system, a crucial neuronal circuit that senses and responds to fluctuations in central and circulating factors that inform about the nutritional status of the organism. Indeed, the activity of these two subsets of neurons is influenced by local (NPY, serotonin, GABA, etc.) and peripheral (leptin, insulin, ghrelin) signals, as well as by nutrients such as glucose and free fatty acids. Numerous pharmacological and genetic studies indicate that the divergent physiological roles of these two populations of neurons are largely the consequence of the release and action of α-MSH and AgRP neuropeptides. α-MSH is an endogenous agonist of MCR3 and 4, thus providing an anorexigenic tone by suppressing appetite and increasing thermogenesis (Poggioli et al., 1986; Wirth et al., 2001). In contrast, AgRP is an antagonist of these receptors and therefore counteracts the effects of α-MSH signaling on food intake and body weight (Ollmann et al., 1997). In addition, the orexigenic actions of AgRP neurons are also mediated by the release of NPY, which binds to specific receptors, and by direct GABAergic synapsis onto POMC neurons (Cowley et al., 2001).

In summary, current evidence indicates that a local ARC circuit constituted by "first order" POMC and AgRP neurons plays a critical role in sensing, integrating, and responding to humoral signals that report on energy status. These neurons engage downstream "second order" multi-level neurocircuits that will produce precise effector responses. The global integration of these signals culminates in the generation of coordinated behavioral, autonomic, and neuroendocrine responses to regulate appetite, energy expenditure, and body weight (Schneeberger et al., 2014).

Leptin and Ghrelin: Key Hormones Regulating Energy Homeostasis

Leptin and ghrelin are prototypical examples of metabolic signals of energy surfeit and deficit respectively, and POMC and AgRP neurons are direct targets of both hormones (Cheung et al., 1997; Elias et al., 1999; Willesen et al., 1999; Cowley et al., 2001). Leptin exerts its anorexigenic effects by increasing *Pomc* expression and processing into α-MSH (Schwartz et al., 1997; Thornton et al., 1997; Mizuno et al., 1998), and by inhibiting both *Npy* and *AgRP* transcription (Stephens et al., 1995; Schwartz et al., 1996; Mizuno and Mobbs, 1999). Leptin also increases the electrical activity of POMC neurons, thereby leading to α-MSH release (Cowley et al., 2001; Claret et al., 2007; Hill et al., 2008; Al-Qassab et al., 2009). In addition to its agonism/antagonism effects on MCRs, leptin attenuates the inhibitory GABAergic tone of AgRP neurons onto POMC neurons (Cowley et al., 2001). Similarly, recent data showed that leptin also acts on non-AgRP presynaptic GABAergic neurons by reducing the inhibitory input on POMC neurons (Vong et al., 2011). Overall, these effects result in reduced food intake and increased energy expenditure.

Under conditions of negative energy balance, circulating ghrelin levels are increased. Evidence indicates that the orexigenic effects of ghrelin are largely mediated by AgRP neurons (Chen et al., 2004b; Luquet et al., 2007; Wang et al., 2014). Consistently, ghrelin enhances *Npy* and *AgRP* transcript expression (Kamegai et al., 2001; Nakazato et al., 2001). The release of AgRP and NPY hyperpolarizes neighboring POMC neurons, thus reducing α-MSH release (Roseberry et al., 2004; Smith et al., 2007; Cyr et al., 2013). Furthermore, electrophysiology studies have shown that ghrelin activates AgRP neurons and increases the number of inhibitory synapses onto POMC neurons (Cowley et al., 2003; Yang et al., 2011; Atasoy et al., 2012). Collectively, these events lead to the simultaneous activation of AgRP neurons and inhibition of POMC neurons, thus enhancing the orexigenic output.

Mitochondrial Function in Hypothalamic ARC Neurons

Neurons are highly energy-demanding, and thus adequate mitochondrial performance is essential for the growth, survival, and function of these cells (Zhu et al., 2012). Mitochondrial ATP production and Ca^{2+} buffering/release are fundamental for a myriad of neuronal functions, including synapse assembly, action potential generation, and synaptic transmission, amongst others. Given their particular and intricate morphology, neurons require the distribution of mitochondria to distal areas in order to cover the high energy demands associated with a number of specialized functions. Thus, mitochondrial function and dynamics must be tightly regulated in order to temporally and spatially satisfy the bioenergetic needs of neurons.

Despite the paramount importance of the regulation of systemic energy balance and metabolism by mitochondria in hypothalamic neurons, few studies have addressed this issue. An important aspect to note is the diametrically different bioenergetic patterns of POMC and AgRP neurons, which are largely the consequence of their divergent physiological functions. Negative energy balance acutely activates AgRP neurons and promotes mitochondrial uncoupling activity associated with elevated mitochondrial density (Coppola et al., 2007; Dietrich et al., 2013). Under these conditions, ghrelin-induced β-oxidation constitutes the main energy supply to maintain AgRP neuron activity. This is achieved through an axis formed by the AMP-activated protein kinase (AMPK) and the muscle isoform of carnitine O-palmitoyltransferase 1 (CPT1-M) (Andrews et al., 2008; Lopez et al., 2008) which allows the uptake of long-chain fatty acyl CoAs by the mitochondria and the subsequent β-oxidation. A key component of this process is uncoupling protein 2 (UCP2), a mitochondrial protein that mediates proton leak, thereby limiting ATP and ROS production (Mailloux and Harper, 2011). Hypothalamic UCP2 expression is induced by fasting (Coppola et al., 2007), and ghrelin-driven feeding by AgRP requires UCP2 (Andrews et al., 2008). In line with these observations, fasting and ghrelin increase mitochondrial proliferation, synaptic plasticity, and electric activity of AgRP neurons in a UCP2-dependent manner (Coppola et al., 2007; Andrews et al., 2008). Under conditions of positive energy balance, when circulating leptin and glucose levels are high, POMC neurons increase their firing rate while AgRP neurons remain silent (Claret et al., 2007; Parton et al., 2007). Consistently, feeding conditions are associated with increased mitochondrial number in POMC neurons (Diano et al., 2011). The current model suggests that cellular glucose metabolism in POMC neurons generates a high proton gradient, concomitant with elevated ATP and ROS production. ATP would inactivate ATP-sensitive potassium (K_{ATP}) channels and depolarize POMC neurons (Ibrahim et al., 2003). In addition, enhanced ROS levels would activate POMC neurons, further contributing to satiety (Diano et al., 2011). Mitochondrial UCP2 may be a key integrator of these processes, as its activity may limit ATP and/or ROS production and thereby modulate neuronal activity.

Collectively, these lines of evidence support the notion that mitochondrial processes and intermediates in ARC hypothalamic neurons play fundamental roles in sensing and integrating metabolic cues and also mediate neuronal function and associated behavior.

Role of Mitochondrial Fusion Proteins on Hypothalamic ARC Neurons

Recent research suggests that mitochondrial dynamics, in addition to constitute a key quality control mechanism, is also implicated in sensing nutrient fluctuations and promoting bioenergetic adaptations to meet the cellular metabolic needs. In general terms, physiological processes associated with enhanced energy demand and reduced energy supply (acute stress, starvation, etc.) are characterized by mitochondrial fusion and coupled respiration. In contrast, physiological situations associated with decreased energy demand and increased supply (high nutrient levels, obesity, type 2 diabetes) correlate with mitochondrial fission and decreased coupling (Liesa and Shirihai, 2013; Gao et al., 2014). Given that hypothalamic POMC and AgRP neurons are metabolic transceivers, it is reasonable to speculate that mitochondrial dynamics is an integral part of the molecular mechanisms by which these neurons sense the energy/nutritional milieu and mediate specific physiological actions to maintain energy homeostasis.

Two recent studies, one from our research group, have investigated mitochondrial dynamics and the role of fusion proteins Mfn1 and 2 in POMC and AgRP neurons upon energy balance control *in vivo* (Schneeberger et al., 2013). Electron microscopy studies under fasting conditions showed decreased mitochondria number but unaltered morphology in POMC neurons, while AgRP neurons exhibited elevated mitochondrial density and reduced size suggesting enhanced fission. High-fat diet (HFD) administration reduced mitochondria number but increased their size and elongation in AgRP neurons, in line with increased fusion (Dietrich et al., 2013). In contrast, POMC neuron mitochondrial elongation and network complexity was reduced, indicating elevated fission (Schneeberger et al., 2013) (**Figure 4**). Together, these results demonstrate specific patterns of mitochondrial dynamics in response to nutrient challenges in POMC and AgRP neurons, which is consistent with their divergent physiological functions and fuel usage.

Remarkably, HFD feeding reduced the number of mitochondria-ER contacts in POMC neurons by ~50%, a defect

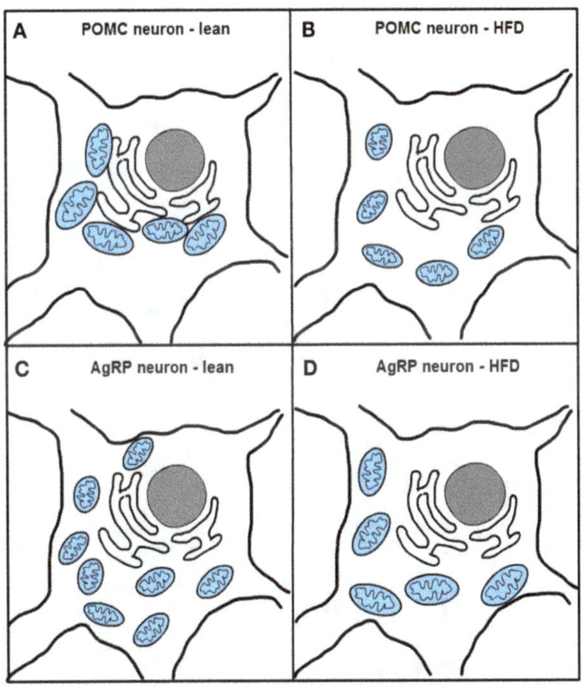

FIGURE 4 | Excess nutrient availability alters ER-mitochondria contacts and mitochondrial dynamics in POMC and AgRP neurons. High-fat diet (HFD) administration increases mitochondrial fragmentation and impairs ER-mitochondria contacts in POMC neurons **(A,B)**. In contrast, AgRP neurons under HFD conditions show increased fusion and unaltered ER-mitochondria contacts **(C,D)**.

that was not observed in the AgRP subpopulation (**Figure 4**). Recent reports have shown that Mfn2 is implicated in the tethering of mitochondria with ER (de Brito and Scorrano, 2008) and in the modulation of ER stress responses (Papanicolaou et al., 2012; Sebastian et al., 2012; Munoz et al., 2013). Indeed, under diet-induced obesity (DIO) conditions hypothalamic Mfn2 expression was reduced and its overexpression in the ARC was able to ameliorate the metabolic disturbances and reduce ER stress markers in the hypothalamus of DIO mice (Schneeberger et al., 2013). Consistent with these observations, conditional deletion of Mfn2 in POMC neurons resulted in a marked obesogenic phenotype as a consequence of loss of mitochondria-ER contacts and early development of ER stress-induced leptin resistance (**Figure 5**). In recent years, hypothalamic ER stress has emerged as a causal factor in the development of leptin resistance and obesity (Zhang et al., 2008; Ozcan et al., 2009) and this study established Mfn2 as a key molecular determinant connecting these processes. Interestingly, the number of mitochondria-ER junctions in POMC neurons may be a potential readout of leptin sensitivity (Schneeberger et al., 2013; Long et al., 2014). The specificity of this dramatic obese phenotype was demonstrated by the lack of energy balance abnormalities in mice lacking the homologous Mfn1 in the same population of neurons (Schneeberger et al., 2013).

Dietrich and associates (Dietrich et al., 2013) also used genetic conditional approaches to investigate the roles of Mfn1 and Mfn2 in AgRP neurons. The metabolic alterations observed in these mouse models were minimal under chow diet conditions (only females showed a slight metabolic improvement). However, a significant observation was that administration of HFD did not lead to the mitochondrial fusion in AgRP-specific knockout mice, suggesting that Mfn1- and Mfn2-mediated fusion was required for the bioenergetic adaptations of this population of neurons to positive energy balance (Schneeberger et al., 2013). This could be the consequence of reduced firing rate and increased number of silent AgRP neurons seen these dietary conditions.

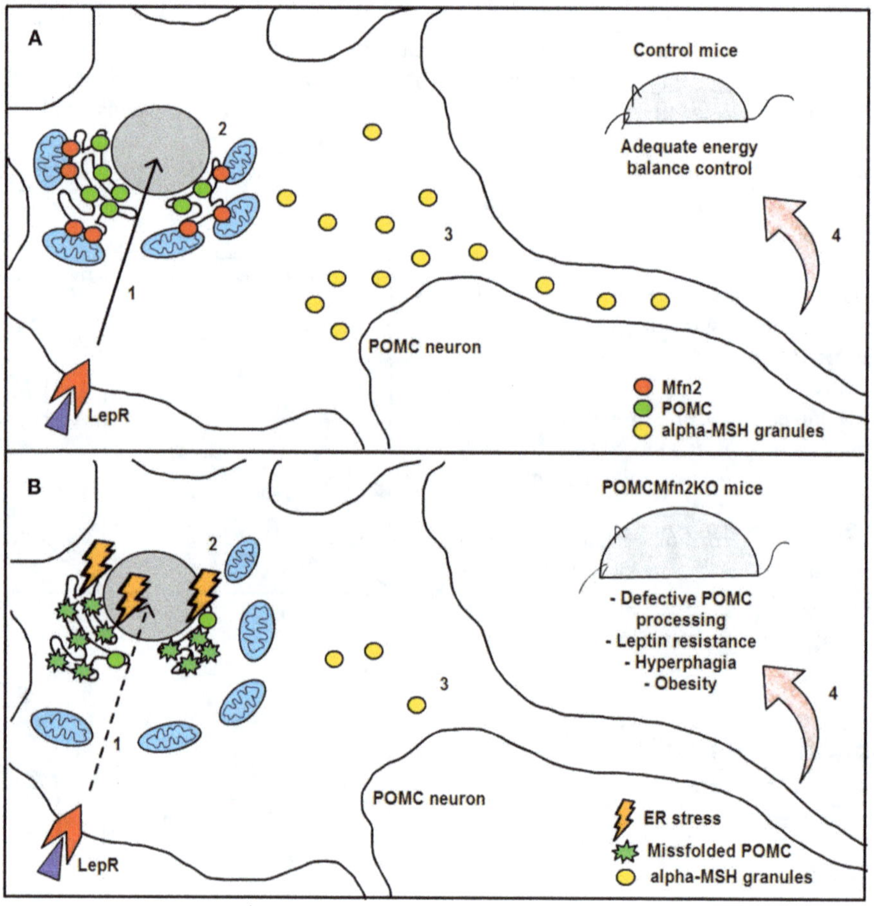

FIGURE 5 | Graphical summary of the consequences of Mfn2 loss in POMC neurons. (A) Under normal physiological conditions, leptin signaling in POMC neurons is adequately transmitted, thereby enhancing POMC transcription in the nucleus (1) and subsequent synthesis in the ER (2). POMC precursor is sorted into secretory granules and processed into α-MSH (3). This neuropeptide is then released into target areas by POMC neuron axonal terminals thus mediating the anorexigenic effects of leptin (4). **(B)** Deletion of Mfn2 specifically in POMC neurons causes loss of ER-mitochondria contacts, thus leading to ER stress which interferes with proper POMC folding (2). Missfolded POMC precursor can not be adequately sorted or processed into α-MSH (3). As a consequence, leptin signaling (1) and leptin-mediated anorexigenic effects are blunted (4). LepR; leptin receptor; Mfn2: mitofusin 2; POMC: proopiomelanocortin; α.MSH: alpha-melanocyte stimulating hormone.

Collectively, and in line with previous studies (Chen et al., 2007; Papanicolaou et al., 2011, 2012; Lee et al., 2012; Pham et al., 2012), these results reinforce the idea of non-overlapping physiological roles for mitofusin proteins and neuron-specific functions. For example, Mfn2 in POMC neurons is particularly involved in maintaining mitochondria-ER contacts and in the modulation of the cellular responses to ER stress, while in AgRP neurons mediates mitochondrial dynamics. It is interesting to note that in other neuronal types, but not in POMC and AgRP neurons, mitofusin proteins are essential for neuron survival and axon growth (Chen et al., 2007; Lee et al., 2012; Pham et al., 2012). The precise description of the basis of such divergent cell-specific biological functions will be of capital importance to understand the role of mitochondrial dynamics in hypothalamic neurons upon the regulation of energy balance and metabolism. These mechanisms will be also important to design potential targeted therapeutical approaches to counteract highly prevalent metabolic disorders such as obesity and type-2 diabetes.

Future Perspectives

A major current medical need is the efficient treatment of prevalent diseases such as obesity, type 2 diabetes, Alzheimer's disease, Parkinson's disease, or Huntington disease. In this respect, it is relevant to identify druggable proteins that participate in the pathophysiology of those disorders, and that permit to stop the progression of the disease or to ameliorate many of the alterations associated to them.

With the turning of the century we have learnt that alterations in genes relevant in mitochondrial dynamics are sufficient to develop diseases, leading to certain forms of CMT and ADOA. Furthermore, data obtained in the last years support the view that alterations in mitochondrial dynamics may be involved in the pathogenesis of neurodegenerative diseases, and in the hypothalamic dysfunctions leading to dysregulated energy balance. Ample evidence indicates that some neurodegenerative disorders are associated with altered metabolic and appetitive behaviors that may be explained by abnormal hypothalamic function. Although it is tempting to speculate that such perturbations are the consequence of defective mitochondrial dynamics, to date direct experimental evidence has not been provided. Certainly, there is a need to fully demonstrate the role of mitochondrial dynamics in the pathogenesis of metabolic and neurodegenerative diseases, and its potential link, by using more sophisticated mouse models and in humans. In spite of these difficulties, we hope that the thorough understanding of the mechanisms that control mitochondrial dynamics, and the interaction between mitochondrial and endoplasmic reticulum will permit to enter into a phase in which some of the mitochondrial dynamics proteins or regulators are amenable for pharmacological manipulation.

Acknowledgments

This study was supported by research grants from the MINECO (SAF2013-40987R), *Generalitat de Catalunya* (2014SGR48), CIBERDEM (*Instituto de Salud Carlos III*), INTERREG IV-B-SUDOE-FEDER (DIOMED, SOE1/P1/E178), National R+D+I Plan (*Ministerio de Ciencia e Innovación*; MICINN) (PI13/01604 and PI10/01074) cofunded by the *Instituto Salud Carlos III* (ISCIII) and ERDF. MC is a recipient of a Miguel Servet contract (MICINN-ISCIII, CP09/00233). AZ is recipient of an ICREA Acadèmia (*Generalitat de Catalunya*). Some of these grants have been co-financed by the European Regional Development Fund "A way to build Europe." This work was carried out in part at the Esther Koplowitz Centre, Barcelona.

References

Akepati, V. R., Muller, E. C., Otto, A., Strauss, H. M., Portwich, M., and Alexander, C. (2008). Characterization of OPA1 isoforms isolated from mouse tissues. *J. Neurochem.* 106, 372–383. doi: 10.1111/j.1471-4159.2008.05401.x

Alavi, M. V., Bette, S., Schimpf, S., Schuettauf, F., Schraermeyer, U., Wehrl, H. F., et al. (2007). A splice site mutation in the murine Opa1 gene features pathology of autosomal dominant optic atrophy. *Brain* 130, 1029–1042. doi: 10.1093/brain/awm005

Al-Qassab, H., Smith, M. A., Irvine, E. E., Guillermet-Guibert, J., Claret, M., Choudhury, A. I., et al. (2009). Dominant role of the p110beta isoform of PI3K over p110alpha in energy homeostasis regulation by POMC and AgRP neurons. *Cell Metab.* 10, 343–354. doi: 10.1016/j.cmet.2009.09.008

Amati-Bonneau, P., Valentino, M. L., Reynier, P., Gallardo, M. E., Bornstein, B., Boissière, A., et al. (2008). OPA1 mutations induce mitochondrial DNA instability and optic atrophy 'plus' phenotypes. *Brain* 131, 338–351. doi: 10.1093/brain/awm298

Amiott, E. A., Lott, P., Soto, J., Kang, P. B., McCaffery, J. M., DiMauro, S., et al. (2008). Mitochondrial fusion and function in Charcot-Marie-Tooth type 2A patient fibroblasts with mitofusin 2 mutations. *Exp. Neurol.* 211, 115–127. doi: 10.1016/j.expneurol.2008.01.010

Ammar, N., Nelis, E., Merlini, L., Barisic, N., Amouri, R., Ceuterick, C., et al. (2003). Identification of novel GDAP1 mutations causing autosomal recessive Charcot-Marie-Tooth disease. *Neuromuscul. Disord.* 13, 720–728. doi: 10.1016/S0960-8966(03)00093-2

Andrews, Z. B., Liu, Z. W., Walllingford, N., Erion, D. M., Borok, E., Friedman, J. M., et al. (2008). UCP2 mediates ghrelin's action on NPY/AgRP neurons by lowering free radicals. *Nature* 454, 846–851. doi: 10.1038/nature07181

Area-Gomez, E., Del Carmen Lara Castillo, M., Tambini, M. D., Guardia-Laguarta, C., de Groof, A. J., Madra, M., et al. (2012). Upregulated function of mitochondria-associated ER membranes in Alzheimer disease. *EMBO J.* 31, 4106–4123. doi: 10.1038/emboj.2012.202

Atasoy, D., Betley, J. N., Su, H. H., and Sternson, S. M. (2012). Deconstruction of a neural circuit for hunger. *Nature* 488, 172–177. doi: 10.1038/nature11270

Bach, D., Pich, S., Soriano, F. X., Vega, N., Baumgartner, B., Oriola, J., et al. (2003). Mitofusin-2 determines mitochondrial network architecture and mitochondrial metabolism. A novel regulatory mechanism altered in obesity. *J. Biol. Chem.* 278, 17190–17197. doi: 10.1074/jbc.M212754200

Baloh, R. H., Schmidt, R. E., Pestronk, A., and Milbrandt, J. (2007). Altered axonal mitochondrial transport in the pathogenesis of charcot-marie-tooth disease from mitofusin 2 mutations. *J. Neurosci.* 27, 422–430. doi: 10.1523/JNEUROSCI.4798-06.2007

Baricault, L., Segui, B., Guegand, L., Olichon, A., Valette, A., Larminat, F., et al. (2007). OPA1 cleavage depends on decreased mitochondrial ATP level and bivalent metals. *Exp. Cell Res.* 313, 3800–3808. doi: 10.1016/j.yexcr.2007.08.008

Baris, O., Delettre, C., Amati-Bonneau, P., Surget, M.-O., Charlin, J.-F., Catier, A., et al. (2003). Fourteen novel OPA1 mutations in autosomal dominant optic atrophy including two de novo mutations in sporadic optic atrophy. *Hum. Mutat.* 21, 656. doi: 10.1002/humu.9152

Barsoum, M. J., Yuan, H., Gerencser, A. A., Liot, G., Kushnareva, Y., Graber, S., et al. (2006). Nitric oxide-induced mitochondrial fission is regulated by dynamin-related GTPases in neurons. *EMBO J.* 25, 3900–3911. doi: 10.1038/sj.emboj.7601253

Baxter, R. V., Ben Othmane, K., Rochelle, J. M., Stajich, J. E., Hulette, C., Dew-Knight, S., et al. (2002). Ganglioside-induced differentiation-associated protein-1 is mutant in Charcot-Marie-Tooth disease type 4A/8q21. *Nat. Genet.* 30, 21–22. doi: 10.1038/ng796

Bereiter-Hahn, J., and Voth, M. (1994). Dynamics of mitochondria in living cells: shape changes, dislocations, fusion, and fission of mitochondria. *Microsc. Res. Tech.* 27, 198–219. doi: 10.1002/jemt.1070270303

Berger, P., Young, P., and Suter, U. (2002). Molecular cell biology of Charcot-Marie-Tooth disease. *Neurogenetics* 4, 1–15. doi: 10.1007/s10048-002-0130-z

Berridge, M. J. (2002). The endoplasmic reticulum: a multifunctional signaling organelle. *Cell Calcium* 32, 235–249. doi: 10.1016/S0143416002001823

Bleazard, W., McCaffery, J. M., King, E. J., Bale, S., Mozdy, A., Tieu, Q., et al. (1999). The dynamin-related GTPase Dnm1 regulates mitochondrial fission in yeast. *Nat. Cell Biol.* 1, 298–304. doi: 10.1038/13014

Boerkoel, C. F., Takashima, H., Nakagawa, M., Izumo, S., Armstrong, D., Butler, I., et al. (2003). CMT4A: identification of a hispanic GDAP1 founder mutation. *Ann. Neurol.* 53, 400–405. doi: 10.1002/ana.10505

Brouillet, E., Hantraye, P., Ferrante, R. J., Dolan, R., Leroy-Willig, A., Kowall, N. W., et al. (1995). Chronic mitochondrial energy impairment produces selective striatal degeneration and abnormal choreiform movements in primates. *Proc. Natl. Acad. Sci. U.S.A.* 92, 7105–7109. doi: 10.1073/pnas.92.15.7105

Cardenas, C., Miller, R. A., Smith, I., Bui, T., Molgo, J., Muller, M., et al. (2010). Essential regulation of cell bioenergetics by constitutive InsP3 receptor Ca2+ transfer to mitochondria. *Cell* 142, 270–283. doi: 10.1016/j.cell.2010.06.007

Cassereau, J., Chevrollier, A., Gueguen, N., Desquiret, V., Verny, C., Nicolas, G., et al. (2011). Mitochondrial dysfunction and pathophysiology of Charcot-Marie-Tooth disease involving GDAP1 mutations. *Exp. Neurol.* 227, 31–41. doi: 10.1016/j.expneurol.2010.09.006

Cereghetti, G. M., Stangherlin, A., Martins De Brito, O., Chang, C. R., Blackstone, C., Bernardi, P., et al. (2008). Dephosphorylation by calcineurin regulates translocation of Drp1 to mitochondria. *Proc. Natl. Acad. Sci. U.S.A.* 105, 15803–15808. doi: 10.1073/pnas.0808249105

Chami, M., Oules, B., Szabadkai, G., Tacine, R., Rizzuto, R., and Paterlini-Brechot, P. (2008). Role of SERCA1 truncated isoform in the proapoptotic calcium transfer from ER to mitochondria during ER stress. *Mol. Cell.* 32, 641–651. doi: 10.1016/j.molcel.2008.11.014

Chan, N. C., Salazar, A. M., Pham, A. H., Sweredoski, M. J., Kolawa, N. J., Graham, R. L., et al. (2011). Broad activation of the ubiquitin-proteasome system by Parkin is critical for mitophagy. *Hum. Mol. Genet.* 20, 1726–1737. doi: 10.1093/hmg/ddr048

Chang, C. R., and Blackstone, C. (2007). Cyclic AMP-dependent protein kinase phosphorylation of Drp1 regulates its GTPase activity and mitochondrial morphology. *J. Biol. Chem.* 282, 21583–21587. doi: 10.1074/jbc.C700083200

Chen, H., and Chan, D. C. (2005). Emerging functions of mammalian mitochondrial fusion and fission. *Hum. Mol. Genet.* 14, R283–R289. doi: 10.1093/hmg/ddi270

Chen, H., Chomyn, A., and Chan, D. C. (2005). Disruption of fusion results in mitochondrial heterogeneity and dysfunction. *J. Biol. Chem.* 280, 26185–26192. doi: 10.1074/jbc.M503062200

Chen, H., Detmer, S. A., Ewald, A. J., Griffin, E. E., Fraser, S. E., and Chan, D. C. (2003). Mitofusins Mfn1 and Mfn2 coordinately regulate mitochondrial fusion and are essential for embryonic development. *J. Cell Biol.* 160, 189–200. doi: 10.1083/jcb.200211046

Chen, H., McCaffery, J. M., and Chan, D. C. (2007). Mitochondrial fusion protects against neurodegeneration in the cerebellum. *Cell* 130, 548–562. doi: 10.1016/j.cell.2007.06.026

Chen, H. Y., Trumbauer, M. E., Chen, A. S., Weingarth, D. T., Adams, J. R., Frazier, E. G., et al. (2004b). Orexigenic action of peripheral ghrelin is mediated by neuropeptide Y and agouti-related protein. *Endocrinology* 145, 2607–2612. doi: 10.1210/en.2003-1596

Chen, K. H., Dasgupta, A., Ding, J., Indig, F. E., Ghosh, P., and Longo, D. L. (2014). Role of mitofusin 2 (Mfn2) in controlling cellular proliferation. *FASEB J.* 28, 382–394. doi: 10.1096/fj.13-230037

Chen, K. H., Guo, X., Ma, D., Guo, Y., Li, Q., Yang, D., et al. (2004a). Dysregulation of HSG triggers vascular proliferative disorders. *Nat. Cell Biol.* 6, 872–883. doi: 10.1038/ncb1161

Cheung, C. C., Clifton, D. K., and Steiner, R. A. (1997). Proopiomelanocortin neurons are direct targets for leptin in the hypothalamus. *Endocrinology* 138, 4489–4492. doi: 10.1210/endo.138.10.5570

Cho, D.-H., Nakamura, T., Fang, J., Cieplak, P., Godzik, A., Gu, Z., et al. (2009). S-Nitrosylation of Drp1 mediates β-amyloid-related mitochondrial fission and neuronal injury. *Science* 324, 102–105. doi: 10.1126/science.1171091

Chung, K. W., Kim, S. B., Park, K. D., Choi, K. G., Lee, J. H., Eun, H. W., et al. (2006). Early onset severe and late-onset mild Charcot–Marie–Tooth disease with mitofusin 2 (MFN2) mutations. *Brain* 129, 2103–2118. doi: 10.1093/brain/awl174

Cipolat, S., De Brito, O. M., Dal Zilio, B., and Scorrano, L. (2004). OPA1 requires mitofusin 1 to promote mitochondrial fusion. *Proc. Natl. Acad. Sci. U.S.A.* 101, 15927–15932. doi: 10.1073/pnas.0407043101

Claret, M., Smith, M. A., Batterham, R. L., Selman, C., Choudhury, A. I., Fryer, L. G., et al. (2007). AMPK is essential for energy homeostasis regulation and glucose sensing by POMC and AgRP neurons. *J. Clin. Invest.* 117, 2325–2336. doi: 10.1172/JCI31516

Cogliati, S., Frezza, C., Soriano, M. E., Varanita, T., Quintana-Cabrera, R., Corrado, M., et al. (2013). Mitochondrial cristae shape determines respiratory chain supercomplexes assembly and respiratory efficiency. *Cell* 155, 160–171. doi: 10.1016/j.cell.2013.08.032

Coppola, A., Liu, Z. W., Andrews, Z. B., Paradis, E., Roy, M. C., Friedman, J. M., et al. (2007). A central thermogenic-like mechanism in feeding regulation: an interplay between arcuate nucleus T3 and UCP2. *Cell Metab.* 5, 21–33. doi: 10.1016/j.cmet.2006.12.002

Cortese, J. D., Voglino, L. A., and Hackenbrock, C. R. (1998). Novel fluorescence membrane fusion assays reveal GTP-dependent fusogenic properties of outer mitochondrial membrane-derived proteins. *Biochim. Biophys. Acta* 1371, 185–198. doi: 10.1016/S0005-2736(97)00266-6

Costa, V., Giacomello, M., Hudec, R., Lopreiato, R., Ermak, G., Lim, D., et al. (2010). Mitochondrial fission and cristae disruption increase the response of cell models of Huntington's disease to apoptotic stimuli. *EMBO Mol. Med.* 2, 490–503. doi: 10.1002/emmm.201000102

Cowley, M. A., Smart, J. L., Rubinstein, M., Cerdan, M. G., Diano, S., Horvath, T. L., et al. (2001). Leptin activates anorexigenic POMC neurons through a neural network in the arcuate nucleus. *Nature* 411, 480–484. doi: 10.1038/35078085

Cowley, M. A., Smith, R. G., Diano, S., Tschop, M., Pronchuk, N., Grove, K. L., et al. (2003). The distribution and mechanism of action of ghrelin in the CNS demonstrates a novel hypothalamic circuit regulating energy homeostasis. *Neuron* 37, 649–661. doi: 10.1016/S0896-6273(03)00063-1

Cribbs, J. T., and Strack, S. (2007). Reversible phosphorylation of Drp1 by cyclic AMP-dependent protein kinase and calcineurin regulates mitochondrial fission and cell death. *EMBO Rep.* 8, 939–944. doi: 10.1038/sj.embor.7401062

Cuesta, A., Pedrola, L., Sevilla, T., Garcia-Planells, J., Chumillas, M. J., Mayordomo, F., et al. (2002). The gene encoding ganglioside-induced differentiation-associated protein 1 is mutated in axonal Charcot-Marie-Tooth type 4A disease. *Nat. Genet.* 30, 22–25. doi: 10.1038/ng798

Cyr, N. E., Toorie, A. M., Steger, J. S., Sochat, M. M., Hyner, S., Perello, M., et al. (2013). Mechanisms by which the orexigen NPY regulates anorexigenic alpha-MSH and TRH. *Am. J. Physiol. Endocrinol. Metab.* 304, E640–E650. doi: 10.1152/ajpendo.00448.2012

Davies, V. J., Hollins, A. J., Piechota, M. J., Yip, W., Davies, J. R., White, K. E., et al. (2007). Opa1 deficiency in a mouse model of autosomal dominant optic atrophy impairs mitochondrial morphology, optic nerve structure and visual function. *Hum. Mol. Genet.* 16, 1307–1318. doi: 10.1093/hmg/ddm079

de Brito, O. M., and Scorrano, L. (2008). Mitofusin 2 tethers endoplasmic reticulum to mitochondria. *Nature* 456, 605–610. doi: 10.1038/nature07534

Delettre, C., Griffoin, J. M., Kaplan, J., Dollfus, H., Lorenz, B., Faivre, L., et al. (2001). Mutation spectrum and splicing variants in the OPA1 gene. *Hum. Genet.* 109, 584–591. doi: 10.1007/s00439-001-0633-y

Delettre, C., Lenaers, G., Griffoin, J. M., Gigarel, N., Lorenzo, C., Belenguer, P., et al. (2000). Nuclear gene OPA1, encoding a mitochondrial dynamin-related protein, is mutated in dominant optic atrophy. *Nat. Genet.* 26, 207–210. doi: 10.1038/79936

De Sandre-Giovannoli, A., Chaouch, M., Boccaccio, I., Bernard, R., Delague, V., Grid, D., et al. (2003). Phenotypic and genetic exploration of severe demyelinating and secondary axonal neuropathies resulting from GDAP1 nonsense and splicing mutations. *J. Med. Genet.* 40:e87. doi: 10.1136/jmg.40.7.e87

Detmer, S. A., and Chan, D. C. (2007). Complementation between mouse Mfn1 and Mfn2 protects mitochondrial fusion defects caused by CMT2A disease mutations. *J. Cell Biol.* 176, 405–414. doi: 10.1083/jcb.200611080

Detmer, S. A., Velde, C. V., Cleveland, D. W., and Chan, D. C. (2008). Hindlimb gait defects due to motor axon loss and reduced distal muscles in a transgenic mouse model of Charcot–Marie–Tooth type 2A. *Hum. Mol. Genet.* 17, 367–375. doi: 10.1093/hmg/ddm314

DeVay, R. M., Dominguez-Ramirez, L., Lackner, L. L., Hoppins, S., Stahlberg, H., and Nunnari, J. (2009). Coassembly of Mgm1 isoforms requires cardiolipin and mediates mitochondrial inner membrane fusion. *J. Cell Biol.* 186, 793–803. doi: 10.1083/jcb.200906098

Diano, S., Liu, Z. W., Jeong, J. K., Dietrich, M. O., Ruan, H. B., Kim, E., et al. (2011). Peroxisome proliferation-associated control of reactive oxygen species sets melanocortin tone and feeding in diet-induced obesity. *Nat. Med.* 17, 1121–1127. doi: 10.1038/nm.2421

Dietrich, M. O., Liu, Z. W., and Horvath, T. L. (2013). Mitochondrial dynamics controlled by mitofusins regulate Agrp neuronal activity and diet-induced obesity. *Cell* 155, 188–199. doi: 10.1016/j.cell.2013.09.004

Dohm, J. A., Lee, S. J., Hardwick, J. M., Hill, R. B., and Gittis, A. G. (2004). Cytosolic domain of the human mitochondrial fission protein fis1 adopts a TPR fold. *Proteins Struct. Funct. Bioinformatics* 54, 153–156. doi: 10.1002/prot.10524

Dyck, P. J., and Lambert, E. H. (1968). Lower motor and primary sensory neuron diseases with peroneal muscular atrophy: I. Neurologic, genetic, and electrophysiologic findings in hereditary polyneuropathies. *Arch. Neurol.* 18, 603–618. doi: 10.1001/archneur.1968.00470360025002

Ehses, S., Raschke, I., Mancuso, G., Bernacchia, A., Geimer, S., Tondera, D., et al. (2009). Regulation of OPA1 processing and mitochondrial fusion by m-AAA protease isoenzymes and OMA1. *J. Cell Biol.* 187, 1023–1036. doi: 10.1083/jcb.200906084

Elias, C. F., Aschkenasi, C., Lee, C., Kelly, J., Ahima, R. S., Bjorbaek, C., et al. (1999). Leptin differentially regulates NPY and POMC neurons projecting to the lateral hypothalamic area. *Neuron* 23, 775–786. doi: 10.1016/S0896-6273(01)80035-0

Engelfried, K., Vorgerd, M., Hagedorn, M., Haas, G., Gilles, J., Epplen, J., et al. (2006). Charcot-Marie-Tooth neuropathy type 2A: novel mutations in the mitofusin 2 gene (MFN2). *BMC Med. Genet.* 7:53. doi: 10.1186/1471-235 0-7-53

Eura, Y., Ishihara, N., Oka, T., and Mihara, K. (2006). Identification of a novel protein that regulates mitochondrial fusion by modulating mitofusin (Mfn) protein function. *J. Cell Sci.* 119, 4913–4925. doi: 10.1242/jcs.03253

Eura, Y., Ishihara, N., Yokota, S., and Mihara, K. (2003). Two mitofusin proteins, mammalian homologues of FZO, with distinct functions are both required for mitochondrial fusion. *J. Biochem.* 134, 333–344. doi: 10.1093/jb/mvg150

Exner, N., Treske, B., Paquet, D., Holmstrom, K., Schiesling, C., Gispert, S., et al. (2007). Loss-of-function of human PINK1 results in mitochondrial pathology and can be rescued by parkin. *J. Neurosci.* 27, 12413–12418. doi: 10.1523/JNEUROSCI.0719-07.2007

Ferreira, I. L., Resende, R., Ferreiro, E., Rego, A. C., and Pereira, C. F. (2010). Multiple defects in energy metabolism in Alzheimer's disease. *Curr. Drug Targets* 11, 1193–1206. doi: 10.2174/1389450111007011193

Ferré, M., Amati-Bonneau, P., Tourmen, Y., Malthièry, Y., and Reynier, P. (2005). eOPA1: an online database for OPA1 mutations. *Hum. Mutat.* 25, 423–428. doi: 10.1002/humu.20161

Frezza, C., Cipolat, S., Martins de Brito, O., Micaroni, M., Beznoussenko, G. V., Rudka, T., et al. (2006). OPA1 controls apoptotic cristae remodeling independently from mitochondrial fusion. *Cell* 126, 177–189. doi: 10.1016/j.cell.2006.06.025

Friedman, J. R., Lackner, L. L., West, M., DiBenedetto, J. R., Nunnari, J., and Voeltz, G. K. (2011). ER tubules mark sites of mitochondrial division. *Science* 334, 358–362. doi: 10.1126/science.1207385

Gandre-Babbe, S., and van der Bliek, A. M. (2008). The novel tail-anchored membrane protein Mff controls mitochondrial and peroxisomal fission in mammalian cells. *Mol. Biol. Cell.* 19, 2402–2412. doi: 10.1091/mbc.E07-12-1287

Gao, A. W., Canto, C., and Houtkooper, R. H. (2014). Mitochondrial response to nutrient availability and its role in metabolic disease. *EMBO Mol. Med.* 6, 580–589. doi: 10.1002/emmm.201303782

Gegg, M. E., Cooper, J. M., Chau, K. Y., Rojo, M., Schapira, A. H., and Taanman, J. W. (2010). Mitofusin 1 and mitofusin 2 are ubiquitinated in a PINK1/parkin-dependent manner upon induction of mitophagy. *Hum. Mol. Genet.* 19, 4861–4870. doi: 10.1093/hmg/ddq419

Gomez-Lazaro, M., Bonekamp, N. A., Galindo, M. F., Jordan, J., and Schrader, M. (2008). 6-Hydroxydopamine (6-OHDA) induces Drp1-dependent mitochondrial fragmentation in SH-SY5Y cells. *Free Radic. Biol. Med.* 44, 1960–1969. doi: 10.1016/j.freeradbiomed.2008.03.009

Griparic, L., Kanazawa, T., and van der Bliek, A. M. (2007). Regulation of the mitochondrial dynamin-like protein Opa1 by proteolytic cleavage. *J. Cell Biol.* 178, 757–764. doi: 10.1083/jcb.200704112

Griparic, L., van der Wel, N. N., Orozco, I. J., Peters, P. J., and van der Bliek, A. M. (2004). Loss of the intermembrane space protein Mgm1/OPA1 induces swelling and localized constrictions along the lengths of mitochondria. *J. Biol. Chem.* 279, 18792–18798. doi: 10.1074/jbc.M400920200

Grunewald, A., Gegg, M. E., Taanman, J. W., King, R. H., Kock, N., Klein, C., et al. (2009). Differential effects of PINK1 nonsense and missense mutations on mitochondrial function and morphology. *Exp. Neurol.* 219, 266–273. doi: 10.1016/j.expneurol.2009.05.027

Hales, K. G., and Fuller, M. T. (1997). Developmentally regulated mitochondrial fusion mediated by a conserved, novel, predicted GTPase. *Cell* 90, 121–129. doi: 10.1016/S0092-8674(00)80319-0

Harder, Z., Zunino, R., and McBride, H. (2004). Sumo1 conjugates mitochondrial substrates and participates in mitochondrial fission. *Curr. Biol.* 14, 340–345. doi: 10.1016/j.cub.2004.02.004

Hayashi, T., and Su, T. P. (2007). Sigma-1 receptor chaperones at the ER-mitochondrion interface regulate Ca(2+) signaling and cell survival. *Cell* 131, 596–610. doi: 10.1016/j.cell.2007.08.036

Head, B., Griparic, L., Amiri, M., Gandre-Babbe, S., and van der Bliek, A. M. (2009). Inducible proteolytic inactivation of OPA1 mediated by the OMA1 protease in mammalian cells. *J. Cell Biol.* 187, 959–966. doi: 10.1083/jcb.200906083

Hernandez-Alvarez, M. I., Paz, J. C., Sebastian, D., Munoz, J. P., Liesa, M., Segales, J., et al. (2013). Glucocorticoid modulation of mitochondrial function in hepatoma cells requires the mitochondrial fission protein Drp1. *Antioxid. Redox Signal.* 19, 366–378. doi: 10.1089/ars.2011.4269

Hill, J. W., Williams, K. W., Ye, C., Luo, J., Balthasar, N., Coppari, R., et al. (2008). Acute effects of leptin require PI3K signaling in hypothalamic proopiomelanocortin neurons in mice. *J. Clin. Invest.* 118, 1796–1805. doi: 10.1172/JCI32964

Hoozemans, J. J. M., Veerhuis, R., Van Haastert, E. S., Rozemuller, J. M., Baas, F., Eikelenboom, P., et al. (2005). The unfolded protein response is activated in Alzheimer's disease. *Acta Neuropathol.* 110, 165–172. doi: 10.1007/s00401-005-1038-0

Hoyt, C. (1980). Autosomal dominant optic atrophy. A spectrum of disability. *Ophthalmology* 87, 245–251. doi: 10.1016/S0161-6420(80)35247-0

Hudson, G., Amati-Bonneau, P., Blakely, E. L., Stewart, J. D., He, L., Schaefer, A. M., et al. (2008). Mutation of OPA1 causes dominant optic atrophy with external ophthalmoplegia, ataxia, deafness and multiple mitochondrial DNA deletions: a novel disorder of mtDNA maintenance. *Brain* 131, 329–337. doi: 10.1093/brain/awm272

Ibrahim, N., Bosch, M. A., Smart, J. L., Qiu, J., Rubinstein, M., Ronnekleiv, O. K., et al. (2003). Hypothalamic proopiomelanocortin neurons are glucose responsive and express K(ATP) channels. *Endocrinology* 144, 1331–1340. doi: 10.1210/en.2002-221033

Ingerman, E., Perkins, E. M., Marino, M., Mears, J. A., McCaffery, J. M., Hinshaw, J. E., et al. (2005). Dnm1 forms spirals that are structurally tailored to fit mitochondria. *J. Cell Biol.* 170, 1021–1027. doi: 10.1083/jcb.200506078

Ishihara, N., Eura, Y., and Mihara, K. (2004). Mitofusin 1 and 2 play distinct roles in mitochondrial fusion reactions via GTPase activity. *J. Cell Sci.* 117, 6535–6546. doi: 10.1242/jcs.01565

Ishihara, N., Fujita, Y., Oka, T., and Mihara, K. (2006). Regulation of mitochondrial morphology through proteolytic cleavage of OPA1. *EMBO J.* 25, 2966–2977. doi: 10.1038/sj.emboj.7601184

Ishihara, N., Nomura, M., Jofuku, A., Kato, H., Suzuki, S. O., Masuda, K., et al. (2009). Mitochondrial fission factor Drp1 is essential for embryonic development and synapse formation in mice. *Nat. Cell Biol.* 11, 958–966. doi: 10.1038/ncb1907

Iwasawa, R., Mahul-Mellier, A. L., Datler, C., Pazarentzos, E., and Grimm, S. (2011). Fis1 and Bap31 bridge the mitochondria-ER interface to establish a platform for apoptosis induction. *EMBO J.* 30, 556–568. doi: 10.1038/emboj.2010.346

Jahani-Asl, A., Pilon-Larose, K., Xu, W., MacLaurin, J. G., Park, D. S., McBride, H. M., et al. (2011). The mitochondrial inner membrane GTPase, optic atrophy 1 (Opa1), restores mitochondrial morphology and promotes neuronal survival following excitotoxicity. *J. Biol. Chem.* 286, 4772–4782. doi: 10.1074/jbc.M110.167155

Jofuku, A., Ishihara, N., and Mihara, K. (2005). Analysis of functional domains of rat mitochondrial Fis1, the mitochondrial fission-stimulating protein. *Biochem. Biophys. Res. Commun.* 333, 650–659. doi: 10.1016/j.bbrc.2005.05.154

Johnston, P., Gaster, R., Smith, V., and Tripathi, R. (1979). A clinicopathologic study of autosomal dominant optic atrophy. *Am. J. Ophthalmol.* 88, 868–875. doi: 10.1016/0002-9394(79)90565-8

Johnston, R. L., Seller, M. J., Behnam, J. T., Burdon, M. A., and Spalton, D. J. (1999). Dominant optic atrophy: refining the clinical diagnostic criteria in light of genetic linkage studies. *Ophthalmology* 106, 123–128. doi: 10.1016/S0161-6420(99)90013-1

Kamegai, J., Tamura, H., Shimizu, T., Ishii, S., Sugihara, H., and Wakabayashi, I. (2001). Chronic central infusion of ghrelin increases hypothalamic neuropeptide Y and Agouti-related protein mRNA levels and body weight in rats. *Diabetes* 50, 2438–2443. doi: 10.2337/diabetes.50.11.2438

Karbowski, M., Neutzner, A., and Youle, R. J. (2007). The mitochondrial E3 ubiquitin ligase MARCH5 is required for Drp1 dependent mitochondrial division. *J. Cell Biol.* 178, 71–84. doi: 10.1083/jcb.200611064

Karren, M. A., Coonrod, E. M., Anderson, T. K., and Shaw, J. M. (2005). The role of Fis1p-Mdv1p interactions in mitochondrial fission complex assembly. *J. Cell Biol.* 171, 291–301. doi: 10.1083/jcb.200506158

Kijima, K., Numakura, C., Izumino, H., Umetsu, K., Nezu, A., Shiiki, T., et al. (2005). Mitochondrial GTPase mitofusin 2 mutation in Charcot–Marie–Tooth neuropathy type 2A. *Hum. Genet.* 116, 23–27. doi: 10.1007/s00439-004-1199-2

Kim, I., Rodriguez-Enriquez, S., and Lemasters, J. J. (2007). Selective degradation of mitochondria by mitophagy. *Arch. Biochem. Biophys.* 462, 245–253. doi: 10.1016/j.abb.2007.03.034

Kim, J. Y., Hwang, J.-M., Ko, H. S., Seong, M.-W., Park, B.-J., and Park, S. S. (2005). Mitochondrial DNA content is decreased in autosomal dominant optic atrophy. *Neurology* 64, 966–972. doi: 10.1212/01.WNL.0000157282.76715.B1

Kjer, P., Jensen, O., and Klinken, L. (1983). Histopathology of eye, optic nerve and brain in a case of dominant optic atrophy. *Acta Ophthalmol.* 61, 300–312. doi: 10.1111/j.1755-3768.1983.tb01424.x

Koshiba, T., Detmer, S. A., Kaiser, J. T., Chen, H., McCaffery, J. M., and Chan, D. C. (2004). Structural basis of mitochondrial tethering by mitofusin complexes. *Science* 305, 858–862. doi: 10.1126/science.1099793

Lackner, L. L., Horner, J. S., and Nunnari, J. (2009). Mechanistic analysis of a dynamin effector. *Science* 325, 874–877. doi: 10.1126/science.1176921

Lawson, V. H., Graham, B. V., and Flanigan, K. M. (2005). Clinical and electrophysiologic features of CMT2A with mutations in the mitofusin 2 gene. *Neurology* 65, 197–204. doi: 10.1212/01.wnl.0000168898.76071.70

Leboucher, G. P., Tsai, Y. C., Yang, M., Shaw, K. C., Zhou, M., Veenstra, T. D., et al. (2012). Stress-induced phosphorylation and proteasomal degradation of mitofusin 2 facilitates mitochondrial fragmentation and apoptosis. *Mol. Cell.* 47, 547–557. doi: 10.1016/j.molcel.2012.05.041

Lee, J. Y., Kapur, M., Li, M., Choi, M. C., Choi, S., Kim, H. J., et al. (2014). MFN1 deacetylation activates adaptive mitochondrial fusion and protects metabolically challenged mitochondria. *J. Cell Sci.* 127, 4954–4963. doi: 10.1242/jcs.157321

Lee, S., Sterky, F. H., Mourier, A., Terzioglu, M., Cullheim, S., Olson, L., et al. (2012). Mitofusin 2 is necessary for striatal axonal projections of midbrain dopamine neurons. *Hum. Mol. Genet.* 21, 4827–4835. doi: 10.1093/hmg/dds352

Lee, Y. J., Jeong, S. Y., Karbowski, M., Smith, C. L., and Youle, R. J. (2004). Roles of the mammalian mitochondrial fission and fusion mediators Fis1, Drp1, Opa1 in apoptosis. *Mol. Biol. Cell.* 15, 5001–5011. doi: 10.1091/mbc.E04-04-0294

Legesse-Miller, A., Massol, R. H., and Kirchhausen, T. (2003). Constriction and Dnm1p recruitment are distinct processes in mitochondrial fission. *Mol. Biol. Cell.* 14, 1953–1963. doi: 10.1091/mbc.E02-10-0657

Lelliott, C. J., Medina-Gomez, G., Petrovic, N., Kis, A., Feldmann, H. M., Bjursell, M., et al. (2006). Ablation of PGC-1beta results in defective mitochondrial activity, thermogenesis, hepatic function, and cardiac performance. *PLoS Biol.* 4:e369. doi: 10.1371/journal.pbio.0040369

Li, J., Li, Y., Jiao, J., Wang, J., Qin, D., and Li, P. (2014). Mitofusin 1 is negatively regulated by microRNA 140 in cardiomyocyte apoptosis. *Mol. Cell. Biol.* 34, 1788–1799. doi: 10.1128/MCB.00774-13

Li, Z., Okamoto, K., Hayashi, Y., and Sheng, M. (2004). The importance of dendritic mitochondria in the morphogenesis and plasticity of spines and synapses. *Cell* 119, 873–887. doi: 10.1016/j.cell.2004.11.003

Liesa, M., Borda-d'Agua, B., Medina-Gomez, G., Lelliott, C. J., Paz, J. C., Rojo, M., et al. (2008). Mitochondrial fusion is increased by the nuclear coactivator PGC-1beta. *PLoS ONE* 3:e3613. doi: 10.1371/journal.pone.0003613

Liesa, M., and Shirihai, O. S. (2013). Mitochondrial dynamics in the regulation of nutrient utilization and energy expenditure. *Cell Metab.* 17, 491–506. doi: 10.1016/j.cmet.2013.03.002

Loiseau, D., Chevrollier, A., Verny, C., Guillet, V., Gueguen, N., Pou de Crescenzo, M. A., et al. (2007). Mitochondrial coupling defect in Charcot-Marie-Tooth type 2A disease. *Ann. Neurol.* 61, 315–323. doi: 10.1002/ana.21086

Lokireddy, S., Wijesoma, I. W., Teng, S., Bonala, S., Gluckman, P. D., McFarlane, C., et al. (2012). The ubiquitin ligase Mul1 induces mitophagy in skeletal muscle in response to muscle-wasting stimuli. *Cell Metab.* 16, 613–624. doi: 10.1016/j.cmet.2012.10.005

Long, L., Toda, C., Jeong, J. K., Horvath, T. L., and Diano, S. (2014). PPARgamma ablation sensitizes proopiomelanocortin neurons to leptin during high-fat feeding. *J. Clin. Invest.* 124, 4017–4027. doi: 10.1172/JCI76220

Lopez, M., Lage, R., Saha, A. K., Perez-Tilve, D., Vazquez, M. J., Varela, L., et al. (2008). Hypothalamic fatty acid metabolism mediates the orexigenic action of ghrelin. *Cell Metab.* 7, 389–399. doi: 10.1016/j.cmet.2008.03.006

Lopez Del Amo, V., Seco-Cervera, M., Garcia-Gimenez, J. L., Whitworth, A. J., Pallardo, F. V., and Galindo, M. I. (2015). Mitochondrial defects and neuromuscular degeneration caused by altered expression of Drosophila Gdap1: implications for the Charcot-Marie-Tooth neuropathy. *Hum. Mol. Genet.* 24, 21–36. doi: 10.1093/hmg/ddu416

Loson, O. C., Song, Z., Chen, H., and Chan, D. C. (2013). Fis1, Mff, MiD49, and MiD51 mediate Drp1 recruitment in mitochondrial fission. *Mol. Biol. Cell.* 24, 659–667. doi: 10.1091/mbc.E12-10-0721

Luquet, S., Phillips, C. T., and Palmiter, R. D. (2007). NPY/AgRP neurons are not essential for feeding responses to glucoprivation. *Peptides* 28, 214–225. doi: 10.1016/j.peptides.2006.08.036

Lutz, A. K., Exner, N., Fett, M. E., Schlehe, J. S., Kloos, K., Lammermann, K., et al. (2009). Loss of parkin or PINK1 function increases Drp1-dependent mitochondrial fragmentation. *J. Biol. Chem.* 284, 22938–22951. doi: 10.1074/jbc.M109.035774

Mailloux, R. J., and Harper, M. E. (2011). Uncoupling proteins and the control of mitochondrial reactive oxygen species production. *Free Radic. Biol. Med.* 51, 1106–1115. doi: 10.1016/j.freeradbiomed.2011.06.022

Martin, O. J., Lai, L., Soundarapandian, M. M., Leone, T. C., Zorzano, A., Keller, M. P., et al. (2014). A role for peroxisome proliferator-activated receptor gamma coactivator-1 in the control of mitochondrial dynamics during postnatal cardiac growth. *Circ. Res.* 114, 626–636. doi: 10.1161/CIRCRESAHA.114.302562

Martorell-Riera, A., Segarra-Mondejar, M., Munoz, J. P., Ginet, V., Olloquequi, J., Perez-Clausell, J., et al. (2014). Mfn2 downregulation in excitotoxicity causes mitochondrial dysfunction and delayed neuronal death. *EMBO J.* 33, 2388–2407. doi: 10.15252/embj.201488327

Mears, J. A., Lackner, L. L., Fang, S., Ingerman, E., Nunnari, J., and Hinshaw, J. E. (2011). Conformational changes in Dnm1 support a contractile mechanism for mitochondrial fission. *Nat. Struct. Mol. Biol.* 18, 20–26. doi: 10.1038/nsmb.1949

Meeusen, S., McCaffery, J. M., and Nunnari, J. (2004). Mitochondrial fusion intermediates revealed *in vitro*. *Science* 305, 1747–1752. doi: 10.1126/science.1100612

Misaka, T., Miyashita, T., and Kubo, Y. (2002). Primary structure of a dynamin-related mouse mitochondrial GTPase and its distribution in brain, subcellular localization, and effect on mitochondrial morphology. *J. Biol. Chem.* 277, 15834–15842. doi: 10.1074/jbc.M109260200

Mizuno, T. M., Kleopoulos, S. P., Bergen, H. T., Roberts, J. L., Priest, C. A., and Mobbs, C. V. (1998). Hypothalamic pro-opiomelanocortin mRNA is reduced by fasting and [corrected] in ob/ob and db/db mice, but is stimulated by leptin. *Diabetes* 47, 294–297. doi: 10.2337/diab.47.2.294

Mizuno, T. M., and Mobbs, C. V. (1999). Hypothalamic agouti-related protein messenger ribonucleic acid is inhibited by leptin and stimulated by fasting. *Endocrinology* 140, 814–817. doi: 10.1210/en.140.2.814

Mozdy, A. D., McCaffery, J. M., and Shaw, J. M. (2000). Dnm1p Gtpase-mediated mitochondrial fission is a multi-step process requiring the novel integral membrane component Fis1p. *J. Cell Biol.* 151, 367–380. doi: 10.1083/jcb.151.2.367

Munoz, J. P., Ivanova, S., Sanchez-Wandelmer, J., Martinez-Cristobal, P., Noguera, E., Sancho, A., et al. (2013). Mfn2 modulates the UPR and mitochondrial function via repression of PERK. *EMBO J.* 32, 2348–2361. doi: 10.1038/emboj.2013.168

Nakazato, M., Murakami, N., Date, Y., Kojima, M., Matsuo, H., Kangawa, K., et al. (2001). A role for ghrelin in the central regulation of feeding. *Nature* 409, 194–198. doi: 10.1038/35051587

Narendra, D. P., Jin, S. M., Tanaka, A., Suen, D.-F., Gautier, C. A., Shen, J., et al. (2010). PINK1 is selectively stabilized on impaired mitochondria to activate parkin. *PLoS Biol.* 8:e1000298. doi: 10.1371/journal.pbio.1000298

Nelis, E., Erdem, S., Van den Bergh, P. Y. K., Belpaire–Dethiou, M.-C., Ceuterick, C., Van Gerwen, V., et al. (2002). Mutations in GDAP1. *Neurology* 59, 1865–1872. doi: 10.1212/01.WNL.0000036272.36047.54

Niemann, A., Ruegg, M., La Padula, V., Schenone, A., and Suter, U. (2005). Ganglioside-induced differentiation associated protein 1 is a regulator of the mitochondrial network: new implications for Charcot-Marie-Tooth disease. *J. Cell Biol.* 170, 1067–1078. doi: 10.1083/jcb.200507087

Nunnari, J., Marshall, W., Straight, A., Murray, A., Sedat, J., and Walter, P. (1997). Mitochondrial transmission during mating in *Saccharomyces cerevisiae* is determined by mitochondrial fusion and fission and the intramitochondrial segregation of mitochondrial DNA. *Mol. Biol. Cell* 8, 1233–1242. doi: 10.1091/mbc.8.7.1233

Olichon, A., Baricault, L., Gas, N., Guillou, E., Valette, A., Belenguer, P., et al. (2003). Loss of OPA1 perturbates the mitochondrial inner membrane structure and integrity, leading to cytochrome c release and apoptosis. *J. Biol. Chem.* 278, 7743–7746. doi: 10.1074/jbc.C200677200

Olichon, A., Elachouri, G., Baricault, L., Delettre, C., Belenguer, P., and Lenaers, G. (2007). OPA1 alternate splicing uncouples an evolutionary conserved function in mitochondrial fusion from a vertebrate restricted function in apoptosis. *Cell Death Differ.* 14, 682–692. doi: 10.1038/sj.cdd.4402048

Olichon, A., Emorine, L. J., Descoins, E., Pelloquin, L., Brichese, L., Gas, N., et al. (2002). The human dynamin-related protein OPA1 is anchored to the mitochondrial inner membrane facing the inter-membrane space. *FEBS Lett.*. 523, 171–176. doi: 10.1016/S0014-5793(02)02985-X

Olichon, A., Guillou, E., Delettre, C., Landes, T., Arnauné-Pelloquin, L., Emorine, L. J., et al. (2006). Mitochondrial dynamics and disease, OPA1. *Biochim. Biophys. Acta* 1763, 500–509. doi: 10.1016/j.bbamcr.2006.04.003

Ollmann, M. M., Wilson, B. D., Yang, Y. K., Kerns, J. A., Chen, Y., Gantz, I., et al. (1997). Antagonism of central melanocortin receptors *in vitro* and *in vivo* by agouti-related protein. *Science* 278, 135–138. doi: 10.1126/science.278.5335.135

Otera, H., Wang, C., Cleland, M. M., Setoguchi, K., Yokota, S., Youle, R. J., et al. (2010). Mff is an essential factor for mitochondrial recruitment of Drp1 during mitochondrial fission in mammalian cells. *J. Cell Biol.* 191, 1141–1158. doi: 10.1083/jcb.201007152

Ozcan, L., Ergin, A. S., Lu, A., Chung, J., Sarkar, S., Nie, D., et al. (2009). Endoplasmic reticulum stress plays a central role in development of leptin resistance. *Cell Metab.* 9, 35–51. doi: 10.1016/j.cmet.2008.12.004

Palmer, C. S., Osellame, L. D., Laine, D., Koutsopoulos, O. S., Frazier, A. E., and Ryan, M. T. (2011). MiD49 and MiD51, new components of the mitochondrial fission machinery. *EMBO Rep.* 12, 565–573. doi: 10.1038/embor.2011.54

Panov, A. V., Gutekunst, C. A., Leavitt, B. R., Hayden, M. R., Burke, J. R., Strittmatter, W. J., et al. (2002). Early mitochondrial calcium defects in Huntington's disease are a direct effect of polyglutamines. *Nat. Neurosci.* 5, 731–736. doi: 10.1038/nn884

Papanicolaou, K. N., Khairallah, R. J., Ngoh, G. A., Chikando, A., Luptak, I., O'Shea, K. M., et al. (2011). Mitofusin-2 maintains mitochondrial structure and contributes to stress-induced permeability transition in cardiac myocytes. *Mol. Cell. Biol.* 31, 1309–1328.

Papanicolaou, K. N., Ngoh, G. A., Dabkowski, E. R., O'Connell, K. A., Ribeiro, R. F. Jr., Stanley, W. C., et al. (2012). Cardiomyocyte deletion of mitofusin-1 leads to mitochondrial fragmentation and improves tolerance to ROS-induced mitochondrial dysfunction and cell death. *Am. J. Physiol. Heart Circ. Physiol.* 302, H167–H179.

Park, Y. Y., and Cho, H. (2012). Mitofusin 1 is degraded at G2/M phase through ubiquitylation by MARCH5. *Cell Div.* 7, 25. doi: 10.1186/1747-1028-7-25

Park, Y. Y., Lee, S., Karbowski, M., Neutzner, A., Youle, R. J., and Cho, H. (2010). Loss of MARCH5 mitochondrial E3 ubiquitin ligase induces cellular senescence through dynamin-related protein 1 and mitofusin 1. *J. Cell Sci.* 123, 619–626. doi: 10.1242/jcs.061481

Parone, P. A., Da Cruz, S., Tondera, D., Mattenberger, Y., James, D. I., Maechler, P., et al. (2008). Preventing mitochondrial fission impairs mitochondrial function and leads to loss of mitochondrial DNA. *PLoS ONE* 3:e3257. doi: 10.1371/journal.pone.0003257

Parton, L. E., Ye, C. P., Coppari, R., Enriori, P. J., Choi, B., Zhang, C. Y., et al. (2007). Glucose sensing by POMC neurons regulates glucose homeostasis and is impaired in obesity. *Nature* 449, 228–232. doi: 10.1038/nature06098

Pesch, U. E. A., Leo-Kottler, B., Mayer, S., Jurklies, B., Kellner, U., Apfelstedt-Sylla, E., et al. (2001). OPA1 mutations in patients with autosomal dominant optic atrophy and evidence for semi-dominant inheritance. *Hum. Mol. Genet.* 10, 1359–1368. doi: 10.1093/hmg/10.13.1359

Pham, A. H., Meng, S., Chu, Q. N., and Chan, D. C. (2012). Loss of Mfn2 results in progressive, retrograde degeneration of dopaminergic neurons in the nigrostriatal circuit. *Hum. Mol. Genet.* 21, 4817–4826. doi: 10.1093/hmg/dds311

Pich, S., Bach, D., Briones, P., Liesa, M., Camps, M., Testar, X., et al. (2005). The Charcot-Marie-Tooth type 2A gene product, Mfn2, up-regulates fuel oxidation through expression of OXPHOS system. *Hum. Mol. Genet.* 14, 1405–1415. doi: 10.1093/hmg/ddi149

Pickrell, A. M., and Youle, R. J. (2015). The roles of PINK1, parkin, and mitochondrial fidelity in parkinson's disease. *Neuron* 85, 257–273. doi: 10.1016/j.neuron.2014.12.007

Pitts, K. R., Yoon, Y., Krueger, E. W., and McNiven, M. A. (1999). The dynamin-like protein DLP1 is essential for normal distribution and morphology of the endoplasmic reticulum and mitochondria in mammalian cells. *Mol. Biol. Cell.* 10, 4403–4417. doi: 10.1091/mbc.10.12.4403

Poggioli, R., Vergoni, A. V., and Bertolini, A. (1986). ACTH-(1-24) and alpha-MSH antagonize feeding behavior stimulated by kappa opiate agonists. *Peptides* 7, 843–848. doi: 10.1016/0196-9781(86)90104-X

Poole, A. C., Thomas, R. E., Yu, S., Vincow, E. S., and Pallanck, L. (2010). The mitochondrial fusion-promoting factor mitofusin is a substrate of the PINK1/parkin pathway. *PLoS ONE* 5:e10054. doi: 10.1371/journal.pone.0010054

Poston, C. N., Krishnan, S. C., and Bazemore-Walker, C. R. (2013). In-depth proteomic analysis of mammalian mitochondria-associated membranes (MAM). *J. Proteomics* 79, 219–230. doi: 10.1016/j.jprot.2012.12.018

Quiros, P. M., Ramsay, A. J., Sala, D., Fernandez-Vizarra, E., Rodriguez, F., Peinado, J. R., et al. (2012). Loss of mitochondrial protease OMA1 alters processing of the GTPase OPA1 and causes obesity and defective thermogenesis in mice. *EMBO J.* 31, 2117–2133. doi: 10.1038/emboj.2012.70

Reddy, P. H., Reddy, T. P., Manczak, M., Calkins, M. J., Shirendeb, U., and Mao, P. (2011). Dynamin-related protein 1 and mitochondrial fragmentation in neurodegenerative diseases. *Brain Res. Rev.* 67, 103–118. doi: 10.1016/j.brainresrev.2010.11.004

Rojo, M., Legros, F., Chateau, D., and Lombès, A. (2002). Membrane topology and mitochondrial targeting of mitofusins, ubiquitous mammalian homologs of the transmembrane GTPase Fzo. *J. Cell Sci.* 115, 1663–1674.

Roseberry, A. G., Liu, H., Jackson, A. C., Cai, X., and Friedman, J. M. (2004). Neuropeptide Y-mediated inhibition of proopiomelanocortin neurons in the arcuate nucleus shows enhanced desensitization in ob/ob mice. *Neuron* 41, 711–722. doi: 10.1016/S0896-6273(04)00074-1

Rui, Y., Tiwari, P., Xie, Z., and Zheng, J. Q. (2006). Acute impairment of mitochondrial trafficking by beta-amyloid peptides in hippocampal neurons. *J. Neurosci.* 26, 10480–10487. doi: 10.1523/JNEUROSCI.3231-06.2006

Sandebring, A., Thomas, K. J., Beilina, A., van der Brug, M., Cleland, M. M., Ahmad, R., et al. (2009). Mitochondrial alterations in PINK1 deficient cells are influenced by calcineurin-dependent dephosphorylation of dynamin-related protein 1. *PLoS ONE* 4:e5701. doi: 10.1371/journal.pone.0005701

Santel, A., Frank, S., Gaume, B., Herrler, M., Youle, R. J., and Fuller, M. T. (2003). Mitofusin-1 protein is a generally expressed mediator of mitochondrial fusion in mammalian cells. *J. Cell Sci.* 116, 2763–2774. doi: 10.1242/jcs.00479

Sarzi, E., Angebault, C., Seveno, M., Gueguen, N., Chaix, B., Bielicki, G., et al. (2012). The human OPA1delTTAG mutation induces premature age-related systemic neurodegeneration in mouse. *Brain* 135, 3599–3613. doi: 10.1093/brain/aws303

Satoh, M., Hamamoto, T., Seo, N., Kagawa, Y., and Endo, H. (2003). Differential sublocalization of the dynamin-related protein OPA1 isoforms in mitochondria. *Biochem. Biophys. Res. Commun.* 300, 482–493. doi: 10.1016/S0006-291X(02)02874-7

Scarpulla, R. C., Vega, R. B., and Kelly, D. P. (2012). Transcriptional integration of mitochondrial biogenesis. *Trends Endocrinol. Metab.* 23, 459–466. doi: 10.1016/j.tem.2012.06.006

Schapira, A. H., Bezard, E., Brotchie, J., Calon, F., Collingridge, G. L., Ferger, B., et al. (2006). Novel pharmacological targets for the treatment of Parkinson's disease. *Nat. Rev. Drug Discov.* 5, 845–854. doi: 10.1038/nrd2087

Schapira, A. H., Olanow, C. W., Greenamyre, J. T., and Bezard, E. (2014). Slowing of neurodegeneration in Parkinson's disease and Huntington's disease: future therapeutic perspectives. *Lancet* 384, 545–555. doi: 10.1016/S0140-6736(14)61010-2

Schneeberger, M., Dietrich, M. O., Sebastian, D., Imbernon, M., Castano, C., Garcia, A., et al. (2013). Mitofusin 2 in POMC neurons connects ER stress with leptin resistance and energy imbalance. *Cell* 155, 172–187. doi: 10.1016/j.cell.2013.09.003

Schneeberger, M., Gomis, R., and Claret, M. (2014). Hypothalamic and brainstem neuronal circuits controlling homeostatic energy balance. *J. Endocrinol.* 220, T25–T46. doi: 10.1530/joe-13-0398

Schon, E. A., and Area-Gomez, E. (2010). Is Alzheimer's disease a disorder of mitochondria-associated membranes? *J. Alzheimer's Dis.* 20, S281–S292. doi: 10.3233/JAD-2010-100495

Schwartz, M. W., Baskin, D. G., Bukowski, T. R., Kuijper, J. L., Foster, D., Lasser, G., et al. (1996). Specificity of leptin action on elevated blood glucose levels and hypothalamic neuropeptide Y gene expression in ob/ob mice. *Diabetes* 45, 531–535. doi: 10.2337/diab.45.4.531

Schwartz, M. W., Seeley, R. J., Woods, S. C., Weigle, D. S., Campfield, L. A., Burn, P., et al. (1997). Leptin increases hypothalamic pro-opiomelanocortin mRNA expression in the rostral arcuate nucleus. *Diabetes* 46, 2119–2123. doi: 10.2337/diab.46.12.2119

Sebastian, D., Hernandez-Alvarez, M. I., Segales, J., Sorianello, E., Munoz, J. P., Sala, D., et al. (2012). Mitofusin 2 (Mfn2) links mitochondrial and endoplasmic reticulum function with insulin signaling and is essential for normal glucose homeostasis. *Proc. Natl. Acad. Sci. U.S.A.* 109, 5523–5528. doi: 10.1073/pnas.1108220109

Senderek, J., Bergmann, C., Ramaekers, V. T., Nelis, E., Bernert, G., Makowski, A., et al. (2003). Mutations in the ganglioside–induced differentiation–associated protein–1 (GDAP1) gene in intermediate type autosomal recessive Charcot–Marie–Tooth neuropathy. *Brain* 126, 642–649. doi: 10.1093/brain/awg068

Sevilla, T., Cuesta, A., Chumillas, M. J., Mayordomo, F., Pedrola, L., Palau, F., et al. (2003). Clinical, electrophysiological and morphological findings of Charcot–Marie–Tooth neuropathy with vocal cord palsy and mutations in the GDAP1 gene. *Brain* 126, 2023–2033. doi: 10.1093/brain/awg202

Shirendeb, U., Reddy, A. P., Manczak, M., Calkins, M. J., Mao, P., Tagle, D. A., et al. (2011). Abnormal mitochondrial dynamics, mitochondrial loss and mutant huntingtin oligomers in Huntington's disease: implications for selective neuronal damage. *Hum. Mol. Genet.* 20, 1438–1455. doi: 10.1093/hmg/ddr024

Simmen, T., Aslan, J. E., Blagoveshchenskaya, A. D., Thomas, L., Wan, L., Xiang, Y., et al. (2005). PACS-2 controls endoplasmic reticulum-mitochondria communication and Bid-mediated apoptosis. *EMBO J.* 24, 717–729. doi: 10.1038/sj.emboj.7600559

Simpson, J. C., Wellenreuther, R., Poustka, A., Pepperkok, R., and Wiemann, S. (2000). Systematic subcellular localization of novel proteins identified by large-scale cDNA sequencing. *EMBO Rep.* 1, 287–292. doi: 10.1093/embo-reports/kvd058

Skre, H. (1974). Genetic and clinical aspects of Charcot-Marie-Tooth's disease. *Clin. Genet.* 6, 98–118. doi: 10.1111/j.1399-0004.1974.tb00638.x

Smith, M. A., Hisadome, K., Al-Qassab, H., Heffron, H., Withers, D. J., and Ashford, M. L. (2007). Melanocortins and agouti-related protein modulate the excitability of two arcuate nucleus neuron populations by alteration of resting potassium conductances. *J. Physiol.* 578(Pt 2), 425–38. doi: 10.1113/jphysiol.2006.119479

Song, W., Chen, J., Petrilli, A., Liot, G., Klinglmayr, E., Zhou, Y., et al. (2011). Mutant huntingtin binds the mitochondrial fission GTPase dynamin-related protein-1 and increases its enzymatic activity. *Nat. Med.* 17, 377–382. doi: 10.1038/nm.2313

Song, Z., Chen, H., Fiket, M., Alexander, C., and Chan, D. C. (2007). OPA1 processing controls mitochondrial fusion and is regulated by mRNA splicing, membrane potential, and Yme1L. *J. Cell Biol.* 178, 749–755. doi: 10.1083/jcb.200704110

Sorianello, E., Soriano, F. X., Fernandez-Pascual, S., Sancho, A., Naon, D., Vila-Caballer, M., et al. (2012). The promoter activity of human Mfn2 depends on Sp1 in vascular smooth muscle cells. *Cardiovasc. Res.* 94, 38–47. doi: 10.1093/cvr/cvs006

Soriano, F. X., Liesa, M., Bach, D., Chan, D. C., Palacin, M., and Zorzano, A. (2006). Evidence for a mitochondrial regulatory pathway defined by peroxisome proliferator-activated receptor-gamma coactivator-1 alpha, estrogen-related receptor-alpha, and mitofusin 2. *Diabetes* 55, 1783–1791. doi: 10.2337/db05-0509

Stephens, T. W., Basinski, M., Bristow, P. K., Bue-Valleskey, J. M., Burgett, S. G., Craft, L., et al. (1995). The role of neuropeptide Y in the antiobesity action of the obese gene product. *Nature* 377, 530–532. doi: 10.1038/377530a0

Stojanovski, D., Koutsopoulos, O. S., Okamoto, K., and Ryan, M. T. (2004). Levels of human Fis1 at the mitochondrial outer membrane regulate mitochondrial morphology. *J. Cell Sci.* 117, 1201–1210. doi: 10.1242/jcs.01058

Stone, S. J., and Vance, J. E. (2000). Phosphatidylserine synthase-1 and -2 are localized to mitochondria-associated membranes. *J. Biol. Chem.* 275, 34534–34540. doi: 10.1074/jbc.M002865200

Sugiura, A., Nagashima, S., Tokuyama, T., Amo, T., Matsuki, Y., Ishido, S., et al. (2013). MITOL regulates endoplasmic reticulum-mitochondria contacts via Mitofusin2. *Mol. Cell.* 51, 20–34. doi: 10.1016/j.molcel.2013.04.023

Supnet, C., and Bezprozvanny, I. (2010). Neuronal calcium signaling, mitochondrial dysfunction, and Alzheimer's disease. *J. Alzheimer's Dis.* 20, S487–S498. doi: 10.3233/JAD-2010-100306

Sutendra, G., Dromparis, P., Wright, P., Bonnet, S., Haromy, A., Hao, Z., et al. (2011). The role of Nogo and the mitochondria-endoplasmic reticulum unit in pulmonary hypertension. *Sci. Transl. Med.* 3:88ra55. doi: 10.1126/scitranslmed.3002194

Suter, U., and Scherer, S. S. (2003). Disease mechanisms in inherited neuropathies. *Nat. Rev. Neurosci.* 4, 714–726. doi: 10.1038/nrn1196

Suzuki, M., Jeong, S.-Y., Karbowski, M., Youle, R. J., and Tjandra, N. (2003). The solution structure of human mitochondria fission protein Fis1 reveals a novel TPR-like helix bundle. *J. Mol. Biol.* 334, 445–458. doi: 10.1016/j.jmb.2003.09.064

Szabadkai, G., Bianchi, K., Varnai, P., De Stefani, D., Wieckowski, M. R., Cavagna, D., et al. (2006). Chaperone-mediated coupling of endoplasmic reticulum and mitochondrial Ca2+ channels. *J. Cell Biol.* 175, 901–911. doi: 10.1083/jcb.200608073

Tabrizi, S. J., Cleeter, M. W., Xuereb, J., Taanman, J. W., Cooper, J. M., and Schapira, A. H. (1999). Biochemical abnormalities and excitotoxicity in Huntington's disease brain. *Ann. Neurol.* 45, 25–32.

Taguchi, N., Ishihara, N., Jofuku, A., Oka, T., and Mihara, K. (2007). Mitotic phosphorylation of dynamin-related GTPase Drp1 participates in mitochondrial fission. *J. Biol. Chem.* 282, 11521–11529. doi: 10.1074/jbc.M607279200

Tanaka, A., Cleland, M. M., Xu, S., Narendra, D. P., Suen, D. F., Karbowski, M., et al. (2010). Proteasome and p97 mediate mitophagy and degradation of mitofusins induced by Parkin. *J. Cell Biol.* 191, 1367–1380. doi: 10.1083/jcb.201007013

Thornton, J. E., Cheung, C. C., Clifton, D. K., and Steiner, R. A. (1997). Regulation of hypothalamic proopiomelanocortin mRNA by leptin in ob/ob mice. *Endocrinology* 138, 5063–5066. doi: 10.1210/endo.138.11.5651

Tondera, D., Grandemange, S., Jourdain, A., Karbowski, M., Mattenberger, Y., Herzig, S., et al. (2009). SlP-2 is required for stress-induced mitochondrial hyperfusion. *EMBO J.* 28, 1589–1600. doi: 10.1038/emboj.2009.89

Twig, G., Elorza, A., Molina, A. J., Mohamed, H., Wikstrom, J. D., Walzer, G., et al. (2008). Fission and selective fusion govern mitochondrial segregation and elimination by autophagy. *EMBO J.* 27, 433–446. doi: 10.1038/sj.emboj.7601963

Vance, J. E. (1990). Phospholipid synthesis in a membrane fraction associated with mitochondria. *J. Biol. Chem.* 265, 7248–7256.

Van Der Bliek, A. M. (1999). Functional diversity in the dynamin family. *Trends Cell Biol.* 9, 96–102. doi: 10.1016/S0962-8924(98)01490-1

Verhoeven, K., Claeys, K. G., Züchner, S., Schröder, J. M., Weis, J., Ceuterick, C., et al. (2006). MFN2 mutation distribution and genotype/phenotype correlation in Charcot–Marie–Tooth type 2. *Brain* 129, 2093–2102. doi: 10.1093/brain/awl126

Vong, L., Ye, C., Yang, Z., Choi, B., Chua, S. Jr., and Lowell, B. B. (2011). Leptin action on GABAergic neurons prevents obesity and reduces inhibitory tone to POMC neurons. *Neuron* 71, 142–154. doi: 10.1016/j.neuron.2011.05.028

Votruba, M., Fitzke, F. W., Holder, G. E., Carter, A., Bhattacharya, S. S., and Moore, A. T. (1998). Clinical features in affected individuals from 21 pedigrees with dominant optic atrophy. *Arch. Ophthalmol.* 116, 351–358. doi: 10.1001/archopht.116.3.351

Wang, H., Lim, P. J., Karbowski, M., and Monteiro, M. J. (2009b). Effects of overexpression of huntingtin proteins on mitochondrial integrity. *Hum. Mol. Genet.* 18, 737–752. doi: 10.1093/hmg/ddn404

Wang, H., Song, P., Du, L., Tian, W., Yue, W., Liu, M., et al. (2011). Parkin ubiquitinates Drp1 for proteasome-dependent degradation. *J. Biol. Chem.* 286, 11649–11658. doi: 10.1074/jbc.M110.144238

Wang, Q., Liu, C., Uchida, A., Chuang, J. C., Walker, A., Liu, T., et al. (2014). Arcuate AgRP neurons mediate orexigenic and glucoregulatory actions of ghrelin. *Mol Metab.* 3, 64–72. doi: 10.1016/j.molmet.2013.10.001

Wang, X., Su, B., Lee, H. G., Li, X., Perry, G., Smith, M. A., et al. (2009a). Impaired balance of mitochondrial fission and fusion in Alzheimer's disease. *J. Neurosci.* 29, 9090–9103. doi: 10.1523/JNEUROSCI.1357-09.2009

Wang, X., Su, B., Siedlak, S. L., Moreira, P. I., Fujioka, H., Wang, Y., et al. (2008). Amyloid-beta overproduction causes abnormal mitochondrial dynamics via differential modulation of mitochondrial fission/fusion proteins. *Proc. Natl. Acad. Sci. U.S.A.* 105, 19318–19323. doi: 10.1073/pnas.0804871105

Wasiak, S., Zunino, R., and McBride, H. M. (2007). Bax/Bak promote sumoylation of DRP1 and its stable association with mitochondria during apoptotic cell death. *J. Cell Biol.* 177, 439–450. doi: 10.1083/jcb.200610042

Willesen, M. G., Kristensen, P., and Romer, J. (1999). Co-localization of growth hormone secretagogue receptor and NPY mRNA in the arcuate nucleus of the rat. *Neuroendocrinology* 70, 306–316. doi: 10.1159/000054491

Williams, P. A., Morgan, J. E., and Votruba, M. (2010). Opa1 deficiency in a mouse model of dominant optic atrophy leads to retinal ganglion cell dendropathy. *Brain* 133, 2942–2951. doi: 10.1093/brain/awq218

Wirth, M. M., Olszewski, P. K., Yu, C., Levine, A. S., and Giraudo, S. Q. (2001). Paraventricular hypothalamic alpha-melanocyte-stimulating hormone and MTII reduce feeding without causing aversive effects. *Peptides* 22, 129–134. doi: 10.1016/S0196-9781(00)00367-3

Yaffe, M. P. (1999). The machinery of mitochondrial inheritance and behavior. *Science* 283, 1493–1497. doi: 10.1126/science.283.5407.1493

Yang, Y., Atasoy, D., Su, H. H., and Sternson, S. M. (2011). Hunger states switch a flip-flop memory circuit via a synaptic AMPK-dependent positive feedback loop. *Cell* 146, 992–1003. doi: 10.1016/j.cell.2011.07.039

Yoon, Y., Krueger, E. W., Oswald, B. J., and McNiven, M. A. (2003). The mitochondrial protein hFis1 regulates mitochondrial fission in mammalian cells through an interaction with the dynamin-like protein DLP1. *Mol. Cell. Biol.* 23, 5409–5420. doi: 10.1128/MCB.23.15.5409-5420.2003

Yue, W., Chen, Z., Liu, H., Yan, C., Chen, M., Feng, D., et al. (2014). A small natural molecule promotes mitochondrial fusion through inhibition of the deubiquitinase USP30. *Cell Res.* 24, 482–496. doi: 10.1038/cr.2014.20

Zhang, X., Zhang, G., Zhang, H., Karin, M., Bai, H., and Cai, D. (2008). Hypothalamic IKKbeta/NF-kappaB and ER stress link overnutrition to energy imbalance and obesity. *Cell* 135, 61–73. doi: 10.1016/j.cell.2008.07.043

Zhu, D., Kennerson, M. L., Walizada, G., Züchner, S., Vance, J. M., and Nicholson, G. A. (2005). Charcot–Marie–Tooth with pyramidal signs is genetically heterogeneous: families with and without MFN2 mutations. *Neurology* 65, 496–497. doi: 10.1212/01.wnl.0000171345.62270.29

Zhu, X. H., Qiao, H., Du, F., Xiong, Q., Liu, X., Zhang, X., et al. (2012). Quantitative imaging of energy expenditure in human brain. *Neuroimage* 60, 2107–2117. doi: 10.1016/j.neuroimage.2012.02.013

Ziviani, E., Tao, R. N., and Whitworth, A. J. (2010). Drosophila parkin requires PINK1 for mitochondrial translocation and ubiquitinates mitofusin. *Proc. Natl. Acad. Sci. U.S.A.* 107, 5018–5023. doi: 10.1073/pnas.0913485107

Zuchner, S., Mersiyanova, I. V., Muglia, M., Bissar-Tadmouri, N., Rochelle, J., Dadali, E. L., et al. (2004). Mutations in the mitochondrial GTPase mitofusin 2 cause Charcot-Marie-Tooth neuropathy type 2A. *Nat. Genet.* 36, 449–451. doi: 10.1038/ng1341

Zunino, R., Braschi, E., Xu, L., and McBride, H. M. (2009). Translocation of SenP5 from the nucleoli to the mitochondria modulates DRP1-dependent fission during mitosis. *J. Biol. Chem.* 284, 17783–17795. doi: 10.1074/jbc.M901902200

2

Adaptive Strategies for the Elderly in Inhibiting Irrelevant and Conflict No-Go Trials while Performing the Go/No-Go Task

Shulan Hsieh[1,2*], *Mengyao Wu*[1,3] *and Chien-Hui Tang*[1]

[1] *Cognitive Electrophysiology Laboratory: Control, Aging, Sleep, and Emotion (CASE), Department of Psychology, National Cheng Kung University, Tainan, Taiwan,* [2] *Institute of Allied Health Sciences, National Cheng Kung University, Tainan, Taiwan,* [3] *Department of Occupational Therapy, Shu-Zen Junior College of Medicine and Management, Kaohsiung, Taiwan*

Edited by:
Junfeng Sun,
Shanghai Jiao Tong University, China

Reviewed by:
Noa Fogelson,
Universidade da Coruña, Spain
Xiangfei Hong,
Philips Research, China

***Correspondence:**
Shulan Hsieh
psyhsl@mail.ncku.edu.tw

This study aimed to differentiate whether or not older adults are more prone to distraction or conflict, as induced by irrelevant and conflict no-go stimuli (irNOGO and cfNOGO), respectively. This study also aimed to determine whether or not older adults would devote more effort to withholding a no-go trial in the higher-control demand condition (20% no-go trials' probability) as compared to the lower-control demand condition (50 and 80% no-go trials' probability). A total of 96 individuals were recruited, and each of the three no-go trials' probability conditions included 32 participants (16 younger adults and 16 older adults). Both behavioral and event-related potential (ERP) data were measured. The behavioral results showed that the older adults performed more poorly than the younger adults for the go trials, as reflected by slower reaction times (RTs) and higher numbers of omission errors in the go trials. In contrast, in the no-go trials, the older adults counter-intuitively exhibited similar behavioral performance (i.e., equivalent commission errors) as compared to the younger adults. The ERP data further showed that the older adults (but not the younger adults) exhibited larger P3 peak amplitudes for the irNOGO than cfNOGO trials. Yet, on the other hand, the older adults performed more poorly (i.e., had more commission errors) in the cfNOGO than irNOGO trials. These results seem to suggest that the older adults recruited more control processes in order to conquer the commitment of responses in the no-go trials, especially in the irNOGO trials. This age-related compensatory response of recruiting more control processes was specifically seen in the 20% no-go trial probability condition. This study therefore provides a deeper understanding into how older adults adopt strategies for performing the go/no-go task such as devoting more control processes to inhibiting the irNOGO trials compared to the cfNOGO trials in order to cope with their deficient inhibition ability.

Keywords: event-related potential, distraction, inhibition, no-go, probability

INTRODUCTION

Daily life often requires an individual to produce a certain behavior in an environment that is filled with irrelevant and often distracting information. Hence, to achieve the goal of acting adequately, one has to adaptively overcome the competition brought by the strong, yet inappropriate, momentary tendency to inhibit a prepotent yet unintentional response in order to prevent negative consequences. These adaptive processes are broadly termed *inhibition* or *suppression*, and they have often been hypothesized to involve the frontal lobe functions (e.g., Rogers et al., 1998). Given the importance of inhibition in everyday life, several studies have attempted to address the issue of whether or not elderly people could successfully cope with brain degeneration, particularly in the frontal lobes (Dempster, 1992; Raz, 2000; West, 2000; Dennis and Cabeza, 2008), to achieve the goal of acting adequately in everyday life scenarios.

However, the findings regarding how capable an elderly person can be in performing an inhibition-related task are equivocal: some studies showed that the elderly suffered from generic inhibition deficit, hence, they were incapable of performing any inhibition-related task as compared to the younger adults (Hasher and Zacks, 1988; Bokura et al., 2002; Vallesi et al., 2009; Vallesi, 2011; Lucci et al., 2013; Pires et al., 2014), while some other studies have shown that the elderly could develop some strategies to compensate for their deficiency in achieving the task goal (Cabeza et al., 2002; Phillips and Andrés, 2010; Hsieh and Fang, 2012; Hsieh et al., 2012; Hsieh and Lin, 2014). Many factors such as different experimental settings, different populations, and different types of stimuli and requirements could potentially contribute to the discrepancies. Among these factors, we suggest that task parameters may play a critical role in older adults' performance strategies. Hence, in this study we manipulated two task parameters in a go/no-go task paradigm to address the inhibition proficiency of older adults. We focused specifically on a go/no-go task paradigm because such an inhibition task has been proven to be sensitive to aging (Bokura et al., 2002; Vallesi et al., 2009; Vallesi, 2011; Lucci et al., 2013; Pires et al., 2014). The two-task parameters we manipulated here include a no-go stimulus and a no-go stimulus probability. With regard to the type of no-go stimulus, we incorporated two types of no-go stimuli: irrelevant no-go (irNOGO) and conflict no-go (cfNOGO). The irNOGO stimuli belong to a different semantic category from that of the go stimuli (e.g., numbers vs. letters), which yields an obvious distinction between the target (go) and non-target (no-go) stimuli, even though the no-go stimuli may share a common feature with the go stimuli. For example, both the irNOGO and go stimuli could be either red or blue, but they belong to numbers and letters, respectively. In contrast, the cfNOGO stimuli share the same category (i.e., letters) as the go stimuli. The rationale for this manipulation is that the irNOGO stimuli should be easier to distinguish from the go stimuli; therefore, it is easier inhibit compared to the cfNOGO stimuli. On the other hand, some prior studies in the memory research domain have suggested that older adults were more vulnerable to internal distraction and weakening concentration skills due to their subtle changes in brain activity (e.g., Grady et al., 2006). It is therefore interesting to examine whether or not older adults are also susceptible to external distractions, such as those induced by the irNOGO stimuli in a go/no-go task.

With regard to no-go stimulus probability, we manipulated the probability of no-go trials in a block to be either 20, 50, or 80%. The rationale for the probability manipulation is that with a strong response bias towards go stimuli (20% no-go probability), one can maximize the engagement of executive control to inhibit no-go stimuli (Bruin and Wijers, 2002; Ford et al., 2004). Subsequently, the performance of a go/no-go task may be more sensitive to aging in the condition of this higher demand condition (20% of no-go probability).

With the manipulation of these two task parameters, we could examine whether or not aging results in a selective deficit in which task parameters are sensitive to the effect of aging in only some scenarios. Because no overt response can be recorded for no-go trials in a go/no-go paradigm, a neural imaging approach is needed to uncover the underlying processes of the no-go trials. In this study, we employed the event-related potential (ERP) method, which yields higher temporal resolution and uncovers the underlying neural activity for no-go trials.

Two ERP components are considered in this study that have been demonstrated to be sensitive to a go/no-go task, that is, the stimulus-locked P3 and N2 components (for a review, see Pires et al., 2014). Stimuli that trigger a tendency to make incorrect prepotent responses (e.g., incongruent or no-go stimuli) have been found to be associated with enhanced fronto-central N2 amplitude, which is thought to reflect inhibition (Van Boxtel et al., 2001; Roche et al., 2005) and/or response conflict control processes (Falkenstein et al., 2001; Van Veen and Carter, 2002a,b; Nieuwenhuis et al., 2003). Furthermore, Nieuwenhuis et al. (2003) observed that no-go N2 amplitudes were higher in the high go-prepotency (20% no-go) condition compared with medium (50%) and low go-prepotency (80% no-go) conditions, which supports the conflict theory of N2. Following the N2, there is a positive ERP component that peaks at approximately 250–500 ms for both go (known as the go P3) and no-go (known as the no-go P3) trials. Both go and no-go P3s may reflect context updating (Donchin and Coles, 1988), which is necessary for successful ongoing execution and inhibition of prepotency responses. Specifically, the no-go P3 has been shown to be closely related to inhibition (Roberts et al., 1994; Fallgatter and Strik, 1999; Tekok-Kilic et al., 2001; Smith et al., 2008). Hence, by observing how aging may modulate the no-go N2 and P3 components, we can uncover age-related inhibition and/or conflict processes.

MATERIALS AND METHODS

Participants

A total of 96 individuals were recruited through the internet and local community advertisements; each of the three no-go probability condition blocks included 32 participants (16 younger adults and 16 older adults). For the 20% no-go probability condition, 16 young adults (9 females) had a mean age of 21.31 ± 1.40 years (range 20–25 years) and an average of 15.69 ± 1.25 years of education; the 16 elderly adults (9 females) had a mean age of 66.38 ± 4.57 years (range 61–72 years) and an average of 12.69 ± 2.15 years of education. For the 50% no-go probability condition, the 16 young adults (8 females) had a mean age of 21.31 ± 1.30 years (range 20–25 years) and an average of 15.00 ± 1.10 years of education; the 16 elderly adults (8 females) had a mean age of 67.25 ± 4.74 years (range 60–76 years) and an average of 12.56 ± 3.60 years of education. For the 80% no-go probability condition, the 16 young adults (9 females) had a mean age of 21.63 ± 1.54 years (range 19–24 years) and an average of 15.44 ± 1.21 years of education; the 16 elderly adults (9 females) had a mean age of 68.63 ± 6.08 years (range 61–80 years) and an average of 13.31 ± 2.75 years of education (see **Table 1**).

The 2-way analysis of variance (ANOVAs) on age with two between-subjects factors of age and no-go probability showed a significant main effect of age (young: 21.42 ± 1.38 years vs. old: 67.42 ± 5.09 years, $F_{(1,90)} = 3529.05$, $p < 0.01$), but it did not show a significant main effect of no-go probability or a significant interaction between age and no-go probability (i.e., all $ps > 0.05$). The 2-way ANOVA on years of education showed a significant effect of age (young: 12.85 ± 2.82 years vs. old: 15.38 ± 1.18 years, $F_{(1,90)} = 31.18$, $p < 0.01$). No significant effect of no-go probability or interaction between age and no-go probability was found (all $ps > 0.05$).

All participants provided their written informed consent, and the study protocol was approved by the Institutional Review Board (IRB) of the National Cheng Kung University Hospital, Taiwan. All participants were paid NT $500–1000 (US $15–30) for approximately 3 h of participation. All participants were right-handed, free of neurological and psychological disorders, and had normal or corrected-to-normal vision. The Mini-Mental State Examination (MMSE; Folstein et al., 1975) screened all participants for dementia based on the following screening criteria: 25–30 points = normal; 21–24 points = mild dementia; 14–20 points = moderate dementia; and ≤13 points = severe dementia. For the 20% no-go probability condition, the mean MMSE score was 28.63 ± 0.60 for the younger adults and 27.06 ± 1.14 for the older adults. For the 50% no-go probability condition, the mean MMSE score was 28.50 ± 0.71 for the younger adults and 26.68 ± 1.10 for the older adults. For the 80% no-go probability condition, the mean MMSE score was 28.18 ± 1.01 for the younger adults and 27.19 ± 0.73 for the older adults.

The 2-way ANOVA on the MMSE score showed a significant effect of age (young: 26.98 ± 1.03 vs. old: 28.44 ± 0.81, $F_{(1,90)} = 58.15$, $p < 0.01$) but no significant effect of no-go probability; also, there was no significant interaction between age and no-go probability (all $ps > 0.05$). Since there was a significant effect of age on MMSE scores, this may be a potential confounding variable for the results, i.e., the changes may be due to cognitive decline rather than physiological aging. In order to preclude the possible contribution of cognitive decline in the older group, we have additionally run an analysis of covariance (ANCOVA) using MMSE as a covariate factor. The results of the ANCOVA showed the same patterns as those of the ANOVA reported here. Hence, although the older adults exhibited lower MMSE scores, they did not confound the current findings.

Stimuli

The stimuli were generated using E-Prime software (Psychology Software Tools, Inc., Pittsburgh, PA, USA) and were presented in red or blue against a black background on the center of a computer screen that was placed at a distance of 90 cm from the participant. In this task, go stimuli were red or blue vowels ("A", "E", "I", "U") and no-go stimuli were either red or blue consonants ("L", "N", "P", "Z"; designed as cfNOGO stimuli) or red and blue numbers ("3", "4", "5", "6"; designed as irNOGO stimuli).

Design and Procedure

Each trial began with the presentation of a white fixation cross "+" for a duration of 200 ms, followed by a go or no-go stimulus for a duration of 300 ms. This was then replaced by a black blank screen that awaited a response or until 1800 ms elapsed if no response was recorded. Also, there was an additional waiting duration that varied randomly between 1–1000 ms before the next trial commenced (see **Figure 1**). Participants were required to make (for a go stimulus) or withhold (for a no-go stimulus) a response as soon and as accurately as possible.

The total number of trials in the no-go probability condition block was 960. The probabilities of no-go stimuli were 20% (192 trials), 50% (480 trials), and 80% (768 trials), respectively. Among the no-go trials, cfNOGO and irNOGO stimuli comprised 50% each. There were at least 36 practice trials (more trials if necessary) before each condition block. During the practice session, feedback of "correct" or "incorrect" was given at the end of each trial

TABLE 1 | The demographic information for all participants in all conditions.

	20% no-go		50% no-go		80% no-go	
	Younger	Older	Younger	Older	Younger	Older
Gender (male/female)	7/9	7/9	8/8	8/8	7/9	7/9
Age (year)	21.31 (1.36)	66.38 (4.43)	21.31 (1.26)	67.25 (4.59)	21.63 (1.49)	68.63 (5.88)
Education (year)	15.69 (1.21)	12.69 (2.08)	15.00 (1.06)	12.56 (3.48)	15.44 (1.17)	13.31 (2.66)
BDI	3.44 (2.06)	5.25 (4.71)	4.69 (3.58)	6.69 (3.58)	3.69 (2.17)	4.25 (3.44)
MMSE	28.63 (0.60)	27.06 (1.14)	28.50 (0.71)	26.69 (1.10)	28.19 (1.01)	27.19 (0.73)

BDI, Beck Depression Inventory; MMSE, Mini-Mental State Examination; the value in each cell denotes the mean, and the value in each bracket denotes standard deviation.

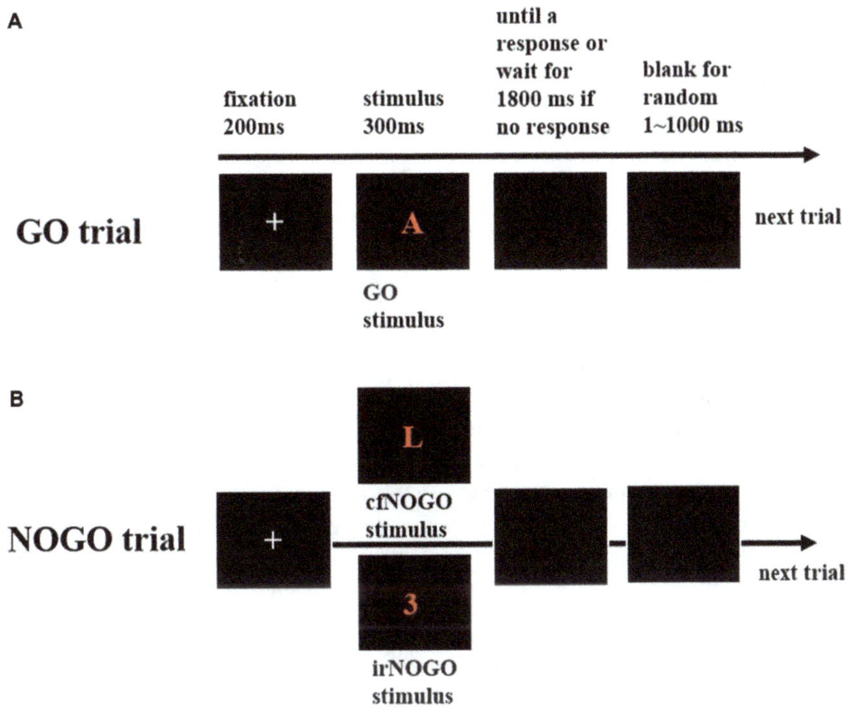

FIGURE 1 | The behavioral paradigm. (A) Schematic representation of the events in a go trial, including a fixation, followed by a go stimulus; **(B)** Schematic representation of the events in a no-go trial, including a fixation, followed by either of the two no-go stimuli, irrelevant (irNOGO) and conflict (cfNOGO).

to facilitate the participants' familiarization with the response rule.

EEG Recording

The participants were seated in a comfortable chair in a sound-attenuated room during the experiment. Electroencephalography (EEG) activity was continuously recorded using Neuroscan SynAmp2 amplifier and Q-Cap (Neuroscan Q-Cap: AgCl-32 electrode cap; Neuroscan, Inc., El Paso, TX, USA) from 32 scalp electrodes. The vertical electrooculogram (EOG) was recorded by two electrodes 2 cm above and 2 cm below the left eye, and the horizontal EOG was recorded by two electrodes 1 cm external to the outer canthus of each eye. A ground electrode was placed on the forehead. The electrodes were initially referenced online to the left mastoid and offline to the average of the left and right mastoids. Electrode impedances were maintained below 5 kΩ. The EEG and EOG signals were amplified and digitized at a sampling rate of 500 Hz, with an online high-pass filter of 0.1 Hz and a low-pass filter of 30 Hz. Ocular artifacts associated with blinks were corrected by the ocular reduction command offered by the Neuroscan software (Neuroscan, Inc., El Paso, TX, USA) and were then further removed via an algorithm (Neuroscan software) that rejected any epoch if the signal was below -50 ± 50 μV, if the drift of the EEG from baseline exceeded -50 ± 50 μV, or if the A/D converts became saturated. The total rejection rate across the various conditions averaged approximately 23, 28 and 24% for each no-go probability condition block, respectively.

Event-Related Potential (ERP) Analysis

We focused on the N2 and P3 components as they have been hypothesized to link inhibition and response conflict control processes. Moreover, because go and no-go trials involve different processes with respect to motor execution, we separated the ERP analyses of go trials from those of no-go trials. In each condition block, stimulus-locked epochs were taken from the continuous EEG signal and time-locked to the onset of the go/no-go stimulus from −50 ms to 800 ms for all recording channels. For each channel, all stimulus-locked epochs were baseline-corrected by obtaining the mean level of activity in the period from 50 ms before to 50 ms after target onset and then subtracting that average from the level of activity at the sample point. The N2 was found to be maximal at the FCz site, whereas the P3 was maximal at the Cz site in this study. Hence, we searched for the peak-to-peak amplitude at the FCz site during the time windows of 150–350 ms (positive dip) and 250–450 ms (negative peak) following the onset of the stimulus and then computed the voltage difference between the positive dip and negative peak as the stimulus-locked N2 peak-to-peak amplitude. Then, we searched for the peak latency and peak amplitude at the Cz site during the time window of 300–750 ms following the onset of the stimulus and then computed the voltage difference between the peak amplitude relative to the baseline as the stimulus-locked P3 peak amplitude and the time point at which the P3 peak amplitude occurred as the P3 peak latency.

Statistical Analysis

The 2-way ANOVAs for the go trials were performed on the behavioral and ERP data, respectively, with two between-subject factors of age and no-go probability. The 3-way ANOVAs for the no-go trials were performed on the behavioral and ERP data, respectively, with two between-subjects factors of age and no-go probability and one within-subject factor of no-go stimulus types. *Post hoc* analysis following the significant effect of no-go probability (with three levels) was performed using Tukey tests. When two (or more) factors in the ANOVA showed a statistically significant interaction, we carried on analyzing the simple main effects which involve the examination of the effect of one factor at one level of the other factor. That is, the data were split for each level of one factor and one-way ANOVAs were conducted. Like any other one-way ANOVA with more than two levels, after the significant F, a *post hoc* Tukey test was conducted to find out which pair (or pairs) of means was (were) statistically different. To overcome the inflation of Type 1 error when a series of simple main effect analyses were conducted, we used the Bonferroni correction to adjust the p value. In addition, in the choice of error term for simple main effect test, we followed the pooled error term approach advised by Howell (2010). That is, Mean Square Error (MSE) from the original factorial ANOVA was used as opposed to MSE from the follow-up one-way ANOVA in calculating the F for the simple main effects. The detailed steps for the calculation are described in Howell's (2010) book (e.g., ps. 483–488 in his book, "*Statistical Methods for Psychology*").

RESULTS

Behavioral Data Analysis

The first trial of each block and trials with RTs faster than 150 ms or slower than 1500 ms were discarded from further analysis. The behavioral results are shown in **Figure 2**, including the go trials' RT (**Figure 2A**) and omission rates (**Figure 2B**) and the no-go trials' commission errors (**Figure 2C**).

Reaction Time (RT) on Go Trials

The 2-way ANOVA on the RTs of the go trials showed that the younger adults generally performed faster than the older adults, $F_{(1,90)} = 63.11$, $p < 0.001$, and that RTs were faster in the 20% no-go probability (high go-prepotency) and the 50% no-go probability (medium go-prepotency) conditions than in the 80% no-go probability (low go-prepotency) condition (no-go probability, $F_{(2,90)} = 21.42$, $p < 0.001$; all Tukey tests: $ps < 0.005$). There was no significant interaction between the two factors, $F_{(2,90)} = 2.61$, $p = 0.08$.

Percentage of Error (PE) on Go Trials: Omission Errors

The 2-way ANOVA on the omission errors of the go trials showed that the younger adults generally performed better (fewer omission errors) than the older adults, $F_{(1,90)} = 15.20$, $p < 0.001$, and that omission errors were fewer in the 20 and 50% no-go probability conditions (3.46 and 3.04%) than in the 80% no-go probability condition (7.70%; $F_{(2,90)} = 4.92$, $p < 0.01$; all Tukey tests: $p < 0.05$). There was no significant interaction between the two factors, $F_{(2,90)} = 0.93$, $p = 0.40$.

Percentage of Error (PE) on No-Go Trials: Commission Errors

The 3-way ANOVA on the commission errors of the no-go trials showed that there was no significant effect of age, $F_{(1,90)} = 2.14$, $p = 0.15$, but there was a significant effect of no-go probability, $F_{(2,90)} = 47.41$, $p < 0.0001$. Commission errors were more frequent in the 20% no-go probability condition (16.53%) than in the 50% (4.13%) and 80% no-go probability conditions (2.95%; all Tukey tests: $ps < 0.05$). There was also a significant effect of no-go stimulus type, $F_{(1,90)} = 88.31$, $p < 0.0001$, showing that irNOGO (4.78%) stimuli elicited fewer commission errors than cfNOGO (10.96%) stimuli. There was also a significant 2-way interaction between no-go probability and no-go stimulus type, $F_{(2,90)} = 26.52$, $p < 0.0001$. Follow-up tests for this interaction showed that the effect of no-go probability was significant on both cfNOGO trials ($F_{(2,90)} = 71.51$, $p < 0.0001$) and irNOGO trials ($F_{(2,90)} = 14.41$, $p < 0.001$), yet there was a larger effect on the cfNOGO trial type. In addition, the simple effect of the no-go stimulus type (fewer commission errors for the irNOGO than cfNOGO trials) was significant only in the 20 and 50% no-go probability conditions.

Summary of Behavioral Data

To summarize, the older adults appeared to perform more poorly than the younger adults on go trials, as reflected by their slower go RTs and higher go omission errors; this age effect was not modulated by no-go probability. In contrast, the older adults counter-intuitively exhibited similar behavioral performance (i.e., equivalent commission errors) as compared to the younger adults. In addition, it appeared to be more difficult for both age groups to withhold a response to cfNOGO stimuli compared to irNOGO stimuli, based on the data of commission errors.

Event-Related Potential (ERP) Data

ERPs associated with each condition and age group at the Fz, FCz, Cz, CPz, and Pz sites as well as topographic maps are shown in **Figures 3A,B** for go trials and **Figures 4A,B** for no-go trials.

P3 Peak Latency on Go Trials

The 2-way ANOVA on the P3 peak latencies of go trials showed that the younger adults exhibited earlier P3 peak latencies than the older adults (young: 526.04 ms vs. old: 596.75 ms), $F_{(1,90)} = 26.63$, $p < 0.0001$, but there was no significant effect of no-go probability, $F_{(2,90)} = 0.81$, $p = 0.45$. There was also no significant 2-way interaction between age and no-go probability, $F_{(2,90)} = 1.11$, $p = 0.34$ (see **Figure 5A**).

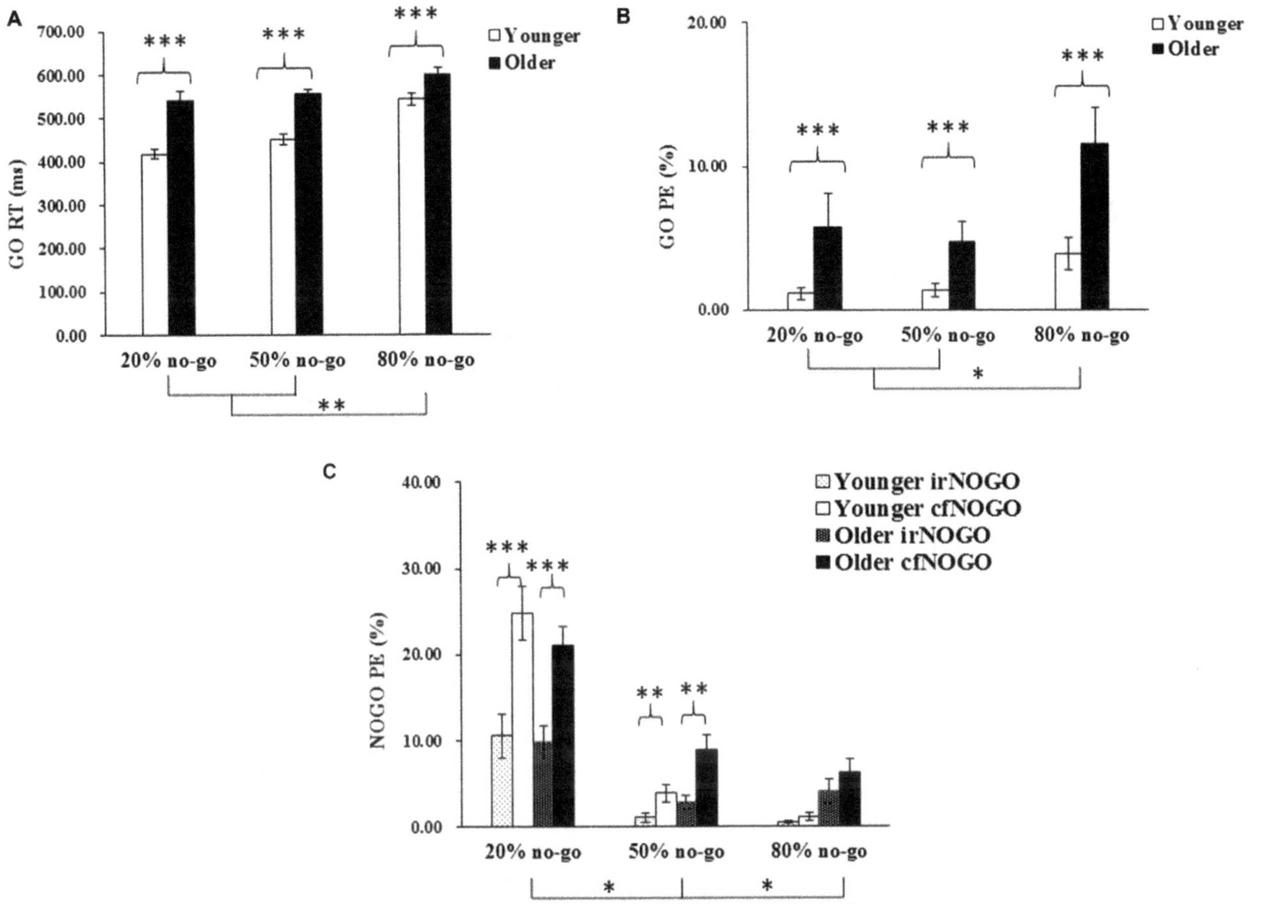

FIGURE 2 | (A) Mean response times (RTs; and standard errors of the mean) of correct responses (in milliseconds) to go stimuli as a function of age and no-go probability condition; **(B)** Mean percentage of errors (PE; and standard errors of the mean) of omitted responses to go stimuli as a function of age and no-go probability condition; **(C)** Mean percentage of errors (PE; and standard errors of the mean) of committed responses to no-go stimuli as a function of age and no-go probability condition. Significant effects are highlighted with $^{*}p < 0.05$, $^{**}p < 0.01$, or $^{***}p < 0.001$.

P3 Peak Amplitude on Go Trials

The 2-way ANOVA on the P3 peak amplitudes of the go trials showed larger P3 peak amplitudes for the younger (12.53 μV) than older (7.01 μV) adults, $F_{(1,90)} = 34.58$, $p < 0.0001$, but no significant main effect of no-go probability, $F_{(2,90)} = 0.79$, $p = 0.46$. Yet, there was a significant 2-way interaction between age and no-go probability, $F_{(2,90)} = 4.94$, $p < 0.01$. A simple effect test following this interaction showed that the significant main effect of no-go probability occurred only for the younger adults, $F_{(2,90)} = 4.80$, $p < 0.05$, but not for the older adults, $F_{(2,90)} = 0.93$, $p = 0.40$, and that the significant effect of age occurred in the 50%, $F_{(1,90)} = 11.49$, $p < 0.005$, and 80%, $F_{(1,90)} = 31.59$, $p < 0.0001$, no-go probability conditions but not in the 20% no-go probability conditions, $F_{(1,90)} = 1.38$, $p = 0.24$ (see **Figure 5B**).

P3 Peak Latency on No-Go Trials

The 3-way ANOVA on the P3 peak latencies of no-go trials showed that the younger adults exhibited earlier P3 peak latencies than the older adults (young: 516.35 ms vs. old: 641.46 ms), $F_{(1,90)} = 162.85$, $p < 0.001$, and that irNOGO stimuli elicited earlier P3 peak latencies than cfNOGO stimuli, $F_{(1,90)} = 30.42$, $p < 0.0001$. There were no significant effect of no-go probability and any interactions (age × type of no-go stimulus: $F_{(1,90)} = 2.03$, $p = 0.16$; no-go probability × type of no-go stimulus: $F_{(2,90)} = 0.08$, $p = 0.93$; age × type of no-go stimulus × no-go probability: $F_{(2,90)} = 0.922$, $p = 0.40$, see **Figure 6A**.

P3 Peak Amplitude on No-Go Trials

The 3-way ANOVA on the P3 peak amplitudes of the no-go stimuli showed that P3 peak amplitudes for the no-go trials were larger in the 20% no-go probability condition than in the 50 and 80% no-go probability conditions, $F_{(2,90)} = 15.58$, $p < 0.0001$ (all Tukey tests: $ps < 0.01$). There was also a significant 2-way interaction between age and no-go stimulus type, $F_{(1,90)} = 13.49$, $p < 0.001$.

A simple effect test on the interaction between age and no-go stimulus type showed that only older adults exhibited larger P3 peak amplitudes for irNOGO stimuli than for cfNOGO stimuli but not for the younger adults (young: $F_{(1,90)} = 1.80$, $p = 0.19$; old: $F_{(1,90)} = 14.83$, $p < 0.001$; see **Figure 6B**).

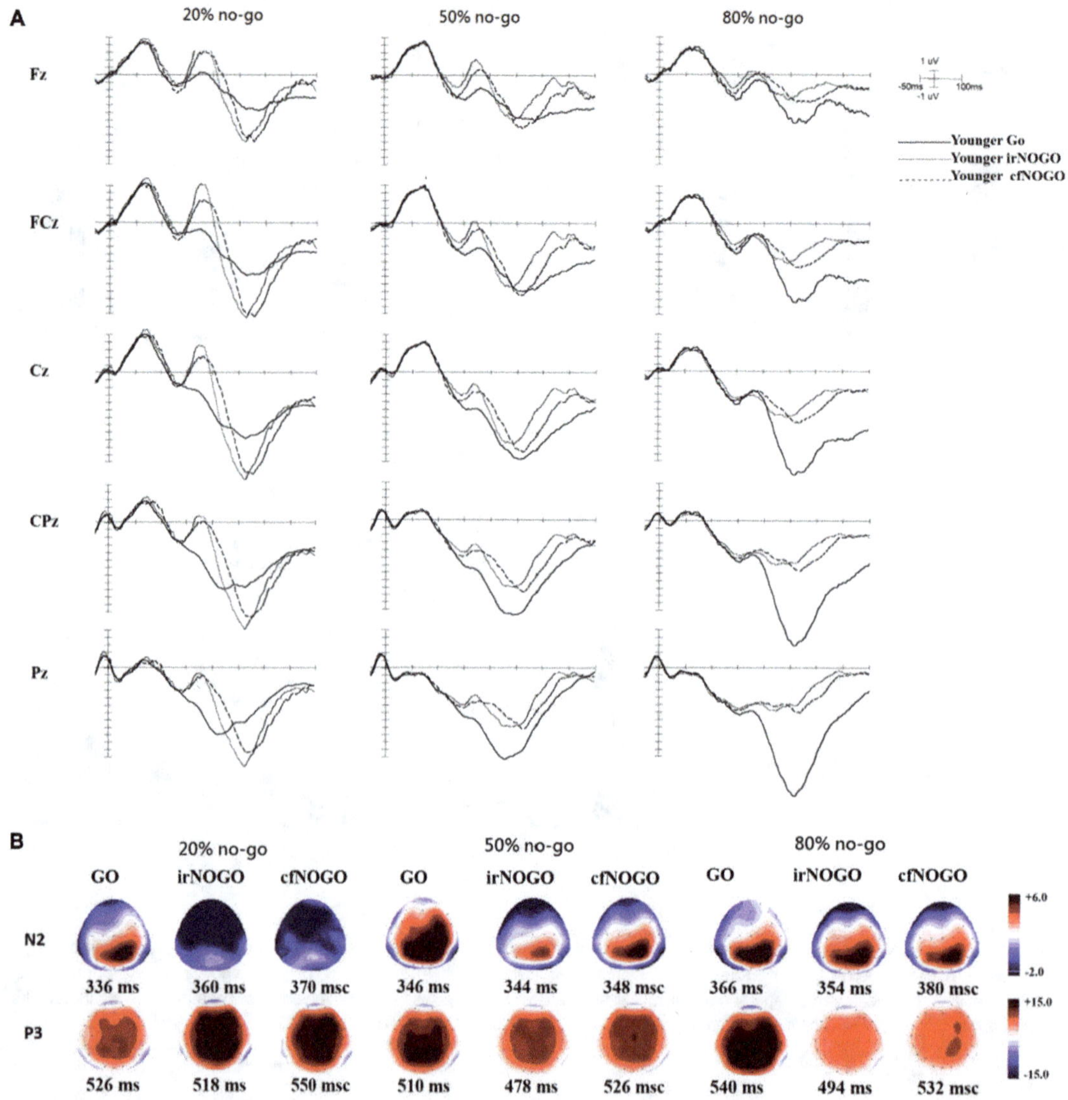

FIGURE 3 | (A) ERP waveforms as a function of no/no-go condition (GO, irNOGO, cfNOGO) and no-go probability condition at five representative electrodes of Fz, FCz, Cz, CPz, and Pz for the younger adults. **(B)** Topographic maps of the GO N2, irNOGO N2, cfNOGO N2, GO P3, irNOGO P3, and cfNOGO P3, separately for each no-go probability condition and for the younger adults. Each map describes the topographic distribution at the peak latency for each condition.

Summary of the P3 Findings

Go P3 Peak Latency and Amplitude

For the go P3 peak latency, there was a significant effect of age that showed an earlier P3 peak latency for the younger adults. As for the go P3 peak amplitude, the significant effect of aging (younger larger than older) occurred only in the 50 and 80% no-go probability conditions. In addition, the significant effect of no-go probability occurred only for the younger adults, i.e., showing smaller go P3 peak amplitudes in the 20% than 80% no-go probability condition but not for the older adults.

No-Go P3 Peak Latency and Amplitude

The significant effect of age was found for the overall no-go P3 peak latency. In addition, both age groups exhibited earlier P3 peak latencies for the irNOGO trials compared to the cfNOGO trials. As for the no-go P3 peak amplitude, there was a significant effect of no-go probability for both age groups, showing larger no-go P3 peak amplitudes in the 20% no-go probability conditions compared to the 50 and 80% no-go probability conditions. More importantly, only the older adults exhibited larger P3 peak amplitudes for the irNOGO trials compared to the cfNOGO trials. These results suggested that while the younger adults exhibited similar no-go P3 peak amplitudes between the irNOGO and cfNOGO trials, the older adults exhibited more prominent P3 peak amplitudes for the irNOGO than cfNOGO trials. Subsequently, this phenomenon resulted in a significant effect of age for the cfNOGO trials but not for the irNOGO trials.

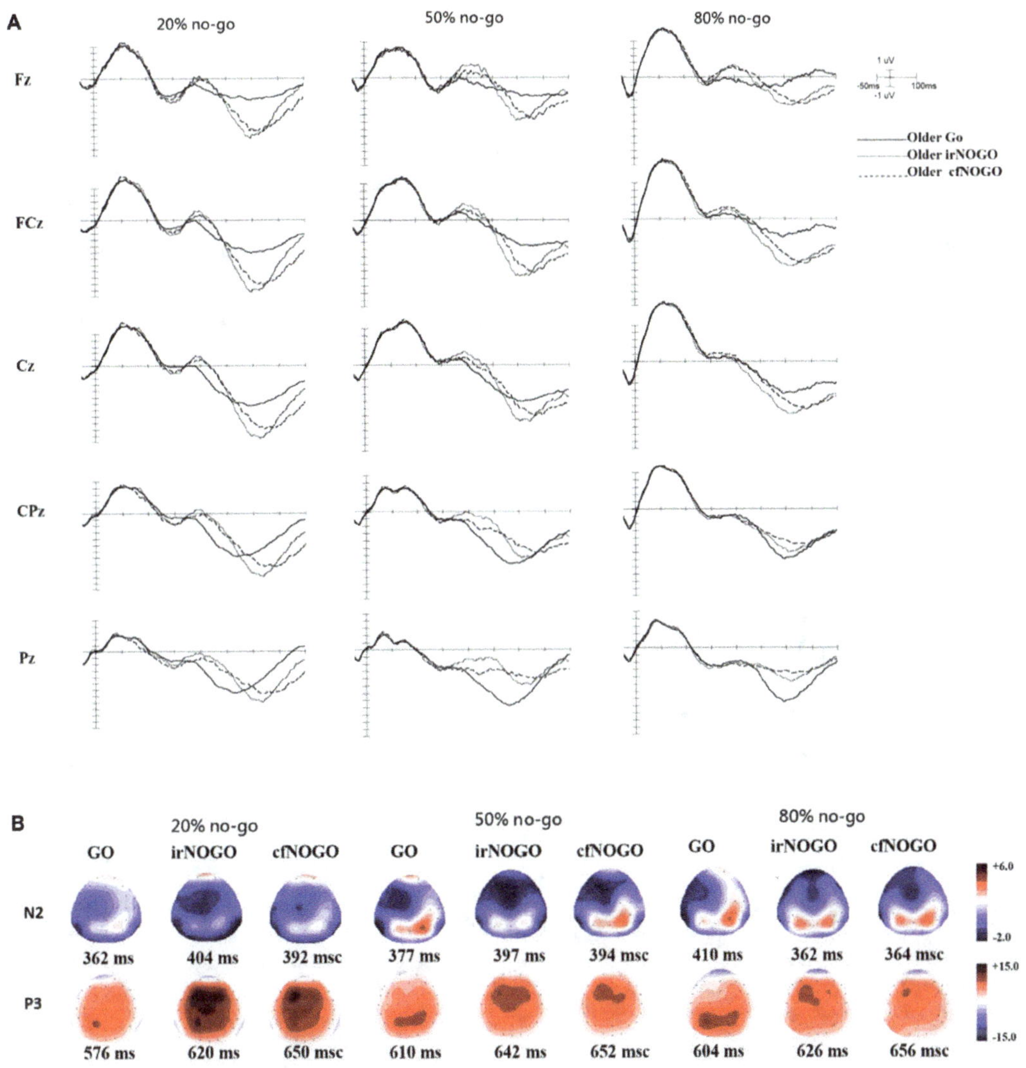

FIGURE 4 | (A) ERP waveforms as a function of no/no-go condition (GO, irNOGO, cfNOGO) and no-go probability condition at five representative electrodes of Fz, FCz, Cz, CPz, and Pz for the older adults. **(B)** Topographic maps of the GO N2, irNOGO N2, cfNOGO N2, GO P3, irNOGO P3, and cfNOGO P3, separately for each no-go probability condition and for the older adults. Each map describes the topographic distribution at the peak latency for each condition.

N2 Peak-to-Peak Amplitude on Go Trials

The 2-way ANOVA on the N2 peak-to-peak amplitudes of the go trials showed no significant effects or interactions (age: $F_{(1,90)} = 1.24, p = 0.27$; no-go probability: $F_{(2,90)} = 1.35, p = 0.27$; age *x* no-go probability: $F_{(2,90)} = 1.89, p = 0.19$; see **Figure 7**).

N2 Peak-to-Peak Amplitude on No-Go Trials

The 3-way ANOVA on the N2 peak-to-peak amplitudes of no-go stimuli showed that the younger adults exhibited larger N2 peak-to-peak amplitudes (−5.97 μV) than the older adults (−4.52 μV), $F_{(1,90)} = 8.24$, $p < 0.01$. Also, N2 peak-to-peak amplitudes were larger in the 20% no-go probability condition compared to the 50% no-go probability condition and amplitudes in the latter condition were larger than amplitudes in the 80% no-go probability condition, $F_{(2,90)} = 33.87$, $p < 0.0001$ (all Tukey tests: *ps* < 0.01). There was also a significant effect of no-go stimulus type, $F_{(1,90)} = 7.61$, $p < 0.01$; this indicates that irNOGO stimuli elicited larger N2 peak-to-peak amplitudes than cfNOGO stimuli. There were significant 2-way interactions between age and no-go probability, $F_{(2,90)} = 3.78$, $p < 0.05$, and between no-go probability and no-go stimulus type, $F_{(2,90)} = 7.34$, $p < 0.005$.

The simple effect test for the interaction between age and no-go probability showed that the effect of age was only significant for the 20% no-go probability condition, where the younger adults exhibited larger N2 peak-to-peak amplitudes than older adults. On the other hand, both age groups exhibited significant effects for the no-go probability on the N2 peak-to-peak amplitude.

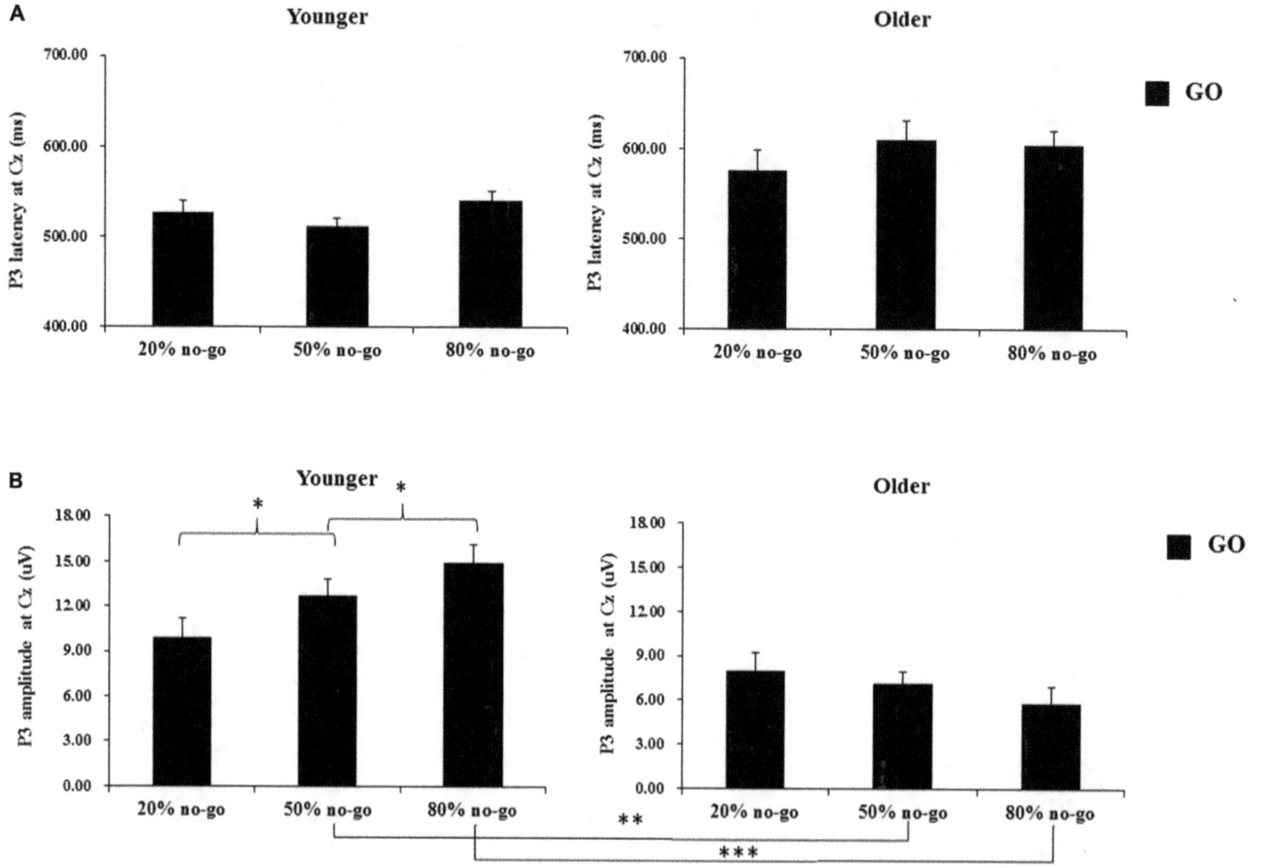

FIGURE 5 | (A) Grand mean P3 peak latencies (in milliseconds) at the Cz site as a function of no-go probability condition for GO trials and for the younger (upper left panel) and older (upper right panel) adults, respectively. Error bars represent standard errors; **(B)** Grand mean P3 peak amplitudes (in μV) at the Cz site as a function of no-go probability condition for GO trials and for the younger (lower left panel) and older (lower right panel) adults, respectively. Error bars represent standard errors. Significant effects are highlighted with *$p < 0.05$, **$p < 0.01$, or ***$p < 0.001$.

The simple effect test on the interaction of no-go probability and no-go stimulus type nevertheless showed a significant main effect of no-go stimulus type (i.e., the irNOGO trials elicited larger N2 amplitudes than cfNOGO trials) in the 20% no-go probability condition, $F_{(1,90)} = 20.03$, $p < 0.0001$, but not for the 50 and 80% no-go probability condition (50%: $F_{(1,90)} = 1.46$, $p = 0.23$; 80%: $F_{(1,90)} = 0.81$, $p = 0.37$). Furthermore, for both the irNOGO and cfNOGO stimuli, the amplitudes were larger in the 20% no-go probability condition than in the 50 and 80% no-go probability condition (all *ps* < 0.05; see **Figure 8**).

Summary of the N2 Findings

Go N2 Peak-to-Peak Amplitude

The significant effect of no-go probability on go N2s occurred only for the younger adults and between the 50 and 80% no-go probability conditions, whereas none of the significant main effects and interactions were found for the older adults.

No-Go N2 Peak-to-Peak Amplitude

The significant effect of age (i.e., the younger adults exhibited larger N2 amplitudes than the older adults) on no-go N2s occurred mainly in the 20% no-go probability condition. In addition, the significant effect of no-go trial type (i.e., irNOGO trials exhibited larger N2 amplitudes than cfNOGO trials) was found only for the 20% no-go probability condition for both age groups. Furthermore, for both the irNOGO and cfNOGO stimuli, the amplitudes were larger in the 20% no-go probability condition than in the 50 and 80% no-go probability conditions.

DISCUSSIONS

The aim of this study was to evaluate whether older adults exhibited selective inhibition deficit by using a go/no-go paradigm with the manipulation of no-go stimulus-type and no-go probability. The current behavioral results showed that the older adults performed more poorly than the younger adults as reflected from their slower RTs and their higher omission errors in the go trials. This age difference was not further modulated by no-go probability, despite the fact that there was a significant effect of no-go probability on both RTs and omission errors. Interestingly, in contrast to the inferior performance on go trials for the older adults compared to the younger adults, the older adults counter-intuitively exhibited similar behavioral

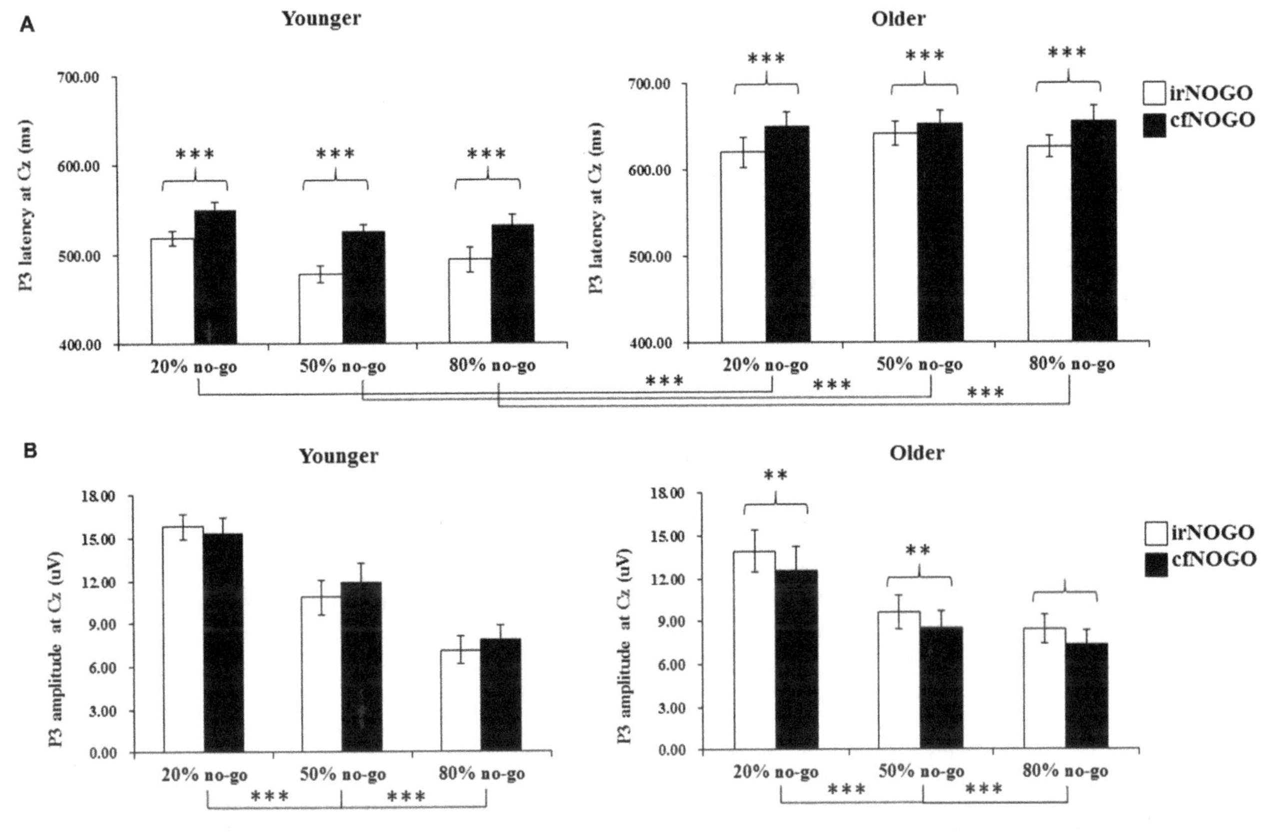

FIGURE 6 | (A) Grand mean P3 peak latencies (in milliseconds) at the Cz site as a function of no-go probability condition for NOGO (irNOGO and cfNOGO) trials and for the younger (upper left panel) and older (upper right panel) adults, respectively. Error bars represent standard errors; **(B)** Grand mean P3 peak amplitudes (in μV) at the Cz site as a function of no-go probability condition for NOGO (irNOGO and cfNOGO) trials and for the younger (lower left panel) and older (lower right panel) adults, respectively. Error bars represent standard errors. Significant effects are highlighted with $^{**}p < 0.01$, or $^{***}p < 0.001$.

performance on no-go trials (i.e., equivalent commission errors) as compared to the younger adults. These results seemed to suggest that the older adults were capable of inhibiting the no-go trials. In addition, based on the no-go commission error data, it appeared to be more difficult for both younger and older adults to withhold a response to cfNOGO stimuli compared to irNOGO stimuli. Yet, since the behavioral no-go performance can only be measured with commission errors, it is interesting to examine whether or not the underlying neural activity for the no-go trials, as reflected by the ERPs, would be also similar, as shown in the behavioral data between the two age groups.

The current ERP data showed that for the younger adults, the cfNOGO stimuli were associated with smaller N2 amplitudes than those of the irNOGO stimuli, specifically for the 20%

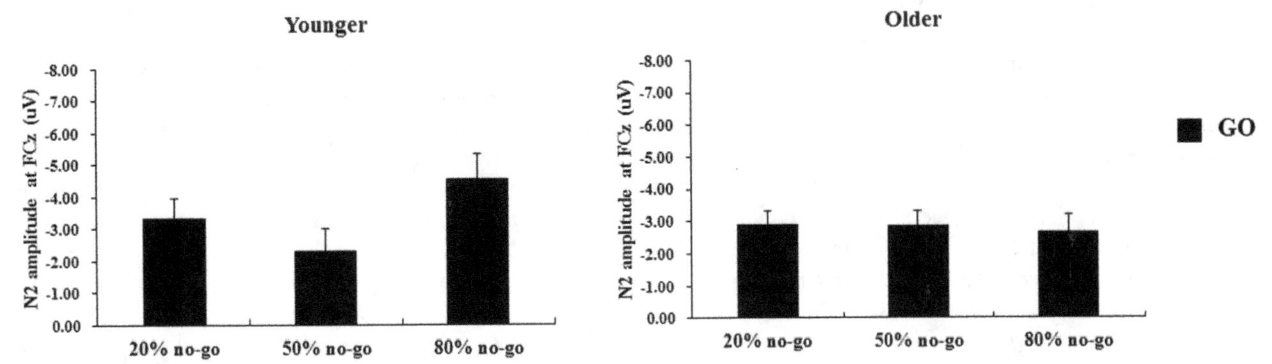

FIGURE 7 | Grand mean N2 peak-to-peak amplitudes (in μV) at the FCz site as a function of no-go probability condition for GO trials and for the younger (left panel) and older (right panel) adults, respectively. Error bars represent standard errors.

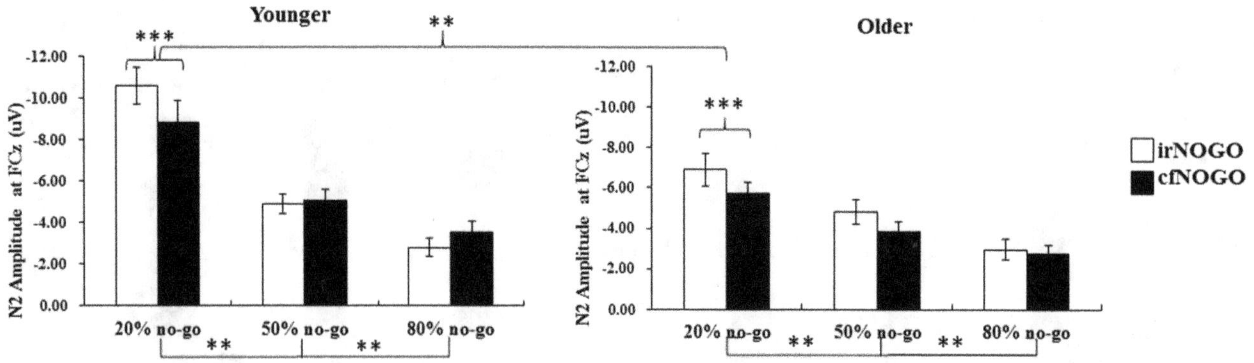

FIGURE 8 | Grand mean N2 peak-to-peak amplitudes (in μV) at the FCz site as a function of no-go probability condition for NOGO (irNOGO and cfNOGO) trials and for the younger (left panel) and older (right panel) adults, respectively. Error bars represent standard errors. Significant effects are highlighted with $^{**}p < 0.01$, or $^{***}p < 0.001$.

no-go probability condition. Previous research has argued that the N2 enhancement of the no-go trials either reflects the operation of a cognitive top-down inhibition mechanism needed to suppress the incorrect tendency to respond or reflects an electrophysiological correlate of conflict between go and no-go response representations that is detected in ACC (Nieuwenhuis et al., 2003). Since the current results showed that the cfNOGO trials were associated with smaller N2 amplitudes and were accompanied with more commission errors than the irNOGO trials (but only for the 20% no-go trial condition), this suggests that either the younger adults experienced less conflict and hence recruited less control processes for the cfNOGO trials than irNOGO trials based on the conflict hypothesis of N2 (Falkenstein et al., 2001; Van Veen and Carter, 2002a,b) or they were less able to inhibit the cfNOGO stimuli based on the inhibition account (Roche et al., 2005). Nevertheless, since we additionally observed that N2 peak-to-peak amplitudes were also modulated by the no-go stimulus probability for the younger adults, the results appeared to be more consistent with the results reported by Nieuwenhuis et al. (2003); see also Smith et al. (2008), who suggested that N2 may reflect response conflict rather than inhibition *per se*.

More importantly, in the current study, the older adults paradoxically exhibited larger P3 amplitudes for the irNOGO than cfNOGO trials, whereas behaviorally they committed more errors in the cfNOGO than irNOGO trials. This seems to suggest that the older adults recruited more control processes in order to conquer the commitment of responses for the no-go trials, especially for the irNOGO trials. The more direct evidence that supports this speculation comes from the correlational analysis between the behavioral performance and P3 amplitudes. The correlation was significant ($r = 0.51$, $p < 0.001$; see **Figure 9**) and showed that better performance (i.e., lower PE) inhibiting the no-go trials was associated with larger the P3 amplitudes in the no-go trials, relative to go trials. This finding was consistent with Vallesi et al. (2009), who showed that the irNOGO trials seemed to be more distracting (and hence cause a larger conflict N2) for the older adults to withhold the response; hence, the older adults needed to recruit more control processes in withholding the response towards the irNOGO trials than the cfNOGO trials, as reflected by their larger no-go P3 peak amplitudes for the irNOGO than cfNOGO trials. However, no such phenomenon was found for the younger adults. This age-related compensatory response (i.e., conquering the irNOGO stimuli with the price of poorer performance of the cfNOGO stimuli) were specifically seen in the 20% no-go trial probability condition. The manipulation of the low probability of no-go trials has proved successful in activating frontal lobe structures associated with executive control in other response inhibition tasks (MacDonald et al., 2000). Hence, in this scenario, the older adults might thus recruit more compensatory responses in withholding the responses towards the no-go trials. This might also explain why there was no age effect seen in the behavioral no-go commission errors due to the compensatory responses.

The current finding that the older adults were more distracted by the irNOGO stimuli than the cfNOGO stimuli appears to be consistent with previous reports in the memory research domain, which suggests that older adults (more pronounced after age 65) suffer from increasing vulnerability to internal distraction and weakening concentration skills due to subtle changes in brain activity (Grady et al., 2006). Grady et al. (2006) found that older adults have difficulty activating brain regions necessary for concentration (e.g., reading) and de-activating or tuning down other regions that are associated with internal thoughts (e.g., thinking about yourself, what you did yesterday). Two key regions of the brain that allow the mind to focus on a single task and tune out unwanted thoughts get out of kilter much earlier in life than previously suspected. When the mind pays strict attention, special neural circuits in the prefrontal cortex become more active, and at the same time, related brain areas in the medial frontal lobe (monitoring more general background activity) slack off. Conversely, when the mind is at rest, the level of brain activity in these two regions is then reversed. Such a seesaw activity pattern can begin to break down during memory tasks starting at about age 40.

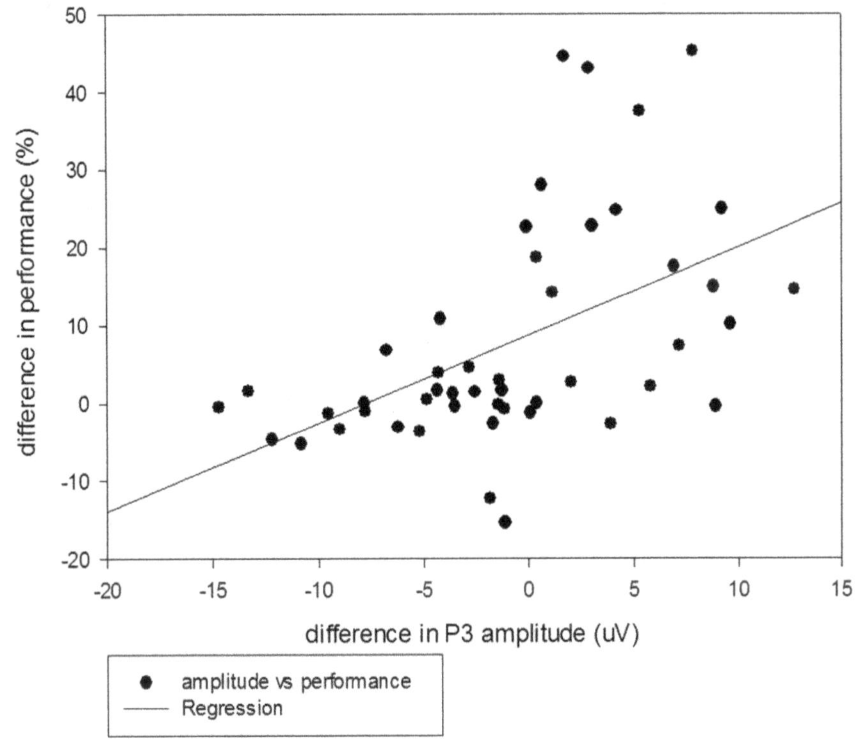

FIGURE 9 | Scatterplot with regression line illustrating the correlation between P3 amplitudes (uV) and behavioral performance (%) for the irNOGO trials relative to GO trials across all three no-go probability conditions for the older adults.

Another interesting finding of this study is that older adults seemed to devote more effort towards no-go trials, since the no-go probability effect was only seen significantly for the no-go trials, whereas the effect of no-go probability was significant for both the go and no-go trials for the younger adults. While the younger adults exhibited the conventional larger P3 amplitudes on go trials in the low go-prepotency condition than in the high go-prepotency condition, the older adults did not show such a pattern. It is therefore not surprising to observe a significant age effect on the go P3 amplitudes in the 50 and 80% no-go probability conditions rather than in the 20% no-go probability condition ($p = 0.24$). On the other hand, the amplitudes of both N2 and P3 on the no-go trials were found to vary significantly as a function of the relative frequency of no-go probability (20, 50 and 80%) conditions for both age groups. These results suggest that the older adults (similarly to the younger adults) when withholding the responses could be influenced by the no-go trials' probability. Given that the older adults were not influenced by the go trials' probability when executing the responses for the go trials but that they were influenced by the no-go trials' probability when withholding the responses on no-go trials, we could suspect that the older adults seemed to devote more effort to the no-go trials since it was more effortful for them to withhold the responses; hence, they were more sensitive to the no-go trials' probability.

Some final issues should be noted. First, this study used a between-subjects design for the factor of no-go probability which might underestimate the effect of no-go probability on the current results, and therefore the current interpretations regarding the interactions with the no-go probability should be treated with caution. Second, although the MMSE scores for the elderly participants in the current study were all within the normal range (on average 26–28), one may be still concerned that these elderly might exhibit an early sign of mild cognitive impairment. Nevertheless, since we have run ANCOVAs using MMSE as a covariate factor and the result patterns remained the same as reported here, we believe that although the older adults exhibited lower MMSE scores, they did not confound the current findings. Third, the topography of the no-go P3 in the older adults (**Figure 4B**) seems to be more frontally distributed compared with the younger adults who showed a more central distribution (**Figure 3B**). This might be a hint toward a posterior-anterior shift in aging (PASA, see Davis et al., 2008). In order to examine if the current findings were consistent with the theory of PASA, we re-ran ANOVAs for the P3 data with an additional factor of electrode sites of FCz, Fz, and Cz. The results of the 4-way ANOVAs showed no significant interactions of electrode sites with all other factors, except its own significant effect; hence, the current data did not seem to show a PASA effect for the elderly. Finally, it has been reported in previous studies that older adults showed similar (Falkenstein et al., 2002) and sometimes stronger no-go P3 amplitudes (Hong et al., 2014) compared with younger adults. However, in this study, it seems that older adults showed smaller no-go P3 amplitudes

(**Figure 6B**). Yet, it is important to note that Falkenstein et al. (2002) and Hong et al. (2014) used the P3 difference wave (P3d: no-go minus go ERPs) rather than the absolute no-go P3 amplitude, as reported in this study. When we subtracted go ERPs from no-go ERPs, we likewise observed similar P3d amplitudes (in 20% condition) and larger P3d amplitudes (in both 50 and 80% conditions) for the older adults compared with the younger adults. We decided to report go and no-go ERPs separately because of the following reasons: (1) go and no-go trials involve different processes with respect to motor execution and (2) we were more interested in contrasting irNOGO and cfNOGO trials.

To conclude, using ERP data the current study revealed that older adults were more prone to distraction induced by irNOGO stimuli, and therefore they exerted more control processes to conquer such distraction. Furthermore, older adults tended to devote more effort to withholding responses towards the no-go trials, especially in the condition where more control demand was needed (e.g., in the 20% no-go trials' probability in this study). This study provided a deeper understanding into how older adults adopted strategies in performing the go/no-go task (e.g., devoting attention to no-go trials in order to cope with their deficient inhibition ability). This interpretation appears to be contradictory to the well-known aging hypothesis of inhibition deficits (Hasher and Zacks, 1988). Yet, given that previous research has already demonstrated that older adults would develop a strategy to cope with some task scenarios, we suggest in the current study that older adults performing the go/no-go task adopted a compensating strategy of paying more attention to the no-go trials.

ETHICS STATEMENT

The study was approved by the Ethical committee of the National Cheng Kung University in accordance with the Declaration of Helsinki. Written informed consent was obtained from all subjects before the experiment.

AUTHOR CONTRIBUTIONS

SH designed the experiment, wrote the grant proposal, guided in executing the experiment, interpreted the data, and wrote the manuscript; MU analyzed the data, plotted the figures; C-HT conducted the experiment and collected the data.

ACKNOWLEDGMENTS

We would like to thank the Ministry of Science Technology (MOST) of the Republic of China, Taiwan for financially supporting this research (Contract No. 101-2410-H-006-046-MY3 and No. 104-2410-H-006-021-MY2). In addition, this research was, in part, supported by the Ministry of Education, Taiwan, R.O.C., The Aim for the Top University Project to the National Cheng Kung University (NCKU). We also wish to thank American Manuscript Editors (AmericanManuscriptEditors.com) for English proofreading.

REFERENCES

Bokura, H., Yamaguchi, S., Matsubara, M., and Kobayashi, S. (2002). Frontal lobe contribution to response inhibition process—an ERP study and aging effect. *Int. Congr. Ser.* 1232, 17–20. doi: 10.1016/s0531-5131(01)00677-x

Bruin, K., and Wijers, A. (2002). Inhibition, response mode and stimulus probability: a comparative event-related potential study. *Clin. Neurophysiol.* 113, 1172–1182. doi: 10.1016/s1388-2457(02)00141-4

Cabeza, R., Anderson, N. D., Locantore, J. K., and McIntosh, A. R. (2002). Aging gracefully: compensatory brain activity in high-performing older adults. *Neuroimage* 17, 1394–1402. doi: 10.1006/nimg.2002.1280

Davis, S. W., Dennis, N. A., Daselaar, S. M., Fleck, M. S., and Cabeza, R. (2008). Que PASA? The posterior-anterior shift in aging. *Cereb. Cortex* 18, 1201–1209. doi: 10.1093/cercor/bhm155

Dempster, F. N. (1992). The rise and fall of the inhibitory mechanism: toward a unified theory of cognitive development and aging. *Dev. Rev.* 12, 45–75. doi: 10.1016/0273-2297(92)90003-k

Dennis, N. A., and Cabeza, R. (2008). "Neuroimaging of healthy cognitive aging," in *The Handbook of Aging and Cognition*, Vol. 3, eds F. I. M. Craik and T. A. Salthouse (Mahwah, NJ: Lawrence Erlbaum Associates), 1–54.

Donchin, E., and Coles, M. G. (1988). Is the P300 component a manifestation of context updating? *Behav. Brain Sci.* 11, 357–374. doi: 10.1017/s0140525x00058027

Falkenstein, M., Hoormann, J., and Hohnsbein, J. (2001). Changes of error-related ERPs with age. *Exp. Brain Res.* 138, 258–262. doi: 10.1007/s002210100712

Falkenstein, M., Hoormann, J., and Hohnsbein, J. (2002). Inhibition-related ERP components: variation with modality, age and time-on-task. *J. Psychophysiol.* 16, 167–175. doi: 10.1027/0269-8803.16.3.167

Fallgatter, A. J., and Strik, W. K. (1999). The NoGo-anteriorization as a neurophysiological standard-index for cognitive response control. *Int. J. Psychophysiol.* 32, 233–238. doi: 10.1016/s0167-8760(99)00018-5

Folstein, M. F., Folstein, S. E., and McHugh, P. R. (1975). "Mini-mental state": a practical method for grading the cognitive state of patients for the clinician. *J. Psychiatr. Res.* 12, 189–198. doi: 10.1016/0022-3956(75)90026-6

Ford, J. M., Gray, M., Whitfield, S. L., Turken, U., Glover, G., Faustman, W. O., et al. (2004). Acquiring and inhibiting prepotent responses in schizophrenia: event-related brain potentials and functional magnetic resonanceimaging. *Arch. Gen. Psychiatry* 61, 119–129. doi: 10.1001/archpsyc.61.2.119

Grady, C. L., Springer, M. V., Hongwanishkul, D., McIntosh, A. R., and Winocur, G. (2006). Age-related changes in brain activity across the adult lifespan. *J. Cogn. Neurosci.* 18, 227–241. doi: 10.1162/jocn.2006.18.2.227

Hasher, L., and Zacks, R. T. (1988). Working memory, comprehension and aging: a review and new view. *Psychol. Learn. Motiv.* 30, 193–225. doi: 10.1016/s0079-7421(08)60041-9

Hong, X., Sun, J., Bengson, J. J., and Tong, S. (2014). Age-related spatiotemporal reorganization during response inhibition. *Int. J. Psychophysiol.* 93, 371–380. doi: 10.1016/j.ijpsycho.2014.05.013

Howell, D. C. (2010). *Statistical Methods for Psychology.* 7th Edn. Belmont, CA: Thomson Wadsworth.

Hsieh, S., and Fang, W. (2012). Elderly adults through compensatory responses can be just as capable as young adults in inhibiting the flanker influence. *Biol. Psychol.* 90, 113–126. doi: 10.1016/j.biopsycho.2012.03.006

Hsieh, S., and Lin, Y.-C. (2014). The boundary condition for observing compensatory responses by the elderly in a flanker-task paradigm. *Biol. Psychol.* 103, 69–82. doi: 10.1016/j.biopsycho.2014.08.008

Hsieh, S., Liang, Y.-C., and Tsai, Y.-C. (2012). Do age-related changes contribute to the flanker effect? *Clin. Neurophysiol.* 123, 960–972. doi: 10.1016/j.clinph.2011.09.013

Lucci, G., Berchicci, M., Spinelli, D., Taddei, F., and Di Russo, F. (2013). The effects of aging on conflict detection. *PLoS One* 8:e56566. doi: 10.1371/journal.pone.0056566

MacDonald, A. W., III, Cohen, J. D., Stenger, V. A., and Carter, C. S. (2000). Dissociating the role of the dorsolateral prefrontal and anterior cingulate cortex in cognitive control. *Science* 288, 1835–1838. doi: 10.1126/science.288.5472.1835

Nieuwenhuis, S., Yeung, N., van den Wildenberg, W., and Ridderinkhof, K. R. (2003). Electrophysiological correlates of anterior cingulate function in a go/no-go task: effects of response conflict and trial type frequency. *Cogn. Affect. Behav. Neurosci.* 3, 17–26. doi: 10.3758/cabn.3.1.17

Phillips, L. H., and Andrés, P. (2010). The cognitive neuroscience of aging: new findings on compensation and connectivity. *Cortex* 46, 421–424. doi: 10.1016/j.cortex.2010.01.005

Pires, L., Leitão, J., Guerrini, C., and Simões, M. R. (2014). Event-related brain potentials in the study of inhibition: cognitive control, source localization and age-related modulations. *Neuropsychol. Rev.* 24, 461–490. doi: 10.1007/s11065-014-9275-4

Raz, N. (2000). "Aging of the brain and its impact on cognitive performance: integration of structural and functional findings," in *Handbook of Aging and Cognition - II*, eds F. I. M. Craik and T. A. Salthouse (Mahwah, NJ: Lawrence Erlbaum Associates Publishers), 1–90.

Roberts, L. E., Rau, H., Lutzenberger, W., and Birbaumer, N. (1994). Mapping P300 waves onto inhibition: Go/No Go discrimination. *Electroencephalogr. Clin. Neurophysiol.* 92, 44–55. doi: 10.1016/0168-5597(94)90006-x

Roche, R. A., Garavan, H., Foxe, J. J., and O'Mara, S. M. (2005). Individual differences discriminate event-related potentials but not performance during response inhibition. *Exp. Brain Res.* 160, 60–70. doi: 10.1007/s00221-004-1985-z

Rogers, R. D., Sahakian, B. J., Hodges, J. R., Polkey, C. E., Kennard, C., and Robbins, T. W. (1998). Dissociating executive mechanisms of task control following frontal lobe damage and Parkinson's disease. *Brain* 121, 815–842. doi: 10.1093/brain/121.5.815

Smith, J. L., Johnstone, S. J., and Barry, R. J. (2008). Movement-related potentials in the Go/NoGo task: the P3 reflects both cognitive and motor inhibition. *Clin. Neurophysiol.* 119, 704–714. doi: 10.1016/j.clinph.2007.11.042

Tekok-Kilic, A., Shucard, J. L., and Shucard, D. W. (2001). Stimulus modality and Go/NoGo effects on P3 during parallel visual and auditory continuous performance tasks. *Psychophysiology* 38, 578–589. doi: 10.1017/s0048577201991279

Vallesi, A. (2011). Targets and non-targets in the aging brain: a go/nogo event-related potential study. *Neurosci. Lett.* 487, 313–317. doi: 10.1016/j.neulet.2010.10.046

Vallesi, A., Stuss, D. T., McIntosh, A. R., and Picton, T. W. (2009). Age-related differences in processing irrelevant information: evidence from event-related potentials. *Neuropsychologia* 47, 577–586. doi: 10.1016/j.neuropsychologia.2008.10.018

Van Boxtel, G. J. M., Van der Molen, M. W., Jennings, J. R., and Brunia, C. H. M. (2001). A psychophysiological analysis of inhibitory motor control in the stop-signal paradigm. *Biol. Psychol.* 58, 229–262. doi: 10.1016/s0301-0511(01)00117-x

Van Veen, V., and Carter, C. S. (2002a). The anterior cingulate as a conflict monitor: fMRI and ERP studies. *Physiol. Behav.* 77, 477–482. doi: 10.1016/s0031-9384(02)00930-7

Van Veen, V., and Carter, C. S. (2002b). The timing of action-monitoring processes in the anterior cingulate cortex. *J. Cogn. Neurosci.* 14, 593–602. doi: 10.1162/08989290260045837

West, R. (2000). In defense of the frontal lobe hypothesis of cognitive aging. *J. Int. Neuropsychol. Soc.* 6, 727–729. doi: 10.1017/s1355617700666109

3

Menopause, Obesity and Inflammation: Interactive Risk Factors for Alzheimer's Disease

*Amy Christensen and Christian J. Pike**

Davis School of Gerontology, University of Southern California, Los Angeles, CA, USA

Edited by:
Paula I. Moreira, University of Coimbra, Portugal

Reviewed by:
Ana I. Duarte, University of Coimbra, Portugal
Lucia Carboni, Alma Mater Studiorum University of Bologna, Italy

***Correspondence:**
Christian J. Pike, Davis School of Gerontology, University of Southern California, 3715 McClintock Avenue, Los Angeles, CA 90089-0191, USA
cjpike@usc.edu

Alzheimer's disease (AD) is a multifactorial neurodegenerative disorder, the development of which is regulated by several environmental and genetic risk factors. Two factors theorized to contribute to the initiation and/or progression of AD pathogenesis are age-related increases in inflammation and obesity. These factors may be particularly problematic in women. The onset of menopause in mid-life elevates the vulnerability of women to AD, an increased risk that is likely associated with the depletion of estrogens. Menopause is also linked with an abundance of additional changes, including increased central adiposity and inflammation. Here, we review the current literature to explore the interactions between obesity, inflammation, menopause and AD.

Keywords: adiposity, aging, Alzheimer's disease, estrogen, hormone therapy, inflammation, obesity

Introduction

Alzheimer's disease (AD) is an age-related neurodegenerative disease that is the leading cause of dementia. The causal factor(s) that drives development and progression of the disease is still debated, though the primary agents are likely β-amyloid protein (Aβ) and the microtubule associated protein tau (LaFerla, 2010; Morris et al., 2014). Aβ is a small, soluble peptide normally found at low levels in brain and bodily fluids. Increased production and/or decreased clearance of Aβ fosters its inherent ability to self-associate into neurotoxic oligomeric forms that become deposited in the brain parenchyma as plaques and in the cerebrovasculature as cerebral amyloid angiopathy (Mucke and Selkoe, 2012). Interestingly, genetic mutations that underlie familial AD yield increased Aβ production or its propensity to aggregate (Tanzi, 2012). Thus, given both the toxic nature of Aβ and its genetic links to the disease, Aβ accumulation is widely theorized to be the key regulator of AD pathogenesis (Hardy and Higgins, 1992; Hardy, 2006). However, increasing evidence indicates an essential role of tau, which undergoes hyperphosphorylation resulting in the formation of neurofibrillary tangles, a hallmark of AD neuropathology found in many dead and dying neurons (Iqbal et al., 2010). Emerging evidence indicates that tau, like Aβ, can be a potent pathogenic protein and that it is capable of spreading pathology in a prion-like manner (Bloom, 2014; Zempel and Mandelkow, 2014).

AD is more than just the accumulation of oligomeric and fibrillar Aβ and abnormally phosphorylated tau. The disease is characterized by many pathologic changes, including hypometabolism (Mosconi et al., 2008; Yao et al., 2011), blood-brain-barrier (BBB) disruption (Zlokovic, 2011), and glial activation (Mrak and Griffin, 2005; Prokop et al., 2013). Sporadic AD, which is not driven by the genetic mutations in familial AD and represents the vast majority of cases, is likely to reflect the interactive effects of normal aging with numerous environmental risk factors and subtle genetic polymorphisms. In turn, these interactions cooperatively disrupt pathways that regulate Aβ, tau, and other AD pathologies. Thus, unraveling AD risk, and perhaps developing successful prevention and intervention strategies, will require understanding the interactions between aging and a set of risk factors.

Two important AD risk factors are obesity and inflammation. Obesity has increased at an alarming rate across westernized countries, with approximately 70% of the US adult population currently classified as either overweight or obese (Ogden et al., 2014). Elevated adiposity increases the risks of numerous conditions, including metabolic syndrome (McGill, 2014), hypertension (Rahmouni, 2014), cardiovascular disease (Rocha and Libby, 2009), and AD (Jayaraman and Pike, 2014). One consequence of obesity that may underlie its pathogenic roles is chronic inflammation, which is observed both in brain and systemically. Inflammation is independently associated with AD and numerous other age-related disorders (Michaud et al., 2013; Bettcher and Kramer, 2014). A wealth of genetic, epidemiological, and experimental findings identifies pro-inflammatory pathways as significant regulators of various AD pathologies (Wyss-Coray and Rogers, 2012). Interestingly, risk factors can affect men and women differently. For example, the apolipoprotein E ε4 allele (ApoE4), the most significant genetic risk factor for late-onset AD, affects women much more strongly than men (Altmann et al., 2014). The enhanced vulnerability of aging women to some conditions, including increased risk of osteoporosis, cardiovascular disease and perhaps AD, is related to depletion of estrogens at menopause. Here, we consider the roles of obesity and inflammation in AD pathogenesis with a specific emphasis on women, who are disproportionately affected by AD.

AD and Obesity

Obesity is a precursor condition for numerous disorders, including cardiovascular disease, metabolic syndrome, and type 2 diabetes (T2D; Bonomini et al., 2015; Kim and Feldman, 2015). More recently, obesity and its associated comorbid conditions have been identified as significant risk factors for both cognitive decline and the development of AD (Jayaraman and Pike, 2014). A growing literature suggests that the insulin resistance and dysregulation of insulin signaling associated with T2D are precursors to both cognitive impairment and AD (Yaffe et al., 2004; Profenno et al., 2010). T2D in humans has been shown to increase the rate of age-related mental decline (Hassing et al., 2004), and those with T2D have been shown to develop cognitive impairment earlier than those without this risk factor (Cigolle et al., 2011). Further, adults with T2D have a significantly increased risk of AD (Luchsinger et al., 2004; Biessels et al., 2006; Profenno et al., 2010). Similarly, obesity appears to significantly increase AD risk, particularly when it is present during middle age (Kivipelto et al., 2005; Beydoun et al., 2008; Fitzpatrick et al., 2009; Xu et al., 2011). In contrast to most of the literature, a recent study with a very large sample size reported that midlife obesity (measured as body mass index, BMI) reduces dementia risk (Qizilbash et al., 2015). The absence of concordance among several well-controlled studies suggests that the relationship between obesity and AD is more complex than simply an increase in adiposity. For example, some studies suggest that dementia risk is not adversely affected by BMI *per se*, but rather by central obesity specifically (Whitmer et al., 2008; Gustafson et al., 2009; Luchsinger et al., 2012), which is often closely associated with adverse health effects including cardiovascular disease. In fact, cardiovascular outcomes are predicted better by measures of central obesity and often poorly by BMI (Yusuf et al., 2005; Dallongeville et al., 2012). Age is also an important consideration, as obesity in late life appears to reduce rather than increase AD risk (Fitzpatrick et al., 2009; Gustafson et al., 2009). Collectively, these observations suggest that central obesity in midlife induces changes that may create a neural environment conducive to initial development of AD pathology.

In general agreement with the human literature, experimental studies in mouse models of AD demonstrate that diet-induced obesity (DIO) significantly exacerbates AD-like neuropathology and worsens cognitive impairment (Julien et al., 2010; Herculano et al., 2013). Short-term high fat diet in an AD mouse model was shown to cause mild metabolic dysfunction and significant cognitive impairment, although no changes were observed in levels of Aβ, a key protein in AD pathogenesis (Herculano et al., 2013). High fat and high sucrose diets have also been shown to affect tau accumulation, processing and hyperphosphorylation (Julien et al., 2010; Orr et al., 2014; Takalo et al., 2014). In 3 × Tg-AD mice, longer-term administration of a high fat diet (16 weeks) impaired cognitive performance in both male and female mice (Barron et al., 2013). In line with the behavioral deficits, both male and female 3 × Tg-AD mice showed increased Aβ burden in the hippocampus. Male and female non-transgenic rodents both exhibit decreased cognitive performance after exposure to high fat diet (Molteni et al., 2002; Farr et al., 2008; Granholm et al., 2008). In some cases, male mice are more vulnerable to diet-induced cognitive impairment (Hwang et al., 2010). Since males typically exhibit significantly more robust metabolic deficits in response to high-fat diets (Barron et al., 2013), this may suggest that some aspects of obesity-induced cognitive impairment are related to metabolic disturbances, including insulin resistance. However, since even short-term exposure (9 days) to diets high in fat (Murray et al., 2009) results in impaired spatial memory in rats, more immediate effects of diet must also contribute to cognitive deficits. Diets high in sugars can also yield negative outcomes in AD mouse models (Cao et al., 2007; Orr et al., 2014) and wild-type rats (Hsu et al., 2015). Together, these studies show that exposure to obesity-inducing diets results in both rapid and long-term neural changes that impair cognitive performance and accelerate development of AD-like pathology.

The mechanism(s) by which obesity increases AD risk and cognitive deficits is unknown, although numerous possibilities have been proposed (Jayaraman et al., 2014). One widely discussed concept is that AD risk is linked with changes in glucose metabolism and insulin signaling (Blázquez et al., 2014; de la Monte and Tong, 2014). Consistent with this position, a reduction in brain glucose metabolism has been shown to be a preclinical symptom of AD (Mosconi, 2005). This reduction appears to be associated with altered insulin signaling. In obese patients, insulin resistance results in an elevated release of peripheral insulin, but insulin concentrations in the brain are reduced, likely due to a decrease in insulin transport across the BBB (Craft, 2007). Although insulin levels are decreased centrally, the situation is further exacerbated by altered insulin signaling in the brain that is less effective than under normal conditions (Anthony et al., 2006). Interestingly, intranasal administration of insulin has been shown to improve hippocampal dependent memory in patients with early stages of AD (Reger et al., 2008; Claxton et al., 2015). Perhaps in contrast to these observations, DIO in female 3 × Tg-AD mice accelerated Aβ accumulation and behavioral impairment in the absence of apparent changes in peripheral insulin levels and sensitivity (Barron et al., 2013). Collectively, these data suggest that obesity-induced insulin resistance and/or impaired insulin signaling can contribute to AD neuropathology although additional factors also play significant roles.

Other than insulin-related deficits induced by obesity, increased adiposity has other systemic effects that may contribute to induction and progression of AD. For example, increased adiposity elevates neuroinflammation (Thaler and Schwartz, 2010; Thaler et al., 2012; Jayaraman et al., 2014; Aguilar-Valles et al., 2015), which has been implicated as a pathologic mechanism in AD (Johnston et al., 2011; Verri et al., 2012; Wyss-Coray and Rogers, 2012). Systemic and central inflammation will be discussed in greater detail below. However, cerebrovascular inflammation in particular has been widely associated with both obesity (Tucsek et al., 2014) and AD (Yu et al., 2012; Takeda et al., 2013). In fact, vascular inflammation may precede AD, as a transgenic rodent model of obesity and AD showed cerebrovascular inflammation and cognitive deficits prior to the deposition of Aβ (Takeda et al., 2010). In this model, cerebral amyloid angiopathy was much greater in obese animals compared to lean ones. Other vascular risk factors that are associated with obesity, including hyperlipidemia and hypertension, have also been identified as AD risk factors (Kivipelto et al., 2005). Thus, the mechanisms by which obesity increases AD risk are presumably multifactorial and likely modulated by a constellation of interactive risk factors and comorbidities.

AD and Inflammation

Although inflammation has been implicated in AD pathogenesis for many years, the importance of its role has been increasingly appreciated in the past few years. As has been discussed in other recent reviews (Mandrekar-Colucci and Landreth, 2010; Wyss-Coray and Rogers, 2012), multiple lines of evidence link inflammation as a key contributor to both the initiation and progression of AD and identify it as a compelling therapeutic target. Much of the recent focus on inflammation comes from the linkage to AD of polymorphisms in genes that are expressed by microglia and or play a role in innate immune responses (Tanzi, 2012). Included in this list are CD33 (Bertram et al., 2008; Hollingworth et al., 2011; Naj et al., 2011) and triggering receptor expressed on myeloid cells 2 (TREM2; Leavy, 2015), which are expressed in microglia and contribute to phagocytosis and Aβ clearance. Other immune-related factors linked to AD are CR1 and clusterin (Harold et al., 2009; Lambert et al., 2009), components of the complement system.

Microglia are the key mediators of neuroinflammation, functioning as the brain's resident macrophages. In their role as brain immune sentinels, microglia constantly survey the neural environment for both normal and pathological disruptions. In their normal state, microglia are clearly beneficial, utilizing phagocytosis to remove unwanted or unneeded materials and to regulate homeostatic processes such as synaptic remodeling (Chen and Trapp, 2015). Further, they may have important neurotrophic roles as suggested by their secretion of brain-derived neurotrophic factor and insulin-like growth factor 1 (Parkhurst et al., 2013; Suh et al., 2013). When activated under more pathological conditions, microglia exhibit a wide range of responses that continue to be defined (Colton, 2009). Among these responses, microglia alter their phagocytic activities and can secrete large amounts of pro-inflammatory cytokines. Cytokine secretion can be aggravated when microglia are primed by an initial activating insult (Teeling and Perry, 2009). This type of priming response may contribute to interactions among comorbid conditions such as obesity. In this case, a high fat diet that results in obesity may represent the first hit on the microglia and Aβ accumulation the second, yielding an exaggerated response that may drive pathology.

The AD brain is characterized by extensive gliosis, including activation and increased numbers of both astrocytes and microglia as well as elevated levels of inflammatory cytokines. Aβ plaques, once formed, are rapidly (within 1–2 days) surrounded by microglia (Meyer-Luehmann et al., 2008). Aβ has been shown to promote the release of inflammatory cytokines from microglia (Wyss-Coray and Rogers, 2012). Interestingly, increased pro-inflammatory factors can result in greater amyloid precursor protein production, leading to even more Aβ release and creating a vicious cycle that further promotes AD pathology (Karran et al., 2011). This progression of pathology appears to yield multiple states of microglial activation and deactivation that presumably vary in their effects on discrete AD pathologies (Colton, 2009). For example, initial exposures of microglia to Aβ, while the microglia are in their resting anti-inflammatory state, can result in effective Aβ clearance. However, this insult induces an activation state associated with the release of pro-inflammatory cytokines like tumor necrosis factor α (TNFα) and interleukin 1β (IL-1β). After microglia achieve a pro-inflammatory state, they may be less able to effectively phagocytose extracellular Aβ (Koenigsknecht-Talboo and Landreth, 2005). Similarly, microglia in an AD mouse model mice were shown to be anti-inflammatory early in the disease, but to be activated later after the pathology had progressed (Jimenez et al., 2008).

Obesity and Inflammation

It has been more than two decades since the link between inflammation and insulin resistance was first shown with an increase in TNFα levels in obese rodents (Hotamisligil et al.,

1993). Confirming an active rather than passive role in pathology, neutralization of TNFα in obese rats resulted in a restored response to insulin. This and other early studies spawned intense study on the role of numerous inflammatory factors in obesity, metabolic syndrome, and T2D. It is now clear that not only is chronic low grade inflammation a symptom of metabolic disorders, but also that both peripheral (Hotamisligil, 2006) and central (Thaler and Schwartz, 2010) inflammation contribute to the development and progression of obesity and its comorbidities.

Visceral fat, also known as central or abdominal fat, is thought to have the greatest correlation with metabolic dysfunction (Kissebah et al., 1982; Nieves et al., 2003). An increase in body weight results in a corresponding increase in the number of mature macrophages found in adipose tissue. Macrophages invade and surround necrotic adipocytes and secrete excess pro- and anti-inflammatory cytokines, including TNFα and interleukin 6 (IL-6). The release of proinflammatory cytokines by macrophages is thought to contribute to the glucose disruptions and insulin resistance that is seen in obese individuals. Indeed, if macrophages are specifically ablated, insulin and glucose homeostasis can be rapidly restored and levels of inflammatory cytokines in adipose tissue, muscle and serum reduced (Patsouris et al., 2008). Further, adipocytes themselves secrete leptin and IL-6 after the macrophage infiltration and further increase the inflammatory response due in obesity. Adipose tissue is a highly active immunological organ that contributes to the increased inflammatory response to weight gain.

The role of inflammation in obesity also includes key contributions from the brain. Obesity-induced increases in peripheral and circulating cytokine levels likely affect the brain in multiple ways. However, available evidence suggests that central inflammation begins prior to the onset of obesity and appears to contribute to the process (Thaler et al., 2013). Much of the data on central inflammation and obesity has been generated from DIO paradigms, in which increased adiposity results from maintaining rodents on high-fat diets. DIO recapitulates much of the human obesity condition and can be modified to include specialized fats and/or sugars. Rodent DIO models have shown that both central and peripheral inflammation are induced with high fat diet (De Souza et al., 2005; Milanski et al., 2009; Thaler et al., 2012). Inflammation in the hypothalamus in response to high fat diet occurs within hours and persists for a few days before subsiding only to return after about 2 weeks (Thaler et al., 2012). Peripheral inflammation takes longer to develop and usually coincides with an increase in adipose tissue mass. Interestingly, mice with IL-1β, IL-6, or TNFα receptor knocked out show a worsening rather than a reduction in both obesity and metabolic syndrome, suggesting that inflammation is not the only contributing factor to these afflictions.

Inflammatory cytokines, which are elevated by obesity in both adipose tissue and brain, appear to be involved in both promoting inflammation and mediating many of its deleterious effects. In the hypothalamus, DIO induces inflammation within 3 days of the initiation of high fat diet in rodent (Thaler et al., 2012). Short-term high fat diet results in an upregulation of activated microglia and astrocytes. In humans, increased gliosis that is similar to that characteristic of injury is seen in the medial basal hypothalamus of obese patients (Thaler et al., 2012). Consistent with their role in adverse neural outcomes, cortical glia cultured from obese mice retain their inflammatory phenotype and impair neuron survival and growth *in vitro* (Jayaraman et al., 2014). Numerous inflammatory factors have been shown to be upregulated by obesity, including IL-1β, IL-6, TNFα and interleukin 18 (IL-18; Vandanmagsar et al., 2011), but which ones are central the relationship between obesity and AD are unclear. Here, we consider a few of the factors that are affected by obesity with an emphasis on those that also have been implicated in AD.

Leptin

Leptin is an adipokine that modulates appetite and informs the brain about the availability of stored energy. Although leptin is thought of as a peptide hormone, it bears remarkable similarity to inflammatory cytokines, especially interleukin 2 (IL-2). Further, the leptin receptor is homologous to the type 1 cytokine receptors. Leptin secretion increases with increasing adiposity (Considine et al., 1996). In the hypothalamus, leptin regulates appetite. High levels of leptin normally induce satiety. However, obese individuals develop leptin resistance, attenuating its ability to properly regulate appetite. The increase in adipose tissue in obese individuals initially results in elevated leptin release, but the response to leptin is blunted and the satiety signal is not recognized. The mechanisms that underlie leptin resistance have not been fully elucidated, but it may be the result of disrupted leptin signaling pathways, decreased leptin transport across the BBB, or increased inflammation in the hypothalamus (Park and Ahima, 2015).

In addition to regulating appetite, leptin is a regulator of inflammation and the immune system. Leptin regulates both innate and adaptive immune responses and generally increases levels of pro-inflammatory cytokines (Conde et al., 2014). Initial evidence of this link emerged from the observation that mice with deficiencies in leptin signaling (*ob/ob* or *db/db*) exhibit impaired immune responses (Lord et al., 1998). On the other hand, leptin exposure increases the proliferation and activation of T lymphocytes and promotes a T helper 1 phenotype (Martín-Romero et al., 2000). Similarly, leptin activates components of the innate immune response. For example, leptin increases activation of monocytes, including their production of cytokines such as TNFα and IL-6 (Santos-Alvarez et al., 1999). Also, leptin can induce the expression of nitric oxide and prostaglandin estrogen 17β-estradiol (E2) in cultured macrophages (Raso et al., 2002). With signaling capacity both peripherally and centrally and release modulated by fat mass, leptin is well positioned to function as a mediator of interactions between the brain and peripheral inflammatory responses (Carlton et al., 2012), particularly in the context of obesity (Aguilar-Valles et al., 2015).

Leptin resistance is predicted to foster AD pathogenesis as normal leptin signaling is associated with reduced AD risk. Persons with mild cognitive impairment or AD show lower plasma levels of leptin than cognitively normal controls (Johnston et al., 2014). Cerebrospinal fluid (CSF) leptin levels can remain stable with progression to AD, but a reduction in leptin signaling in hippocampus suggests AD is associated with attenuation of leptin actions (Maioli et al., 2015). Conversely, in a prospective study, elevated leptin levels were associated with greater cerebral brain volume and reduced dementia risk (Lieb et al., 2009). In experimental AD models, leptin administration has been shown to have therapeutic effects on both Aβ deposition (Fewlass et al., 2004) and tau phosphorylation (Greco et al., 2008). Such protective pathways may become dysfunctional in the AD brain, where leptin levels are elevated but expression of its receptor is downregulated (Bonda et al., 2014). Further, the leptin receptor protein was found localized to neurons containing neurofibrillary tangles and within plaques, a situation expected to disrupt its signaling capability. Indeed, phosphorylation of the leptin receptor, which is required for its activation, was reduced when the leptin receptor was found in tangle-bearing neurons (Bonda et al., 2014). Collectively, available data indicate that a loss of beneficial leptin signaling can contribute to AD, suggesting that leptin resistance may be a mechanism by which obesity affects AD risk.

TNFα

TNFα appears to be produced exclusively by macrophages in adipose tissue with no contribution from adipocytes (Weisberg et al., 2003). Both TNFα protein and mRNA are robustly upregulated in obesity, an increase that has been shown to correlate with the development of insulin resistance (Hotamisligil et al., 1995). An increase in abdominal adipose tissue in particular has been shown to correlate with increased TNFα release (Tsigos et al., 1999). After weight loss, a decrease in TNFα protein in adipose tissue and a decrease in serum insulin is observed (Hotamisligil et al., 1995).

The neural effects of TNFα, which is produced in brain by neurons and glia, can be both desirable and detrimental. Transiently elevated levels of TNFα are beneficial. For example, TNFα can recruit astrocytes and microglia to sites of injury and activate a glial response (Flynn et al., 2003). However, TNFα also exerts negative effects on neural plasticity, such as reducing levels of long-term potentiation (Beattie et al., 2002; Ferguson et al., 2008). Increased TNFα is also thought to promote AD pathogenesis. For instance, *in vitro* and *in vivo* evidence indicate that TNFα increases Aβ levels by increasing expression of BACE1, an enzyme that drives Aβ production (Yamamoto et al., 2007). Further, TNFα has been shown to inhibit the transport of Aβ out of the brain and into peripheral circulation where it can be eliminated (López et al., 2008). TNFα-mediated increases in Aβ can lead to a vicious cycle. Aβ not only increases expression of TNFα (Meda et al., 1995; Akama and Van Eldik, 2000) but also is able to activate the TNFα receptor TNFRI, which is upregulated in AD brains compared to normal controls (Li et al., 2004; Cheng et al., 2010). Further, Aβ-induced generation of TNFα is implicated in the neurotoxic effects of Aβ (Xie et al., 2002). Conversely, reducing TNFα may be neuroprotective. For example, TNFRI knockout in AD transgenic mice diminishes AD-like neuropathology (He et al., 2007).

IL-6

Both adipocytes and macrophages can generate and secrete IL-6 from adipose tissue. Greater adiposity results in increased IL-6 secretion. Serum IL-6 concentrations have been positively correlated with obesity, insulin resistance (Bastard et al., 2000; Kern et al., 2001), T2D (Pradhan et al., 2001), and cardiovascular disease (Plutzky, 2001). Multiple studies in both mice and humans have linked IL-6 to T2D as the cytokine with the strongest association with metabolic dysfunction (Kern et al., 2001; Pradhan et al., 2001). Although IL-6 production is associated with visceral fat (Fontana et al., 2007), the relationship between IL-6 and obesity is not straightforward. For example, IL-6 knockout mice develop obesity, elevated leptin, and altered glucose homeostasis with aging (Wallenius et al., 2002), suggesting that long-term IL-6 depletion can contribute to metabolic dysfunction. IL-6 administered peripherally in knockout mice, reduces body weight and leptin levels. However, IL-6 treatment is also associated with deleterious effects in several paradigms. For example, in mouse hepatocytes and a human hepatocarcinoma model, IL-6 disrupts insulin signaling by decreasing insulin's ability to activate Akt, a critical part of insulin's modulation of downstream metabolic effects (Senn et al., 2002).

As with several other pro-inflammatory cytokines, chronic elevation of IL-6 results in negative neural consequences. Cross-sectional and longitudinal data indicate that elevated plasma IL-6 in mid-life is associated with significant cognitive decline (Singh-Manoux et al., 2014). Several IL-6 genetic variants have been shown to significantly regulate AD risk (Papassotiropoulos et al., 1999; Chen et al., 2012; Flex et al., 2014). IL-6 has consistently been shown to be elevated in the brains, especially near Aβ plaques, and in the CSF of AD patients (Bauer et al., 1991; Blum-Degen et al., 1995). The astrogliosis and microgliosis triggered by AD results in increased IL-6 release from both of these cell types (Erta et al., 2012). IL-6 has been implicated in AD pathogenesis through several different mechanisms. For example, cultured cortical neurons show more damage when treated with both Aβ and IL-6. Further, in cultured hippocampal neurons, IL-6 has been shown to increase tau phosphorylation (Quintanilla et al., 2004).

AD, Menopause and Hormone Therapy

Since women are disproportionately affected by AD, there has been considerable interest in understanding differences in estrogen across the lifespan associated with AD risk. One approach to investigating this idea is to consider the effects of pregnancies, which yield a net decrease in lifetime estrogen exposure (Bernstein et al., 1985; Hankinson et al., 1995). Several studies have shown that women who have birthed children are more likely to suffer from cognitive impairment and AD than nulliparous women (Ptok et al., 2002; McLay et al., 2003; Colucci et al., 2006; Beeri et al., 2009). Men with or without children show no change in AD risk, so the difference cannot be due to environmental factors associated with child rearing (Ptok et al., 2002). Nulliparous women are therefore seemingly protected from cognitive decline by their greater lifetime exposure to estrogens.

Another approach to address this issue is to consider the potential effects of estrogen loss on AD risk. Most studies have found that surgical menopause *prior* to the development of natural menopause significantly increases risks for cognitive decline and AD (Rocca et al., 2007, 2011; Phung et al., 2010; Bove et al., 2014). Conversely, oophorectomy *after* the age of natural menopause does not appear to significantly alter AD risk (Rocca et al., 2011; Imtiaz et al., 2014). The implication of these studies is that early loss of sex steroid hormones can accelerate the development of AD. However, although brain levels of estrogens are lower in women with AD than age-matched women without neurologic disease, this relationship has been reported for only for women older than age 80 years (Yue et al., 2005; Rosario et al., 2011). Thus, while low estrogen appears to be associated with AD, the timing of this relationship with respect to disease onset remains unsettled.

If the depletion of ovarian sex steroid hormones at menopause is a risk factor for AD, then maintenance of hormones would be predicted to reduce AD risk. Consistent with this idea, AD risk has been reported to be lowest in postmenopausal women with the highest endogenous E2 levels and greatest in those with low E2 levels (Manly et al., 2000). Another approach is to consider how AD risk is affected by treatment with estrogen-based HT. Initial observational studies generally found significantly reduced risk of AD in women with a history of hormone therapy (HT) use (Henderson et al., 1994, 1996), findings that were supported by subsequent prospective studies (Tang et al., 1996; Kawas et al., 1997; Zandi et al., 2002). Human studies have been mirrored by experiments in transgenic mouse models of AD, in which ovariectomy (OVX) induced loss of sex steroid hormones increases and treatment with E2 generally reduces AD-like neuropathology (Zheng et al., 2002; Yue et al., 2005; Carroll et al., 2007; Zhao et al., 2011).

Despite the apparent benefits of estrogen-based HT in reducing AD risk, discrepant clinical findings have demonstrated neural risks and questioned its benefits. Most importantly, results of the Women's Health Initiative (WHI), a large double-blinded, placebo-controlled clinical trial, indicated increased rather than reduced dementia in subjects randomized to HT treatment (Shumaker et al., 2003, 2004). There are numerous factors that may contribute to the discordance of estrogen's benefits across the many human and rodent paradigms, including formulation of the treatment, continuous vs. discontinuous delivery, and route of administration. Perhaps the most significant issue is the timing of treatment, with initiation of HT near the onset of menopause hypothesized to be critical for its neural efficacy (Maki, 2006). In the WHI, the mean age of subjects was about 65 years old, many years past the average onset of menopause at age 51. Studies in which HT was initiated at or near menopause have generally reported benefits rather than risks. For example, in a Danish study in which middle aged women were randomized to HT and placebo treatment groups, beneficial effects on cognitive function were observed more than 10 years after the cessation of the 2–3 year HT regimen (Bagger et al., 2005). This finding suggests that using HT, even for a short time during menopause, may have a positive effect on cognition much later. Similar results have been found for AD risk: HT is associated with decreased risk if delivered near menopause but has no benefit or even increases risk when started several years after menopause (Henderson et al., 2005; Whitmer et al., 2011; Shao et al., 2012). More work will be required to fully elucidate the relationship between HT and AD risk, but emerging results seem to suggest that short-term HT near menopause onset may offer a reasonable strategy to impede development of dementia.

Efficacy of HT is also likely to be modulated by genetic factors. The most significant genetic risk factor for late-onset AD is the ε4 allele of ApoE4. ApoE4 regulates lipid trafficking and may play a role in the removal of Aβ from the brain (Näslund et al., 1995; Leduc et al., 2011). HT may be differentially effective in women based on their ApoE status. In mice, E2 is able to reduce inflammatory markers in cultures from ApoE3, but not ApoE4 mice (Brown et al., 2008). One study showed that HT around menopause is more effective in preventing cognitive decline in ApoE4-negative women than those with even a single ApoE4 allele (Yaffe et al., 2000). Further, the ApoE4 genotype may increase the risk of AD more in females than males (Farrer et al., 1997; Bretsky et al., 1999). Increased AD risk in ApoE4 carriers requires only one ApoE4 allele in females with no further risk increase in homozygotes, whereas significant male risk appears to require two ApoE4 copies (Payami et al., 1996). A more recent study showed that both male and female ApoE4 carriers were at greater risk of AD with even one ApoE4 allele, but that the risk for female carriers was significantly greater (Altmann et al., 2014). How interactions between ApoE, HT and AD are modulated by obesity, inflammation, and other factors that drive AD pathogenesis remains to be determined.

Menopause and Adiposity

The shift from young adulthood into middle age is associated with increasing proportions of women that are overweight and/or obese (Ogden et al., 2014). This weight gain likely reflects multifaceted consequences of aging. There is evidence that depletion of sex steroid hormones during menopause can contribute to weight gain, although body weight also predicts subsequent changes in hormone levels (Guthrie et al., 1999; Sternfeld et al., 2004; Wildman et al., 2012). Significant increases in central fat have been reported with greater waist circumference after the last menstrual period (Poehlman et al., 1995; Björkelund et al., 1996; Ho et al., 2010). This increase in adiposity associated with menopause is linked with increased risks for obesity (Rachoń and Teede, 2010), metabolic syndrome (Carr, 2003; Cho et al., 2008) and T2D (Wajchenberg, 2000). Although increasing age may partially account for the increase T2D incidence in postmenopausal women (Janssen et al., 2008), the change in fat distribution has also been shown to be a contributing cause (Barrett-Connor et al., 1996; Tchernof et al., 1998; Sites et al., 2000).

Studies in both humans (menopause) and rodents (reproductive senescence) indicate that age-related ovarian hormone loss contributes to changes in the distribution of adipose tissue. The significant decrease in estrogen and progesterone that results from follicular depletion yields a more androgenic pattern of fat distribution—an increase in central or abdominal adiposity. OVX in mice, a model of surgical menopause, can result in a significant increase in body weight (Stubbins et al., 2012). This elevated weight results from a decrease in energy expenditure, as opposed to increases in calorie consumption, and promotes insulin resistance, increased adipocyte size, and peripheral inflammation (Rogers et al., 2009). Treatment of mice with the E2 results in reductions in all of these outcomes.

In postmenopausal women, estrogen-based HT has been shown to decrease some of these metabolic effects in addition to restoring a more gynoid pattern of fat distribution (Barrett-Connor et al., 1996; Salpeter et al., 2006). HT can attenuate central adiposity when administered to early postmenopausal women (Haarbo et al., 1991; Ahtiainen et al., 2012). Additionally, HT may decrease total weight gain during menopause, especially in non-obese women (Kristensen et al., 1999). Further, HT has been shown to increase the effectiveness of concurrent lifestyle and pharmaceutical treatments for some obesity-related comorbidities (Golden et al., 2013).

The mechanisms by which E2 reduces obesity and risk of T2D remain to be fully elucidated. Paradoxically, risk of maternal insulin resistance is highest in late pregnancy when E2 levels are high (Ryan and Enns, 1988), yet low E2 levels after menopause have been linked with T2D (Carr, 2003; Meyer et al., 2011). Aromatase knockout mice, which cannot synthesize E2, are obese and insulin resistant (Jones et al., 2000). Estrogen receptor α (ERα) is likely to play a role in regulation of obesity as ERα knockout mice are more obese and glucose intolerant than wild-type females (Heine et al., 2000; Bryzgalova et al., 2006). Further, both peripheral and central E2 administrations have been shown to act through different pathways with similar overall outcomes of reductions in insulin resistance, glucose dysregulation and adiposity (Yonezawa et al., 2012). Peripheral and central E2 administration resulted in decreased adipocyte size and reduced expression of macrophage markers, although peripheral E2 treatment elicited greater changes. Only peripheral E2 administration decreased adipose expression of the pro-inflammatory cytokine TNFα. Central and peripheral E2 administration both increased energy expenditure, but central E2 caused much greater spontaneous locomotor activity. Thus, E2 likely regulates adiposity and metabolic outcomes by actions on several tissues. How these actions are affected by aging likely underlies the interactions between menopause, obesity and the efficacy of HT.

Inflammation and Menopause

There are extensive literatures on the relationships between estrogens and other sex steroid hormones and regulation of inflammation. In general, one can reasonably argue that estrogens function as potent anti-inflammatory factors. Thus, depletion of E2 at menopause results in elevated pro-inflammatory cytokines and may place tissues throughout the body at increased risk of inflammation and diseases associated with inflammation (Pfeilschifter et al., 2002). However, this is an extensive and complex literature as estrogens regulate several aspects of immune function and inflammation (Straub, 2007) and thus can protect against some conditions but promote others (Gilliver, 2010). The relationships between estrogens, menopause, and inflammation-related disorders have been well described in numerous reviews for several conditions, including cardiovascular disease (Camilleri et al., 2012; Knowlton and Lee, 2012), osteoarthritis (Martín-Millán and Castañeda, 2013), and rheumatoid arthritis (Islander et al., 2011). Thus, although estrogens can be broadly defined as anti-inflammatory, the effects of estrogen loss and estrogen-based HT depend upon the tissue, cell type, and context.

How menopause affects neuroinflammation has not been well studied. However, as with other tissues, the brain exhibits a generally pro-inflammatory phenotype with increasing age. In a study that examined changes in gene expression across age in adult human brain, male and female brains exhibited significant differences in the number of genes changing expression (higher in males), the patterns of changes in terms of gene function, and the brain region-specific nature of the changes (Berchtold et al., 2008). Of particular interest to the current topic, women exhibited greater proportional age-related increases in expression of genes associated with immune and inflammatory functions. Further, both women and men showed increased expression of these genes in hippocampus and entorhinal cortex (both of which are strongly affected in AD), but only women had significant increases in other brain regions (Berchtold et al., 2008), suggesting a more global pro-inflammatory condition in the aging female brain.

Like the human brain, the rodent female brain shows increased inflammation with aging that is regulated, in part, by estrogen status. For example, the frontal cortex of middle-aged female rats shows increased expression of several microglial and immune function genes as a consequence of both aging and estrogen-deprivation (Sárvári et al., 2012). Importantly, the authors also found a strongly overlapping pattern of gene expression changes in the frontal cortex of older postmenopausal women relative to younger premenopausal women. Confirming a protective role of estrogens, treatment of OVX middle-aged rats with E2 or ER-specific agonists significantly decreased expression of several microglial and immune function genes in the frontal cortex (Sárvári et al., 2011). This relationship extends to pro-inflammatory cytokines such as TNFα and IL-1β, which show increased hippocampal expression in female mice as consequences of both aging and OVX-induced estrogen depletion (Benedusi et al., 2012). The age-related increase in the pro-inflammatory state of the brain can be exacerbated by inflammatory challenges. For example, the increased hippocampal expression of cytokines induced by high cholesterol diet is significantly worsened in reproductively senescent female rats, an effect that can be attenuated by estradiol treatment (Lewis et al., 2010). However, the ability of E2 to protect against elevated cytokine levels can significantly diminish, and in some cases reverse, in aged female brain (Nordell et al., 2003). Collectively, these observations indicate that both aging and menopause contribute to increasing levels of neuroinflammation, which are predicted to cooperatively interact in the promotion of inflammation neural diseases such as AD.

Conclusion

AD neuropathology is characterized and likely driven by the accumulation of Aβ and abnormally phosphorylated tau. The development of these and other components of AD

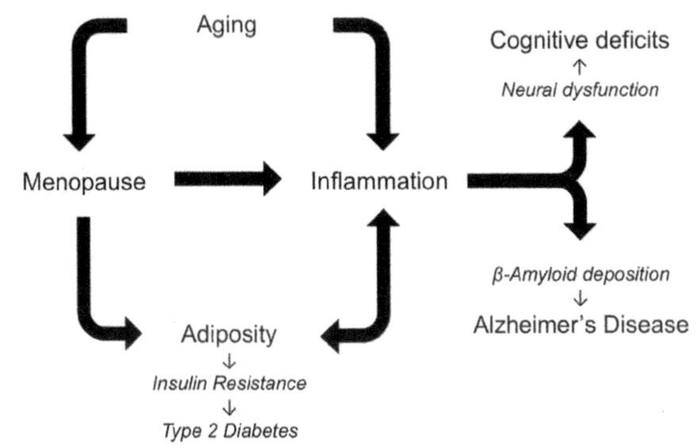

FIGURE 1 | Alzheimer's disease (AD) is a multifactorial disorder in which multiple risk factors are theorized to interact in regulating pathogenesis. As depicted in the diagram an essential factor in AD is increasing age, which is also associated with elevated inflammation and, in women, menopause. The loss of estrogens at menopause increases central adiposity, which in turn increases inflammation and predisposes women to metabolic syndrome, insulin resistance, and AD. Individually and cooperatively, aging, menopause, adiposity, and inflammation lead to cognitive deficits and AD.

neuropathology result from the interactive effects of several risk factors (**Figure 1**). Most importantly, AD is dependent upon aging. The negative outcomes of all genetic and environmental risk factors of AD require advancing age. In women, chronological aging is also tied to reproductive aging that is manifested as menopause in mid-life. Menopause results in cessation of the ovarian cycle and its cyclical production of estrogens and progesterone, sex steroid hormones with numerous protective roles against AD (Pike et al., 2009). Beyond protective actions against specific aspects of AD neuropathology, estrogens function throughout the body to guard against the development of increasing central adiposity and inflammation, both of which are implicated in the initiation and progression of AD. Of course, aging is also associated with significant increases in inflammation and central obesity, independent of estrogen levels. Thus, women are simultaneously exposed to the consequences of both chronological and reproductive aging, both of which can function as drivers of AD, obesity, and inflammation.

Estrogen-based HT initiated prior to the end of menopause has been shown to be effective in combating both the increased adiposity and the cognitive decline associated with aging. Although HT can exhibit adverse side effects, especially in those women who may be predisposed, emerging results suggest that relatively short-term HT initiated near the onset of menopause is likely to yield largely beneficial effects for most women. Much more research will need to be done to determine precisely which genetic or environmental factors define the target population.

Inflammation is another seemingly invariant consequence of aging. In females, inflammation is further increased by the loss of estrogens at menopause. As with many other age-related diseases, AD is linked with elevated inflammation during aging by abundant data from several fields. Several specific inflammatory factors have been linked to both obesity and AD including leptin, TNF-α and IL-6. Since estrogens protect against both the development and deleterious consequences of inflammation across many tissues, depletion of estrogens at menopause is theorized to contribute to women's vulnerability to AD. Age-related increases in adiposity and changes in the distribution of fat to central depots further increase the risk of obesity, which promotes downstream conditions including insulin resistance, metabolic syndrome and T2D. Thus, a highly interactive set of relationships develops in women: the cumulative effects of aging, menopause, adiposity, and inflammation result in increased risk for neural dysfunction and AD pathogenesis (**Figure 1**). Certainly this set of factors is incomplete, as new data continue to identify additional factors, including bioenergetics, that not only are altered during reproductive aging but also can promote AD (Yin et al., 2015). Continued research is needed to address many unresolved issues about these pathological interactions, including how they are modified by genetic risk factors such as Apolipoprotein E (ApoE) and the extent to which they can be effectively attenuated by estrogen-based HT.

Acknowledgments

This work was supported by NIH grant AG026572 (RD Brinton and CJP/Project 3).

References

Aguilar-Valles, A., Inoue, W., Rummel, C., and Luheshi, G. N. (2015). Obesity, adipokines and neuroinflammation. *Neuropharmacology* 96, 124–134. doi: 10.1016/j.neuropharm.2014.12.023

Ahtiainen, M., Alen, M., Pöllänen, E., Pulkkinen, S., Ronkainen, P. H., Kujala, U. M., et al. (2012). Hormone therapy is associated with better body composition and adipokine/glucose profiles: a study with monozygotic co-twin control design. *Menopause* 19, 1329–1335. doi: 10.1097/gme.0b013e31825a3344

Akama, K. T., and Van Eldik, L. J. (2000). Beta-amyloid stimulation of inducible nitric-oxide synthase in astrocytes is interleukin-1beta- and tumor necrosis factor-alpha (TNFalpha)-dependent and involves a TNFalpha receptor-associated factor- and NFkappaB-inducing kinase-dependent signaling mechanism. *J. Biol. Chem.* 275, 7918–7924. doi: 10.1074/jbc.275.11.7918

Altmann, A., Tian, L., Henderson, V. W., Greicius, M. D., and Alzheimer's Disease Neuroimaging Initiative Investigators. (2014). Sex modifies the APOE-related risk of developing Alzheimer disease. *Ann. Neurol.* 75, 563–573. doi: 10.1002/ana.24135

Anthony, K., Reed, L. J., Dunn, J. T., Bingham, E., Hopkins, D., Marsden, P. K., et al. (2006). Attenuation of insulin-evoked responses in brain networks controlling appetite and reward in insulin resistance: the cerebral basis for impaired control of food intake in metabolic syndrome? *Diabetes* 55, 2986–2992. doi: 10.2337/db06-0376

Bagger, Y. Z., Tankó, L. B., Alexandersen, P., Qin, G., Christiansen, C., and PERF Study Group. (2005). Early postmenopausal hormone therapy may prevent cognitive impairment later in life. *Menopause* 12, 12–17. doi: 10.1097/00042192-200512010-00005

Barrett-Connor, E., Schrott, H. G., Greendale, G., Kritz-Silverstein, D., Espeland, M. A., Stern, M. P., et al. (1996). Factors associated with glucose and insulin levels in healthy postmenopausal women. *Diabetes Care* 19, 333–340. doi: 10.2337/diacare.19.4.333

Barron, A. M., Rosario, E. R., Elteriefi, R., and Pike, C. J. (2013). Sex-specific effects of high fat diet on indices of metabolic syndrome in 3xTg-AD mice: implications for Alzheimer's disease. *PLoS One* 8:e78554. doi: 10.1371/journal.pone.0078554

Bastard, J. P., Jardel, C., Bruckert, E., Blondy, P., Capeau, J., Laville, M., et al. (2000). Elevated levels of interleukin 6, are reduced in serum and subcutaneous adipose tissue of obese women after weight loss. *J. Clin. Endocrinol. Metab.* 85, 3338–3342. doi: 10.1210/jc.85.9.3338

Bauer, J., Strauss, S., Schreiter-Gasser, U., Ganter, U., Schlegel, P., Witt, I., et al. (1991). Interleukin-6 and alpha-2-macroglobulin indicate an acute-phase state in Alzheimer's disease cortices. *FEBS Lett.* 285, 111–114. doi: 10.1016/0014-5793(91)80737-n

Beattie, M. S., Hermann, G. E., Rogers, R. C., and Bresnahan, J. C. (2002). Cell death in models of spinal cord injury. *Prog. Brain Res.* 137, 37–47. doi: 10.1016/s0079-6123(02)37006-7

Beeri, M. S., Rapp, M., Schmeidler, J., Reichenberg, A., Purohit, D. P., Perl, D. P., et al. (2009). Number of children is associated with neuropathology of Alzheimer's disease in women. *Neurobiol. Aging* 30, 1184–1191. doi: 10.1016/j.neurobiolaging.2007.11.011

Benedusi, V., Meda, C., Della Torre, S., Monteleone, G., Vegeto, E., and Maggi, A. (2012). A lack of ovarian function increases neuroinflammation in aged mice. *Endocrinology* 153, 2777–2788. doi: 10.1210/en.2011-1925

Berchtold, N. C., Cribbs, D. H., Coleman, P. D., Rogers, J., Head, E., Kim, R., et al. (2008). Gene expression changes in the course of normal brain aging are sexually dimorphic. *Proc. Natl. Acad. Sci. U S A* 105, 15605–15610. doi: 10.1073/pnas.0806883105

Bernstein, L., Pike, M. C., Ross, R. K., Judd, H. L., Brown, J. B., and Henderson, B. E. (1985). Estrogen and sex hormone-binding globulin levels in nulliparous and parous women. *J. Natl. Cancer Inst.* 74, 741–745.

Bertram, L., Lange, C., Mullin, K., Parkinson, M., Hsiao, M., Hogan, M. F., et al. (2008). Genome-wide association analysis reveals putative Alzheimer's disease susceptibility loci in addition to APOE. *Am. J. Hum. Genet.* 83, 623–632. doi: 10.1016/j.ajhg.2008.10.008

Bettcher, B. M., and Kramer, J. H. (2014). Longitudinal inflammation, cognitive decline and Alzheimer's disease: a mini-review. *Clin. Pharmacol. Ther.* 96, 464–469. doi: 10.1038/clpt.2014.147

Beydoun, M. A., Lhotsky, A., Wang, Y., Dal Forno, G., An, Y., Metter, E. J., et al. (2008). Association of adiposity status and changes in early to mid-adulthood with incidence of Alzheimer's disease. *Am. J. Epidemiol.* 168, 1179–1189. doi: 10.1093/aje/kwn229

Biessels, G. J., De Leeuw, F. E., Lindeboom, J., Barkhof, F., and Scheltens, P. (2006). Increased cortical atrophy in patients with Alzheimer's disease and type 2, diabetes mellitus. *J. Neurol. Neurosurg. Psychiatry* 77, 304–307. doi: 10.1136/jnnp.2005.069583

Björkelund, C., Lissner, L., Andersson, S., Lapidus, L., and Bengtsson, C. (1996). Reproductive history in relation to relative weight and fat distribution. *Int. J. Obes. Relat. Metab. Disord.* 20, 213–219.

Blázquez, E., Velázquez, E., Hurtado-Carneiro, V., and Ruiz-Albusac, J. M. (2014). Insulin in the brain: its pathophysiological implications for states related with central insulin resistance, type 2, diabetes and Alzheimer's disease. *Front. Endocrinol. (Lausanne)* 5:161. doi: 10.3389/fendo.2014.00161

Bloom, G. S. (2014). Amyloid-β and tau: the trigger and bullet in Alzheimer disease pathogenesis. *JAMA Neurol.* 71, 505–508. doi: 10.1001/jamaneurol.2013.5847

Blum-Degen, D., Müller, T., Kuhn, W., Gerlach, M., Przuntek, H., and Riederer, P. (1995). Interleukin-1 beta and interleukin-6 are elevated in the cerebrospinal fluid of Alzheimer's and de novo Parkinson's disease patients. *Neurosci. Lett.* 202, 17–20. doi: 10.1016/0304-3940(95)12192-7

Bonda, D. J., Stone, J. G., Torres, S. L., Siedlak, S. L., Perry, G., Kryscio, R., et al. (2014). Dysregulation of leptin signaling in Alzheimer disease: evidence for neuronal leptin resistance. *J. Neurochem.* 128, 162–172. doi: 10.1111/jnc.12380

Bonomini, F., Rodella, L. F., and Rezzani, R. (2015). Metabolic syndrome, aging and involvement of oxidative stress. *Aging Dis.* 6, 109–120. doi: 10.14336/ad.2014.0305

Bove, R., Secor, E., Chibnik, L. B., Barnes, L. L., Schneider, J. A., Bennett, D. A., et al. (2014). Age at surgical menopause influences cognitive decline and Alzheimer pathology in older women. *Neurology* 82, 222–229. doi: 10.1212/WNL.0000000000000033

Bretsky, P. M., Buckwalter, J. G., Seeman, T. E., Miller, C. A., Poirier, J., Schellenberg, G. D., et al. (1999). Evidence for an interaction between apolipoprotein E genotype, gender and Alzheimer disease. *Alzheimer Dis. Assoc. Disord.* 13, 216–221. doi: 10.1097/00002093-199910000-00007

Brown, C. M., Choi, E., Xu, Q., Vitek, M. P., and Colton, C. A. (2008). The APOE4 genotype alters the response of microglia and macrophages to 17beta-estradiol. *Neurobiol. Aging* 29, 1783–1794. doi: 10.1016/j.neurobiolaging.2007.04.018

Bryzgalova, G., Gao, H., Ahren, B., Zierath, J. R., Galuska, D., Steiler, T. L., et al. (2006). Evidence that oestrogen receptor-alpha plays an important role in the regulation of glucose homeostasis in mice: insulin sensitivity in the liver. *Diabetologia* 49, 588–597. doi: 10.1007/s00125-005-0105-3

Camilleri, G., Borg, M., Brincat, S., Schembri-Wismayer, P., Brincat, M., and Calleja-Agius, J. (2012). The role of cytokines in cardiovascular disease in menopause. *Climacteric* 15, 524–530. doi: 10.3109/13697137.2012.700743

Cao, D., Lu, H., Lewis, T. L., and Li, L. (2007). Intake of sucrose-sweetened water induces insulin resistance and exacerbates memory deficits and amyloidosis in a transgenic mouse model of Alzheimer disease. *J. Biol. Chem.* 282, 36275–36282. doi: 10.1074/jbc.m703561200

Carlton, E. D., Demas, G. E., and French, S. S. (2012). Leptin, a neuroendocrine mediator of immune responses, inflammation and sickness behaviors. *Horm. Behav.* 62, 272–279. doi: 10.1016/j.yhbeh.2012.04.010

Carr, M. C. (2003). The emergence of the metabolic syndrome with menopause. *J. Clin. Endocrinol. Metab.* 88, 2404–2411. doi: 10.1210/jc.2003-030242

Carroll, J. C., Rosario, E. R., Chang, L., Stanczyk, F. Z., Oddo, S., LaFerla, F. M., et al. (2007). Progesterone and estrogen regulate Alzheimer-like neuropathology in female 3xTg-AD mice. *J. Neurosci.* 27, 13357–13365. doi: 10.1523/jneurosci.2718-07.2007

Chen, S. Y., Chen, T. F., Lai, L. C., Chen, J. H., Sun, Y., Wen, L. L., et al. (2012). Sequence variants of interleukin 6, (IL-6) are significantly associated with a decreased risk of late-onset Alzheimer's disease. *J. Neuroinflammation* 9:21. doi: 10.1186/1742-2094-9-21

Chen, Z., and Trapp, B. D. (2015). Microglia and neuroprotection. *J. Neurochem.* doi: 10.1111/jnc.13062 [Epub ahead of print].

Cheng, X., Yang, L., He, P., Li, R., and Shen, Y. (2010). Differential activation of tumor necrosis factor receptors distinguishes between brains from Alzheimer's disease and non-demented patients. *J. Alzheimers Dis.* 19, 621–630. doi: 10.3233/JAD-2010-1253

Cho, G. J., Lee, J. H., Park, H. T., Shin, J. H., Hong, S. C., Kim, T., et al. (2008). Postmenopausal status according to years since menopause as an independent risk factor for the metabolic syndrome. *Menopause* 15, 524–529. doi: 10.1097/gme.0b013e3181559860

Cigolle, C. T., Lee, P. G., Langa, K. M., Lee, Y. Y., Tian, Z., and Blaum, C. S. (2011). Geriatric conditions develop in middle-aged adults with diabetes. *J. Gen. Intern. Med.* 26, 272–279. doi: 10.1007/s11606-010-1510-y

Claxton, A., Baker, L. D., Hanson, A., Trittschuh, E. H., Cholerton, B., Morgan, A., et al. (2015). Long-acting intranasal insulin detemir improves cognition for adults with mild cognitive impairment or early-stage Alzheimer's disease dementia. *J. Alzheimers Dis.* 44, 897–906. doi: 10.3233/JAD-141791

Colton, C. A. (2009). Heterogeneity of microglial activation in the innate immune response in the brain. *J. Neuroimmune Pharmacol.* 4, 399–418. doi: 10.1007/s11481-009-9164-4

Colucci, M., Cammarata, S., Assini, A., Croce, R., Clerici, F., Novello, C., et al. (2006). The number of pregnancies is a risk factor for Alzheimer's disease. *Eur. J. Neurol.* 13, 1374–1377. doi: 10.1111/j.1468-1331.2006.01520.x

Conde, J., Scotece, M., Abella, V., López, V., Pino, J., Gómez-Reino, J. J., et al. (2014). An update on leptin as immunomodulator. *Expert Rev. Clin. Immunol.* 10, 1165–1170. doi: 10.1586/1744666x.2014.942289

Considine, R. V., Sinha, M. K., Heiman, M. L., Kriauciunas, A., Stephens, T. W., Nyce, M. R., et al. (1996). Serum immunoreactive-leptin concentrations in normal-weight and obese humans. *N. Engl. J. Med.* 334, 292–295. doi: 10.1056/NEJM199602013340503

Craft, S. (2007). Insulin resistance and Alzheimer's disease pathogenesis: potential mechanisms and implications for treatment. *Curr. Alzheimer Res.* 4, 147–152. doi: 10.2174/156720507780362137

Dallongeville, J., Bhatt, D. L., Steg, P. H., Ravaud, P., Wilson, P. W., Eagle, K. A., et al. (2012). Relation between body mass index, waist circumference and cardiovascular outcomes in 19,579 diabetic patients with established vascular disease: the REACH registry. *Eur. J. Prev. Cardiol.* 19, 241–249. doi: 10.1177/1741826710394305

de la Monte, S. M., and Tong, M. (2014). Brain metabolic dysfunction at the core of Alzheimer's disease. *Biochem. Pharmacol.* 88, 548–559. doi: 10.1016/j.bcp.2013.12.012

De Souza, C. T., Araujo, E. P., Bordin, S., Ashimine, R., Zollner, R. L., Boschero, A. C., et al. (2005). Consumption of a fat-rich diet activates a proinflammatory response and induces insulin resistance in the hypothalamus. *Endocrinology* 146, 4192–4199. doi: 10.1210/en.2004-1520

Erta, M., Quintana, A., and Hidalgo, J. (2012). Interleukin-6, a major cytokine in the central nervous system. *Int. J. Biol. Sci.* 8, 1254–1266. doi: 10.7150/ijbs.4679

Farr, S. A., Yamada, K. A., Butterfield, D. A., Abdul, H. M., Xu, L., Miller, N. E., et al. (2008). Obesity and hypertriglyceridemia produce cognitive impairment. *Endocrinology* 149, 2628–2636. doi: 10.1210/en.2007-1722

Farrer, L. A., Cupples, L. A., Haines, J. L., Hyman, B., Kukull, W. A., Mayeux, R., et al. (1997). Effects of age, sex and ethnicity on the association between apolipoprotein E genotype and Alzheimer diseaseA meta-analysis. APOE and Alzheimer disease meta analysis consortium. *J.AMA* 278, 1349–1356. doi: 10.1001/jama.1997.03550160069041

Ferguson, A. R., Christensen, R. N., Gensel, J. C., Miller, B. A., Sun, F., Beattie, E. C., et al. (2008). Cell death after spinal cord injury is exacerbated by rapid TNF alpha-induced trafficking of GluR2-lacking AMPARs to the plasma membrane. *J. Neurosci.* 28, 11391–11400. doi: 10.1523/JNEUROSCI.3708-08.2008

Fewlass, D. C., Noboa, K., Pi-Sunyer, F. X., Johnston, J. M., Yan, S. D., and Tezapsidis, N. (2004). Obesity-related leptin regulates Alzheimer's Abeta. *FASEB J.* 18, 1870–1878. doi: 10.1096/fj.04-2572com

Fitzpatrick, A. L., Kuller, L. H., Lopez, O. L., Diehr, P., O'Meara, E. S., Longstreth, W. T., et al. (2009). Midlife and late-life obesity and the risk of dementia: cardiovascular health study. *Arch. Neurol.* 66, 336–342. doi: 10.1001/archneurol.2008.582

Flex, A., Giovannini, S., Biscetti, F., Liperoti, R., Spalletta, G., Straface, G., et al. (2014). Effect of proinflammatory gene polymorphisms on the risk of Alzheimer's disease. *Neurodegener. Dis.* 13, 230–236. doi: 10.1159/000353395

Flynn, G., Maru, S., Loughlin, J., Romero, I. A., and Male, D. (2003). Regulation of chemokine receptor expression in human microglia and astrocytes. *J. Neuroimmunol.* 136, 84–93. doi: 10.1016/s0165-5728(03)00009-2

Fontana, L., Eagon, J. C., Trujillo, M. E., Scherer, P. E., and Klein, S. (2007). Visceral fat adipokine secretion is associated with systemic inflammation in obese humans. *Diabetes* 56, 1010–1013. doi: 10.2337/db06-1656

Gilliver, S. C. (2010). Sex steroids as inflammatory regulators. *J. Steroid Biochem. Mol. Biol.* 120, 105–115. doi: 10.1016/j.jsbmb.2009.12.015

Golden, S. H., Kim, C., Barrett-Connor, E., Nan, B., Kong, S., Goldberg, R., et al. (2013). The association of elective hormone therapy with changes in lipids among glucose intolerant postmenopausal women in the diabetes prevention program. *Metabolism* 62, 1313–1322. doi: 10.1016/j.metabol.2013.04.005

Granholm, A. C., Bimonte-Nelson, H. A., Moore, A. B., Nelson, M. E., Freeman, L. R., and Sambamurti, K. (2008). Effects of a saturated fat and high cholesterol diet on memory and hippocampal morphology in the middle-aged rat. *J. Alzheimers Dis.* 14, 133–145.

Greco, S. J., Sarkar, S., Johnston, J. M., Zhu, X., Su, B., Casadesus, G., et al. (2008). Leptin reduces Alzheimer's disease-related tau phosphorylation in neuronal cells. *Biochem. Biophys. Res. Commun.* 376, 536–541. doi: 10.1016/j.bbrc.2008.09.026

Gustafson, D. R., Bäckman, K., Waern, M., Ostling, S., Guo, X., Zandi, P., et al. (2009). Adiposity indicators and dementia over 32, years in Sweden. *Neurology* 73, 1559–1566. doi: 10.1212/WNL.0b013e3181c0d4b6

Guthrie, J. R., Dennerstein, L., and Dudley, E. C. (1999). Weight gain and the menopause: a 5-year prospective study. *Climacteric* 2, 205–211. doi: 10.3109/13697139909038063

Haarbo, J., Marslew, U., Gotfredsen, A., and Christiansen, C. (1991). Postmenopausal hormone replacement therapy prevents central distribution of body fat after menopause. *Metabolism* 40, 1323–1326. doi: 10.1016/0026-0495(91)90037-w

Hankinson, S. E., Colditz, G. A., Hunter, D. J., Manson, J. E., Willett, W. C., Stampfer, M. J., et al. (1995). Reproductive factors and family history of breast cancer in relation to plasma estrogen and prolactin levels in postmenopausal women in the Nurses' Health Study (United States). *Cancer Causes Control* 6, 217–224. doi: 10.1007/bf00051793

Hardy, J. (2006). Alzheimer's disease: the amyloid cascade hypothesis: an update and reappraisal. *J. Alzheimers Dis.* 9, 151–153.

Hardy, J. A., and Higgins, G. A. (1992). Alzheimer's disease: the amyloid cascade hypothesis. *Science* 256, 184–185. doi: 10.1126/science.1566067

Harold, D., Abraham, R., Hollingworth, P., Sims, R., Gerrish, A., Hamshere, M. L., et al. (2009). Genome-wide association study identifies variants at CLU and PICALM associated with Alzheimer's disease. *Nat. Genet.* 41, 1088–1093. doi: 10.1038/ng.440

Hassing, L. B., Hofer, S. M., Nilsson, S. E., Berg, S., Pedersen, N. L., McClearn, G., et al. (2004). Comorbid type 2, diabetes mellitus and hypertension exacerbates cognitive decline: evidence from a longitudinal study. *Age Ageing* 33, 355–361. doi: 10.1093/ageing/afh100

He, P., Zhong, Z., Lindholm, K., Berning, L., Lee, W., Lemere, C., et al. (2007). Deletion of tumor necrosis factor death receptor inhibits amyloid beta generation and prevents learning and memory deficits in Alzheimer's mice. *J. Cell Biol.* 178, 829–841. doi: 10.1083/jcb.200705042

Heine, P. A., Taylor, J. A., Iwamoto, G. A., Lubahn, D. B., and Cooke, P. S. (2000). Increased adipose tissue in male and female estrogen receptor-alpha knockout mice. *Proc. Natl. Acad. Sci. U S A* 97, 12729–12734. doi: 10.1073/pnas.97.23.12729

Henderson, V. W., Benke, K. S., Green, R. C., Cupples, L. A., Farrer, L. A., and Group, M. S. (2005). Postmenopausal hormone therapy and Alzheimer's disease risk: interaction with age. *J. Neurol. Neurosurg. Psychiatry* 76, 103–105. doi: 10.1136/jnnp.2003.024927

Henderson, V. W., Paganini-Hill, A., Emanuel, C. K., Dunn, M. E., and Buckwalter, J. G. (1994). Estrogen replacement therapy in older women. Comparisons between Alzheimer's disease cases and nondemented control subjects. *Arch. Neurol.* 51, 896–900. doi: 10.1001/archneur.1994.00540210068014

Henderson, V. W., Watt, L., and Buckwalter, J. G. (1996). Cognitive skills associated with estrogen replacement in women with Alzheimer's disease. *Psychoneuroendocrinology* 21, 421–430. doi: 10.1016/0306-4530(95)00060-7

Herculano, B., Tamura, M., Ohba, A., Shimatani, M., Kutsuna, N., and Hisatsune, T. (2013). beta-alanyl-L-histidine rescues cognitive deficits caused by feeding a high fat diet in a transgenic mouse model of Alzheimer's disease. *J. Alzheimers Dis.* 33, 983–997. doi: 10.3233/JAD-2012-121324

Ho, S. C., Wu, S., Chan, S. G., and Sham, A. (2010). Menopausal transition and changes of body composition: a prospective study in Chinese perimenopausal women. *Int. J. Obes. (Lond)* 34, 1265–1274. doi: 10.1038/ijo.2010.33

Hollingworth, P., Harold, D., Sims, R., Gerrish, A., Lambert, J. C., Carrasquillo, M. M., et al. (2011). Common variants at ABCA7, MS4A6A/MS4A4E, EPHA1, CD33 and CD2AP are associated with Alzheimer's disease. *Nat. Genet.* 43, 429–435. doi: 10.1038/ng.803

Hotamisligil, G. S. (2006). Inflammation and metabolic disorders. *Nature* 444, 860–867. doi: 10.1038/nature05485

Hotamisligil, G. S., Arner, P., Caro, J. F., Atkinson, R. L., and Spiegelman, B. M. (1995). Increased adipose tissue expression of tumor necrosis factor-alpha in human obesity and insulin resistance. *J. Clin. Invest.* 95, 2409–2415. doi: 10.1172/jci117936

Hotamisligil, G. S., Shargill, N. S., and Spiegelman, B. M. (1993). Adipose expression of tumor necrosis factor-alpha: direct role in obesity-linked insulin resistance. *Science* 259, 87–91. doi: 10.1126/science.7678183

Hsu, T. M., Konanur, V. R., Taing, L., Usui, R., Kayser, B. D., Goran, M. I., et al. (2015). Effects of sucrose and high fructose corn syrup consumption on spatial memory function and hippocampal neuroinflammation in adolescent rats. *Hippocampus* 25, 227–239. doi: 10.1002/hipo.22368

Hwang, L. L., Wang, C. H., Li, T. L., Chang, S. D., Lin, L. C., Chen, C. P., et al. (2010). Sex differences in high-fat diet-induced obesity, metabolic alterations and learning and synaptic plasticity deficits in mice. *Obesity (Silver Spring)* 18, 463–469. doi: 10.1038/oby.2009.273

Imtiaz, B., Tuppurainen, M., Tiihonen, M., Kivipelto, M., Soininen, H., Hartikainen, S., et al. (2014). Oophorectomy, hysterectomy and risk of Alzheimer's disease: a nationwide case-control study. *J. Alzheimers Dis.* 42, 575–581. doi: 10.3233/JAD-140336

Iqbal, K., Liu, F., Gong, C. X., and Grundke-Iqbal, I. (2010). Tau in Alzheimer disease and related tauopathies. *Curr. Alzheimer Res.* 7, 656–664. doi: 10.2174/156720510793611592

Islander, U., Jochems, C., Lagerquist, M. K., Forsblad-d'Elia, H., and Carlsten, H. (2011). Estrogens in rheumatoid arthritis; the immune system and bone. *Mol. Cell. Endocrinol.* 335, 14–29. doi: 10.1016/j.mce.2010.05.018

Janssen, I., Powell, L. H., Crawford, S., Lasley, B., and Sutton-Tyrrell, K. (2008). Menopause and the metabolic syndrome: the study of women's health across the nation. *Arch. Intern. Med.* 168, 1568–1575. doi: 10.1001/archinte.168.14.1568

Jayaraman, A., Lent-Schochet, D., and Pike, C. J. (2014). Diet-induced obesity and low testosterone increase neuroinflammation and impair neural function. *J. Neuroinflammation* 11:162. doi: 10.1186/s12974-014-0162-y

Jayaraman, A., and Pike, C. J. (2014). Alzheimer's disease and type 2, diabetes: multiple mechanisms contribute to interactions. *Curr. Diab. Rep.* 14:476. doi: 10.1007/s11892-014-0476-2

Jimenez, S., Baglietto-Vargas, D., Caballero, C., Moreno-Gonzalez, I., Torres, M., Sanchez-Varo, R., et al. (2008). Inflammatory response in the hippocampus of PS1M146L/APP751SL mouse model of Alzheimer's disease: age-dependent switch in the microglial phenotype from alternative to classic. *J. Neurosci.* 28, 11650–11661. doi: 10.1523/JNEUROSCI.3024-08.2008

Johnston, H., Boutin, H., and Allan, S. M. (2011). Assessing the contribution of inflammation in models of Alzheimer's disease. *Biochem. Soc. Trans.* 39, 886–890. doi: 10.1042/BST0390886

Johnston, J. M., Hu, W. T., Fardo, D. W., Greco, S. J., Perry, G., Montine, T. J., et al. (2014). Low plasma leptin in cognitively impaired ADNI subjects: gender differences and diagnostic and therapeutic potential. *Curr. Alzheimer Res.* 11, 165–174. doi: 10.2174/1567205010666131212114156

Jones, M. E., Thorburn, A. W., Britt, K. L., Hewitt, K. N., Wreford, N. G., Proietto, J., et al. (2000). Aromatase-deficient (ArKO) mice have a phenotype of increased adiposity. *Proc. Natl. Acad. Sci. U S A* 97, 12735–12740. doi: 10.1073/pnas.97.23.12735

Julien, C., Tremblay, C., Phivilay, A., Berthiaume, L., Emond, V., Julien, P., et al. (2010). High-fat diet aggravates amyloid-beta and tau pathologies in the 3xTg-AD mouse model. *Neurobiol. Aging* 31, 1516–1531. doi: 10.1016/j.neurobiolaging.2008.08.022

Karran, E., Mercken, M., and De Strooper, B. (2011). The amyloid cascade hypothesis for Alzheimer's disease: an appraisal for the development of therapeutics. *Nat. Rev. Drug Discov.* 10, 698–712. doi: 10.1038/nrd3505

Kawas, C., Resnick, S., Morrison, A., Brookmeyer, R., Corrada, M., Zonderman, A., et al. (1997). A prospective study of estrogen replacement therapy and the risk of developing Alzheimer's disease: the Baltimore longitudinal study of aging. *Neurology* 48, 1517–1521. doi: 10.1212/wnl.48.6.1517

Kern, P. A., Ranganathan, S., Li, C., Wood, L., and Ranganathan, G. (2001). Adipose tissue tumor necrosis factor and interleukin-6 expression in human obesity and insulin resistance. *Am. J. Physiol. Endocrinol. Metab.* 280, E745–E751.

Kim, B., and Feldman, E. L. (2015). Insulin resistance as a key link for the increased risk of cognitive impairment in the metabolic syndrome. *Exp. Mol. Med.* 47:e149. doi: 10.1038/emm.2015.3

Kissebah, A. H., Vydelingum, N., Murray, R., Evans, D. J., Hartz, A. J., Kalkhoff, R. K., et al. (1982). Relation of body fat distribution to metabolic complications of obesity. *J. Clin Endocrinol Metab* 54, 254–260. doi: 10.1210/jcem-54-2-254

Kivipelto, M., Ngandu, T., Fratiglioni, L., Viitanen, M., Kåreholt, I., Winblad, B., et al. (2005). Obesity and vascular risk factors at midlife and the risk of dementia and Alzheimer disease. *Arch. Neurol.* 62, 1556–1560. doi: 10.1001/archneur.62.10.1556

Knowlton, A. A., and Lee, A. R. (2012). Estrogen and the cardiovascular system. *Pharmacol. Ther.* 135, 54–70. doi: 10.1016/j.pharmthera.2012.03.007

Koenigsknecht-Talboo, J., and Landreth, G. E. (2005). Microglial phagocytosis induced by fibrillar beta-amyloid and IgGs are differentially regulated by proinflammatory cytokines. *J. Neurosci.* 25, 8240–8249. doi: 10.1523/jneurosci.1808-05.2005

Kristensen, K., Pedersen, S. B., Vestergaard, P., Mosekilde, L., and Richelsen, B. (1999). Hormone replacement therapy affects body composition and leptin differently in obese and non-obese postmenopausal women. *J. Endocrinol.* 163, 55–62. doi: 10.1677/joe.0.1630055

LaFerla, F. M. (2010). Pathways linking Abeta and tau pathologies. *Biochem. Soc. Trans.* 38, 993–995. doi: 10.1042/BST0380993

Lambert, J. C., Heath, S., Even, G., Campion, D., Sleegers, K., Hiltunen, M., et al. (2009). Genome-wide association study identifies variants at CLU and CR1 associated with Alzheimer's disease. *Nat. Genet.* 41, 1094–1099. doi: 10.1038/ng.439

Leavy, O. (2015). Neuroimmunology: TREM2 in Alzheimer disease. *Nat. Rev. Immunol.* 15:201. doi: 10.1038/nri3842

Leduc, V., Domenger, D., De Beaumont, L., Lalonde, D., Belanger-Jasmin, S., and Poirier, J. (2011). Function and comorbidities of apolipoprotein e in Alzheimer's disease. *Int. J. Alzheimers Dis.* 2011:974361. doi: 10.4061/2011/974361

Lewis, D. K., Bake, S., Thomas, K., Jezierski, M. K., and Sohrabji, F. (2010). A high cholesterol diet elevates hippocampal cytokine expression in an age and estrogen-dependent manner in female rats. *J. Neuroimmunol.* 223, 31–38. doi: 10.1016/j.jneuroim.2010.03.024

Li, R., Strohmeyer, R., Liang, Z., Lue, L. F., and Rogers, J. (2004). CCAAT/enhancer binding protein delta (C/EBPdelta) expression and elevation in Alzheimer's disease. *Neurobiol. Aging* 25, 991–999. doi: 10.1016/j.neurobiolaging.2003.10.016

Lieb, W., Beiser, A. S., Vasan, R. S., Tan, Z. S., Au, R., Harris, T. B., et al. (2009). Association of plasma leptin levels with incident Alzheimer disease and MRI measures of brain aging. *JAMA* 302, 2565–2572. doi: 10.1001/jama.2009.1836

López, S., Bermúdez, B., Pacheco, Y. M., Villar, J., Abia, R., and Muriana, F. J. (2008). Distinctive postprandial modulation of beta cell function and insulin sensitivity by dietary fats: monounsaturated compared with saturated fatty acids. *Am. J. Clin. Nutr.* 88, 638–644.

Lord, G. M., Matarese, G., Howard, J. K., Baker, R. J., Bloom, S. R., and Lechler, R. I. (1998). Leptin modulates the T-cell immune response and reverses starvation-induced immunosuppression. *Nature* 394, 897–901. doi: 10.1038/29795

Luchsinger, J. A., Cheng, D., Tang, M. X., Schupf, N., and Mayeux, R. (2012). Central obesity in the elderly is related to late-onset Alzheimer disease. *Alzheimer Dis. Assoc. Disord.* 26, 101–105. doi: 10.1097/WAD.0b013e318222f0d4

Luchsinger, J. A., Tang, M. X., Shea, S., and Mayeux, R. (2004). Hyperinsulinemia and risk of Alzheimer disease. *Neurology* 63, 1187–1192. doi: 10.1212/01.wnl.0000140292.04932.87

Maioli, S., Lodeiro, M., Merino-Serrais, P., Falahati, F., Khan, W., Puerta, E., et al. (2015). Alterations in brain leptin signalling in spite of unchanged CSF leptin levels in Alzheimer's disease. *Aging Cell* 14, 122–129. doi: 10.1111/acel.12281

Maki, P. M. (2006). Potential importance of early initiation of hormone therapy for cognitive benefit. *Menopause* 13, 6–7. doi: 10.1097/01.gme.0000194822.76774.30

Mandrekar-Colucci, S., and Landreth, G. E. (2010). Microglia and inflammation in Alzheimer's disease. *CNS Neurol. Disord. Drug Targets* 9, 156–167. doi: 10.2174/187152710791012071

Manly, J. J., Merchant, C. A., Jacobs, D. M., Small, S. A., Bell, K., Ferin, M., et al. (2000). Endogenous estrogen levels and Alzheimer's disease among postmenopausal women. *Neurology* 54, 833–837. doi: 10.1212/wnl.54.4.833

Martín-Millán, M., and Castañeda, S. (2013). Estrogens, osteoarthritis and inflammation. *Joint Bone Spine* 80, 368–373. doi: 10.1016/j.jbspin.2012.11.008

Martín-Romero, C., Santos-Alvarez, J., Goberna, R., and Sánchez-Margalet, V. (2000). Human leptin enhances activation and proliferation of human circulating T lymphocytes. *Cell Immunol.* 199, 15–24. doi: 10.1006/cimm.1999.1594

McGill, A. T. (2014). Past and future corollaries of theories on causes of metabolic syndrome and obesity related co-morbidities part 2: a composite unifying theory review of human-specific co-adaptations to brain energy consumption. *Arch. Public Health* 72:31. doi: 10.1186/2049-3258-72-31

McLay, R. N., Maki, P. M., and Lyketsos, C. G. (2003). Nulliparity and late menopause are associated with decreased cognitive decline. *J. Neuropsychiatry Clin. Neurosci.* 15, 161–167. doi: 10.1176/appi.neuropsych.15.2.161

Meda, L., Cassatella, M. A., Szendrei, G. I., Otvos, L. Jr., Baron, P., Villalba, M., et al. (1995). Activation of microglial cells by beta-amyloid protein and interferon-gamma. *Nature* 374, 647–650. doi: 10.1038/374647a0

Meyer, M. R., Clegg, D. J., Prossnitz, E. R., and Barton, M. (2011). Obesity, insulin resistance and diabetes: sex differences and role of oestrogen receptors. *Acta Physiol. (Oxf.)* 203, 259–269. doi: 10.1111/j.1748-1716.2010.02237.x

Meyer-Luehmann, M., Spires-Jones, T. L., Prada, C., Garcia-Alloza, M., de Calignon, A., Rozkalne, A., et al. (2008). Rapid appearance and local toxicity of amyloid-beta plaques in a mouse model of Alzheimer's disease. *Nature* 451, 720–724. doi: 10.1038/nature06616

Michaud, M., Balardy, L., Moulis, G., Gaudin, C., Peyrot, C., Vellas, B., et al. (2013). Proinflammatory cytokines, aging and age-related diseases. *J. Am. Med. Dir. Assoc.* 14, 877–882. doi: 10.1016/j.jamda.2013.05.009

Milanski, M., Degasperi, G., Coope, A., Morari, J., Denis, R., Cintra, D. E., et al. (2009). Saturated fatty acids produce an inflammatory response predominantly through the activation of TLR4 signaling in hypothalamus: implications for the pathogenesis of obesity. *J. Neurosci.* 29, 359–370. doi: 10.1523/JNEUROSCI.2760-08.2009

Molteni, R., Barnard, R. J., Ying, Z., Roberts, C. K., and Gómez-Pinilla, F. (2002). A high-fat, refined sugar diet reduces hippocampal brain-derived neurotrophic factor, neuronal plasticity and learning. *Neuroscience* 112, 803–814. doi: 10.1016/s0306-4522(02)00123-9

Morris, G. P., Clark, I. A., and Vissel, B. (2014). Inconsistencies and controversies surrounding the amyloid hypothesis of Alzheimer's disease. *Acta Neuropathol. Commun.* 2:135. doi: 10.1186/s40478-014-0135-5

Mosconi, L. (2005). Brain glucose metabolism in the early and specific diagnosis of Alzheimer's disease. FDG-PET studies in MCI and AD. *Eur. J. Nucl. Med. Mol. Imaging* 32, 486–510. doi: 10.1007/s00259-005-1762-7

Mosconi, L., Pupi, A., and De Leon, M. J. (2008). Brain glucose hypometabolism and oxidative stress in preclinical Alzheimer's disease. *Ann. N Y Acad. Sci.* 1147, 180–195. doi: 10.1196/annals.1427.007

Mrak, R. E., and Griffin, W. S. (2005). Glia and their cytokines in progression of neurodegeneration. *Neurobiol. Aging* 26, 349–354. doi: 10.1016/j.neurobiolaging.2004.05.010

Mucke, L., and Selkoe, D. J. (2012). Neurotoxicity of amyloid beta-protein: synaptic and network dysfunction. *Cold Spring Harb. Perspect. Med.* 2:a006338. doi: 10.1101/cshperspect.a006338

Murray, A. J., Knight, N. S., Cochlin, L. E., McAleese, S., Deacon, R. M., Rawlins, J. N., et al. (2009). Deterioration of physical performance and cognitive function in rats with short-term high-fat feeding. *FASEB J.* 23, 4353–4360. doi: 10.1096/fj.09-139691

Naj, A. C., Jun, G., Beecham, G. W., Wang, L. S., Vardarajan, B. N., Buros, J., et al. (2011). Common variants at MS4A4/MS4A6E, CD2AP, CD33 and EPHA1 are associated with late-onset Alzheimer's disease. *Nat. Genet.* 43, 436–441. doi: 10.1038/ng.801

Näslund, J., Thyberg, J., Tjernberg, L. O., Wernstedt, C., Karlstrom, A. R., Bogdanovic, N., et al. (1995). Characterization of stable complexes involving apolipoprotein E and the amyloid beta peptide in Alzheimer's disease brain. *Neuron* 15, 219–228. doi: 10.1016/0896-6273(95)90079-9

Nieves, D. J., Cnop, M., Retzlaff, B., Walden, C. E., Brunzell, J. D., Knopp, R. H., et al. (2003). The atherogenic lipoprotein profile associated with obesity and insulin resistance is largely attributable to intra-abdominal fat. *Diabetes* 52, 172–179. doi: 10.2337/diabetes.52.1.172

Nordell, V. L., Scarborough, M. M., Buchanan, A. K., and Sohrabji, F. (2003). Differential effects of estrogen in the injured forebrain of young adult and reproductive senescent animals. *Neurobiol. Aging* 24, 733–743. doi: 10.1016/s0197-4580(02)00193-8

Ogden, C. L., Carroll, M. D., Kit, B. K., and Flegal, K. M. (2014). Prevalence of childhood and adult obesity in the United States, 2011–2012. *JAMA* 311, 806–814. doi: 10.1001/jama.2014.732

Orr, M. E., Salinas, A., Buffenstein, R., and Oddo, S. (2014). Mammalian target of rapamycin hyperactivity mediates the detrimental effects of a high sucrose diet on Alzheimer's disease pathology. *Neurobiol. Aging* 35, 1233–1242. doi: 10.1016/j.neurobiolaging.2013.12.006

Papassotiropoulos, A., Bagli, M., Jessen, F., Bayer, T. A., Maier, W., Rao, M. L., et al. (1999). A genetic variation of the inflammatory cytokine interleukin-6 delays the initial onset and reduces the risk for sporadic Alzheimer's disease. *Ann. Neurol.* 45, 666–668. doi: 10.1002/1531-8249(199905)45:5<666::aid-ana18>3.0.co;2-3

Park, H. K., and Ahima, R. S. (2015). Physiology of leptin: energy homeostasis, neuroendocrine function and metabolism. *Metabolism* 64, 24–34. doi: 10.1016/j.metabol.2014.08.004

Parkhurst, C. N., Yang, G., Ninan, I., Savas, J. N., Yates, J. R. IIII, Lafaille, J. J., et al. (2013). Microglia promote learning-dependent synapse formation through brain-derived neurotrophic factor. *Cell* 155, 1596–1609. doi: 10.1016/j.cell.2013.11.030

Patsouris, D., Li, P. P., Thapar, D., Chapman, J., Olefsky, J. M., and Neels, J. G. (2008). Ablation of CD11c-positive cells normalizes insulin sensitivity in obese insulin resistant animals. *Cell Metab.* 8, 301–309. doi: 10.1016/j.cmet.2008.08.015

Payami, H., Zareparsi, S., Montee, K. R., Sexton, G. J., Kaye, J. A., Bird, T. D., et al. (1996). Gender difference in apolipoprotein E-associated risk for familial Alzheimer disease: a possible clue to the higher incidence of Alzheimer disease in women. *Am. J. Hum. Genet.* 58, 803–811.

Pfeilschifter, J., Köditz, R., Pfohl, M., and Schatz, H. (2002). Changes in proinflammatory cytokine activity after menopause. *Endocr. Rev.* 23, 90–119. doi: 10.1210/er.23.1.90

Phung, T. K., Waltoft, B. L., Laursen, T. M., Settnes, A., Kessing, L. V., Mortensen, P. B., et al. (2010). Hysterectomy, oophorectomy and risk of dementia: a nationwide historical cohort study. *Dement. Geriatr. Cogn. Disord.* 30, 43–50. doi: 10.1159/000314681

Pike, C. J., Carroll, J. C., Rosario, E. R., and Barron, A. M. (2009). Protective actions of sex steroid hormones in Alzheimer's disease. *Front. Neuroendocrinol.* 30, 239–258. doi: 10.1016/j.yfrne.2009.04.015

Plutzky, J. (2001). Inflammatory pathways in atherosclerosis and acute coronary syndromes. *Am. J. Cardiol.* 88, 10K–15K. doi: 10.1016/s0002-9149(01)01924-5

Poehlman, E. T., Toth, M. J., and Gardner, A. W. (1995). Changes in energy balance and body composition at menopause: a controlled longitudinal study. *Ann. Intern. Med.* 123, 673–675. doi: 10.7326/0003-4819-123-9-199511010-00005

Pradhan, A. D., Manson, J. E., Rifai, N., Buring, J. E., and Ridker, P. M. (2001). C-reactive protein, interleukin 6 and risk of developing type 2, diabetes mellitus. *JAMA* 286, 327–334. doi: 10.1001/jama.286.3.327

Profenno, L. A., Porsteinsson, A. P., and Faraone, S. V. (2010). Meta-analysis of Alzheimer's disease risk with obesity, diabetes and related disorders. *Biol. Psychiatry* 67, 505–512. doi: 10.1016/j.biopsych.2009.02.013

Prokop, S., Miller, K. R., and Heppner, F. L. (2013). Microglia actions in Alzheimer's disease. *Acta Neuropathol.* 126, 461–477. doi: 10.1007/s00401-013-1182-x

Ptok, U., Barkow, K., and Heun, R. (2002). Fertility and number of children in patients with Alzheimer's disease. *Arch. Womens Ment. Health.* 5, 83–86. doi: 10.1007/s00737-002-0142-6

Qizilbash, N., Gregson, J., Johnson, M. E., Pearce, N., Douglas, I., Wing, K., et al. (2015). BMI and risk of dementia in two million people over two decades: a retrospective cohort study. *Lancet Diabetes Endocrinol.* 3, 431–436. doi: 10.1016/s2213-8587(15)00033-9

Quintanilla, R. A., Orellana, D. I., González-Billault, C., and Maccioni, R. B. (2004). Interleukin-6 induces Alzheimer-type phosphorylation of tau protein by deregulating the cdk5/p35 pathway. *Exp. Cell Res.* 295, 245–257. doi: 10.1016/j.yexcr.2004.01.002

Rachoń, D., and Teede, H. (2010). Ovarian function and obesity—interrelationship, impact on women's reproductive lifespan and treatment options. *Mol. Cell. Endocrinol.* 316, 172–179. doi: 10.1016/j.mce.2009.09.026

Rahmouni, K. (2014). Obesity-associated hypertension: recent progress in deciphering the pathogenesis. *Hypertension* 64, 215–221. doi: 10.1161/hypertensionaha.114.00920

Raso, G. M., Pacilio, M., Esposito, E., Coppola, A., Di Carlo, R., and Meli, R. (2002). Leptin potentiates IFN-gamma-induced expression of nitric oxide synthase and cyclo-oxygenase-2 in murine macrophage J774A.1. *Br. J. Pharmacol.* 137, 799–804. doi: 10.1038/sj.bjp.0704903

Reger, M. A., Watson, G. S., Green, P. S., Wilkinson, C. W., Baker, L. D., Cholerton, B., et al. (2008). Intranasal insulin improves cognition and modulates beta-amyloid in early AD. *Neurology* 70, 440–448. doi: 10.1212/01.WNL.0000265401.62434.36

Rocca, W. A., Bower, J. H., Maraganore, D. M., Ahlskog, J. E., Grossardt, B. R., de Andrade, M., et al. (2007). Increased risk of cognitive impairment or dementia in women who underwent oophorectomy before menopause. *Neurology* 69, 1074–1083. doi: 10.1212/01.wnl.0000276984.19542.e6

Rocca, W. A., Grossardt, B. R., and Shuster, L. T. (2011). Oophorectomy, menopause, estrogen treatment and cognitive aging: clinical evidence for a window of opportunity. *Brain Res.* 1379, 188–198. doi: 10.1016/j.brainres.2010.10.031

Rocha, V. Z., and Libby, P. (2009). Obesity, inflammation and atherosclerosis. *Nat. Rev. Cardiol.* 6, 399–409. doi: 10.1038/nrcardio.2009.55

Rogers, N. H., Perfield, J. W. 2nd, Strissel, K. J., Obin, M. S., and Greenberg, A. S. (2009). Reduced energy expenditure and increased inflammation are early events in the development of ovariectomy-induced obesity. *Endocrinology* 150, 2161–2168. doi: 10.1210/en.2008-1405

Rosario, E. R., Chang, L., Head, E. H., Stanczyk, F. Z., and Pike, C. J. (2011). Brain levels of sex steroid hormones in men and women during normal aging and in Alzheimer's disease. *Neurobiol. Aging* 32, 604–613. doi: 10.1016/j.neurobiolaging.2009.04.008

Ryan, E. A., and Enns, L. (1988). Role of gestational hormones in the induction of insulin resistance. *J. Clin. Endocrinol. Metab.* 67, 341–347. doi: 10.1210/jcem-67-2-341

Salpeter, S. R., Walsh, J. M., Ormiston, T. M., Greyber, E., Buckley, N. S., and Salpeter, E. E. (2006). Meta-analysis: effect of hormone-replacement therapy on components of the metabolic syndrome in postmenopausal women. *Diabetes Obes. Metab.* 8, 538–554. doi: 10.1111/j.1463-1326.2005.00545.x

Santos-Alvarez, J., Goberna, R., and Sánchez-Margalet, V. (1999). Human leptin stimulates proliferation and activation of human circulating monocytes. *Cell. Immunol.* 194, 6–11. doi: 10.1006/cimm.1999.1490

Sárvári, M., Hrabovszky, E., Kalló, I., Solymosi, N., Likó, I., Berchtold, N., et al. (2012). Menopause leads to elevated expression of macrophage-associated genes in the aging frontal cortex: rat and human studies identify strikingly similar changes. *J. Neuroinflammation* 9:264. doi: 10.1186/1742-2094-9-264

Sárvári, M., Hrabovszky, E., Kalló, I., Solymosi, N., Tóth, K., Likó, I., et al. (2011). Estrogens regulate neuroinflammatory genes via estrogen receptors alpha and beta in the frontal cortex of middle-aged female rats. *J. Neuroinflammation* 8:82. doi: 10.1186/1742-2094-8-82

Senn, J. J., Klover, P. J., Nowak, I. A., and Mooney, R. A. (2002). Interleukin-6 induces cellular insulin resistance in hepatocytes. *Diabetes* 51, 3391–3399. doi: 10.2337/diabetes.51.12.3391

Shao, H., Breitner, J. C., Whitmer, R. A., Wang, J., Hayden, K., Wengreen, H., et al. (2012). Hormone therapy and Alzheimer disease dementia: new findings from the Cache County Study. *Neurology* 79, 1846–1852. doi: 10.1212/WNL.0b013e318271f823

Shumaker, S. A., Legault, C., Kuller, L., Rapp, S. R., Thal, L., Lane, D. S., et al. (2004). Conjugated equine estrogens and incidence of probable dementia and mild cognitive impairment in postmenopausal women: women's health initiative memory study. *JAMA* 291, 2947–2958. doi: 10.1001/jama.291.24.2947

Shumaker, S. A., Legault, C., Rapp, S. R., Thal, L., Wallace, R. B., Ockene, J. K., et al. (2003). Estrogen plus progestin and the incidence of dementia and mild cognitive impairment in postmenopausal women: the women's health initiative memory study: a randomized controlled trial. *JAMA* 289, 2651–2662. doi: 10.1001/jama.289.20.2651

Singh-Manoux, A., Dugravot, A., Brunner, E., Kumari, M., Shipley, M., Elbaz, A., et al. (2014). Interleukin-6 and C-reactive protein as predictors of cognitive decline in late midlife. *Neurology* 83, 486–493. doi: 10.1212/wnl.0000000000000665

Sites, C. K., Calles-Escandon, J., Brochu, M., Butterfield, M., Ashikaga, T., and Poehlman, E. T. (2000). Relation of regional fat distribution to insulin sensitivity in postmenopausal women. *Fertil. Steril.* 73, 61–65. doi: 10.1016/s0015-0282(99)00453-7

Sternfeld, B., Wang, H., Quesenberry, C. P. Jr., Abrams, B., Everson-Rose, S. A., Greendale, G. A., et al. (2004). Physical activity and changes in weight and waist circumference in midlife women: findings from the study of women's health across the nation. *Am. J. Epidemiol.* 160, 912–922. doi: 10.1093/aje/kwh299

Straub, R. H. (2007). The complex role of estrogens in inflammation. *Endocr. Rev.* 28, 521–574. doi: 10.1210/er.2007-0001

Stubbins, R. E., Holcomb, V. B., Hong, J., and Nunez, N. P. (2012). Estrogen modulates abdominal adiposity and protects female mice from obesity and impaired glucose tolerance. *Eur. J. Nutr.* 51, 861–870. doi: 10.1007/s00394-011-0266-4

Suh, H. S., Zhao, M. L., Derico, L., Choi, N., and Lee, S. C. (2013). Insulin-like growth factor 1 and 2, (IGF1, IGF2) expression in human microglia: differential regulation by inflammatory mediators. *J. Neuroinflammation* 10:37. doi: 10.1186/1742-2094-10-37

Takalo, M., Haapasalo, A., Martiskainen, H., Kurkinen, K. M., Koivisto, H., Miettinen, P., et al. (2014). High-fat diet increases tau expression in the brain of T2DM and AD mice independently of peripheral metabolic status. *J. Nutr. Biochem.* 25, 634–641. doi: 10.1016/j.jnutbio.2014.02.003

Takeda, S., Sato, N., Ikimura, K., Nishino, H., Rakugi, H., and Morishita, R. (2013). Increased blood-brain barrier vulnerability to systemic inflammation in an Alzheimer disease mouse model. *Neurobiol. Aging* 34, 2064–2070. doi: 10.1016/j.neurobiolaging.2013.02.010

Takeda, S., Sato, N., Uchio-Yamada, K., Sawada, K., Kunieda, T., Takeuchi, D., et al. (2010). Diabetes-accelerated memory dysfunction via cerebrovascular inflammation and Abeta deposition in an Alzheimer mouse model with diabetes. *Proc. Natl. Acad. Sci. U S A* 107, 7036–7041. doi: 10.3410/f.2820960.2486058

Tang, M. X., Jacobs, D., Stern, Y., Marder, K., Schofield, P., Gurland, B., et al. (1996). Effect of oestrogen during menopause on risk and age at onset of Alzheimer's disease. *Lancet* 348, 429–432. doi: 10.1016/s0140-6736(96)03356-9

Tanzi, R. E. (2012). The genetics of Alzheimer disease. *Cold Spring Harb. Perspect. Med.* 2:a006296. doi: 10.1101/cshperspect.a006296

Tchernof, A., Calles-Escandon, J., Sites, C. K., and Poehlman, E. T. (1998). Menopause, central body fatness and insulin resistance: effects of hormone-replacement therapy. *Coron. Artery Dis.* 9, 503–511. doi: 10.1097/00019501-199809080-00006

Teeling, J. L., and Perry, V. H. (2009). Systemic infection and inflammation in acute CNS injury and chronic neurodegeneration: underlying mechanisms. *Neuroscience* 158, 1062–1073. doi: 10.1016/j.neuroscience.2008.07.031

Thaler, J. P., Guyenet, S. J., Dorfman, M. D., Wisse, B. E., and Schwartz, M. W. (2013). Hypothalamic inflammation: marker or mechanism of obesity pathogenesis? *Diabetes* 62, 2629–2634. doi: 10.2337/db12-1605

Thaler, J. P., and Schwartz, M. W. (2010). Minireview: inflammation and obesity pathogenesis: the hypothalamus heats up. *Endocrinology* 151, 4109–4115. doi: 10.1210/en.2010-0336

Thaler, J. P., Yi, C. X., Schur, E. A., Guyenet, S. J., Hwang, B. H., Dietrich, M. O., et al. (2012). Obesity is associated with hypothalamic injury in rodents and humans. *J. Clin. Invest.* 122, 153–162. doi: 10.1172/JCI59660

Tsigos, C., Kyrou, I., Chala, E., Tsapogas, P., Stavridis, J. C., Raptis, S. A., et al. (1999). Circulating tumor necrosis factor alpha concentrations are higher in abdominal versus peripheral obesity. *Metabolism* 48, 1332–1335. doi: 10.1016/s0026-0495(99)90277-9

Tucsek, Z., Toth, P., Sosnowska, D., Gautam, T., Mitschelen, M., Koller, A., et al. (2014). Obesity in aging exacerbates blood-brain barrier disruption, neuroinflammation and oxidative stress in the mouse hippocampus: effects on expression of genes involved in beta-amyloid generation and Alzheimer's disease. *J. Gerontol. A Biol. Sci. Med. Sci.* 69, 1212–1226. doi: 10.1093/gerona/glt177

Vandanmagsar, B., Youm, Y. H., Ravussin, A., Galgani, J. E., Stadler, K., Mynatt, R. L., et al. (2011). The NLRP3 inflammasome instigates obesity-induced inflammation and insulin resistance. *Nat. Med.* 17, 179–188. doi: 10.1038/nm.2279

Verri, M., Pastoris, O., Dossena, M., Aquilani, R., Guerriero, F., Cuzzoni, G., et al. (2012). Mitochondrial alterations, oxidative stress and neuroinflammation in Alzheimer's disease. *Int. J. Immunopathol. Pharmacol.* 25, 345–353.

Wajchenberg, B. L. (2000). Subcutaneous and visceral adipose tissue: their relation to the metabolic syndrome. *Endocr. Rev.* 21, 697–738. doi: 10.1210/er.21.6.697

Wallenius, V., Wallenius, K., Ahren, B., Rudling, M., Carlsten, H., Dickson, S. L., et al. (2002). Interleukin-6-deficient mice develop mature-onset obesity. *Nat. Med.* 8, 75–79. doi: 10.1038/nm0102-75

Weisberg, S. P., McCann, D., Desai, M., Rosenbaum, M., Leibel, R. L., Ferrante, A. W. Jr., et al. (2003). Obesity is associated with macrophage accumulation in adipose tissue. *J. Clin. Invest.* 112, 1796–1808. doi: 10.1172/jci200319246

Whitmer, R. A., Gustafson, D. R., Barrett-Connor, E., Haan, M. N., Gunderson, E. P., and Yaffe, K. (2008). Central obesity and increased risk of dementia more than three decades later. *Neurology* 71, 1057–1064. doi: 10.1212/01.wnl.0000306313.89165.ef

Whitmer, R. A., Quesenberry, C. P., Zhou, J., and Yaffe, K. (2011). Timing of hormone therapy and dementia: the critical window theory revisited. *Ann. Neurol.* 69, 163–169. doi: 10.1002/ana.22239

Wildman, R. P., Tepper, P. G., Crawford, S., Finkelstein, J. S., Sutton-Tyrrell, K., Thurston, R. C., et al. (2012). Do changes in sex steroid hormones precede or follow increases in body weight during the menopause transition? Results from the study of women's health across the nation. *J. Clin. Endocrinol. Metab.* 97, E1695–E1704. doi: 10.1210/jc.2012-1614

Wyss-Coray, T., and Rogers, J. (2012). Inflammation in Alzheimer disease-a brief review of the basic science and clinical literature. *Cold Spring Harb. Perspect. Med.* 2:a006346. doi: 10.1101/cshperspect.a006346

Xie, Z., Wei, M., Morgan, T. E., Fabrizio, P., Han, D., Finch, C. E., et al. (2002). Peroxynitrite mediates neurotoxicity of amyloid beta-peptide1-42- and lipopolysaccharide-activated microglia. *J. Neurosci.* 22, 3484–3492.

Xu, W. L., Atti, A. R., Gatz, M., Pedersen, N. L., Johansson, B., and Fratiglioni, L. (2011). Midlife overweight and obesity increase late-life dementia risk: a population-based twin study. *Neurology* 76, 1568–1574. doi: 10.1212/WNL.0b013e3182190d09

Yaffe, K., Blackwell, T., Kanaya, A. M., Davidowitz, N., Barrett-Connor, E., and Krueger, K. (2004). Diabetes, impaired fasting glucose and development of cognitive impairment in older women. *Neurology* 63, 658–663. doi: 10.1212/01.wnl.0000134666.64593.ba

Yaffe, K., Haan, M., Byers, A., Tangen, C., and Kuller, L. (2000). Estrogen use, APOE and cognitive decline: evidence of gene-environment interaction. *Neurology* 54, 1949–1954. doi: 10.1212/wnl.54.10.1949

Yamamoto, M., Kiyota, T., Horiba, M., Buescher, J. L., Walsh, S. M., Gendelman, H. E., et al. (2007). Interferon-gamma and tumor necrosis factor-alpha regulate amyloid-beta plaque deposition and beta-secretase expression in Swedish mutant APP transgenic mice. *Am. J. Pathol.* 170, 680–692. doi: 10.2353/ajpath.2007.060378

Yao, J., Rettberg, J. R., Klosinski, L. P., Cadenas, E., and Brinton, R. D. (2011). Shift in brain metabolism in late onset Alzheimer's disease: implications for biomarkers and therapeutic interventions. *Mol. Aspects Med.* 32, 247–257. doi: 10.1016/j.mam.2011.10.005

Yin, F., Yao, J., Sancheti, H., Feng, T., Melcangi, R. C., Morgan, T. E., et al. (2015). The perimenopausal aging transition in the female rat brain: decline in bioenergetic systems and synaptic plasticity. *Neurobiol. Aging* 36, 2282–2295. doi: 10.1016/j.neurobiolaging.2015.03.013

Yonezawa, R., Wada, T., Matsumoto, N., Morita, M., Sawakawa, K., Ishii, Y., et al. (2012). Central versus peripheral impact of estradiol on the impaired glucose metabolism in ovariectomized mice on a high-fat diet. *Am. J. Physiol. Endocrinol. Metab.* 303, E445–E456. doi: 10.1152/ajpendo.00638.2011

Yu, D., Corbett, B., Yan, Y., Zhang, G. X., Reinhart, P., Cho, S. J., et al. (2012). Early cerebrovascular inflammation in a transgenic mouse model of Alzheimer's disease. *Neurobiol. Aging* 33, 2942–2947. doi: 10.1016/j.neurobiolaging.2012.02.023

Yue, X., Lu, M., Lancaster, T., Cao, P., Honda, S., Staufenbiel, M., et al. (2005). Brain estrogen deficiency accelerates Abeta plaque formation in an Alzheimer's disease animal model. *Proc. Natl. Acad. Sci. U S A* 102, 19198–19203. doi: 10.1073/pnas.0505203102

Yusuf, S., Hawken, S., Ounpuu, S., Bautista, L., Franzosi, M. G., Commerford, P., et al. (2005). Obesity and the risk of myocardial infarction in 27,000 participants from 52, countries: a case-control study. *Lancet* 366, 1640–1649. doi: 10.1016/S0140-6736(05)67663-5

Zandi, P. P., Carlson, M. C., Plassman, B. L., Welsh-Bohmer, K. A., Mayer, L. S., Steffens, D. C., et al. (2002). Hormone replacement therapy and incidence of Alzheimer disease in older women: the Cache County Study. *JAMA* 288, 2123–2129. doi: 10.1001/jama.288.17.2123

Zempel, H., and Mandelkow, E. (2014). Lost after translation: missorting of Tau protein and consequences for Alzheimer disease. *Trends Neurosci.* 37, 721–732. doi: 10.1016/j.tins.2014.08.004

Zhao, L., Yao, J., Mao, Z., Chen, S., Wang, Y., and Brinton, R. D. (2011). 17beta-Estradiol regulates insulin-degrading enzyme expression via an ERbeta/PI3-K pathway in hippocampus: relevance to Alzheimer's prevention. *Neurobiol. Aging* 32, 1949–1963. doi: 10.1016/j.neurobiolaging.2009.12.010

Zheng, H., Xu, H., Uljon, S. N., Gross, R., Hardy, K., Gaynor, J., et al. (2002). Modulation of A(beta) peptides by estrogen in mouse models. *J. Neurochem.* 80, 191–196. doi: 10.1046/j.0022-3042.2001.00690.x

Zlokovic, B. V. (2011). Neurovascular pathways to neurodegeneration in Alzheimer's disease and other disorders. *Nat. Rev. Neurosci.* 12, 723–738. doi: 10.1038/nrn3114

4

Age-Related Differences in the Modulation of Small-World Brain Networks during a Go/NoGo Task

Xiangfei Hong[1,2], *Yuelu Liu*[3], *Junfeng Sun*[2] *and Shanbao Tong*[2*]

[1] *Shanghai Key Laboratory of Psychotic Disorders, Shanghai Mental Health Center, Shanghai Jiao Tong University School of Medicine, Shanghai, China,* [2] *School of Biomedical Engineering, Shanghai Jiao Tong University, Shanghai, China,* [3] *Center for Mind and Brain, University of California, Davis, CA, USA*

Edited by:
Jean Mariani,
Université Pierre et Marie Curie, France

Reviewed by:
Tamer Demiralp,
Istanbul University, Turkey
Laura Lorenzo-López,
University of A Coruña, Spain

Correspondence:
Shanbao Tong
stong@sjtu.edu.cn

Although inter-regional phase synchrony of neural oscillations has been proposed as a plausible mechanism for response control, little is known about the possible effects due to normal aging. We recorded multi-channel electroencephalography (EEG) from healthy younger and older adults in a Go/NoGo task, and examined the aging effects on synchronous brain networks with graph theoretical analysis. We found that in both age groups, brain networks in theta, alpha or beta band for either response execution (Go) or response inhibition (NoGo) condition showed prominent small-world property. Furthermore, small-world property of brain networks showed significant differences between different task conditions. Further analyses of node degree suggested that frontal-central theta band phase synchrony was enhanced during response inhibition, whereas during response execution, increased phase synchrony was observed in beta band over central-parietal regions. More interestingly, these task-related modulations on brain networks were well preserved and even more robust in older adults compared with younger adults. Taken together, our findings not only suggest that response control involves synchronous brain networks in functionally-distinct frequency bands, but also indicate an increase in the recruitment of brain network resources due to normal aging.

Keywords: aging, graph theory, induced activity, phase synchrony, response inhibition

INTRODUCTION

Response inhibition, the ability to inhibit a prepotent tendency of behavioral response, is a core component of human cognitive control functions (Diamond, 2013). Previous electroencephalography (EEG) studies regularly focused on the event-related potentials (ERPs) evoked by Go and NoGo (or Stop) stimuli in Go/NoGo (or Stop-Signal) response control paradigm. Two ERP components, i.e., N2 and P3, were consistently identified in the ERP waves elicited by the NoGo (or Stop) stimuli compared with the Go stimuli, typically observed over frontal-central cortex after ~200 ms and ~300 ms post-stimulus onset, respectively. Such ERP components were usually interpreted as the neural markers of response inhibition (Falkenstein et al., 1999; Albert et al., 2013; Huster et al., 2013), and were also shown to be sensitive to normal aging (Hong et al., 2014).

Besides the analysis of ERP, frequency or time-frequency domain analysis on oscillatory EEG power during Go/NoGo tasks has also been reported in several studies. For example, states or tasks that require an increased level of cognitive control, i.e., NoGo condition, always evoked higher power of theta oscillations during 200–600 ms post-stimulus period over the frontal-central scalp (Kirmizi-Alsan et al., 2006; Huster et al., 2013; Ergen et al., 2014). As a widely replicated finding, frontal theta activity was recently proposed to be a plausible mechanism for cognitive control functions (Cavanagh and Frank, 2014). While during movement execution tasks (Go condition), decreased power of alpha and beta oscillations over the sensorimotor areas was a common finding in the literature (Leocani et al., 1997; Pfurtscheller and Lopes da Silva, 1999).

Although ERP and frequency-domain analyses have been the dominating techniques in previous EEG research on Go/NoGo tasks, recent studies began to focus on the neural oscillations from the perspective of inter-regional phase synchrony in different frequency bands, and suggested an important role of large-scale neural synchrony in response inhibition (Serrien et al., 2005; Moore et al., 2008; Tallet et al., 2009; Brier et al., 2010; Muller and Anokhin, 2012; Anguera et al., 2013b; Cavanagh and Frank, 2014). For example, one recent study suggested that the effective inhibition of a prepotent response should be associated with an increase of the theta-band phase synchrony between the frontal and parietal cortices in a Go/NoGo task (Muller and Anokhin, 2012), and another study reported inhibition-specific changes in beta-band phase coherence between cerebral motor areas in a stop task (Tallet et al., 2009).

In spite of accumulating studies reporting the role of phase synchrony among healthy young adults, the influences of normal aging during an active inhibitory state have been scarce in the literature. Nonetheless, there have been phase synchrony studies that mainly focused on the pathological aging population, i.e., Alzheimer's disease, showing the reduced phase synchrony during either the resting state (Uhlhaas and Singer, 2006; Stam et al., 2007, 2009; Knyazeva et al., 2010) or task states such as working memory (Pijnenburg et al., 2004) compared with normal elders. More interestingly, a recent study showed an increase of frontal-posterior theta-band phase coherence in healthy older adults following cognitive training that resulted in performance benefits (Anguera et al., 2013a). However, although such findings consistently implied a close relationship between cognitive control and neural synchrony during cognitive aging, a comprehensive and direct comparison of neural synchrony between healthy young and old adults from the perspective of large-scale neural synchrony is still lacking.

We inferred that there might be different possibilities on the results. On one hand, inspired by previous findings that the decline in cognitive ability was always accompanied with reduced neural synchrony during pathological aging (Uhlhaas and Singer, 2006), one may infer that the cognitive decline during normal aging would implicate a reduction in the ability to modulate neural synchrony for older adults compared with younger adults. Yet alternatively, from the perspective of compensatory mechanisms of cognitive aging, older adults might recruit additional brain activation to partially compensate the cognitive decline (Cabeza et al., 2002; Rajah and D'Esposito, 2005; Park and Reuter-Lorenz, 2009; Grady, 2012), which would lead to the enhancement of the neural synchrony in older adults. Nonetheless, in either case, investigating the effects of normal aging on neural synchrony during a cognitive control tasks would provide valuable insights for understanding the age-related changes in neural mechanisms of cognitive control functions.

In this study, we aimed to study the influence of normal aging on neural synchrony during response control. To this end, we recorded multi-channel EEG from healthy younger and older adults in a Go/NoGo response control task. Frequency-domain analysis was performed to examine task-related modulations on oscillatory EEG power, which could provide useful information for the comparison with existing literature. After that, functional brain networks were constructed based on phase synchrony analysis (Sun et al., 2012). Graph theory was then used to analyze the topological organizations of oscillatory brain networks during Go and NoGo conditions (Bullmore and Sporns, 2009; Rubinov and Sporns, 2010). We expected to observe the task-related modulations on brain networks between response execution (Go) and response inhibition (NoGo) conditions in functionally-distinct frequency bands, i.e., theta, alpha and beta bands (Tallet et al., 2009; Brier et al., 2010; Muller and Anokhin, 2012; Anguera et al., 2013b). Furthermore, we compared the task-modulated brain networks between younger and older adults to investigate age-related differences in neural synchrony during response inhibition and execution.

MATERIALS AND METHODS

Participants

We recruited 23 healthy younger (mean ± standard deviation; age: 21.4 ± 2 years; range: 18–25 years; 7 females; all right-handed) and 18 healthy older adults (mean ± standard deviation; age: 61 ± 6 years; range: 50–70 years; 11 females; all right-handed) as participants. All participants reported normal or corrected-to-normal vision, without a history of neurological or psychiatric disorders. All older participants went through the Mini-Mental Status Examination (mean score: 28/30; range: ≥26; Folstein et al., 1975) with normal cognition. A minimum of 9 years of school education was required for each participant. All participants gave their written informed consents before the experiment, and were financially compensated for the experiment regardless of their performance. The experimental protocols were approved by the institutional Ethical Committee of Shanghai Jiao Tong University, complying with the Declaration of Helsinki.

Stimuli and Procedures

A modified visual Go/NoGo task was adopted in this study. Before each trial, a black central crosshair (1.38° by 1.38°) and two lateral black location markers (2.39° by 2.39°, located 9.05° from the vertical meridian, and 7.2° below the horizontal meridian) were constantly presented on a white background. Participants were instructed to always maintain fixation on the crosshair whenever it was displayed. Each trial began with a 200 ms central black arrow cue pointing to either the left (50%) or the right (50%). Subjects were required to covertly attend the left or the right location according to the cue and ignore the other location. The target stimulus (1.67° by 1.67°), either a plus sign (50%) or the letter "x" (50%), was presented for 200 ms inside either the left (50%) or the right (50%) location marker after a random cue-target interval (CTI: jittered between 1000–1200 ms). Subjects were required to respond only to the plus sign presented in the attended location (Go trials) as quickly and accurately as possible with the right index finger, and refrain from responding to the letter "x" presented in the attended location marker (NoGo trials). Targets presented in the unattended location marker were to be ignored completely. A fixed inter-trial interval of 2600 ms was presented between the target offset and the cue onset of the next trial. For the Go trials, responses within 1600 ms after the target offset were recorded as valid trials.

Participants were comfortably seated in a sound attenuated room during the experiment. All stimuli were presented on a 19 inch LCD display (Dell: P190SB) placed 60 cm in front of the participant. The experimental paradigm was implemented in E-Prime (Version: 2.0, Psychology Software Tools, Inc., Sharpsburg, PA, USA), and behavioral responses were recorded with the Serial Response Box™ included in the E-Prime toolkit. Each block consisted of 60 trials lasting for about 5 min. To minimize subject fatigue, a short (2–3 min) break was included between two successive blocks. All subjects went through a training block to get familiar with the experimental procedures. After the training, all younger subjects completed eight blocks of formal experiment trials and older subjects completed six blocks, considering the fact that the elders are more likely to develop mental fatigue that could affect the brain activity (Sun et al., 2014). To eliminate potential differences due to unequal trial numbers in the two groups, further EEG analyses only included data from the first six blocks in the younger group.

EEG Recording and Preprocessing

Continuous EEG signals were recorded from 32 scalp electrodes (30 recording channels: Fp1, Fp2, F3, F4, F7, F8, Fz, FC1, FC2, FC5, FC6, C3, C4, Cz, T7, T8, CP1, CP2, CP5, CP6, P3, P4, P7, P8, 171 Pz, O1, O2, Oz, TP9, TP10; recording reference: FCz; ground: AFz) using the BrainAmp MR Plus amplifier and EasyCap™ (Brain Products GmbH, Gilching, Germany). Two additional electrodes were placed on the outer left canthus and above the right eye to record horizontal electrooculogram (HEOG) and vertical electrooculogram (VEOG), respectively. EEG signals were amplified and sampled at 1000 Hz with 0.016–100 Hz online band-pass filtering. Impedance of each electrode was maintained below 10 kΩ during the recording.

EEG preprocessing was performed in the Matlab-based (MathWorks, MA, USA) EEGLAB (Delorme and Makeig, 2004) and ERPLAB toolboxes (Lopez-Calderon and Luck, 2014). Raw continuous EEG data first went through a two-way, zero phase shift, Butterworth filter (band-pass: 0.1–40 Hz; roll-off slope: 12 dB/oct), followed by a Parks McClellan notch filter to eliminate remaining noise at 50 Hz. Independent component analysis was performed to remove the ocular artifacts (Jung et al., 2000). Continuous EEG data were then re-referenced to the average of bilateral mastoid electrodes (TP9 and TP10), and segmented into epochs from −200 to 800 ms referring to the target onsets. Epochs with physical artifact in any EEG channel were marked as bad epochs according to the following criteria: (1) the maximal absolute value of voltage difference within a moving window (width: 200 ms; step: 50 ms) exceeding 150 μV; and (2) the maximal absolute value of voltage at any time point exceeding 100 μV. Furthermore, EEG epochs with overt eye movements or blinks that might prevent subjects from recognizing the targets were marked as bad epochs according to the following criteria: (1) the maximal absolute value of voltage difference in the HEOG channel within a moving window (width: 400 ms; step: 10 ms) exceeding 40 μV; and (2) the maximal absolute value of voltage difference in the VEOG channel at any time point around the target (−200 to 200 ms post-stimulus) exceeding 50 μV. After that, all EEG epochs were further visually inspected and all bad epochs were excluded in subsequent analyses.

In this study, the 200–700 ms post-stimulus period was chosen for the following analysis of EEG spectral power and phase synchrony, considering that: (1) our previous study has shown that this window covers the processes related to response inhibition, as suggested by the ERP components (N2 and P3) observed during this window (Hong et al., 2014); (2) from the computational perspective, our previous research based on surrogate tests has shown that an epoch of 500 ms yields optimal results for phase synchrony analysis in EEG theta, alpha and beta bands (Sun et al., 2012). For the sake of comparison, the last 500 ms of inter-trial interval (−500 to 0 pre-cue) was selected as the Baseline condition, which was included in the following analysis as reference.

It has been widely agreed that the event-related EEG includes both evoked and induced activities (Pfurtscheller and Lopes da Silva, 1999; Bastiaansen and Hagoort, 2003). The evoked activity, directly driven by the stimulus and both time- and phase-locked to it, can be extracted from the ongoing EEG by a straightforward averaging of EEG epochs, resulting in the ERP. The induced activity, on the other hand, is largely rhythmic (oscillatory) in nature, refers to oscillations caused or modulated by stimuli or state changes that do not directly drive the rhythm, so that they are time-locked, but not necessarily phase-locked, to the eliciting event. Moreover, previous studies have suggested to remove evoked activity when analyzing induced activity (Dietl et al., 1999; Doppelmayr et al., 2000; Gruber et al., 2002; Deiber et al., 2009). In this study, we are only interested in induced activity, because evoked activity (ERP, N2 and P3 components) has been analyzed and reported in our previous study (Hong et al., 2014). Therefore, ERP activity from each task condition (Go, NoGo) was subtracted from EEG epochs of the same condition for each subject to eliminate the contributions from evoked activity before subsequent analyses of

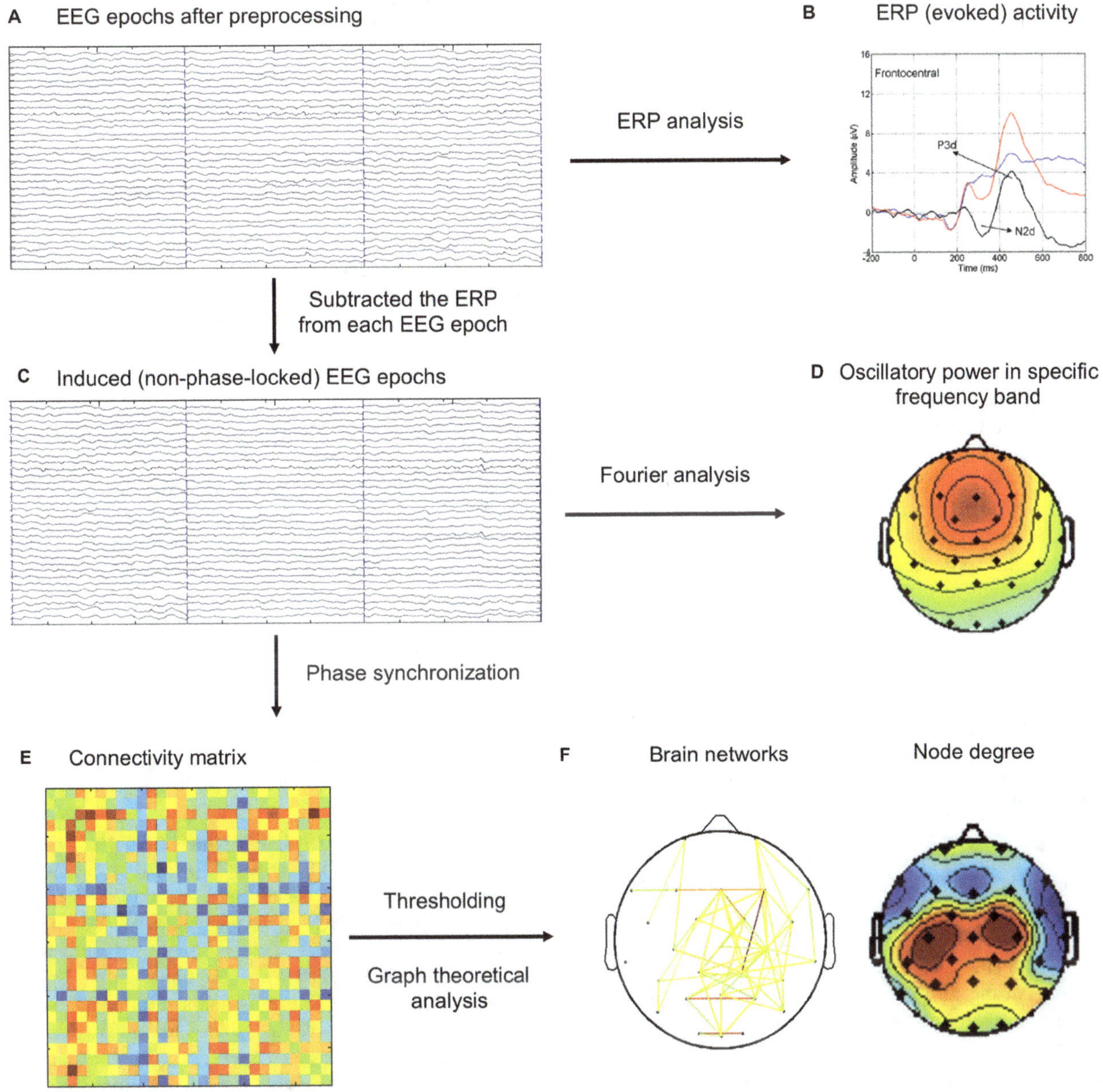

FIGURE 1 | The schematic diagram for the brain network analysis. (A) Electroencephalography (EEG) epochs after preprocessing steps. **(B)** The event-related potentials (ERPs) were computed by averaging the same type of EEG epochs (Go, NoGo), which was reported in our previous study (Hong et al., 2014). **(C)** ERP activity was subtracted from EEG epochs. **(D)** Frequency-domain analysis of oscillatory power using Fourier analysis. **(E)** Phase synchronization (PS) index was computed for each pair of channels in each trial, and the connectivity matrix was averaged across the same type of EEG epochs (Baseline, Go, NoGo). **(F)** Different thresholds were applied on the connectivity matrix to construct brain networks, which were then analyzed using graph theoretical metrics.

induced activity. The flowchart of EEG analysis was illustrated in **Figure 1**.

EEG Spectral Power Analysis

To analyze the modulation of EEG band power during the Go/NoGo task, we computed fast Fourier transform for the 200–700 ms post-stimulus period with Hamming window for each electrode, and then averaged the spectra across all trials of the same experimental condition (Baseline, NoGo, Go). To eliminate the inter-subject variance, task-related power change was computed as the percentage change of spectral power between different task conditions (Hong et al., 2013).

Phase Synchronization Analysis

Phase synchronization (PS) has been successfully used to analyze rhythmic synchrony in oscillatory neural signals (Sun et al., 2012; Hong et al., 2013; Yan et al., 2013). The strength of phase synchrony can be quantified by PS index (PSI), which is based on the instantaneous phase (IP) of oscillations. For an epoch of real-value narrow-band EEG signal $s(t)$, its IP can be defined as:

$$\phi(t) = \arg[z(t)] = arctan\frac{\tilde{s}(t)}{s(t)} \quad (1)$$

where,

$$z(t) = s(t) + j\tilde{s}(t) \quad (2)$$

is the analytic signal of $s(t)$, and

$$\tilde{s}(t) = \frac{1}{\pi}\text{P.V.}\int_{-\infty}^{\infty}\frac{s(\tau)}{t-\tau}d\tau \quad (3)$$

is the Hilbert transform of $s(t)$ (P.V. denotes that the integral is taken in the sense of Cauchy principal value). Let $\phi_1(t)$ and $\phi_2(t)$ denote the IPs of two narrow-band EEG waves from two EEG channels during the same period. If the IP difference, i.e., $|m\phi_1(t) - n\phi_2(t)|$, is bounded by a constant, this pair of EEG waves are deemed to be in m:n PS, where m and n are positive integers (Tass et al., 1998; Wacker and Witte, 2011). In this study, we followed the approach adopted in recent studies of phase synchrony and only focused on the 1:1 PS (Sun et al., 2012; Hong et al., 2013; Yan et al., 2013). In this case, the PSI (ρ) can be quantified as the mean phase coherence of the IP difference, i.e.,

$$\rho = \sqrt{\langle\cos[\phi_1(t) - \phi_2(t)]\rangle_t^2 + \langle\sin[\phi_1(t) - \phi_2(t)]\rangle_t^2} \quad (4)$$

where $\langle\cdot\rangle_t$ denotes the average over time. The value of PSI (ρ) is in the range of [0 1], with $\rho = 0$ indicating no PS at all and $\rho = 1$ indicating perfect PS.

In this study, the PS analysis for each EEG epoch was performed as follows: (1) filtering the EEG epochs into different frequency bands (theta: 4–8 Hz; alpha: 8–13 Hz; beta: 13–30 Hz); (2) computing the IP of the sub-band EEG signals according to Eq (1) for each epoch; (3) computing the PSI between each pair of electrodes using Eq (4); and (4) assigning the PSIs into an association matrix (28 × 28 in this study), with element in the ith row and j^{th} column, ρ_{ij}, representing the PSI between channel i and channel j. Finally, we averaged PSI matrices from all epochs under the same experimental conditions (Baseline, Go, NoGo) for each subject and obtained three PSI matrices (Baseline, Go, NoGo) in each frequency band for each subject.

Graph Theoretical Analysis

In graph theoretical analysis, each channel is defined as a node, and the connectivity strength between two nodes is designated as the edge that connects them. The association matrix ($\{\rho_{ij}\}$) was converted into a weighted graph ($\{w_{ij}\}$) by applying a threshold (T) to eliminate those weak and spurious connections, i.e.,

$$w_{ij} = \begin{cases} \rho_{ij}, & \text{if} \geq T \\ 0, & \text{otherwise.} \end{cases} \quad (5)$$

where w_{ij} denotes the connectivity strength between node i and node j. The threshold value T was determined via a commonly used approach which explores the brain graph as a function of the changing threshold (Bullmore and Bassett, 2011; Hong et al., 2013; Yan et al., 2013). Previous studies have shown that the efficient organization of brain networks is typically observed in relatively sparse networks with network densities (the ratio between the existing edge number and maximal possible edge number) being less than 0.5, and that the maximal cost-efficiency of brain networks are typically reached at a network density of around 0.3 (Achard and Bullmore, 2007; Bassett et al., 2009; Bullmore and Bassett, 2011; Bullmore and Sporns, 2012; Jin et al., 2012). Therefore, in this study, we constructed connectivity graphs under a series of edge numbers (K) ranging from 60–180 with a step of 20. Specifically, for a given edge number K, the threshold (T) was assigned as the Kth largest value among all PSIs. The corresponding network density hence ranged approximately from 0.16 to 0.48.

The degree of a node, defined as the total connectivity strength of the corresponding node, was used to describe the importance of that node in the graph. Nodes with high degrees are regarded as hubs and are likely to play an important role in network communications (Bullmore and Sporns, 2009; Bullmore and Bassett, 2011). For weighted networks, the degree of node i (D_i) is quantified as:

$$D_i = \sum_{j\in N} w_{ij} \quad (6)$$

where N denotes the set of all nodes in the network.

Recent research has shown that brain networks typically exhibit the so-called "small-world" property, which is thought to reflect an efficient organization with an optimal compromise between local segregation and global integration (Bassett et al., 2006; Achard and Bullmore, 2007; Jin et al., 2012). In this study, we will compare the small-world property of functional brain networks between young and old adults within different frequency bands to explore age-related reorganizations during the response inhibition task. Generally, small-world networks are characterized as networks with significantly greater local segregation but approximately the same level of global integration compared with random networks (Watts and Strogatz, 1998; Rubinov and Sporns, 2010; Bullmore and Sporns, 2012). Clustering coefficient is a measure indicating the level of local segregation of a network (Rubinov and Sporns, 2010). For a weighted network, the clustering coefficient is defined as the average clustering coefficient between all nodes in the network (Onnela et al., 2005),

$$C = \frac{1}{n}\sum_{i\in N} C_i = \frac{1}{n}\sum_{i\in N}\left[\frac{1}{D_i(D_i-1)}\sum_{j,h\in N}\left(w_{ij}w_{ih}w_{jh}\right)^{1/3}\right] \quad (7)$$

where n is number of nodes in the graph and D_i is the degree for node i as defined in Eq (6) Characteristic path length, on the other hand, describes the level of global integration of a network (Rubinov and Sporns, 2010). It is defined as the average shortest path length between all pairs of nodes (Latora and Marchiori, 2001),

$$L = \frac{1}{\frac{1}{n(n-1)} \sum_{i \neq j \in N} \frac{1}{d_{ij}}} \quad (8)$$

where d_{ij} denotes the shortest path length between node i and node j.

To examine the small-world property of functional brain networks, the clustering coefficient and characteristic path length were compared with those from 20 size-matched random networks generated from randomly rewiring the original brain networks (Maslov and Sneppen, 2002). This procedure yielded the normalized clustering coefficient $\gamma = C/C_{rand}$ and characteristic path length $\lambda = L/L_{rand}$, where C_{rand} and L_{rand} denote the average clustering coefficient and characteristic path length of the 20 random networks, respectively. The small-world property can then be quantified by the small-worldness index (Humphries and Gurney, 2008),

$$\sigma = \frac{\gamma}{\lambda} \quad (9)$$

For a typical small-world network, σ is greater than 1 ($\gamma > 1$, $\lambda \approx 1$). Note that the graph theoretical analysis was performed in Matlab with Brain Connectivity Toolbox (Rubinov and Sporns, 2010).

Statistical Analysis

For the analysis of C and L, we used the normalized values, i.e., γ and λ, to eliminate possible influences from connectivity strength (Rubinov et al., 2009), and performed the statistical analysis under different network density levels. It should be noted that: (1) the purpose of constructing brain graphs under a series of network density levels was to cover the *real* network density level that has been suggested to be located in the pre-defined range as much as possible; (2) the brain graphs under different network density levels are far from independent graphs, and thus the correction for multiple comparisons, i.e., Bonferroni correction, is not appropriate here (Stam et al., 2007; Rubinov et al., 2009; Jin et al., 2012; Hong et al., 2013; Li et al., 2015). Instead of the correction for p-values, in this study, we did not treat the results as significant unless the $p < 0.05$ significance level was observed under at least 3 (out of 7) different network density levels. For the statistical analysis of node degree, we chose a specific threshold around the median edge density of 0.3 (120 edges; network density: 120/378 = 0.3175) that is typically regarded as the most economical network density level (Achard and Bullmore, 2007; Bassett et al., 2009; Bullmore and Bassett, 2011). Statistical significance of network measures were assessed by the repeated-measures analysis of variance (ANOVA), independent-samples t-test and paired-samples t-test (two-tailed). Statistical analysis was performed in SPSS 16.0.

RESULTS

Behavioral Performance

The behavioral results have been reported elsewhere (Hong et al., 2014). Briefly, the overall accuracy including both Go and NoGo trials was marginally higher for younger adults compared with older adults (younger: 99.52% ± 0.08% vs. older: 98.91% ± 0.31%; $t_{(18.027)} = 1.893$, $p = 0.074$). Older adults responded more slowly to Go targets than younger adults (younger: 477.56 ± 10.74 ms vs. older: 556.49 ± 28.46 ms; $t_{(20.582)} = -2.595$, $p = 0.017$). Furthermore, the analysis of false alarm rate (FAR) to NoGo-targets at the attended location showed no significant differences between the two groups (younger: 0.52% ± 0.13% vs. older: 1.17% ± 0.50%; $t_{(18.115)} = -1.250$, $p > 0.2$). Taken together, behavioral results suggested that although the response was slower due to aging, both younger and older adults showed satisfactory and comparable inhibitory performances in the Go/NoGo task.

EEG Spectral Power Modulation

As shown in **Figure 2**, both younger and older adults showed increased frontal-central theta power during NoGo condition than Baseline condition and Go condition. In alpha and beta band, there were power decreases over central-parietal areas during Go condition than Baseline condition and NoGo condition, and such decreases were stronger in the older group than the younger group. Overall, our results replicated previous studies on EEG band power modulation during Go/NoGo tasks (Leocani et al., 1997; Pfurtscheller and Lopes da Silva, 1999; Kirmizi-Alsan et al., 2006; Huster et al., 2013; Cavanagh and Frank, 2014; Ergen et al., 2014).

Brain Network Results

Small-World Property

The normalized clustering coefficient (γ), characteristic path length (λ) and small-worldness index (σ) for younger and older adults within the theta, alpha and beta frequency bands are illustrated in **Figure 3**. Statistical significance was tested by two-way repeated-measures ANOVA with Task (Baseline, Go and NoGo) as a within-group factor and Age (younger, older) as a between-group factor. The statistical results for γ, λ and σ are included in **Tables 1–3**, respectively. The major findings include:

1. Theta band: Main effect of Task was observed for γ ($p < 0.05$ under all 7 network density levels), λ ($p < 0.05$ under 3 network density levels) and σ ($p < 0.05$ under all 7 network density levels). Follow-up analysis suggested that both age groups showed larger γ ($p < 0.05$ under all 7 network density levels), smaller λ ($p < 0.05$ under 5 network density levels) and larger σ ($p < 0.05$ under all 7 network density levels) during Go condition than NoGo condition. Furthermore, the difference in σ between Go condition and NoGo condition was larger in older adults than that in younger adults, as indicated by significant interaction between

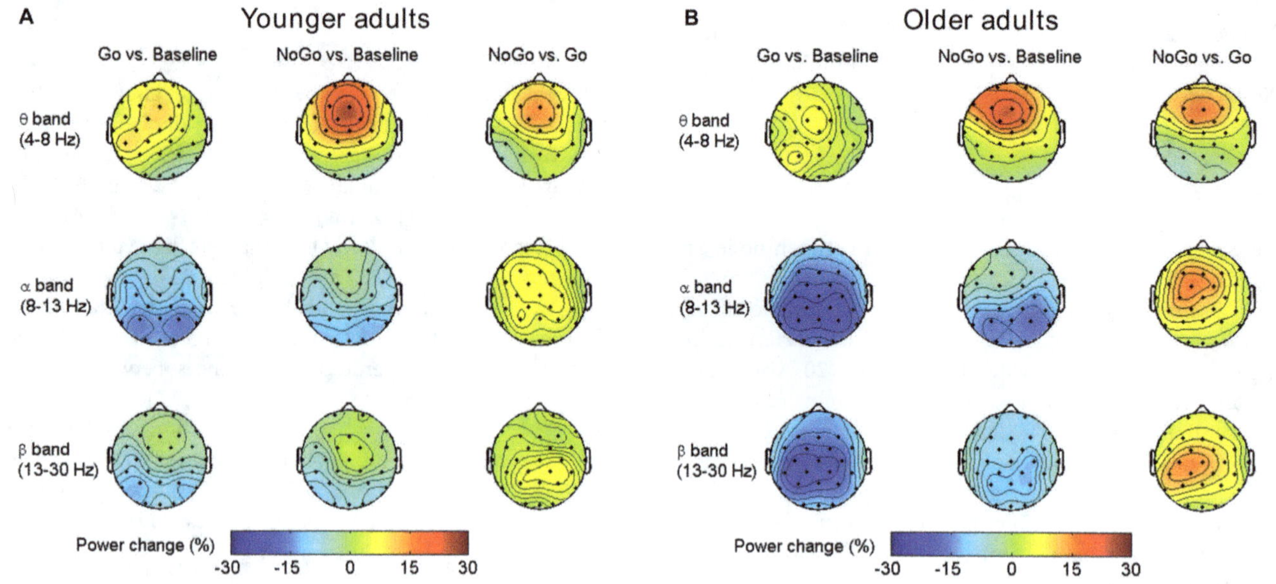

FIGURE 2 | Group-averaged task-related oscillatory power changes in different frequency bands for the younger group (A) and older group (B).

Task (Go, NoGo) and Age (younger, older; $p < 0.05$ under 4 network density levels). In addition, older adults showed larger γ and σ than younger adults during both Go and NoGo conditions ($p < 0.05$ under all 7 network density levels).

2. Alpha band: Main effect of Task was observed for γ ($p < 0.05$ under all 7 network density levels) and σ ($p < 0.05$ under all 7 network density levels). Follow-up analysis suggested that both age groups showed smaller γ ($p < 0.05$ under 4 network density levels) and σ ($p < 0.05$ under 3 network density levels) during Go condition than NoGo condition. However, there were no stable main effects or interactions related to Age under different network density levels in the alpha band.
3. Beta band: Main effect of Task was observed for γ ($p < 0.05$ under all 7 network density levels) and σ ($p < 0.05$ under all 7 network density levels). Follow-up analysis suggested that both age groups showed smaller γ ($p < 0.05$ under all 7 network density levels) and smaller σ (significant under 6 network density levels) during Go than NoGo condition. Furthermore, older adults showed smaller λ than younger adults during both Go and NoGo conditions ($p < 0.05$ under all 7 network density levels).

In summary, both younger and older adults showed stable task-related modulations of functional brain networks in theta, alpha and beta bands during the Go/NoGo task. Furthermore, age-related differences were observed in both theta and beta band brain networks. Older adults showed stronger task-related modulations of theta band brain networks than younger adults. In alpha band, however, no stable age-related differences were observed between the two age groups.

Node Degree Distribution

The differences in node degree between different task conditions (Baseline, Go, NoGo) were tested by paired-samples *t*-test in each age group separately. The statistical *t*-maps under the edge number of 120 (31.75% network density) are presented in **Figure 4**. Consistent with the small-world property, task-related modulations on node degree could also be clearly observed in theta, alpha and beta bands. In theta band, the frontal-central nodes showed an increase of degree during NoGo condition than Go condition. In beta band, higher node degree was observed during Go condition than NoGo condition among the central-parietal nodes. While in alpha band, such difference between Go condition and NoGo condition was much smaller than that in theta and beta bands.

To quantitatively analyze the task- and age-related effects on node degree in theta and beta band brain networks, we defined two regions of interest (ROIs) based on the *t*-maps in **Figure 4**: (1) the frontal-central ROI (channels Fp1, Fp2, F3, F4, C3, C4, F7, F8, Fz, Cz, FC1, FC2, FC5, FC6); and (2) the central-parietal ROI (channels C3, C4, P3, P4, Cz, Pz, CP1, CP2, CP5, CP6). The node degree within each ROI was averaged in theta and beta bands, respectively. The ROI-averaged node degree was then subject to a three-way ANOVA with Task (Baseline, Go, NoGo) as a within-group factor and Age (younger, older) as a between-group factor (**Figure 5A**). In theta band, we observed a main effect of Task ($F_{(2,76)} = 9.736$, $p < 0.001$) on frontal-central node degree. Follow-up analysis suggested that for younger adults, the task-modulated effects on frontal-central node degree were marginally significant (Go vs. NoGo: $t_{(22)} = -2.004$, $p = 0.058$). For the older adults, in contrast, such task-modulated effects were highly significant (Go vs. Baseline: $t_{(16)} = -2.725$, $p = 0.015$; Go vs. NoGo: $t_{(16)} = -5.174$,

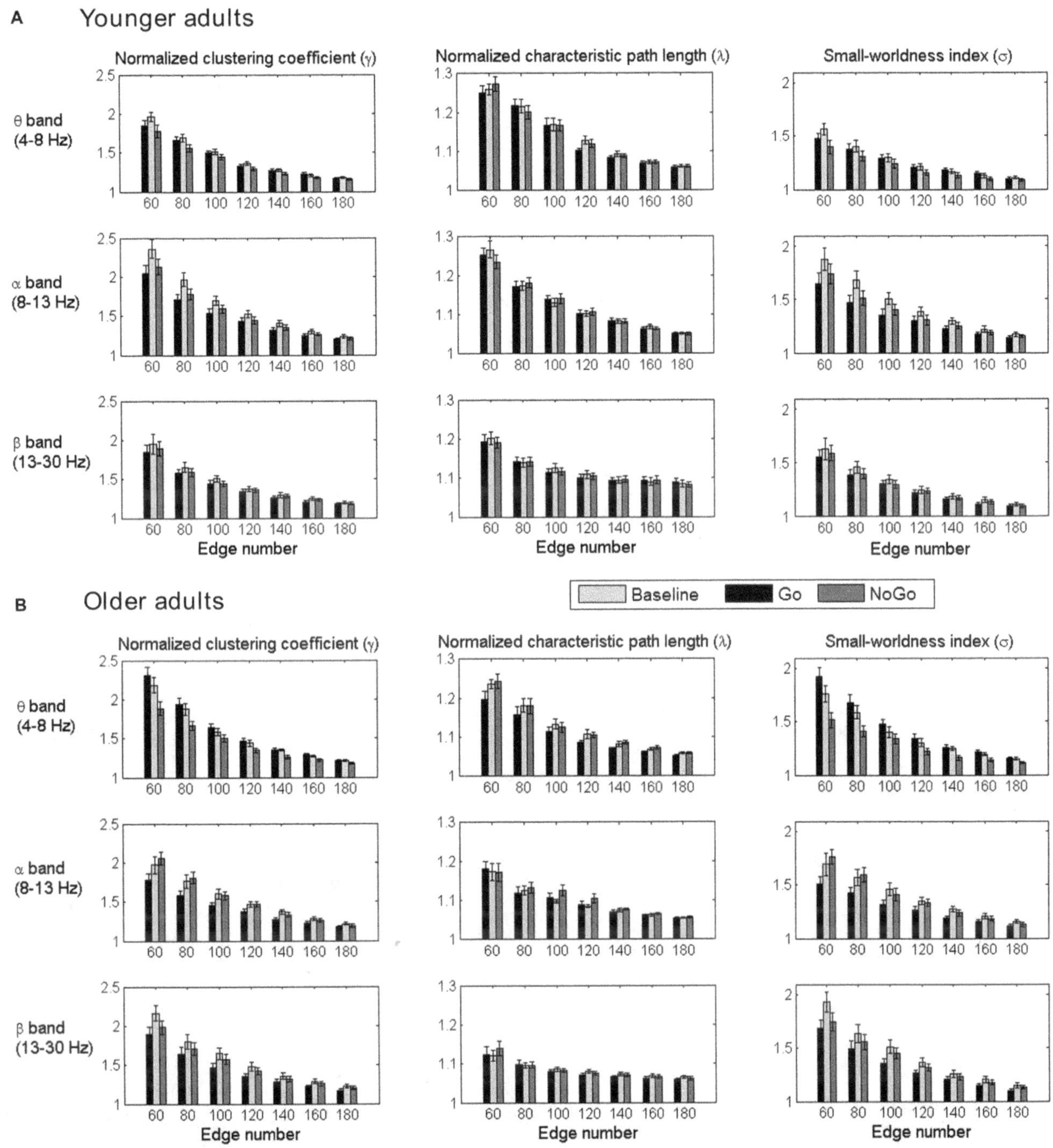

FIGURE 3 | Group-averaged normalized clustering coefficient (γ), characteristic path length (λ) and small-worldness index (σ) of the brain networks for all task conditions (Baseline, Go, NoGo) in the younger group (A) and older group (B) under different network density levels. Error bars indicate the standard error of the mean (SEM).

$p < 0.001$). In beta band, there was a main effect of Task ($F_{(2,76)} = 52.488, p < 0.001$) and a significant interaction of GNG × Age ($F_{(2,76)} = 10.217, p < 0.001$) on the central-parietal node degree. Follow-up analysis suggested that the task-modulated effects on central-parietal node degree were significant in either the younger (Go vs. Baseline: $t_{(22)} = 4.604, p < 0.001$; NoGo vs. Baseline: $t_{(22)} = 2.632, p = 0.015$; Go vs. NoGo: $t_{(22)} = 2.307, p = 0.031$) or the older (Go vs. Baseline: $t_{(16)} = 7.674, p < 0.001$; NoGo vs. Baseline: $t_{(16)} = 4.404, p < 0.001$; Go vs. NoGo: $t_{(16)} = 5.205, p < 0.001$) group.

To further characterize the age-related differences in task-modulated effects on node degree, we calculated

TABLE 1 | Results of two-way repeated-measures ANOVA (Task: Baseline vs. Go vs. NoGo; Age: younger vs. older) on normalized clustering coefficient (observed/random).

Frequency band	Edge number	Factors: Task	Factors: Age	Factors: Task × Age
Theta (4–8 Hz)	60	**$F = 10.019, p < 0.001$**	**$F = 8.262, p = 0.007$**	**$F = 4.057, p = 0.021$**
	80	**$F = 11.458, p < 0.001$**	**$F = 8.367, p = 0.006$**	$F = 2.045, p = 0.136$
	100	**$F = 4.609, p = 0.013$**	**$F = 4.258, p = 0.046$**	$F = 0.966, p = 0.385$
	120	**$F = 8.959, p < 0.001$**	**$F = 7.485, p = 0.009$**	$F = 1.565, p = 0.216$
	140	**$F = 11.839, p < 0.001$**	**$F = 6.873, p = 0.013$**	$F = 1.198, p = 0.307$
	160	**$F = 10.436, p < 0.001$**	**$F = 11.981, p = 0.001$**	$F = 0.316, p = 0.730$
	180	**$F = 5.444, p = 0.006$**	**$F = 12.504, p = 0.001$**	$F = 0.878, p = 0.420$
Alpha (8–13 Hz)	60	**$F = 6.712, p = 0.002$**	$F = 3.883, p = 0.056$	$F = 2.640, p = 0.078$
	80	**$F = 9.112, p < 0.001$**	$F = 2.568, p = 0.083$	$F = 1.182, p = 0.284$
	100	**$F = 7.107, p = 0.003$**	$F = 0.940, p = 0.339$	$F = 0.537, p = 0.587$
	120	**$F = 4.966, p = 0.013$**	$F = 0.361, p = 0.551$	$F = 1.402, p = 0.252$
	140	**$F = 10.138, p < 0.001$**	$F = 0.832, p = 0.367$	$F = 0.267, p = 0.767$
	160	**$F = 7.474, p = 0.001$**	$F = 0.225, p = 0.638$	$F = 0.185, p = 0.831$
	180	**$F = 5.794, p = 0.007$**	$F = 0.671, p = 0.418$	$F = 0.058, p = 0.944$
Beta (13–30 Hz)	60	**$F = 9.988, p < 0.001$**	$F = 0.702, p = 0.407$	$F = 2.320, p = 0.105$
	80	**$F = 9.379, p = 0.001$**	$F = 1.363\ p = 0.250$	$F = 1.129, p = 0.329$
	100	**$F = 18.344, p < 0.001$**	$F = 1.960, p = 0.170$	**$F = 5.175, p = 0.008$**
	120	**$F = 14.281, p < 0.001$**	$F = 1.449, p = 0.236$	**$F = 4.024, p = 0.022$**
	140	**$F = 14.111, p < 0.001$**	$F = 1.062, p = 0.309$	$F = 1.502, p = 0.229$
	160	**$F = 23.374, p < 0.001$**	$F = 0.588, p = 0.448$	$F = 1.599, p = 0.209$
	180	**$F = 16.803, p < 0.001$**	$F = 0.179, p = 0.675$	**$F = 5.812, p = 0.004$**

Significant results are marked as bold.

TABLE 2 | Results of two-way repeated-measures ANOVA (Task: Baseline vs. Go vs. NoGo; Age: younger vs. older) on normalized characteristic path length (observed/random).

Frequency band	Edge number	Factors: Task	Factors: Age	Factors: Task × Age
Theta (4–8 Hz)	60	**$F = 3.390, p = 0.039$**	$F = 3.583, p = 0.066$	$F = 0.746, p = 0.478$
	80	$F = 0.435, p = 0.649$	$F = 3.324, p = 0.076$	$F = 1.175, p = 0.314$
	100	$F = 0.472, p = 0.626$	**$F = 6.299, p = 0.016$**	$F = 0.261, p = 0.771$
	120	**$F = 6.260, p = 0.003$**	$F = 3.153, p = 0.084$	$F = 0.195, p = 0.823$
	140	$F = 3.030, p = 0.071$	$F = 2.075, p = 0.158$	$F = 0.757, p = 0.472$
	160	$F = 2.570, p = 0.095$	$F = 0.803, p = 0.376$	$F = 1.145, p = 0.324$
	180	**$F = 7.533, p = 0.002$**	$F = 0.944, p = 0.337$	$F = 1.041, p = 0.358$
Alpha(8-13 Hz)	60	$F = 0.510, p = 0.602$	**$F = 13.099, p = 0.001$**	$F = 0.404, p = 0.669$
	80	$F = 0.874, p = 0.421$	**$F = 10.463, p = 0.003$**	$F = 0.038, p = 0.962$
	100	$F = 3.224, p = 0.059$	$F = 4.034, p = 0.052$	$F = 0.886, p = 0.417$
	120	$F = 2.228, p = 0.115$	$F = 1.567, p = 0.218$	$F = 0.889, p = 0.415$
	140	$F = 0.241, p = 0.692$	$F = 1.516, p = 0.226$	$F = 0.504, p = 0.606$
	160	$F = 0.499, p = 0.532$	$F = 0.291, p = 0.592$	$F = 1.344, p = 0.267$
	180	$F = 0.044, p = 0.957$	$F = 1.215, p = 0.277$	$F = 1.061, p = 0.351$
Beta (13–30 Hz)	60	$F = 0.151, p = 0.860$	**$F = 11.322, p = 0.002$**	$F = 0.747, p = 0.477$
	80	$F = 0.196, p = 0.822$	**$F = 9.128, p = 0.004$**	$F = 0.014, p = 0.986$
	100	$F = 2.905, p = 0.061$	**$F = 8.689, p = 0.005$**	$F = 0.262, p = 0.770$
	120	$F = 1.815, p = 0.170$	**$F = 8.787, p = 0.005$**	$F = 0.017, p = 0.983$
	140	**$F = 3.998, p = 0.039$**	**$F = 6.597, p = 0.014$**	$F = 2.248, p = 0.113$
	160	$F = 0.480, p = 0.561$	**$F = 5.083, p = 0.030$**	$F = 2.580, p = 0.082$
	180	$F = 0.504, p = 0.579$	**$F = 4.710, p = 0.036$**	$F = 1.525, p = 0.224$

Significant results are marked as bold.

the relative changes of ROI-averaged node degree between Go condition and NoGo condition, and then compared the relative changes between the two groups using independent-samples t-test. Older adults showed significantly larger relative changes of node degree than younger adults in both the theta (frontal-central ROI, $t_{(38)} = 2.228$, $p = 0.032$) and the beta (central-parietal ROI, $t_{(38)} = -2.540$, $p = 0.015$) bands. **Figure 5B** illustrates the main connections that have different strengths between different task conditions. Apparently, in theta band brain network, NoGo condition evoked stronger cortical connections than Go condition within

TABLE 3 | Results of two-way repeated-measures ANOVA (Task: Baseline vs. Go vs. NoGo; Age: younger vs. older) on small-worldness index.

		Factors		
Frequency band	**Edge number**	**Task**	**Age**	**Task × Age**
Theta (4–8 Hz)	60	**$F = 13.507, p < 0.001$**	**$F = 13.344, p = 0.001$**	**$F = 5.809, p = 0.004$**
	80	**$F = 9.625, p < 0.001$**	**$F = 10.069, p = 0.003$**	**$F = 3.175, p = 0.047$**
	100	**$F = 4.505, p = 0.014$**	**$F = 6.705, p = 0.014$**	$F = 1.215, p = 0.302$
	120	**$F = 9.402, p < 0.001$**	**$F = 7.839, p = 0.008$**	$F = 1.403, p = 0.252$
	140	**$F = 12.770, p < 0.001$**	**$F = 7.145, p = 0.011$**	$F = 1.741, P = 0.182$
	160	**$F = 11.397, p < 0.001$**	**$F = 10.748, p = 0.002$**	$F = 0.540, p = 0.585$
	180	**$F = 5.956, p = 0.004$**	**$F = 12.059, p = 0.001$**	$F = 1.101, p = 0.338$
Alpha (8–13 Hz)	60	**$F = 5.778, p = 0.005$**	$F = 0.787, p = 0.381$	$F = 1.460, p = 0.239$
	80	**$F = 7.094, p = 0.003$**	$F = 0.069, p = 0.794$	$F = 2.152, p = 0.123$
	100	**$F = 7.320, p = 0.002$**	$F = 0.140, p = 0.711$	$F = 0.253, p = 0.777$
	120	**$F = 4.774, p = 0.015$**	$F = 0.068, p = 0.796$	$F = 0.823, p = 0.443$
	140	**$F = 9.117, p = 0.001$**	$F = 0.357, p = 0.554$	$F = 0.146, p = 0.865$
	160	**$F = 6.219, p = 0.003$**	$F = 0.135, p = 0.716$	$F = 0.048, p = 0.954$
	180	**$F = 5.470, p = 0.010$**	$F = 0.874, p = 0.356$	$F = 0.069, p = 0.934$
Beta (13–30 Hz)	60	**$F = 9.399, p < 0.001$**	$F = 3.040, p = 0.089$	$F = 2.955, p = 0.058$
	80	**$F = 10.485, p < 0.001$**	$F = 3.289, p = 0.078$	$F = 1.314, p = 0.275$
	100	**$F = 15.622, p < 0.001$**	**$F = 4.638, p = 0.038$**	**$F = 5.972, p = 0.004$**
	120	**$F = 10.008, p < 0.001$**	$F = 4.010, p = 0.052$	**$F = 3.300, p = 0.042$**
	140	**$F = 11.703, p < 0.001$**	$F = 3.106, p = 0.086$	$F = 0.900, p = 0.411$
	160	**$F = 20.484, p < 0.001$**	$F = 2.518, p = 0.121$	$F = 0.520, p = 0.597$
	180	**$F = 13.819, p < 0.001$**	$F = 2.815, p = 0.066$	$F = 1.714, p = 0.198$

Significant results are marked as bold.

frontal-central area (**Figures 5Bk,l**), while in beta band brain network, Go condition evoked stronger cortical connections than NoGo condition within central-parietal area (**Figures 5Bm,n**).

DISCUSSION

We present a thorough analysis on the task-related modulations on induced EEG activities as well as the effects caused by normal aging during a Go/NoGo task. Behaviorally, both younger and older adults showed high accuracy and negligible FARs in the Go/NoGo task, suggesting a sufficient level of inhibitory performance. Fourier analysis revealed an increase in frontal-central theta power during NoGo condition, and decreased central-parietal alpha and beta power during Go condition, which replicated previous findings in the literature. For the graph theoretical analysis on oscillatory brain networks, both age groups showed classic small-world brain networks in theta, alpha and beta bands, and older adults showed stronger task-modulated effects on small-world property than younger adults. Meanwhile, such frequency-specific modulation of brain networks were spatially segregated, indicating the differences of brain network between response inhibition and response execution. Specifically, theta-band brain network showed larger frontal-central node degree in NoGo condition than that in Go condition, whereas beta-band brain network showed larger central-parietal node degree in Go condition than that in NoGo condition. Moreover, these task-related modulations on node degree were also stronger in older adults than younger adults. Taken together, our findings indicate that the topological organization of oscillatory brain networks in theta and beta bands might serve as a hallmark for response inhibition and execution, which might become stronger and more robust due to normal aging.

Task-Related Effects on Oscillatory Brain Networks

It is commonly agreed that small-worldness implies both high local clustering and short path length, which reflects an optimal balance between local segregation and global integration of brain networks (Watts and Strogatz, 1998; Bassett and Bullmore, 2006; Rubinov and Sporns, 2010). Several studies have documented the small-world organization of oscillatory brain networks in simple motor tasks, i.e., finger or foot movements, and resting state (Bassett et al., 2006; De Vico Fallani et al., 2008; Jin et al., 2012). In this study, we further demonstrated the small-worldness of brain networks in a Go/NoGo task that requires high-level cognitive computations. More importantly, we found that the index of small-worldness (σ) was significantly different between Go condition and NoGo condition. Although previous research failed to observe significantly different small-worldness index between simple motor tasks and the resting state, there seemed to be an overall trend of decreasing small-worldness indices during a finger-tapping task compared with resting state in the beta band network (Jin et al., 2012). These results were in line with our findings of the decreased small-worldness index in Go condition than Baseline condition and NoGo condition in beta band network. In theta band, however, we observed an increase of small-worldness index in Go condition than NoGo condition. These findings indicate that the theta and beta band brain networks play different functional roles in the Go/NoGo task, which is concordant with the literature, that is, the theta-band phase synchrony is more likely to be involved in inhibitory process (NoGo; Brier et al., 2010; Muller and Anokhin, 2012;

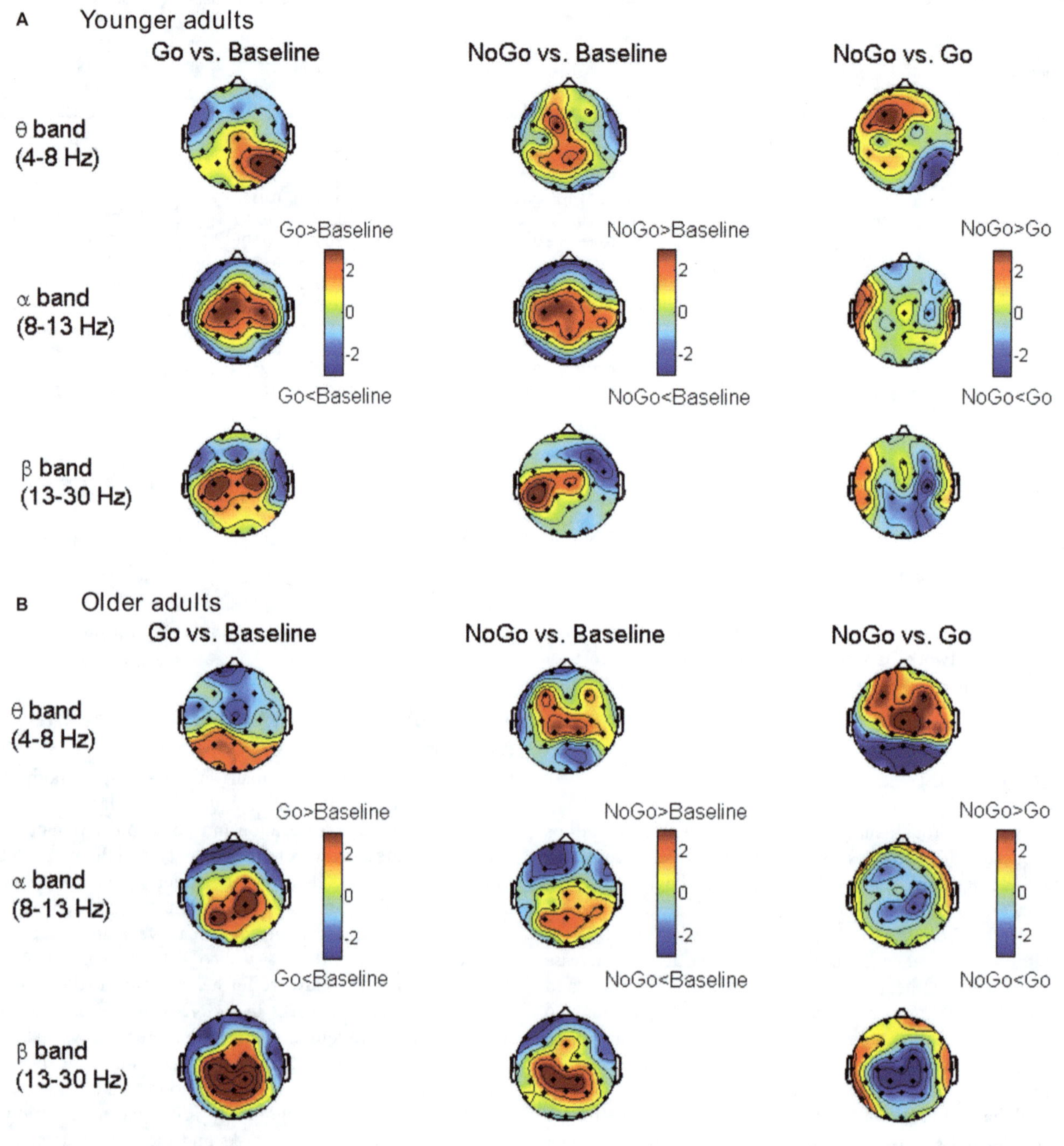

FIGURE 4 | Topographic maps for *t*-values of the node degree between different task conditions for the younger group (A) and older group (B) in different frequency bands. The results are illustrated under the network density level of 120 edges.

Anguera et al., 2013b), while the beta-band phase synchrony plays a major role in motor production (Go; Aoki et al., 2001; Brovelli et al., 2004; Jin et al., 2012).

The quantitative analysis of node degree further supported that theta- and beta-band phase synchrony played different functional roles in the Go/NoGo task. In theta band brain network, response inhibition significantly enhanced the frontal-central node degree (**Figure 5A**). This finding coincides well with the current understanding of theta oscillations, that is, frontal theta phase synchrony is commonly enhanced when more cognitive control is required (Cavanagh and Frank, 2014). On the other hand, in beta band brain network, response execution significantly enhanced the central-parietal node degree (**Figure 5B**), indicating that motor response is associated with the increase of beta-band synchrony which enhances

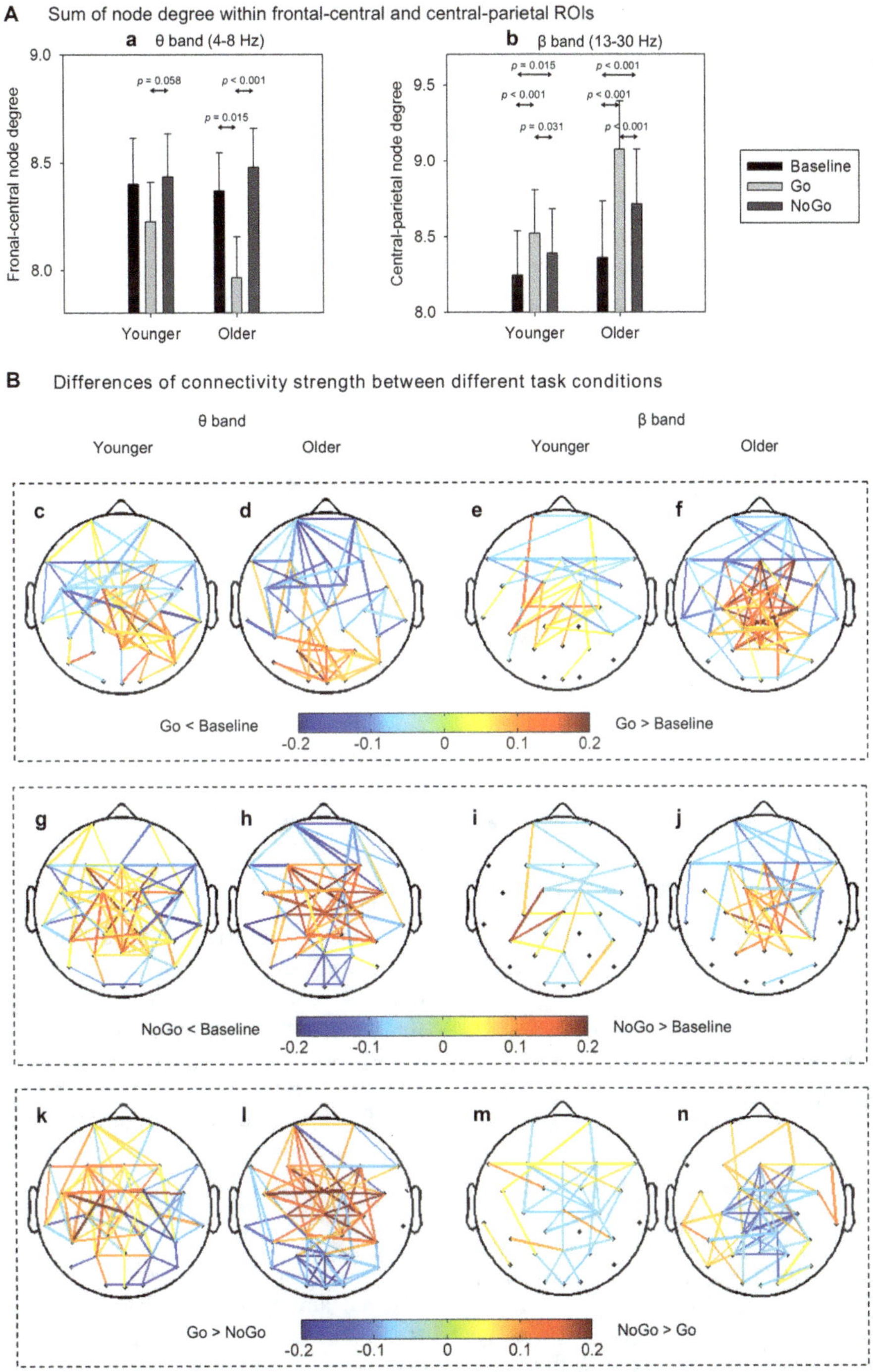

FIGURE 5 | (A) Group-averaged node degree within the frontal-central (theta band) and central-parietal (beta band) regions of interest (ROIs). Error bars indicate SEM. **(B)** Group-averaged differences of connectivity strength between different task conditions. Only the connections with absolute differences greater than 0.05 are shown in the figure. The results are illustrated under the network density level of 120 edges.

cortical connections with or within the sensorimotor areas (Mima et al., 2000; Bassett et al., 2006; Jin et al., 2012).

In theta band network, task-modulated effects on small-worldness manifested in significantly decreased clustering coefficient and increased characteristic path length in NoGo condition than that in Go condition. In the beta band network, however, the task-modulated effects on small-worldness index was only presented in the significant changes in clustering coefficient (**Figure 3**). Given that clustering coefficient and characteristic path length represent local segregation and global integration of complex networks, respectively (Watts and Strogatz, 1998; Rubinov and Sporns, 2010; Bullmore and Bassett, 2011), our findings suggest that theta band brain network involved more distant cortical connections than beta band brain network. Furthermore, this inference was also supported by the differences in connectivity strength between Go condition and NoGo condition. Specifically, task-related changes (NoGo > Go) in theta band brain network involved relatively large-scale cortical connections, including the frontal, central and parietal areas (**Figures 5Bk,l**), whereas in beta band brain network, task-related changes (Go > NoGo) in cortical connections were primarily concentrated around the sensorimotor area (**Figures 5Bm,n**).

Aging Effects on Oscillatory Brain Networks

Compared with younger adults, the small-worldness as well as task-modulated effects were well preserved in older adults. Furthermore, the task-modulated effects on node degree distribution in theta and beta band brain network were more prominent in older adults than younger adults (**Figure 5A**). There have been neuroimaging evidences that older adults could recruit more frontal activation than younger adults in cognitive control tasks, i.e., the Go/NoGo task, reflecting a functional compensation (Rajah and D'Esposito, 2005; Park and Reuter-Lorenz, 2009; Spreng et al., 2010; Heilbronner and Münte, 2013; Hong et al., 2014). Therefore, it could be inferred that normal aging not only increases the functional activation in specific regions, but also enhances the brain functional connections, which might indicate the recruitment of additional resources, and such findings are consistent with recent functional connectivity study based on functional magnetic resonance imaging (fMRI; Geerligs et al., 2014). Collectively, our findings clearly show that normal aging does not reduce, but rather enhances the neural synchrony during cognitively demanding tasks, which could shed new light on the neural mechanisms of cognitive aging when combined with the previously reported decrease in neural synchrony due to pathological aging (Pijnenburg et al., 2004; Uhlhaas and Singer, 2006; Stam et al., 2007, 2009; Knyazeva et al., 2010).

An attention-cueing Go/NoGo task with cue-target design, rather than a simple Go/NoGo task was used in this study. In such cue-target paradigm, Go/NoGo stimuli were always preceded by an instructive cue that led to increased response preparation in order to get a fast response to Go-stimulus. In this case, a prepared response had to be aborted when a NoGo-stimulus appeared at the cued location, which led to a robust response inhibition process (Bruin et al., 2001; Smith et al., 2006, 2007). Consistently, significant inhibition-related ERP components had been reported in our previous study (Hong et al., 2014). Moreover, since this study focused on response inhibition and execution, attention-related cognitive process and brain activity was not included here, which though, had been reported elsewhere (Hong et al., 2015).

In this study, the averaged ERP activity was subtracted from EEG signals before PS analysis to eliminate the effects from evoked activities that are phase-locked to the stimulus onset, i.e., N2 and P3 components. The N2 and P3 components have been widely reported to be the neural marker of response inhibition (Falkenstein et al., 1999; Albert et al., 2013; Huster et al., 2013; Hong et al., 2014). Since the ERP waves have subtracted before phase synchrony and brain network analysis, our findings suggest that task-modulated brain network constructed from induced (non-phase-locked) EEG activity could serve as another possible neural marker that is independent of conventional ERP markers. Moreover, such marker of brain network could be well preserved and even become stronger during normal aging.

One limitation in this study should be noted. Following a common approach in the literature (Dietl et al., 1999; Doppelmayr et al., 2000; Gruber et al., 2002; Deiber et al., 2009), we subtracted the averaged ERP from EEG epochs to eliminate the effects from evoked activity in this study. Such approach is based on the assumption that the same ERP is present in each single trial, which however, may be problematic. Unfortunately, extracting precise ERP activity at single trial level is still a highly challenging task, and currently there is still lack of widely accepted method in this field. Future work is required to address this limitation.

To conclude, by employing graph theoretical analysis, we thoroughly investigated the age-related differences in synchronous neural network within functionally-distinct frequency bands in a Go/NoGo task. This study explicitly demonstrated a close relationship between the frequency-specific neural synchrony and response inhibition as well as response execution. Our findings could also provide important implications into the current understanding of the neural mechanisms of cognitive aging from the perspective of synchronous brain networks.

AUTHOR CONTRIBUTIONS

XH, YL, JS and ST designed research; XH performed research; XH, YL and JS analyzed data; XH, YL and ST wrote the article.

ACKNOWLEDGMENTS

This work was supported by National Natural Science Foundation of China (No. 61571295) and Science and Technology Commission of the Shanghai Municipality (No. 13dz2260500). XH was supported by China Scholarship Council (201206230034). JS was supported in part by Med-X Research Fund of Shanghai Jiao Tong University (YG2012MS09). We thank Yixue Li for assistance with the data collection.

REFERENCES

Achard, S., and Bullmore, E. (2007). Efficiency and cost of economical brain functional networks. *PLoS Comput. Biol.* 3:e17. doi: 10.1371/journal.pcbi.0030017

Albert, J., López-Martin, S., Hinojosa, J. A., and Carretiá, L. (2013). Spatiotemporal characterization of response inhibition. *Neuroimage* 76, 272–281. doi: 10.1016/j.neuroimage.2013.03.011

Anguera, J. A., Boccanfuso, J., Rintoul, J. L., Al-Hashimi, O., Faraji, F., Janowich, J., et al. (2013a). Video game training enhances cognitive control in older adults. *Nature* 501, 97–101. doi: 10.1038/nature12486

Anguera, J. A., Lyman, K., Zanto, T. P., Bollinger, J., and Gazzaley, A. (2013b). Reconciling the influence of task-set switching and motor inhibition processes on stop signal after-effects. *Front. Psychol.* 4:649. doi: 10.3389/fpsyg.2013.00649

Aoki, F., Fetz, E. E., Shupe, L., Lettich, E., and Ojemann, G. A. (2001). Changes in power and coherence of brain activity in human sensorimotor cortex during performance of visuomotor tasks. *Biosystems* 63, 89–99. doi: 10.1016/s0303-2647(01)00149-6

Bassett, D. S., and Bullmore, E. (2006). Small-world brain networks. *Neuroscientist* 12, 512–523. doi: 10.1177/1073858406293182

Bassett, D. S., Bullmore, E. T., Meyer-Lindenberg, A., Apud, J. A., Weinberger, D. R., and Coppola, R. (2009). Cognitive fitness of cost-efficient brain functional networks. *Proc. Natl. Acad. Sci. U S A* 106, 11747–11752. doi: 10.1073/pnas.0903641106

Bassett, D. S., Meyer-Lindenberg, A., Achard, S., Duke, T., and Bullmore, E. (2006). Adaptive reconfiguration of fractal small-world human brain functional networks. *Proc. Natl. Acad. Sci. U S A* 103, 19518–19523. doi: 10.1073/pnas.0606005103

Bastiaansen, M., and Hagoort, P. (2003). Event-induced theta responses as a window on the dynamics of memory. *Cortex* 39, 967–992. doi: 10.1016/s0010-9452(08)70873-6

Brier, M. R., Ferree, T. C., Maguire, M. J., Moore, P., Spence, J., Tillman, G. D., et al. (2010). Frontal theta and alpha power and coherence changes are modulated by semantic complexity in Go/NoGo tasks. *Int. J. Psychophysiol.* 78, 215–224. doi: 10.1016/j.ijpsycho.2010.07.011

Brovelli, A., Ding, M., Ledberg, A., Chen, Y., Nakamura, R., and Bressler, S. L. (2004). Beta oscillations in a large-scale sensorimotor cortical network: directional influences revealed by Granger causality. *Proc. Natl. Acad. Sci. U S A* 101, 9849–9854. doi: 10.1073/pnas.0308538101

Bruin, K. J., Wijers, A. A., and van Staveren, A. S. (2001). Response priming in a go/nogo task: do we have to explain the go/nogo N2 effect in terms of response activation instead of inhibition? *Clin. Neurophysiol.* 112, 1660–1671. doi: 10.1016/s1388-2457(01)00601-0

Bullmore, E. T., and Bassett, D. S. (2011). Brain graphs: graphical models of the human brain connectome. *Annu. Rev. Clin. Psychol.* 7, 113–140. doi: 10.1146/annurev-clinpsy-040510-143934

Bullmore, E., and Sporns, O. (2009). Complex brain networks: graph theoretical analysis of structural and functional systems. *Nat. Rev. Neurosci.* 10, 186–198. doi: 10.1038/nrn2575

Bullmore, E., and Sporns, O. (2012). The economy of brain network organization. *Nat. Rev. Neurosci.* 13, 336–349. doi: 10.1038/nrn3214

Cabeza, R., Anderson, N. D., Locantore, J. K., and McIntosh, A. R. (2002). Aging gracefully: compensatory brain activity in high-performing older adults. *Neuroimage* 17, 1394–1402. doi: 10.1006/nimg.2002.1280

Cavanagh, J. F., and Frank, M. J. (2014). Frontal theta as a mechanism for cognitive control. *Trends Cogn. Sci.* 18, 414–421. doi: 10.1016/j.tics.2014.04.012

De Vico Fallani, F., Astolfi, L., Cincotti, F., Mattia, D., Marciani, M. G., Tocci, A., et al. (2008). Cortical network dynamics during foot movements. *Neuroinformatics* 6, 23–34. doi: 10.1007/s12021-007-9006-6

Deiber, M. P., Ibañez, V., Missonnier, P., Herrmann, F., Fazio-Costa, L., Gold, G., et al. (2009). Abnormal-induced theta activity supports early directed-attention network deficits in progressive MCI. *Neurobiol. Aging* 30, 1444–1452. doi: 10.1016/j.neurobiolaging.2007.11.021

Delorme, A., and Makeig, S. (2004). EEGLAB: an open source toolbox for analysis of single-trial EEG dynamics including independent component analysis. *J. Neurosci. Methods* 134, 9–21. doi: 10.1016/j.jneumeth.2003.10.009

Diamond, A. (2013). Executive functions. *Annu. Rev. Psychol.* 64, 135–168. doi: 10.1146/annurev-psych-113011-143750

Dietl, T., Dirlich, G., Vogl, L., Lechner, C., and Strian, F. (1999). Orienting response and frontal midline theta activity: a somatosensory spectral perturbation study. *Clin. Neurophysiol.* 110, 1204–1209. doi: 10.1016/s1388-2457(99)00057-7

Doppelmayr, M., Klimesch, W., Schwaiger, J., Stadler, W., and Röhm, D. (2000). The time locked theta response reflects interindividual differences in human memory performance. *Neurosci. Lett.* 278, 141–144. doi: 10.1016/s0304-3940(99)00925-8

Ergen, M., Saban, S., Kirmizi-Alsan, E., Uslu, A., Keskin-Ergen, Y., and Demiralp, T. (2014). Time-frequency analysis of the event-related potentials associated with the Stroop test. *Int. J. Psychophysiol.* 94, 463–472. doi: 10.1016/j.ijpsycho.2014.08.177

Falkenstein, M., Hoormann, J., and Hohnsbein, J. (1999). ERP components in Go/Nogo tasks and their relation to inhibition. *Acta Psychol. (Amst)* 101, 267–291. doi: 10.1016/s0001-6918(99)00008-6

Folstein, M. F., Folstein, S. E., and McHugh, P. R. (1975). "Mini-mental state". A practical method for grading the cognitive state of patients for the clinician. *J. Psychiatr. Res.* 12, 189–198. doi: 10.1016/0022-3956(75)90026-6

Geerligs, L., Saliasi, E., Renken, R. J., Maurits, N. M., and Lorist, M. M. (2014). Flexible connectivity in the aging brain revealed by task modulations. *Hum. Brain Mapp.* 35, 3788–3804. doi: 10.1002/hbm.22437

Grady, C. (2012). The cognitive neuroscience of ageing. *Nat. Rev. Neurosci.* 13, 491–505. doi: 10.1038/nrn3256

Gruber, T., Müller, M. M., and Keil, A. (2002). Modulation of induced gamma band responses in a perceptual learning task in the human EEG. *J. Cogn. Neurosci.* 14, 732–744. doi: 10.1162/08989290260138636

Heilbronner, U., and Münte, T. F. (2013). Rapid event-related near-infrared spectroscopy detects age-related qualitative changes in the neural correlates of response inhibition. *Neuroimage* 65, 408–415. doi: 10.1016/j.neuroimage.2012.09.066

Hong, X., Sun, J., Bengson, J. J., Mangun, G. R., and Tong, S. (2015). Normal aging selectively diminishes alpha lateralization in visual spatial attention. *Neuroimage* 106, 353–363. doi: 10.1016/j.neuroimage.2014.11.019

Hong, X., Sun, J., Bengson, J. J., and Tong, S. (2014). Age-related spatiotemporal reorganization during response inhibition. *Int. J. Psychophysiol.* 93, 371–380. doi: 10.1016/j.ijpsycho.2014.05.013

Hong, X., Sun, J., and Tong, S. (2013). Functional brain networks for sensory maintenance in top-down selective attention to audiovisual inputs. *IEEE Trans. Neural Syst. Rehabil. Eng.* 21, 734–743. doi: 10.1109/TNSRE.2013.2272219

Humphries, M. D., and Gurney, K. (2008). Network 'small-world-ness': a quantitative method for determining canonical network equivalence. *PLoS One* 3:e0002051. doi: 10.1371/journal.pone.0002051

Huster, R. J., Enriquez-Geppert, S., Lavallee, C. F., Falkenstein, M., and Herrmann, C. S. (2013). Electroencephalography of response inhibition tasks: functional networks and cognitive contributions. *Int. J. Psychophysiol.* 87, 217–233. doi: 10.1016/j.ijpsycho.2012.08.001

Jin, S. H., Lin, P., and Hallett, M. (2012). Reorganization of brain functional small-world networks during finger movements. *Hum. Brain Mapp.* 33, 861–872. doi: 10.1002/hbm.21253

Jung, T. P., Makeig, S., Westerfield, M., Townsend, J., Courchesne, E., and Sejnowski, T. J. (2000). Removal of eye activity artifacts from visual event-related potentials in normal and clinical subjects. *Clin. Neurophysiol.* 111, 1745–1758. doi: 10.1016/s1388-2457(00)00386-2

Kirmizi-Alsan, E., Bayraktaroglu, Z., Gurvit, H., Keskin, Y. H., Emre, M., and Demiralp, T. (2006). Comparative analysis of event-related potentials during Go/NoGo and CPT: decomposition of electrophysiological markers of response inhibition and sustained attention. *Brain Res.* 1104, 114–128. doi: 10.1016/j.brainres.2006.03.010

Knyazeva, M. G., Jalili, M., Brioschi, A., Bourquin, I., Fornari, E., Hasler, M., et al. (2010). Topography of EEG multivariate phase synchronization in early Alzheimer's disease. *Neurobiol. Aging* 31, 1132–1144. doi: 10.1016/j.neurobiolaging.2008.07.019

Latora, V., and Marchiori, M. (2001). Efficient behavior of small-world networks. *Phys. Rev. Lett.* 87:198701. doi: 10.1103/physrevlett.87.198701

Leocani, L., Toro, C., Manganotti, P., Zhuang, P., and Hallett, M. (1997). Event-related coherence and event-related desynchronization/synchronization in the 10 Hz and 20 Hz EEG during self-paced movements. *Electroencephalogr. Clin. Neurophysiol.* 104, 199–206. doi: 10.1016/s0168-5597(96)96051-7

Li, Y., Cao, D., Wei, L., Tang, Y., and Wang, J. (2015). Abnormal functional connectivity of EEG gamma band in patients with depression during emotional face processing. *Clin. Neurophysiol.* 126, 2078–2089. doi: 10.1016/j.clinph.2014.12.026

Lopez-Calderon, J., and Luck, S. J. (2014). ERPLAB: an open-source toolbox for the analysis of event-related potentials. *Front. Hum. Neurosci.* 8:213. doi: 10.3389/fnhum.2014.00213

Maslov, S., and Sneppen, K. (2002). Specificity and stability in topology of protein networks. *Science* 296, 910–913. doi: 10.1016/j.ijpsycho.2014.05.013

Mima, T., Matsuoka, T., and Hallett, M. (2000). Functional coupling of human right and left cortical motor areas demonstrated with partial coherence analysis. *Neurosci. Lett.* 287, 93–96. doi: 10.1016/s0304-3940(00)01165-4

Moore, R. A., Gale, A., Morris, P. H., and Forrester, D. (2008). Alpha power and coherence primarily reflect neural activity related to stages of motor response during a continuous monitoring task. *Int. J. Psychophysiol.* 69, 79–89. doi: 10.1016/j.ijpsycho.2008.03.003

Muller, V., and Anokhin, A. P. (2012). Neural synchrony during response production and inhibition. *PLoS One* 7:e38931. doi: 10.1371/journal.pone.0038931

Onnela, J. P., Saramäki, J., Kertész, J., and Kaski, K. (2005). Intensity and coherence of motifs in weighted complex networks. *Phys. Rev. E Stat. Nonlin. Soft. Matter Phys.* 71:065103. doi: 10.1103/physreve.71.065103

Park, D. C., and Reuter-Lorenz, P. (2009). The adaptive brain: aging and neurocognitive scaffolding. *Annu. Rev. Psychol.* 60, 173–196. doi: 10.1146/annurev.psych.59.103006.093656

Pfurtscheller, G., and Lopes da Silva, F. H. (1999). Event-related EEG/MEG synchronization and desynchronization: basic principles. *Clin. Neurophysiol.* 110, 1842–1857. doi: 10.1016/s1388-2457(99)00141-8

Pijnenburg, Y. A., v d Made, Y., van Cappellen van Walsum, A. M., Knol, D. L., Scheltens, P., and Stam, C. J. (2004). EEG synchronization likelihood in mild cognitive impairment and Alzheimer's disease during a working memory task. *Clin. Neurophysiol.* 115, 1332–1339. doi: 10.1016/j.clinph.2003.12.029

Rajah, M. N., and D'Esposito, M. (2005). Region-specific changes in prefrontal function with age: a review of PET and fMRI studies on working and episodic memory. *Brain* 128, 1964–1983. doi: 10.1093/brain/awh608

Rubinov, M., Knock, S. A., Stam, C. J., Micheloyannis, S., Harris, A. W., Williams, L. M., et al. (2009). Small-world properties of nonlinear brain activity in schizophrenia. *Hum. Brain Mapp.* 30, 403–416. doi: 10.1002/hbm.20517

Rubinov, M., and Sporns, O. (2010). Complex network measures of brain connectivity: uses and interpretations. *Neuroimage* 52, 1059–1069. doi: 10.1016/j.neuroimage.2009.10.003

Serrien, D. J., Orth, M., Evans, A. H., Lees, A. J., and Brown, P. (2005). Motor inhibition in patients with Gilles de la Tourette syndrome: functional activation patterns as revealed by EEG coherence. *Brain* 128, 116–125. doi: 10.1093/brain/awh318

Smith, J. L., Johnstone, S. J., and Barry, R. J. (2006). Effects of pre-stimulus processing on subsequent events in a warned Go/NoGo paradigm: response preparation, execution and inhibition. *Int. J. Psychophysiol.* 61, 121–133. doi: 10.1016/j.ijpsycho.2005.07.013

Smith, J. L., Johnstone, S. J., and Barry, R. J. (2007). Response priming in the Go/NoGo task: the N2 reflects neither inhibition nor conflict. *Clin. Neurophysiol.* 118, 343–355. doi: 10.1016/j.clinph.2006.09.027

Spreng, R. N., Wojtowicz, M., and Grady, C. L. (2010). Reliable differences in brain activity between young and old adults: a quantitative meta-analysis across multiple cognitive domains. *Neurosci. Biobehav. Rev.* 34, 1178–1194. doi: 10.1016/j.neubiorev.2010.01.009

Stam, C. J., de Haan, W., Daffertshofer, A., Jones, B. F., Manshanden, I., van Cappellen van Walsum, A. M., et al. (2009). Graph theoretical analysis of magnetoencephalographic functional connectivity in Alzheimer's disease. *Brain* 132, 213–224. doi: 10.1093/brain/awn262

Stam, C. J., Jones, B. F., Nolte, G., Breakspear, M., and Scheltens, P. (2007). Small-world networks and functional connectivity in Alzheimer's disease. *Cereb. Cortex* 17, 92–99. doi: 10.1093/cercor/bhj127

Sun, J., Hong, X., and Tong, S. (2012). Phase synchronization analysis of EEG signals: an evaluation based on surrogate tests. *IEEE Trans. Biomed. Eng.* 59, 2254–2263. doi: 10.1109/TBME.2012.2199490

Sun, Y., Lim, J., Meng, J., Kwok, K., Thakor, N., and Bezerianos, A. (2014). Discriminative analysis of brain functional connectivity patterns for mental fatigue classification. *Ann. Biomed. Eng.* 42, 2084–2094. doi: 10.1007/s10439-014-1059-8

Tallet, J., Barral, J., and Hauert, C. A. (2009). Electro-cortical correlates of motor inhibition: a comparison between selective and non-selective stop tasks. *Brain Res.* 1284, 68–76. doi: 10.1016/j.brainres.2009.05.058

Tass, P., Rosenblum, M., Weule, J., Kurths, J., Pikovsky, A., Volkmann, J., et al. (1998). Detection of n:m phase locking from noisy data: application to magnetoencephalography. *Phys. Rev. Lett.* 81, 3291–3294. doi: 10.1142/9789812793782_0004

Uhlhaas, P. J., and Singer, W. (2006). Neural synchrony in brain disorders: relevance for cognitive dysfunctions and pathophysiology. *Neuron* 52, 155–168. doi: 10.1016/j.neuron.2006.09.020

Wacker, M., and Witte, H. (2011). On the stability of the n:m phase synchronization index. *IEEE Trans. Biomed. Eng.* 58, 332–338. doi: 10.1109/TBME.2010.2063028

Watts, D. J., and Strogatz, S. H. (1998). Collective dynamics of 'small-world' networks. *Nature* 393, 440–442. doi: 10.1038/30918

Yan, J., Sun, J., Guo, X., Jin, Z., Li, Y., Li, Z., et al. (2013). Motor imagery cognitive network after left ischemic stroke: study of the patients during mental rotation task. *PLoS One* 8:e77325. doi: 10.1371/journal.pone.0077325

5

An Event-Related Potential Investigation of the Effects of Age on Alerting, Orienting, and Executive Function

David A. S. Kaufman[1], *Christopher N. Sozda*[2,3], *Vonetta M. Dotson*[2] *and William M. Perlstein*[2,3,4,5,6]*

[1] Department of Psychology, Saint Louis University, St. Louis, MO, USA, [2] Department of Clinical and Health Psychology, University of Florida, Gainesville, FL, USA, [3] Malcom Randall Veterans Administration Medical Center, Gainesville, FL, USA, [4] McKnight Brain Institute, University of Florida, Gainesville, FL, USA, [5] Departments of Psychiatry, Saint Louis University, St. Louis, MO, USA, [6] VA RR&D Brain Rehabilitation Research Center of Excellence, Malcom Randall Veterans Administration Medical Center, Gainesville, FL, USA

Edited by:
Junfeng Sun,
Shanghai Jiao Tong University, China

Reviewed by:
Yury (Juri) Kropotov,
The Institute of the Human Brain of Russian Academy of Sciences, Russia
Laura Lorenzo-López,
University of A Coruña, Spain

***Correspondence:**
William M. Perlstein
wmp@phhp.ufl.edu

The present study compared young and older adults on behavioral and neural correlates of three attentional networks (alerting, orienting, and executive control). Nineteen young and 16 older neurologically-healthy adults completed the Attention Network Test (ANT) while behavioral data (reaction time and error rates) and 64-channel event-related potentials (ERPs) were acquired. Significant age-related RT differences were observed across all three networks; however, after controlling for generalized slowing, only the alerting network remained significantly reduced in older compared with young adults. ERP data revealed that alerting cues led to enhanced posterior N1 responses for subsequent attentional targets in young adults, but this effect was weakened in older adults. As a result, it appears that older adults did not benefit fully from alerting cues, and their lack of subsequent attentional enhancements may compromise their ability to be as responsive and flexible as their younger counterparts. N1 alerting deficits were associated with several key neuropsychological tests of attention that were difficult for older adults. Orienting and executive attention networks were largely similar between groups. Taken together, older adults demonstrated behavioral and neural alterations in alerting, however, they appeared to compensate for this reduction, as they did not significantly differ in their abilities to use spatially informative cues to aid performance (e.g., orienting), or successfully resolve response conflict (e.g., executive control). These results have important implications for understanding the mechanisms of age-related changes in attentional networks.

Keywords: ANT, attentional networks, alerting, N1, aging, ERPs

INTRODUCTION

Intact attentional processes are vital for goal-directed behavior, as they guide the allocation of cognitive resources in accordance with changing environmental demands. Research from the past several decades has proposed that attention is comprised of dissociable yet interrelated anatomical and functional neural networks responsible for alerting, orienting, and executive control (Posner and Peterson, 1990; Posner and Fan, 2004). The alerting system helps us to achieve and sustain an alert state (Fernandez-Duque and Posner, 1997), which is thought to facilitate response preparation via enhanced early attentional processing. The orienting system functions to select information from sensory input, and through spatial cuing, can be manipulated to covertly direct attention (Posner, 1980; Fan et al., 2002). Lastly, executive control of attention encompasses higher-order cognitive processes needed to resolve conflict associated with the need to override a prepotent, but contextually inappropriate response (Fan et al., 2002). These executive operations are particularly crucial when situations are novel or difficult, and require response monitoring or inhibition of strong prepotent response tendencies (Fan and Posner, 2004).

In order to probe these different attentional networks, Fan et al. (2002) developed a single-trial computerized task known as the Attention Network Test (ANT). The ANT combines aspects of Posner and Peterson (1990) spatial cuing task with features of the Eriksen Flanker task (Eriksen and Eriksen, 1974), such that target flankers are spatially and/or temporally cued. Moreover, the ANT has been used to characterize the three attentional networks in studies employing behavioral (e.g., Fan et al., 2002), electrophysiological (e.g., Fan et al., 2007; Neuhaus et al., 2007), and hemodynamic (e.g., Fan et al., 2005; Posner et al., 2006) methodologies. Despite the popularity of this task, cautions have been raised about its psychometric properties. A large meta-analysis found poor split-half reliabilities within alerting and orienting network effects, along with significant inter-network correlations between the various networks (MacLeod et al., 2010). Accordingly, these attentional networks may not be as reliable or independent as initially thought, and it is important for researchers to document these psychometric properties when reporting individual study findings.

Several studies have used the ANT to examine how attentional networks are affected by aging processes; however, findings have been mixed. After controlling for the effects of generalized cognitive slowing, older adults have demonstrated weakened alerting effects, relative to younger adults (Jennings et al., 2007; Gamboz et al., 2010). In contrast, when longer cue presentation was employed, Fernandez-Duque and Black (2006) found a significantly larger alerting effect in older compared to young adults. Recent findings did not reveal significantly differing orienting effects between young and older adults (Jennings et al., 2007), a result consistent with prior literature that spatial cueing benefits older adults as much as young adults (Hartley et al., 1990; Folk and Hoyer, 1992; Greenwood et al., 1993). Regarding executive control, no significant conflict-related effects have been observed in several studies comparing older and young adults (Fernandez-Duque and Black, 2006; Jennings et al., 2007). In contrast, a more recent study suggests age-related changes may occur in the executive control network (Zhou et al., 2011). Taken together, it remains unclear whether age-related attentional declines may be confounded by cognitive slowing (Verhaeghen and De Meersman, 1998; Verhaeghen and Cerella, 2002), or other cognitive disruptions beyond slowed speed of information processing (Hartley, 1993).

Electrophysiological methodologies have provided further insight about the underlying neural mechanisms of attentional networks. In particular, studies of attentional processes (e.g., Fan et al., 2007; Neuhaus et al., 2007, 2010) have employed scalp-recorded brain event-related potentials (ERPs), which provide unmatched temporal sensitivity for examining neural correlates. Despite recent electrophysiological investigations, the alerting network has received the least focus of the three attentional networks in the literature. With the goal of examining effects of alerting cues on subsequent attentional processing, one study reported significant increases in N1 amplitude evoked by targets that followed alerting cues (Neuhaus et al., 2010). This posterior N1 component is believed to reflect early attentional facilitation of target processing, which is enhanced by valid cues that reliably predict target location (Hillyard et al., 1998).

With respect to orienting of visual attention, researchers have also observed increased amplitude of posterior negativity beginning approximately 100 ms following validly cued target stimuli (Harter et al., 1989; Hopf and Mangun, 2000; Nobre et al., 2000; Talsma et al., 2005). These results have been replicated using the ANT (Neuhaus et al., 2010), and are presumed to reflect the successful shift of selective visual attention from one stimuli to another in response to validly cued stimuli (Mangun, 1995; Hillyard et al., 1998). Neuroimaging findings suggest activation within a dorsal fronto-parietal network is strongly associated with orienting of attention (e.g., Fan et al., 2005).

Executive aspects of attention can be measured many different ways, with researchers typically targeting higher-order cognitive processes involved in conflict processing, inhibition, or decision-making. One method that has been frequently studied is the flanker task, in which compatibility of stimuli surrounding target stimuli is manipulated to vary the level of response inhibition needed. ERP investigations using the ANT in healthy young adults have revealed attenuation of posterior positivity following incongruent target stimuli (Neuhaus et al., 2007, 2010). Although the P300 is commonly observed in paradigms that probe attentional resource allocation (see Polich, 2007), it is also susceptible to conflict effects. For example, incongruent Stroop stimuli have been associated with negative deflections occurring during the P300 response time window (approximately 450 ms following stimulus onset). Although these conflict-sensitive N450 components have been shown to exhibit a more frontocentral scalp distribution (van Veen and Carter, 2002; Larson et al., 2009), cognitive/response conflict also appears to affect the more parietal-maximal P300. Consistent with the literature on the N450 component, these negative deflections during the P300 likely reflect anterior cingulate cortex (ACC) mediated conflict-resolution associated with the inhibition of a strong pre-potent response tendency (Fan et al., 2005, 2007; Neuhaus et al., 2010).

While the above results demonstrate the utility of the ANT to elucidate the presence of the three neural attentional networks, no published studies to date have examined the neural correlates of the ANT in *older* adults. Additionally, although a growing body of behavioral literature suggests age-related impairments in each attentional network, findings are mixed and often confounded by generalized slowing in older participants. Consequently, the primary aim of the current study was to use ERPs to supplement behavioral data to determine whether significant between-group neural differences are observed in the presence-and/or absence of significant behavioral deficits, as well as if neural correlates are more closely associated to behavioral findings that are corrected for generalized slowing than when uncorrected. Guided by prior electrophysiological findings of Neuhaus et al. (2007, 2010), ERP components of interest included the posterior N1 (for alerting and orienting networks), and parietal P300 (executive control network) components, which are presumed to reflect phasic alerting, orienting of attention, and processing of response conflict (executive control), respectively.

MATERIALS AND METHODS

Participants

Participants included 19 young (12 females, 7 males; mean age 22.9 ± 4.0 years) and 16 older (8 females, 8 males; mean age 64.8 ± 8.0 years) adults recruited from the community through local advertisements. All participants were right-handed, native-English speakers, and had normal or corrected-to-normal vision. Groups were matched for gender, $\chi 2_{(1)} = 0.62$, $ps > 0.43$. Although older adults reported a higher mean level of educational attainment than young adults, $t_{(33)} = -2.70$, $p < 0.02$, education did not correlate with ANT RT, error-rates, or ERP amplitudes collapsed across conditions (p's > 0.052). Education was significantly correlated with Stroop performance, $r_{(34)} = 0.49$, $p < 0.003$, however, this measure is typically only corrected for age and not education in standard clinical practice. Exclusion criteria included presence of psychiatric illness, learning disability, probable dementia or global cognitive impairment (as determined by a MMSE score <25), neurological disorders, and motor difficulties that would interfere with task performance. All participants provided written informed consent in accordance with procedures established by the University of Florida Health Science Center Institutional Review Board, and received course credit or financial compensation for their study participation.

Procedures

Cognitive and Emotional Assessment

Participants completed the following neuropsychological tests: Mini-Mental State Exam (MMSE; Folstein et al., 1975), Trail Making Test A and B (TMT; Reitan and Wolfson, 1995), Digit-Symbol Coding from the Wechsler Adult Intelligence Scale, 3rd Edition (WAIS-III; Wechsler, 1997), and Stroop Color and Word Test (ST; Golden, 1978). The Beck Depression Inventory-Second Edition (BDI-II; Beck, 1996), Geriatric Depression Scale (GDS; Yesavage et al., 1983), State-Trait Anxiety Inventory (STAI; Speilberger et al., 1983), and modified Apathy Scale (AS; Starkstein et al., 1992), were used to measure symptoms of depression, anxiety, and apathy, respectively. Demographic and neuropsychological characteristics of participants are presented in **Table 1**.

Cognitive Task and Stimuli

Participants completed a computerized experimental task identical to the procedure used by Fan et al. (2002), as depicted in **Figure 1**. Stimuli were programmed and presented using E-Prime (v.1.0, Psychology Software Tools, Inc.,). Briefly, individuals were instructed to focus on a centrally located fixation cross throughout the procedure, and to determine as

TABLE 1 | Demographic and neuropsychological data for young and older participant groups.

	Young Adults		Older Adults			Analysis	
	Mean	SD	Mean	SD	*t*	*p*	Cohen's *d*
Age (years)	22.95	4.0	64.81	8.0	−20.02	<0.001	6.81
Educational level (years)	15.05	1.2	17.13	3.1	−2.70	0.011	0.92
BDI-II score	3.05	3.2	2.88	3.0	0.16	ns	0.05
f GDS score	1.79	2.4	0.94	1.3	1.26	ns	0.43
STAI—State score	26.79	5.2	27.56	7.2	−0.37	ns	0.12
STAI –Trait score	31.10	7.3	28.50	5.2	1.20	ns	0.40
Apathy Scale score	8.10	4.8	8.81	4.6	−0.47	ns	0.15
MMSE Score	28.95	1.0	28.69	1.3	0.69	ns	0.23
Stroop Test—Word-reading	99.26	12.3	107.06	17.4	−1.55	ns	0.53
Stroop Test—Color-naming	74.37	9.0	77.50	13.8	−0.81	ns	0.27
Stroop Test—Color-word	45.31	10.1	46.19	13.4	−0.22	ns	0.08
Stroop Test—Interference	2.99	8.8	1.51	9.3	0.48	ns	0.16
Digit symbol coding (# correct)	89.89	13.1	72.87	11.6	3.95	<0.001	1.38
TMT—Part A (sec)	22.16	4.1	31.06	9.8	−3.61	0.001	1.22
TMT—Part B (sec)	50.53	18.2	67.81	27.9	−2.20	0.035	0.75
TMT—Part B minus Part A (sec)	28.37	16.9	36.75	22.2	−1.27	ns	0.43

BDI-II, Beck Depression Inventory—Second Edition; GDS, Geriatric Depression Scale; STAI, State-Trait Anxiety Inventory; MMSE, Mini-Mental State Exam; TMT, Trail Making Test.

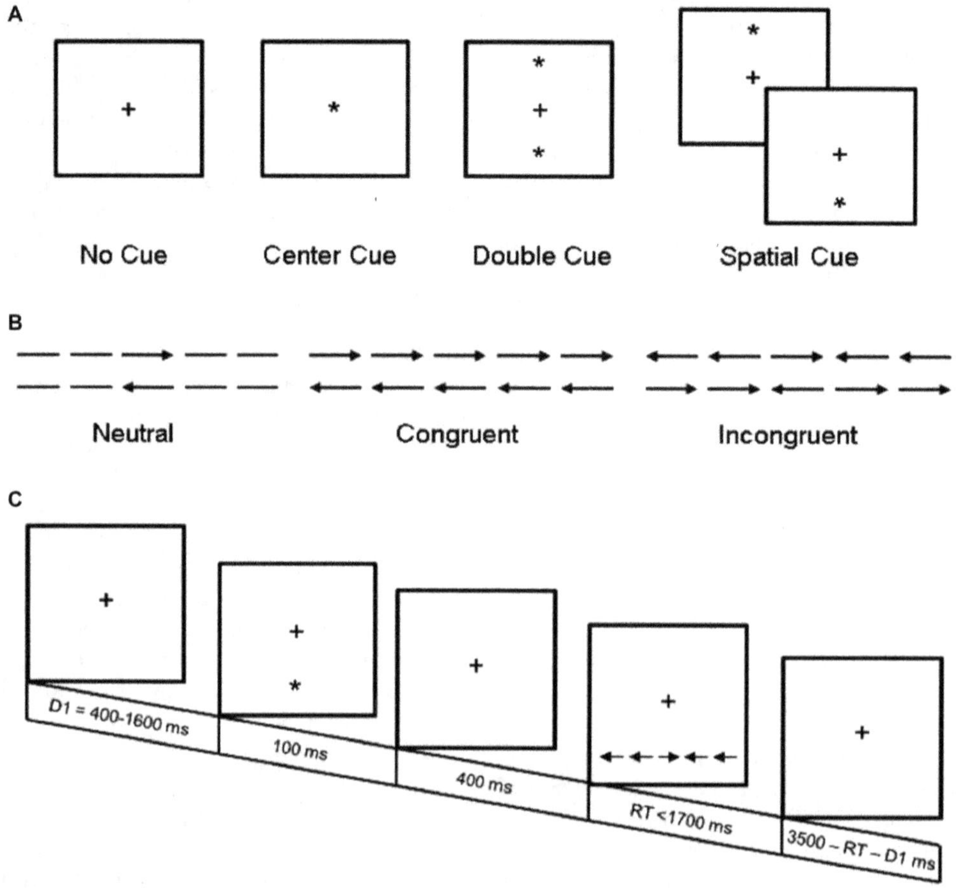

FIGURE 1 | Experimental procedure. (A) The four cue conditions, in which the asterisk cue (*) provides information about the presence (center and double cue) or location (spatial cue) of the upcoming target stimuli; **(B)** The six target stimuli used in the present experiment; and **(C)** An example trial (spatial cue—incongruent target stimuli). Adapted from Fan et al. (2002).

rapidly and accurately as possible whether the target probe, a central arrow, located above or below central fixation pointed left or right. In addition to varying target locations, on 75% of trials the target probe was preceded by different types of cues, and on 67% of trials the target probe was accompanied by congruent or incongruent flankers (which were equally frequent). The task utilized two target locations (above or below central fixation), two target directions (left or right), four cue conditions (no-cue, center-cue, double-cue and spatial-cue), and three flanker conditions (congruent, incongruent, or neutral), yielding 48 different types of trials. Each trial lasted ~4000 ms and consisted of five events: (1) random variable pre-cue fixation (400–1600 ms); (2) warning cue presentation (100 ms); (3) post-cue fixation (400 ms); (4) target and flanker presentation (self-terminating up to 1700 ms); and (5) post-target fixation (3500 ms minus duration of pre-cue fixation minus RT). Participants completed a 24-trial practice block, followed by 3-experimental blocks of 96 pseudo-random trials (2 target locations × 2 target directions × 2 repetitions × 3 flanker conditions × 4 cue conditions). Accuracy and RT feedback were provided to participants only during the practice block.

Electrophysiological Data Acquisition and Reduction

Electroencephalogram (EEG) was recorded from 64 scalp sites using a geodesic sensor net and Electrical Geodesics, Inc., (EGI; Eugene, Oregon) amplifier system (20 K gain, nominal bandpass = 0.10–100 Hz). Reported electrode sites have been renamed from the 64-channel geodesic sensor net to conform to the international 10–10 positions. Electrode placements enabled recording vertical and horizontal eye movements reflecting electro-oculographic (EOG) activity. EEG was digitized continuously at 250 Hz with a 16-bit analog-to-digital converter and referenced to Cz. A right posterior electrode served as common ground, and electrode impedances were maintained below 50 kΩ, consistent with manufacturer recommendations. Following recording, EEG data were adjusted for movement, electromyographic muscle artifact, electro-ocular eye movement, and blink artifacts using spatial filtering methods implemented through Brain Electric Source Analysis (BESA v5.1; Scherg, 1990). Single-trial EEG epochs were excluded from the averaging using threshold criteria that maximized the number of trials accepted from each individual, following the recommendations of Luck (2005). The average voltage threshold used for excluding trials was 113.86 μV

(SD = 16.89), and voltage threshold did not significantly differ between groups, $t_{(33)} = 1.46$, $p = 0.16$. Point-to-point transitions were not allowed to exceed 75 μV. Individual-subject per condition EEG epochs were separately extracted and averaged across trials from the continuous EEG recording, with epochs lasting 1600 ms (300 ms pre-cue to 800 ms post-probe including 400 ms cue-offset–probe-onset interval). Cue-locked target ERP components were examined to observe the sustained effects of cue on subsequent target processing, in replication of methods used previously (Neuhaus et al., 2010). All averaged ERP epochs were digitally filtered at 30 Hz low-pass and baseline-corrected using respective pre-stimulus windows. Peak voltage values for target-related N1 amplitude were measured bilaterally over posterior parietal scalp sites (10–10 system equivalents = P9, PO7, PO8, P10) between 176–216 ms post-target onset. Because of group-related latency differences apparent in P300 grand-average waveforms, ERPs were scored such that mean P300 amplitude was measured from 380–410 ms for young adults and 500–530 ms for older adults at central-posterior electrode sites (10–10 equivalents = CPz, Pz, and POz), averaged 30-ms symmetrically about the peak. The scoring windows for each group were determined by identifying the maximum peak amplitude of P300 within grand-averaged waveforms for each age group.

Data Analyses

Behavioral Performance Data

Statistical analyses were carried out with JMP 7.0.2 (SAS Institute Inc., Cary, NC, USA). Attention network effects and neuropsychological variables were analyzed using one-way mixed-model restricted maximum likelihood analyses of variance (REML ANOVAs; Wolfinger et al., 1994). Median correct-trial RT (Ratcliff, 1993) and arcsine transformed commission-error rates, excluding non-responses (Neter et al., 1985), were analyzed separately using 2-Group (young adults, older adults) × 3-Flanker type (incongruent, neutral, congruent) × 4-Cue type (no, spatial, double, and center) mixed-model REML ANOVAs. In order to follow up on these ANOVA results, attention network effects were calculated using the following cognitive subtractions: *alerting effect* = no-cue RT minus double-cue RT; *orienting effect* = center-cue RT minus spatial cue RT; *executive control (conflict) effect* = incongruent RT minus congruent RT. For ANOVA factors that differed by group, independent t-tests were used to compare attentional network effects between young and older adults. Additionally, to examine whether condition-related RT effects were artificially created due to generalized slowing experienced by older adults, we calculated a z-score transformation of each participant's RT by taking the mean over all conditions for a given individual, subtracting his/her condition mean from the overall mean, and dividing by the overall standard deviation across the overall mean. This method has been proven effective in identifying age-related cognitive effects independent of global slowing (Bush et al., 1993; Faust et al., 1999; Jennings et al., 2007). Finally, split-half reliabilities for each network effect were calculated by correlating data from the first and second halves of trials within each network.

ERP Data

In a manner parallel to the behavioral data, ERP activity from attention networks was analyzed using REML ANOVAs, which included the following factors: Group × Channel (N1 analyses = 10–10 equivalents P9, PO7, PO8, P10; P3 analyses = 10–10 equivalents CPz, Pz, and POz), × Condition (either double cue and no cue, spatial cue and center cue, or congruent probe and incongruent probe, depending on the attention network being analyzed). Selection of electrode sites for analyses of electrophysiological data was based on evaluation of the scalp-distribution maps in which N1 and P300 amplitudes were maximal. Interaction effects were decomposed using least-square means contrasts; and Cohen's-d effect sizes (Cohen, 1988) were calculated using pooled standard deviations for group and/or condition-related effects. ANOVAs were then followed up with the calculation of attention network effects, using the same paired subtractions that were used to generate the behavioral attention network effects. ERP network effects were derived using the following cognitive comparisons: *alerting N1 effect* = double-cue amplitude − no-cue amplitude; *orienting N1 effect* = spatial cue amplitude − center-cue amplitude; *executive control P3 ("conflict") effect* = congruent amplitude − incongruent amplitude. Group differences on these ERP network effects were analyzed using independent t-tests. Mean amplitudes for ERP network effect were then correlated with neuropsychological measures that differentiated young and older adults.

RESULTS

ANT Behavioral Performance

A Group × Flanker type × Cue type ANOVA on correct-trial median RTs revealed a significant main effect of group, $F_{(1,33)} = 38.75$, $p < 0.0001$, reflecting the expected pattern of generalized slowing in older adult participants. As expected, a significant main effect of flanker type, $F_{(2,363)} = 832.73$, $p < 0.0001$, was also observed, reflecting increased slowing when faced with incongruent flankers. Participants responded more quickly as cue types became more informative (no cue RT < center cue RT < double cue RT < spatial cue RT), as evidence by a significant main effect of cue type, $F_{(3,363)} = 137.96$, $p < 0.0001$. Additionally, a significant Group × Flanker type interaction, $F_{(2,363)} = 4.59$, $p < 0.02$, indicated that older adult participants responded significantly more slowly compared to neutral trials for both congruent and incongruent stimuli, whereas young adults only displayed slowing compared to neutral stimuli for incongruent target conditions. A Group × Cue-type interaction, $F_{(3,363)} = 5.20$, $p < 0.002$, indicated that older adults did not benefit from center cues as much as young adults. Flanker type × Cue type, $F_{(6,363)}$ = 1.47, p = 0.19, and Group × Flanker type × Cue type, $F_{(6,363)}$ = 1.54, p = 0.16, interactions were not significant.

Attention network difference scores revealed significant RT differences between groups for alerting (Young = 46 ± 25 ms; Older = 18 ± 32 ms), $F_{(1,33)}$ = 7.69, $p < 0.01$, orienting (Young = 43 ± 27 ms; Older = 87 ± 32 ms), $F_{(1,33)}$ = 19.81, $p < 0.0001$, and executive control (Young = 117 ± 22 ms; Older = 135 ± 29 ms), $F_{(1,33)}$ = 4.32, $p < 0.05$, effects. However, after normalization of RT data to account for generalized slowing experienced by older adults using z-score transformations, significant group differences remained only for the alerting effect, $F_{(1,33)}$ = 8.02, $p < 0.01$. In other words, young adults responded faster following alerting cues, but older adults did not—even after controlling for group differences in overall speed. Group differences in the orienting effect, $F_{(1,33)}$ = 0.39, $ps > 0.53$, and conflict effect $F_{(1,33)}$ = 2.39, $ps > 0.13$, were no longer significant following normalization to control for generalized slowing. Mean attention network effects, z-score transformed attention network effects, and correct-trial median RT data for both groups as a function of flanker type and cue type are summarized in **Table 2**.

Split-half reliabilities on RT data revealed that the conflict effect had the highest internal consistency ($r_{(33)} = 0.41, p < 0.05$), followed by alerting ($r_{(33)}$ = 0.37, $p < 0.05$) and orienting ($r_{(33)} = 0.29, p = 0.09$) effects. When analyzed separately by group, network reliabilities were much lower for older adults than young. Young adults had significant split-half reliabilities for the conflict ($r_{(17)} = 0.54, p < 0.05$) and alerting ($r_{(17)} = 0.48, p < 0.05$) networks, while older adults had no significant reliabilities within networks. Alerting and conflict effects were significantly correlated in younger adults ($r_{(17)} = -0.50$, $p < 0.05$), but no other cross network correlations were significant for task RT.

Regarding task performance accuracy, a Group × Flanker type × Cue type ANOVA revealed a significant main effect of flanker type, $F_{(2,363)}$ = 36.56, $p < 0.0001$, reflecting the expected larger error-rates on incongruent than congruent trials. A significant main effect of cue type $F_{(3,363)} = 4.26, p < 0.006$, was also observed, indicating greater accuracy to targets following spatial cues. The group main effect, $F_{(1,33)}$ = 0.30, p = 0.59, and Group × Congruency interaction, $F_{(2,363)}$ = 2.84, $ps > 0.06$, were not significant, suggesting equal task performance across groups regardless of task difficulty. Finally, a significant Group × Flanker type × Cue-type, $F_{(6,363)}$ = 2.17, $p < 0.05$, revealed that spatial cuing improved accuracy on incongruent trials for young, but not older adults. This finding reveals that conflict processing is improved following spatial cues for young adults only, and may suggest that older adults fail to benefit fully from spatial cueing when increased conflict is present. With regard to task accuracy, attention network difference scores did not differ as a function of group, which is likely attributable to the low error rates seen in both groups. Of additional note, a negative correlation was observed between alerting effect RT and alerting effect error rate for young adults ($r_{(17)}$ = −0.61, $p < 0.01$), suggesting that they exhibited a speed-accuracy tradeoff when engaging the alerting network. This effect was not seen in older adults ($r_{(14)}$ = −0.25, $ps > 0.35$).

ERP Components

As shown in **Table 3**, the average number of trials included in ERPs did not differ significantly between groups for target N1 alerting and orienting components. However, older adults had more trials included in the target P300 conflict component relative to younger adults.

Target N1 Alerting Effect (Double-cue vs. No-cue)

Occipito-parietal waveforms illustrating grand average ERP waveforms for the alerting effect are shown in **Figure 2**. The Group × Condition × Channel ANOVA yielded significant main effects of group, $F_{(1,33)}$ = 10.20, p = 0.0031, channel, $F_{(3,231)}$ = 6.47, p = 0.0003, and condition, $F_{(1,231)}$ = 8.96, p = 0.0031. A significant Group × Channel interaction,

TABLE 2 | Mean (± SD) attention network effects (RT), *Z*-score transformations for attention network effects, and arcsine transformed error rates as a function of flanker-type and group.

	Young Adults		Older Adults			Analysis	
	Mean	SD	Mean	SD	*t*	*p*	Cohen's *d*
Mean RT (ms)	485.16	44.9	646.44	109.6	−5.87	<0.001	1.99
Alerting effect (ms)	46.29	24.9	17.78	32.1	2.77	0.009	1.00
Orienting effect (ms)	43.08	27.0	87.41	31.9	−4.45	<0.001	1.51
Conflict effect (ms)	117.29	22.3	135.41	29.2	−2.08	0.050	0.71
Z-score RT transformations							
Alerting effect	0.68	0.34	0.27	0.50	2.83	0.008	0.98
Orienting effect	0.65	0.40	0.76	0.62	−0.63	0.540	0.21
Conflict effect	1.64	0.36	1.39	0.58	1.54	0.140	0.53
Mean error rates (%)	6.20	12.4	5.40	10.5	−0.73	ns	0.07
Congruent	1.90	6.0	2.40	7.0	0.46	ns	0.08
Incongruent	13.70	16.6	9.60	13.3	−1.59	ns	0.27
Neutral	3.00	8.1	4.20	8.8	0.79	ns	0.14

Alerting, no cue (RT) minus double cue (RT); Orienting, center cue (RT) minus spatial cue (RT); Conflict, incongruent (RT) minus congruent (RT).

TABLE 3 | Mean (± SD) number of ERP segments comprising each component, as a function of group.

	Young Adults		Older Adults		Analysis		
	Mean	SD	Mean	SD	*t*	*p*	Cohen's *d*
ERP Component							
Target N1 Alerting	43.82	10.24	49.66	9.87	−1.71	0.10	0.59
Target N1 Orienting	44.50	10.97	49.53	9.73	−1.42	0.16	0.49
Target P300 Conflict	57.95	13.04	68.63	11.62	−2.53	0.02	0.88

$F_{(3,231)} = 4.04$, $p = 0.0079$, indicated that voltages did not significantly differ between any channels for older adults, however, young adults demonstrated significantly greater voltage fluctuations between channels. A Group × Condition interaction, $F_{(1,231)} = 15.07$, $p < 0.0001$, revealed that young adults demonstrated larger N1 amplitude for double cues relative to no cue, $t_{(18)} = 1.90$, $p = 0.001$, $d = 0.90$, while older adults showed no difference between these two cue conditions, $t_{(15)} = -0.25$, $ps > 0.54$. Attention network difference scores calculated from peak amplitudes supported these ANOVA results with significant N1 alerting amplitude differences between groups, Young = -2.58 ± 2.62 μV; Older = 0.17 ± 1.35 μV, $t_{(33)} = 3.99$, $p < 0.001$, suggesting that young adults demonstrated a strong alerting effect on N1 amplitude, while older adults did not.

Target N1 Orienting Effect (Spatial-cue vs. Center-cue)

Occipito-parietal waveforms illustrating grand average ERP waveforms for the orienting effect are shown in **Figure 3**. The Group × Condition × Channel ANOVA yielded significant main effects of group, $F_{(1,33)} = 14.22$, $p = 0.0006$, condition, $F_{(1,231)} = 8.35$, $p = 0.0042$, and channel, $F_{(3,231)} = 3.59$, $p < 0.015$. The main effect of group reflected significantly smaller N1 amplitude in older compared to young adults, while increased amplitude to spatial vs. center cue was revealed in the main effect of condition. The effect of channel revealed greatest amplitude at PO7 and smallest amplitude at P10. No significant interactions were observed ($ps > 0.09$). Furthermore, attention network difference scores calculated from peak N1 orienting amplitudes revealed no group differences ($p > 0.09$).

Target P300 Conflict Effect (Congruent vs. Incongruent)

Parietal waveforms illustrating conflict-related target processing are illustrated in **Figure 4**. The Group × Condition × Channel ANOVA yielded significant main effects of group, $F_{(1,33)} = 11.90$, $p = 0.0016$, condition, $F_{(1,165)} = 39.32$, $p < 0.0001$, and channel, $F_{(2,165)} = 4.02$, $p < 0.02$. The main effect of group reflected significantly smaller P300 amplitude collapsed across target conditions in older compared to young adults, while reduced amplitude to incongruent vs. congruent cue was revealed in the main effect of condition. The effect of channel revealed greatest amplitude at CPz and smallest amplitude at

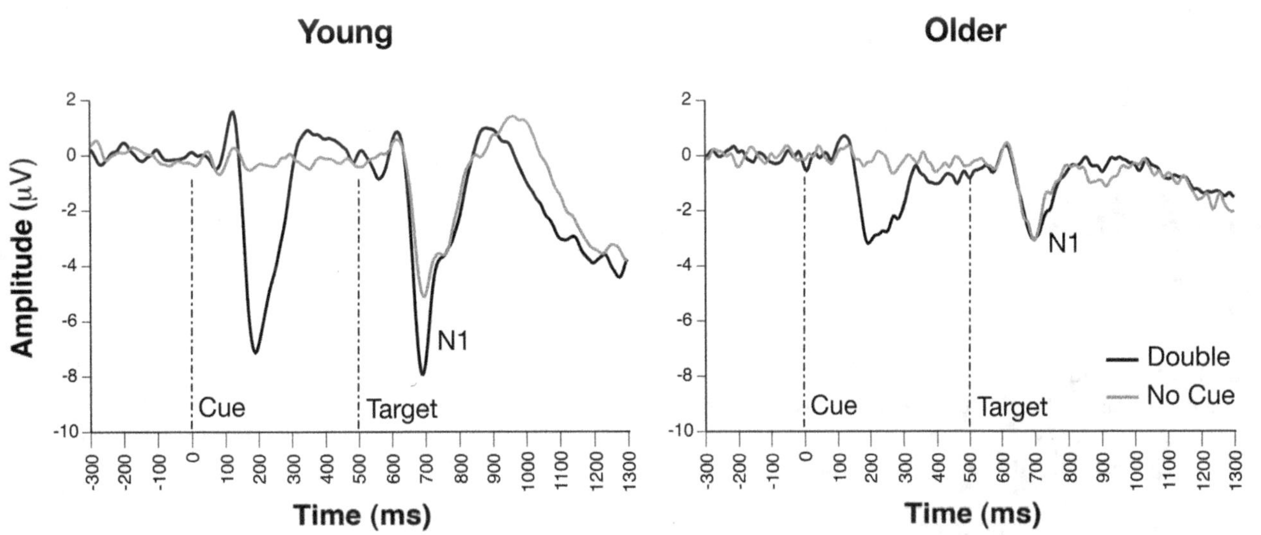

FIGURE 2 | Grand average event-related potential (ERP), waveforms of cue- and probe-locked double and no cue trials, revealing group differences on alerting effects on target-related N1 amplitudes (channel PO7).

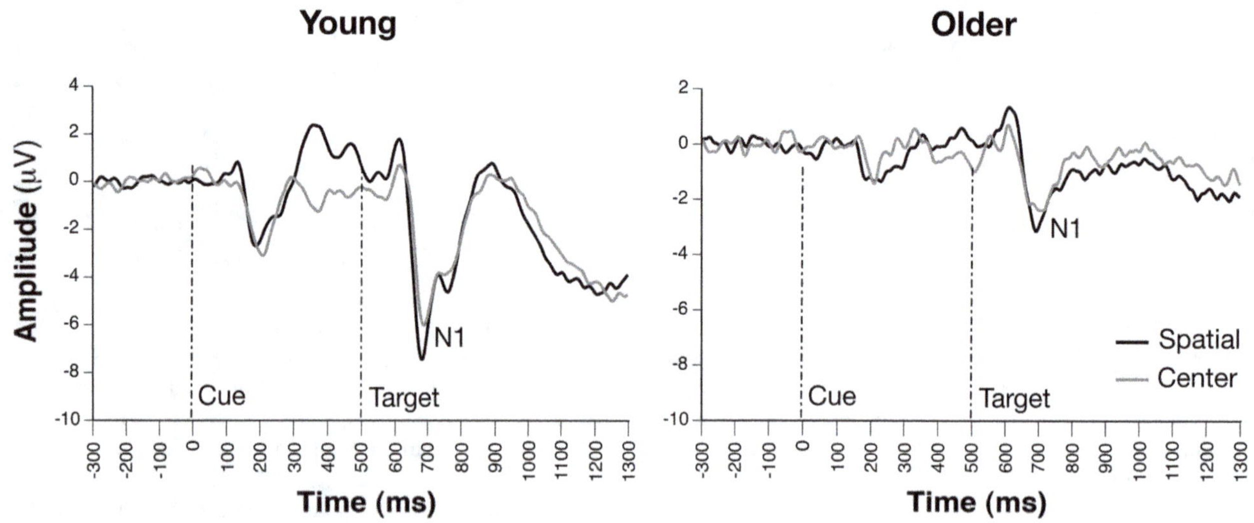

FIGURE 3 | Grand average ERP waveforms of cue- and probe-locked spatial and center cue trials, revealing similar orienting effects on target-related N1 amplitudes between groups (channel PO7).

POz. No significant interactions were observed (*ps* > 0.37). Additionally, attention network difference scores calculated from peak P300 conflict amplitudes revealed no group differences ($p > 0.90$).

Relationships Between Behavioral and ERP Attention Network Effects

Mean N1 alerting amplitude taken from the channel with maximal amplitude (PO7) was not correlated with RT alerting effects (no cue − double cue), but N1 alerting amplitude was significantly correlated with performance on Digit Symbol Coding ($r_{(33)} = -0.50$, $p < 0.01$), Trails A ($r_{(33)} = 0.52$, $p = 0.001$), and Trails B ($r_{(33)} = 0.42$, $p = 0.01$). Mean N1 orienting amplitude (taken from PO7) was not correlated with RT orienting effects (center cue − spatial cue) or any other neuropsychological variables. Mean P300 conflict amplitude (taken from Pz) was not correlated with RT conflict effects (incongruent − congruent) or any other neuropsychological variables.

DISCUSSION

This study employed behavioral measures and high-density ERPs to probe age-related changes in the functioning of three attentional networks (alerting, orienting, and executive control). After controlling for effects of generalized slowing, only the alerting network remained significantly different in older compared with young adults, as suggested by limited facilitation of RT when provided with a double cue compared to no cue. With respect to ERP correlates of alerting, double cues significantly enhanced target-related N1 amplitude relative to the no-cue condition in young adults, consistent with prior findings of enhanced early attentional processing of targets following alerting cues (Neuhaus et al., 2010). While this N1 alerting effect was pronounced in younger adults, it was completely absent in older adults. These results support prior findings that early attentional processes reflected in the N1 are attenuated in older adults (Ford et al., 1995; Golub et al., 2001). Even more importantly, N1 alerting amplitude during the ANT was correlated with performance on three neuropsychological measures of controlled attention (i.e., Digit-Symbol Coding, Trails A and B) that differentiated older and younger adults. These findings reveal a unique vulnerability of the alerting network in aging, and suggest that compromised alerting in older adults is associated with broader difficulties in controlled attention.

While older adults demonstrated difficulty in using alerting cues to prepare for subsequent events, they were not impaired in their ability to use spatially informative cues to aid performance (orienting), or in their ability to successfully resolve response conflict (executive control). These results parallel the findings of other studies (e.g., Jennings et al., 2007; Gamboz et al., 2010) that also found age-related declines in the alerting network but intact functioning in other networks, after generalized slowing was taken into account. With regard to performance accuracy, both young and older participants committed significantly more errors during the more difficult incongruent flanker condition vs. neutral and congruent conditions. However, error rates did not significantly differ between groups, suggesting that older adults successfully inhibited strong prepotent response tendencies as well as their younger peers. Despite this, there were group differences in the relationship between error rate and response time for the alerting effect. While young adults adopted a strong speed-accuracy tradeoff when engaging the alerting network, older adults did not show this tendency. This finding is consistent with prior research on the speed-accuracy tradeoff in aging (Forstmann et al., 2011), which has suggested that older adults

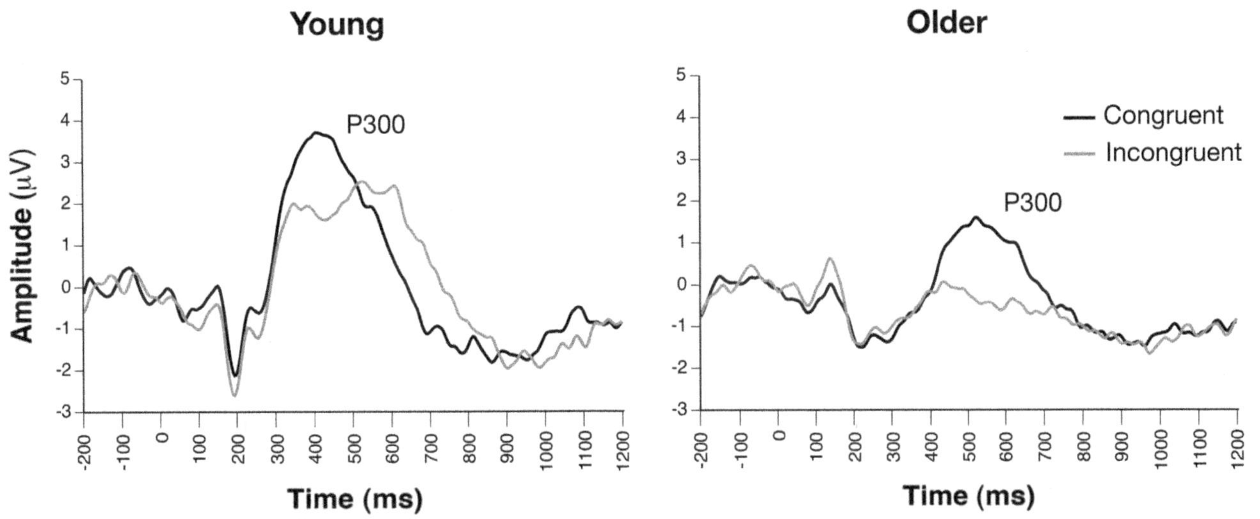

FIGURE 4 | Grand average ERP waveforms of target-locked congruent and incongruent trials, revealing similar conflict effects on target-related P300 amplitudes between groups (channel Pz).

may have difficulty speeding up their response tendencies due to disrupted brain connections (particularly in corticostriatal pathways).

Regarding ERP correlates of visual orienting of attention, spatial cues were found to significantly enhance N1 amplitude vs. center cues in both young and older adult participants. Both groups appeared to engage neural processes underlying the orienting of attention and subsequent processing of target information equally well. These results also imply that valid cueing was beneficial and had a lasting effect on subsequent processing of target stimuli, a result consistent with other ERP examinations of the ANT demonstrating enhanced N1 during attentional orienting (Neuhaus et al., 2010), as well as studies of orienting of visual attention which found similar enhancements in N1-like posterior negativities following validly-cued target stimuli (Harter et al., 1989; Hopf and Mangun, 2000; Nobre et al., 2000; Talsma et al., 2005). Such results also suggest that although older adults may demonstrate less efficient response preparation as evidenced by reduced alerting, they are still able to shift attentional resources under the guidance of spatially informative cues.

Finally, examination of target-related conflict P300 revealed that both young and older adults showed significant and equivalent P300 amplitude reductions to incongruent vs. congruent target stimuli. Older adults did show reduced P300 amplitudes overall, as has been shown previously (e.g., Fjell and Walhovd, 2001); however, this group effect did not interact with target congruency. Thus, older adults engaged similar mechanisms of conflict processing and their cortical systems underlying inhibitory processes were relatively intact. Whereas this study is to the best of our knowledge the first to employ ERPs to examine the ANT in older adults, our young adult data support recent ERP studies of the ANT that have demonstrated P300 reductions to incongruent vs. congruent target stimuli (e.g., Neuhaus et al., 2007, 2010). Similar congruency effects have been observed in Stroop paradigms (Zurrón et al., 2009), which have been interpreted in the context of well-replicated reductions in posterior P300 amplitude as task difficulty increases (Polich, 1987; Katayama and Polich, 1998). Given these consistent findings across different paradigms, it appears that reductions in P300 amplitudes reflect a disrupted allocation of attention that is associated with processing incongruent stimuli relative to congruent stimuli. Importantly, our findings suggest that congruency effects on P300 amplitudes are present in both young and older adults.

Taken together, our findings revealed significant behavioral and neural alterations of the alerting network in older adults. Cues designed to facilitate an alerting response were less effective in older than young adults. While alerting cues enhanced subsequent ERP reflections of attentional processing in younger adults, older adults did not show this effect. In fact, reductions in the N1 alerting effect in older adults help to account for broader age-related neuropsychological declines in attention. By contrast, ERP correlates of orienting and executive control networks reflected generalized amplitude reductions consistent with normal aging. These novel findings reveal that aging does not impact all networks of attention equally, but is uniquely associated with impairments in attentional alerting.

With regard to study limitations, the version of the ANT used in this study did not include an "invalid" spatial cueing condition, which would have enabled us to examine the full complement of engagement *and* disengagement of attentional orienting. Thus, we cannot interpret our results in terms of potential age-related deficits in disengagement (c.f., Shulman et al., 2010). Recently, several investigators have included invalid cues in their ANT paradigms, and have noted both beneficial and detrimental effects on the ability to overcome response conflict following valid and invalid cues, respectively (e.g., Fan et al., 2009). Specifically, whereas valid cues likely enhance prepotent stimulus processing and effective shifting (i.e., orienting) of attention, invalid cueing conditions likely require the re-direction of attentional processes and the use of additional resources for conflict resolution. Consequently, future studies should investigate the differential effects of cue-validity on early ERP components, which have been found to be differentially sensitive to the effects of valid and invalid cueing conditions (e.g., Wright et al., 1995; Talsma et al., 2005). Similarly, the use of vertical, rather than lateralized cueing may have obscured orienting effects, as evidenced by small N1 to the spatial vs. center-cue conditions. Future ERP studies of orienting may benefit from use of lateralized attention network paradigms used in previous behavioral studies (e.g., Greene et al., 2008).

A broader problem associated with the ANT is the use of cognitive subtractions. For example, the alerting effect is typically assumed to reflect a contrast between two similar cognitive states that are differentiated only by cues. However, the condition in which no cue is provided may create additional difficulty for participants, as they do not know which type of stimulus will be presented next (Galvao-Carmona et al., 2014). By contrast, the appearance of the double cue removes uncertainty about the upcoming stimulus, particularly when these cues are always valid. Thus, a differential cognitive load may develop and interact with participant expectations during these trials, rendering a simplistic cognitive subtraction inadequate. In the current study, the additional analysis of ERP correlates in a factorial design produced ANOVA results that supported the findings of the cognitive subtractions, suggesting that the observed alerting effects cannot be dismissed as a simplistic comparison of two conditions.

An additional limitation was that our sample size was relatively small, which may have introduced variability and influenced our ability to detect significant differences. Finally, both groups of participants performed the task with very high accuracy. The near-ceiling performance accuracy precludes our ability to examine task errors on the ANT more fully, given their low frequency and non-normal distribution. Insufficient numbers of trials also hindered our ability to separately examine the neural reflections of each congruency condition as a function of cue condition. Instead, target congruency had to be collapsed across conditions in order to observe the effects of cue, which may have masked potentially meaningful insights about the interactions between cues and subsequent attentional targets.

SUMMARY AND CONCLUSIONS

The current study examined age-related differences on the behavioral and neural correlates of three attentional networks (alerting, orienting, and executive control). Results revealed significant behavioral and ERP alterations in the alerting system of healthy older adults, even after controlling for generalized slowing and amplitude reductions. It appears that older adults had selective difficulty engaging the alerting network of attention, which prevented efficient facilitation of attention and subsequent responding. However, there is good news for those feeling "antsy" about age effects on attentional networks, as older adults did not exhibit behavioral or neural differences in orienting and executive control networks. As such, older adults may not be as efficiently alerted to upcoming information, yet they are equally capable in other aspects of attentional function. As the world's population ages, these results have important implications for our understanding of healthy aging.

ETHICS STATEMENT

The study was approved by the University of Florida, Health Sciences Institutional Review Board.

AUTHOR CONTRIBUTIONS

DASK was responsible for experimental design, data collection, and manuscript preparation. CNS was responsible for data collection, data analysis, and manuscript preparation. VMD was responsible for manuscript preparation. WMP was responsible for manuscript preparation.

REFERENCES

Beck, A. T. (1996). *Beck Depression Inventory - Second Edition (BDI-II).* San Antonio, TX, USA: The Psychological Corporation.

Bush, L., Hess, U., and Wolford, G. (1993). Transformations for within-subject designs: a monte carlo investigation. *Psychol. Bull.* 113, 566–579. doi: 10.1037/0033-2909.113.3.566

Cohen, J. (1988). *Statistical Power Analysis for the Behavioral Sciences.* Hillsdale, NJ: Erlbaum Associates.

Eriksen, B. A., and Eriksen, C. W. (1974). Effects of noise letters upon the identification of a target letter in a nonsearch task. *Percept. Psychophys.* 16, 143–149. doi: 10.3758/bf03203267

Fan, J., Byrne, J., Worden, M. S., Guise, K. G., McCandliss, B. D., Fossella, J., et al. (2007). The relation of brain oscillations to attentional networks. *J. Neurosci.* 27, 6197–6206. doi: 10.1523/JNEUROSCI.1833-07.2007

Fan, J., Gu, X., Guise, K. G., Liu, X., Fossella, J., Wang, H., et al. (2009). Testing the behavioral interaction and integration of attentional networks. *Brain Cogn.* 70, 209–220. doi: 10.1016/j.bandc.2009.02.002

Fan, J., Hof, P. R., Guise, K. G., Fossella, J. A., and Posner, M. I. (2007). The functional integration of the anterior cingulate cortex during conflict processing. *Cereb. Cortex* 187, 796–805. doi: 10.1093/cercor/bhm125

Fan, J., McCandliss, B. D., Fossella, J., Flombaum, J. I., and Posner, M. I. (2005). The activation of attentional networks. *Neuroimage* 26, 471–479. doi: 10.1016/j.neuroimage.2005.02.004

Fan, J., McCandliss, B. D., Sommers, T., Raz, A., and Posner, M. I. (2002). Testing the efficiency and independence of attentional networks. *J. Cogn. Neurosci.* 14, 340–347. doi: 10.1162/089892902317361886

Fan, J., and Posner, M. (2004). Human attentional networks. *Psychiatr. Prax.* 31, S210–S214. doi: 10.1055/s-2004-828484

Faust, M. E., Balota, D. A., Spieler, D. H., and Ferraro, F. R. (1999). Individual differences in information processing rate and amount: implications for group differences in response latency. *Psychol. Bull.* 125, 777–799. doi: 10.1037/0033-2909.125.6.777

Fernandez-Duque, D., and Black, S. E. (2006). Attentional networks in normal aging and Alzheimer's disease. *Neuropsychology* 20, 133–143. doi: 10.1037/0894-4105.20.2.133

Fernandez-Duque, D., and Posner, M. I. (1997). Relating the mechanisms of orienting and alerting. *Neuropsychologia* 35, 477–486. doi: 10.1016/s0028-3932(96)00103-0

Fjell, A. M., and Walhovd, K. B. (2001). P300 and neuropsychological tests as measures of aging: scalp topography and cognitive changes. *Brain Topogr.* 14, 25–40. doi: 10.1023/A:1012563605837

Folk, C. L., and Hoyer, W. J. (1992). Aging and shifts of visual spatial attention. *Psychol. Aging* 7, 453–465. doi: 10.1037/0882-7974.7.3.453

Folstein, M. F., Folstein, S. E., and McHugh, P. R. (1975). "Mini-mental state": a practical method for grading the cognitive state of patients for the clinician. *J. Psychiatr. Res.* 12, 189–198. doi: 10.1016/0022-3956(75)90026-6

Ford, J. M., Roth, W. T., Isaacks, B. G., White, P. M., Hood, S. H., and Pfefferbaum, A. (1995). Elderly men and women are less responsive to startling noises: N1, P3 and blink evidence. *Biol. Psychol.* 39, 57–80. doi: 10.1016/0301-0511(94)00959-2

Forstmann, B. U., Tittgemeyer, M., Wagenmakers, E. J., Derrfus, J., Imperait, E., and Brown, S. (2011). The speed-accuracy tradeoff in the elderly brain: a structural model-based approach. *J. Neurosci.* 31, 17242–17249. doi: 10.1523/JNEUROSCI.0309-11.2011

Galvao-Carmona, A., González-Rosa, J. J., Hidalgo-Muñoz, A. R., Parámo, D., Benétez, M. L., Izquierdo, G., et al. (2014). Disentangling the attention network test: behavioral, event related potentials and neural source analysis. *Front. Hum. Neurosci.* 8:813. doi: 10.3389/fnhum.2014.00813

Gamboz, N., Zamarian, S., and Cavellero, C. (2010). Age-related differences in the attention network test (ANT). *Exp. Aging Res.* 36, 287–305. doi: 10.1080/0361073X.2010.484729

Golden, C. J. (1978). *Stroop Color and Word Test.* Chicago: Stoelting.

Golub, E. J., Miranda, G. G., Johnson, J. K., and Starr, A. (2001). Sensory cortical interactions in aging, mild cognitive impairment and Alzheimer's disease. *Neurobiol. Aging* 22, 755–763. doi: 10.1016/s0197-4580(01)00244-5

Greene, D. J., Barnea, A., Herzberg, K., Rassis, A., Neta, M., Raz, A., et al. (2008). Measuring attention in the hemispheres: the lateralized attention network test (LANT). *Brain Cogn.* 66, 21–31. doi: 10.1016/j.bandc.2007.05.003

Greenwood, P. M., Parasuraman, R., and Haxby, J. V. (1993). Visuospatial attention across the adult lifespan. *Neuropsychologia* 31, 471–485. doi: 10.1016/0028-3932(93)90061-4

Harter, M. R., Miller, S. L., Price, N. J., LaLonde, M. E., and Keyes, A. L. (1989). Neural processes involved in directing attention. *J. Cogn. Neurosci.* 1, 223–237. doi: 10.1162/jocn.1989.1.3.223

Hartley, A. A. (1993). Evidence for the selective preservation of spatial selective attention in old age. *Psychol. Aging* 8, 371–379. doi: 10.1037/0882-7974.8.3.371

Hartley, A. A., Kieley, J. M., and Slabach, E. H. (1990). Age differences and similarities in the effects of cues and prompts. *J. Exp. Psychol. Hum. Percept. Perform.* 16, 523–537. doi: 10.1037/0096-1523.16.3.523

Hillyard, S. A., Vogel, E. K., and Luck, S. J. (1998). Sensory gain control (amplification) as a mechanism of selective attention: electrophysiological and neuroimaging evidence. *Philos. Trans. R. Soc. Lond. B Biol. Sci.* 353, 1257–1270. doi: 10.1098/rstb.1998.0281

Hopf, J. M., and Mangun, G. R. (2000). Shifting attention in space: an electrophysiological analysis using high spatial resolution mapping. *Clin. Neurophysiol.* 111, 1241–1257. doi: 10.1016/s1388-2457(00)00313-8

Jennings, J. M., Dagenbach, D., Engle, C. M., and Funke, L. J. (2007). Age-related changes and the attention network task: an examination of alerting, orienting and executive function. *Neuropsychol. Dev. Cogn. B Aging Neuropsychol. Cogn.* 14, 353–369. doi: 10.1080/13825580600788837

Katayama, J., and Polich, J. (1998). Stimulus context determines P3a and P3b. *Psychophysiology* 35, 23–33. doi: 10.1111/1469-8986.3510023

Larson, M. J., Kaufman, D. A., and Perlstein, W. M. (2009). Neural time course of conflict adaptation effects on the Stroop task. *Neuropsychologia* 47, 663–670. doi: 10.1016/j.neuropsychologia.2008.11.013

Luck, S. J. (2005). *An Introduction to the Event-Related Potential Technique* Cambridge, MA: MIT Press.

MacLeod, J. W., Lawrence, M. A., McConnell, M. M., Eskes, G. A., Klein, R. M., and Shore, D. I. (2010). Appraising the ANT: psychometric and theoretical considerations of the attention network test. *Neuropsychology* 24, 637–651. doi: 10.1037/a0019803

Mangun, G. R. (1995). Neural mechanisms of visual selective attention. *Psychophysiology* 32, 4–18. doi: 10.1111/j.1469-8986.1995.tb03400.x

Neter, J., Wasserman, W., and Kutner, M. H. (1985). *Applied Linear Statistical Models: Regression, Analysis of Variance and Experimental Designs.* 2nd Edn. Homewood, IL: R.D. Irwin.

Neuhaus, A. H., Koehler, S., Opgen-Rhein, C., Urbanek, C., Hahn, E., and Dettling, M. (2007). Selective anterior cingulate cortex deficit during conflict solution in schizophrenia: an event-related potential study. *J. Psychiatr. Res.* 41, 635–644. doi: 10.1016/j.jpsychires.2006.06.012

Neuhaus, A. H., Urbanek, C., Opgen-Rhein, C., Hahn, E., Ta, T. M. T., Koehler, S., et al. (2010). Event-related potentials associated with Attention Network Test. *Int. J. Psychophysiol.* 76, 72–79. doi: 10.1016/j.ijpsycho.2010.02.005

Nobre, A. C., Sebestyen, G. N., and Miniussi, C. (2000). The dynamics of shifting visuospatial attention revealed by event-related potentials. *Neuropsychologia* 38, 964–974. doi: 10.1016/s0028-3932(00)00015-4

Polich, J. (1987). Task difficulty, probability and inter-stimulus interval as determinants of P300 from auditory stimuli. *Electroencephalogr. Clin. Neurophysiol.* 68, 311–320. doi: 10.1016/0168-5597(87)90052-9

Polich, J. (2007). Updating P300: an integrative theory of P3a and P3b. *Clin. Neurophysiol.* 118, 2128–2148. doi: 10.1016/j.clinph.2007.04.019

Posner, M. I. (1980). Orienting of attention. *Q. J. Exp. Psychol.* 32, 3–25.

Posner, M. I., and Fan, J. (2004). "Attention as an organ system," in *Topics in Integrative Neuroscience: From Cells to Cognition*, eds J. R. Pomerantz and M. C. Crair (Cambridge: Cambridge University Press), 31–61.

Posner, M. I., and Peterson, S. E. (1990). The attention system of the human brain. *Annu. Rev. Neurosci.* 13, 25–42. doi: 10.1146/annurev.neuro.13.1.25

Posner, M. I., Sheese, B. E., Odludaş, Y., and Tang, Y. (2006). Analyzing and shaping human attentional networks. *Neural Netw.* 19, 1422–1429. doi: 10.1016/j.neunet.2006.08.004

Ratcliff, R. (1993). Methods for dealing with reaction time outliers. *Psychol. Bull.* 114, 510–532. doi: 10.1037/0033-2909.114.3.510

Reitan, R. M., and Wolfson, D. (1995). Category test and trail making test as measures of frontal lobe functions. *Clin. Neuropsychol.* 9, 50–56. doi: 10.1080/13854049508402057

Scherg, M. (1990). "Fundamentals of dipole source potential analysis," in *Auditory Evoked Magnetic Fields and Electric Potentials. Advances in Audiology*, (Vol. 6) eds F. Grandori and M. Hoke (Basel: Karger), 65–78.

Shulman, G. L., Pope, D. L., Astafiev, S. V., McAvoy, M. P., Snyder, A. Z., and Corbetta, M. (2010). Right hemisphere dominance during spatial selective attention and target detection occurs outside the dorsal frontoparietal network. *J. Neurosci.* 30, 3640–3651. doi: 10.1523/JNEUROSCI.4085-09.2010

Speilberger, C. D., Gorusch, R. L., Lushene, R., Vagg, P. R., and Jacobs, G. A. (1983). *Manual for the State-Trait Anxiety Inventory.* Palo Alto, CA: Consulting Psychologists Press.

Starkstein, S. E., Mayberg, H. S., Preziosi, T. J., Andrezejewski, P., Leiguarda, R., and Robinson, R. G. (1992). Reliability, validity and clinical correlates of apathy in Parkinson's disease. *J. Neuropsychiatry Clin. Neurosci.* 4, 134–139. doi: 10.1176/jnp.4.2.134

Talsma, D., Slagter, H. A., Nieuwenhuis, S., Hage, J., and Kok, A. (2005). The orienting of visuospatial attention: an event-related potential study. *Brain Res. Cogn. Brain Res.* 25, 117–129. doi: 10.1016/j.cogbrainres.2005.04.013

van Veen, V., and Carter, C. S. (2002). The anterior cingulate as a conflict monitor: fMRI and ERP studies. *Physiol. Behav.* 77, 477–482. doi: 10.1016/s0031-9384(02)00930-7

Verhaeghen, P., and Cerella, J. (2002). Aging, executive control and attention: a review of meta-analyses. *Neurosci. Biobehav. Rev.* 26, 849–857. doi: 10.1016/s0149-7634(02)00071-4

Verhaeghen, P., and De Meersman, L. (1998). Aging and the Stroop effect: a meta-analysis. *Psychol. Aging* 13, 120–126. doi: 10.1037/0882-7974.13.1.120

Wechsler, D. A. (1997). *Wechsler Adult Intelligence Scale.* 3rd Edn. San Antonio, TX: The Psychological Corporation.

Wolfinger, R., Tobias, R., and Sall, J. (1994). Computing gaussian likelihoods and their derivatives for general linear mixed models. *SIAM J. Sci. Comput.* 15, 1294–1310. doi: 10.1137/0915079

Wright, M. J., Geffen, G. M., and Geffen, L. B. (1995). Event-related potentials during covert orientation of visual-attention: effects of cue validity and directionality. *Biol. Psychol.* 41, 183–202. doi: 10.1016/0301-0511(95)05128-7

Yesavage, J. A., Brink, T. L., Rose, T. L., Lum, O., Huang, V., Adey, M., et al. (1983). Development and validation of a geriatric depression screening scale: a preliminary report. *J. Psychiatr. Res.* 17, 37–49. doi: 10.1016/0022-3956(82)90033-4

Zhou, S. S., Fan, J., Lee, T. M., Wang, C. Q., and Wang, K. (2011). Age-related differences in attentional networks of alerting and executive control in young, middle-aged, and older Chinese adults. *Brain Cogn.* 75, 205–210. doi: 10.1016/j.bandc.2010.12.003

Zurrón, M., Pousoa, M., Lindína, M., Galdoa, S., and Díaza, F. (2009). Event-related potentials with the Stroop colour-word task: timing of semantic conflict. *Int. J. Psychophysiol.* 72, 246–252. doi: 10.1016/j.ijpsycho.2009.01.002

6

Retrieval Deficiency in Brain Activity of Working Memory in Amnesic Mild Cognitive Impairment Patients: A Brain Event-Related Potentials Study

Bin-Yin Li[1], *Hui-Dong Tang*[1] *and Sheng-Di Chen*[1, 2*]

[1] *Department of Neurology and Collaborative Innovation Center for Brain Science, Rui Jin Hospital Affiliated to Shanghai Jiao Tong University School of Medicine, Shanghai, China,* [2] *Laboratory of Neurodegenerative Diseases and Key Laboratory of Stem Cell Biology, Institute of Health Science, Shanghai Institutes for Biological Sciences, Chinese Academy of Science and Shanghai Jiao Tong University School of Medicine, Shanghai, China*

Edited by:
Chunbo Li,
Shanghai Jiao Tong University School of Medicine, China

Reviewed by:
Yury (Juri) Kropotov,
Institute of the Human Brain of the Russian Academy of Sciences, Russia
Jijun Wang,
Shanghai Mental Health Center, China

****Correspondence:***
Sheng-Di Chen
chen_sd@medmail.com.cn

In the early stage of Alzheimer disease (AD) or mild cognitive impairment (MCI), working memory (WM) deficiency is prominent and could be attributed to failure in encoding, maintenance or retrieval of information. However, evidence for a retention or retrieval deficit remains equivocal. It is also unclear what cognitive mechanism in WM is impaired in MCI or early AD. We enrolled 46 subjects from our Memory Clinics and community, with 24 amnesic MCI patients and 22 normal subjects. After neurological and cognitive assessments, they performed a classic delayed match to sample (DMS) task with simultaneous event-related potential (ERP) recorded. The ERPs in encoding and retrieval epoch during WM were analyzed separately. The latency and amplitude of every ERP component were compared between two groups, and then analyzed to explore their relationship with neuropsychological performance. Finally, the locations of maximal difference in cortex were calculated by standard low-resolution tomographic analysis. A total of five components were found: P1, N1, P2, N2, and P300. The amplitude of P2 and P300 was larger in normal subjects than in MCI patients only during retrieval, not encoding epoch, while the latency did not show statistical difference. The latency and amplitude of P1 and N1 were similar in two groups. P2 amplitude in the retrieval epoch positively correlated with memory test (auditory verbal learning test) and visual spatial score of Chinese Addenbrooke's Cognitive Examination-Revised (ACE-R), while P300 amplitude correlated with ACE-R. The activation difference in P2 time range was maximal at medial frontal gyrus. However, the difference in cortex activation during P300 time range did not show significance. The amplitude of P2 indicated deficiency in memory retrieval process, potentially due to dysfunction of central executive in WM model. Regarding the location of P2 during WM task, medial frontal plays important role in memory retrieval. The findings in the present study suggested that MCI patients have retrieval deficit, probably due to central executive based on medial frontal gyrus. Thus, it may provide new biomarker for early detection and intervention for aMCI.

Keywords: event-related potentials, amnesic mild cognitive impairment, working memory, retrieval, sLORETA

INTRODUCTION

Cognitive decline is usually considered as an age-related phenomenon, which involves a continuous disease course from preclinical state, mild cognitive impairment (MCI) to Alzheimer's disease (AD). Prevalence of MCI in population-based epidemiological studies ranges from 3 to 20% in adults older than 60 or 65 years old (Gauthier et al., 2006; Ravaglia et al., 2008; Jia et al., 2014; Ding et al., 2015). Some MCI patients remain stable or even return to normal over time (Gauthier et al., 2006), while approximately half patients will progress to AD over 4–5 years.

Early detection and intervention for AD is remarkably important. Initially, most researchers agreed that the early and predominant cognitive deficit in AD is episodic memory impairment. However, cognitive processes under this kind of memory and their deficit in early AD were unclear in long period (Germano and Kinsella, 2005). Working memory (WM) provides a new insight into memory theory, which is defined as the capacity to hold information that is absent in mind for brief periods of time (Baddeley, 2012) and is closely related with daily activity performance.

In WM model, it involves at least three processes: information encoding, maintenance, and retrieval. All information-processing steps are regulated and controlled by the central executive. The central executive system is able to allocate attention to concurrent tasks, against potentially distracting irrelevant information. Long-term memory is formed when information is transferred from temporary or short-term storage to permanent episodic representation by rehearsal (Baddeley, 2001).

In early AD, memory complaint could be attributed to encoding, maintenance, and retrieval of information. The inability to encode and retrieve memory is present at the earliest stages of the disease and deteriorates during disease course (Aggarwal et al., 2005). Which part is the most problematic one? It is generally observed that a deficit in the acquisition of new information (encoding) is characteristic of early AD (Pasquier et al., 2001), while evidence for a retention or retrieval deficit in early AD remains equivocal (Grober and Kawas, 1997; Albert et al., 2001). However, all these observation is based on behavioral tests. As poor memory performance could be resulted from any deficit in the information processing, it is still unclear which cognitive mechanism is impaired in AD.

As WM works as a serial process at first a few seconds, event-related potentials (ERPs) provide a high temporal-resolution method to compare time-related cognitive process between different populations. Pinal et al. (2014) assessed the time course of brain activity during encoding and retrieval. Larger N2 amplitude and stronger activation of the left temporal lobe were found after long maintenance periods during information retrieval.

They also (Pinal et al., 2015a) used ERP recording and a delayed match to sample (DMS) task to assess age-related changes in young and old adults during successful information encoding in WM. The result revealed that smaller P2 and P300 amplitudes may signal the existence of an age dependent reduction in the processing resources available, and P2 and N2 latencies were longer in old than in young subjects.

In similar DMS, younger individuals have more posterior regions involved in WM processing, while adulthood has more anterior regions involved (Barriga-Paulino et al., 2015). Functional MRI (fMRI) study provided high spatial-resolution evidence. Galashan et al. (2015) combined EEG and fMRI with the same task, and they found a temporal pattern of source activities starting in occipital and temporal brain regions, followed by a simultaneous engagement of parietal and frontal brain regions and a later activity of a source in pre-supplementary motor area.

To our knowledge, no studies have compared the difference of cognitive process in WM between MCI and normal aging people. The encoding and retrieval deficit in WM also remains controversial in MCI patients. Amnesic MCI (aMCI) is one important type of pre-AD cognitive state with or without disability in other cognitive domains. WM studies in MCI patients revealed increased P200-N200 latencies, as well as an early dysfunction of neural generators within the parietal cortex in two-back paradigm (Missonnier et al., 2005, 2007). However, these studies did not uncover the deficit in information processing of WM. Therefore, we recruited aMCI patients from our memory clinics, and used ERP technique to precisely record time course of brain activity during encoding and retrieval in WM task.

MATERIALS AND METHODS

Subjects

We recruited normal elderly subjects from community and patients with memory complaint for more than 6 months from our Memory Clinics of the Department of Neurology, Rui Jin Hospital from December 2014 to July 2015. All participants were firstly evaluated by memory-disorders specialists and screened by the Mini Mental State Examination (MMSE, Chinese Version; Katzman et al., 1988), Zung Self-rating Anxiety Scale (SAS) and Zung Self-rating Depression scale (SDS). Each patient from memory clinics was subsequently performed blood test for possible causes of memory impairment including thyroid function, syphilis, HIV, folic acid, and vitamin B12, etc. Brain MRI scanning was also done for detecting vascular causes and hippocampus atrophy. Finally, the diagnosis of MCI was based on a detailed medical history, relevant physical and neurological examinations, negative laboratory findings, and neuroimaging studies. Exclusion criteria included evidence of stroke, Parkinson's disease, HIV/AIDS, mood problems, and reversible dementias, as well as treatment with benzodiazepines, antipsychotic, or antiepileptic medications. Patients with poor vision were also excluded.

A total of 46 subjects were finally enrolled. A patient was diagnosed as MCI patients if any of the following criteria were met as proposed by Petersen et al. (1999): memory has become worse gradually, as reported by the subject or his/her caregiver; objective evidence of impaired memory compared with normal controls matched for age, gender, and education; Clinical Dementia Rating global score = 0.5; normal activities of daily living, and not demented. Finally, 24 patients were diagnosed as MCI and 22 subjects from community as normal control (CDR = 0 and normal activities of daily living) by two neurologists independently (Li and Chen; **Table 1**).

Neuropsychological Assessment

A neuropsychological battery for multiple cognitive domains was performed in 35 subjects among 46 subjects by trained researcher who was blind to diagnosis (16 MCI patients and 19 normal subjects). These tests included the Chinese Addenbrooke's Cognitive Examination-Revised (ACE-R) (Fang et al., 2014), the Auditory Verbal Learning Test (AVLT)-Huashan version (Zhao et al., 2012), the Shape Trail Test (STT, including Part A and B), the Rey-Osterrieth Complex Figure Test (CFT), the Stroop Color-Word Test (SCWT), and the Symbol-Digit Modalities Test (SDMT).

Our study received ethical approval from the Research Ethics Committee, Rui Jin Hospital Affiliated to Shanghai Jiao Tong University School of Medicine, Shanghai, China. Written informed consent was obtained from all subjects or their guardians. All subjects were of unrelated Chinese Han descent with education level of secondary school or above, and knew English letter very well.

TABLE 1 | Demographic data and task performance (Mean ± Standard Deviation).

	MCI (n = 24)	Normal control (n = 22)	P
Age	69.27 ± 7.55	69.17 ± 8.91	0.947
Sex (female/all)*	9/24	8/22	0.936
Year of education#	13.33 ± 2.80	14.18 ± 3.09	0.206
MMSE#	26.41 ± 2.12	28.95 ± 0.95	<0.001
Reaction time (ms)#	1166.53 ± 160.33	1079.63 ± 141.08	0.068
Accuracy (%)#	68.58 ± 12.39	75.77 ± 11.37	0.090
ACE-R##	84.50 ± 7.33	93.26 ± 3.61	<0.001
AVLT-Immediate##	5.04 ± 1.13	6.87 ± 1.33	<0.001
AVLT-20 min##	2.81 ± 2.14	6.78 ± 2.68	<0.001
Digit-Symbol##	35.12 ± 10.20	45.44 ± 8.55	0.003
CFT-Copy##	34.75 ± 1.48	35.38 ± 1.24	0.181
CFT-recall##	11.56 ± 8.62	19.53 ± 8.22	0.011
SCWT C/A##	3.38 ± 0.80	3.19 ± 1.10	0.566
STT-A##	68.36 ± 20.07	52.67 ± 17.76	0.020
STT-B##	168.73 ± 43.65	120.43 ± 38.57	0.001

Chi-square test, #Mann-Whitney U-test, ##The total sample size is 35, with 16 subjects in MCI group and 19 subjects in control group. Independent t-test were performed. ACE-R, Addenbrooke's Cognitive Examination-Revised; AVLT, Auditory Verbal Learning Test-Huashan version; STT, Shape Trail Test (including Part A and B); CFT, the Rey-Osterrieth Complex Figure Test (CFT); SCWT, Stroop Color-Word Test.

The Delayed Match to Sample Task

Subjects first took a simple English letter test to make sure everyone knew all 26 letters. Then every subject was asked to complete a DMS task, which employed a visual task with WM. All visual stimuli were white presented on a dark background. In one trial, after a "+" in the middle of screen for 500 ms, one single letters (sample stimulus) randomly selected from 26 letters were displayed in the center of screen for 2000 ms. Subject was asked to keep it in mind. A blank followed the letter lasted for 3000 ms as an interruption. Probe stimulus (six letters randomly selected from 26 letters in a 2 * 3 matrix) was then presented in the middle of screen (**Figure 1**). Subject has to judge whether the letter seen before was among the six letters (press numeric keyboard "1" for "yes," "2," for "no"). The matrix was presented until the subject pressed key or for 2000 ms at maximum. After 5000 ms blank for a rest, a new trial started. Every individual underwent two sequential blocks. One contained 20 trials for practice, and the other contained 100 trials for test. In 50% of trials in each block, the correct answer was "yes," while the left was "no." "YES" and "No" trials were randomized in each block. Not until the subject had accuracy over 50% in practice block could she or he start the test block. The task was programmed and behavioral data (reaction time and accuracy) was recorded by E-Prime 2.0 software (Psychology Software Tools, Inc., Pittsburgh, PA, USA).

Memory storage of the first letters was required in order to compare it with the probe stimuli. The stimuli were large (height of 5.5° visual angle), bright (55 cd/m2), and presented in the middle of a computer monitor in order to make it easy for the subjects to see them. The whole test lasted for about 15–18 min.

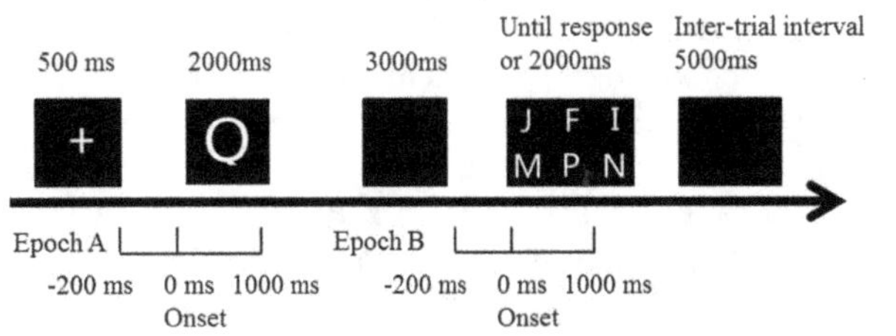

FIGURE 1 | Illustration of the trial time course in the DMS paradigm. Subjects were presented with one single letter (sample stimulus). They had to keep it in mind for a fixed delay (3 s) before judging as quickly and accurately as possible whether it was presented among the presenting six letters (probe stimulus). ERP epoch A (encoding period): extends from 200 ms prior to sample stimulus onset to 1000 ms after. ERP epoch B (retrieval period): extends from 200 ms prior to probe stimulus onset to 1000 ms after.

EEG Recordings and Data Processing

EEG and electro-oculogram (EOG) were recorded with a 32-channel EEG amplifier (BrainAmp by Brain Products, Munich, Germany) using 32 Ag-AgCl electrodes. EEG electrodes were set in a standard EEG cap according to extended 10–20 system with inter-optode distances between 2 and 3 cm. Thirty-two scalp electrodes (Fp1, Fp2, F3, F4, C3, C4, P3, P4, O1, O2, F7, F8, T7, T8, P7, P8, Fz, FCz, Cz, Pz, FC1, FC2, CP1, CP2, FC5, FC6, CP5, CP6, FT9, FT10, TP9, TP10) with reference to bilateral linked ear lobes (TP9, TP10) recorded electrical brain activity while the subject performed the DMS task.

The sampling rate of every channel was 500 Hz, with frequency band-pass from 0.1 to 70 Hz. Artifact criteria were applied to all electrodes. Recorded data were passed through a digital filter with the high cut-off frequency set at 50 Hz and with a low cut-off frequency set at 0.1 Hz. Notch-filter centered at 50 Hz was also applied to minimize electrical line noise. Ocular artifacts were corrected using the Infomax Restricted algorithm in an Independent Component Analysis as implemented in Brain Vision Analyzer 2.0 (Brain Products GmbH). Artifact rejection was followed by semi-automatic check (maximal allowed voltage step: 50 μV/ms; maximal allowed difference of values in intervals: 200 μV; lowest allowed activity in intervals: 0.5 μV). Mean artifact rejection rate for all MCI subjects was >1%. Then data was segmented in two epochs (**Figure 1**). Encoding epoch lasted from 200 ms before presentation of sample stimulus to 1000 ms after, while retrieval epoch lasted from 200 ms before probe stimulus to 1000 ms after. Baseline correction was done with the mean activity in the 200 ms prior to stimulus, and ERPs were based on correct trials.

Statistical Analysis

ERP Component Analysis

Based on the grand-averaged ERP waveforms, five ERP components were searched both in encoding and retrieval, according to the reports reviewed in the introduction section: N1, P1, N2, P2, and P300. We chose electrodes and then calculated peak latency and amplitude on the basis of studies with the same paradigm, as well as choosing the electrodes where amplitude was maximal. The N1 peak was measured as the voltage at the largest negative going peak in the latency window of 150–210 ms after stimulus onset at P7 and P8. The P1 was at the maximum peak in the latency window of 84–140 ms at O1, O2, P7 and P8. The N2 was considered at the most negative peak between 230 and 300 ms at F3, F4, C3, C4, CZ, FZ, FCz, while P2 was between 150 and 250 ms at FC1, FC1, CZ, FZ, FCz. P300 was identified as the maximum positive peak at O1, O1, and Pz between 250 and 450 ms after stimulus onset.

Demographics, Psychometrics and ERPs

The difference of age, education level, MMSE score, reaction time, accuracy and sex between two groups was compared by the Mann-Whitney or Pearson's chi-square test. Reaction time (RT) was defined as the time between the onset of probe stimulus and subject's response, only in the correct trials. ERP components' parameters (latency and amplitude in each component) were compared by independent *t*-test between two groups in both encoding and retrieval epochs. Any statistically significant findings in the comparison lead to deep analysis for behavioral and electrophysiological association. The potential relationship between neuropsychological performance and brain activity was estimated by correlation analysis and linear regression. Pearson's correlation was calculated separately between each cognitive assessment score and ERP components parameters.

Standard Low Resolution Tomography Analysis (s-LORETA)

The sLORETA is a functional imaging method for locating current source and widely used in EPR studies (Pandey et al., 2012). The LORETA algorithm has been identified as an efficient tool for functional mapping, also in encoding or retrieval period of WM studies (Pinal et al., 2015a). We employed sLORETA version that is identical with the one proved validated in previous studies (Pandey et al., 2012), available at: http://www.uzh.ch/keyinst/loreta.htm.

As described in sLORETA manual, a collection of volume elements in brain cortex has been modeled in the digitized Montreal Neurological Institute (MNI) coordinates corrected to the Talairach coordinates. In the study, the averaged waveforms (500 time samples, 1000 ms, post-stimulus) from 32 original recording montages for each subject were converted and saved into ASCII values. Transformation matrix was also constructed from these original data and electrode coordinates. The sLORETA values of each subject were computed for separately using ASCII values, electrode coordinates, and the transformation matrix. Regarding the sLORETA analysis, it compared differences between two groups in the time range of specific waveforms which showed difference in amplitude or latency, and constructed images to localize these differences in the three dimensional (3-D) space within the brain. For each comparison, one single test (Log of ratio of averages) was calculated for time-samples in significant ERP components (based on results from ERPs analysis above) with 5000 random permutations. The resultant values were then plotted in a 3-D brain model and evaluated for the level of significances. We also reported the maximum differences between groups at respective MNI coordinates and Brodmann areas (BA).

RESULTS

Demographics and Task Performance

The age, education years and sex proportion were similar in two groups. The independent Mann-Whitney *U*-test of task performance data (accuracy and RT) revealed marginally significant difference ($p = 0.090$ and 0.068), with a bit lower accuracy and longer reaction time in MCI patients. The MMSE score in MCI group was much lower than control group, consistent with their global cognitive ability and our clinical diagnosis. The matched age and education years in two groups helped to balance cognitive-related factors in the following analysis. Neuropsychological assessment also provided critical difference in cognitive tasks (AVLT, SDMT, CFT) where memory played a major role (**Table 1**).

Brain Activity in Encoding and Retrieval

The number of valid trials used for averaging ERPs in both encoding and retrieval epoch did not differ between two groups (**Tables 2, 3**). In the encoding epoch, no significant effect of group was found in parameters of all five ERPs components (**Figure 2, Table 2**). In the retrieval epoch (**Figure 3**), the independent *t*-test revealed significant effect of group in the amplitude of P2 and P300 components ($p = 0.025$ and 0.038). The P2 and P300 amplitude in aMCI group was smaller than in control group. However, latency of those two components was not significantly affected by the group effect. Regarding the N1, N2, and P1, neither difference in amplitude or latency reached statistically significant between two groups (**Table 3**).

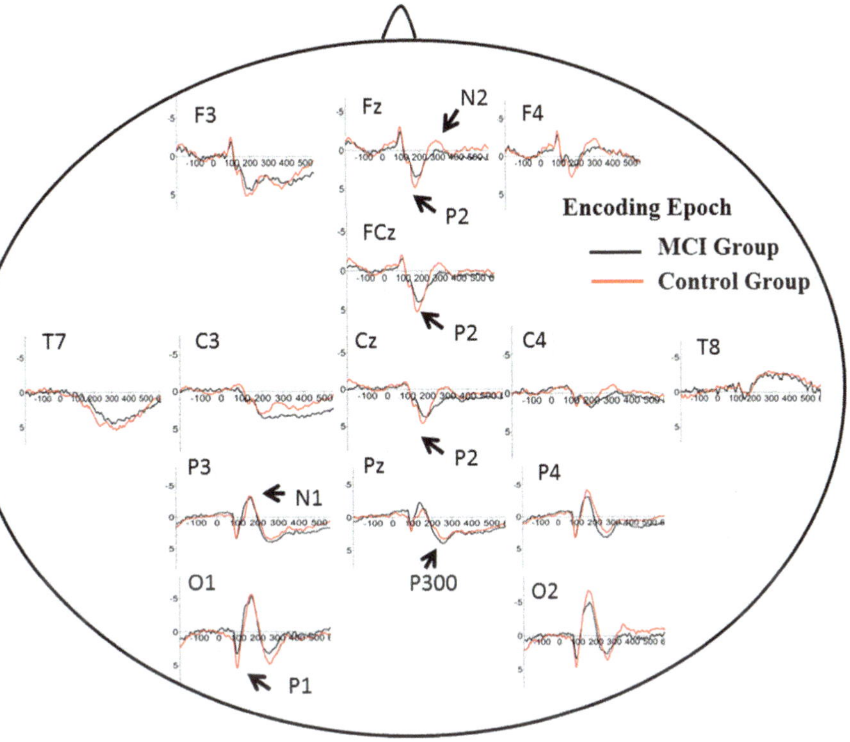

FIGURE 2 | Grand average ERP waveform in aMCI (black line) and normal control group (red line) during retrieval period in WM task. Time was shown in milliseconds where stimulus onset was at 0, and potentials were shown in micro-voltage.

TABLE 2 | Parameters of ERP component in encoding epoch (Mean ± Standard deviation).

Encoding		MCI ($n = 24$)	Normal control ($n = 22$)	p*
Number of valid trials		1643	1637	0.889
P300	Latency	317.69 ± 46.51	312.64 ± 45.17	0.711
	Amplitude	4.37 ± 2.66	4.50 ± 2.88	0.803
P2	Latency	191.65 ± 20.77	182.69 ± 16.59	0.115
	Amplitude	5.02 ± 2.04	5.77 ± 3.22	0.344
N2	Latency	272.55 ± 18.12	269.58 ± 14.36	0.543
	Amplitude	−0.29 ± 2.15	−1.21 ± 2.27	0.164
P1	Latency	79.72 ± 6.38	80.63 ± 8.40	0.676
	Amplitude	4.72 ± 2.65	5.06 ± 2.07	0.638
N1	Latency	173.12 ± 12.08	173.45 ± 12.51	0.928
	Amplitude	−6.27 ± 3.27	−7.21 ± 3.24	0.335

Latency and amplitude were measured in milliseconds (ms) and micro-voltage (μV).
**Independent T-test.*

TABLE 3 | Parameters of ERP component in retrieval epoch (Mean ± Standard deviation).

Retrieval		MCI ($n = 24$)	Normal control ($n = 22$)	p*
Number of valid trials		1642	1604	0.634
P300	Latency	296.67 ± 37.75	306.54 ± 34.80	0.363
	Amplitude	3.72 ± 2.31	5.45 ± 3.14	***0.038***
P2	Latency	195.30 ± 28.33	183.87 ± 21.42	0.165
	Amplitude	4.83 ± 2.62	6.81 ± 3.14	***0.025***
N2	Latency	267.25 ± 19.26	267.58 ± 16.92	0.951
	Amplitude	0.70 ± 2.62	1.21 ± 2.84	0.531
P1	Latency	85.05 ± 7.28	82.91 ± 7.79	0.341
	Amplitude	4.44 ± 2.88	4.01 ± 2.47	0.597
N1	Latency	167.08 ± 14.57	170.08 ± 10.96	0.396
	Amplitude	−4.41 ± 3.52	−5.96 ± 3.13	0.123

Latency and amplitude were measured in milliseconds (ms) and micro-voltage (μV).
**Independent T-test. Bold and italic values are indicated as statistical significance.*

Brain Activity and Cognitive Ability

Among all subjects, a neuropsychological battery for multiple cognitive domains was performed in 35 subjects (16 MCI patients and 19 normal subjects). Based on the results of ERP components analysis, the Pearson's correlation was calculated in all subjects between cognitive assessment score and ERP components parameters (the amplitude of P2 and P300) separately. Regarding P2 amplitude, significant correlation was found in its relationship with AVLT-20 min recall ($r = 0.368$, $p = 0.030$) and scores of visual spatial ability in ACE-R. Scores in AVLT-5 min recall and recognition were marginally significant correlated with P2 amplitude ($r = 0.286$, $p = 0.096$; $r = 0.292$, $p = 0.089$). The amplitude of P300 was correlated with ACE-R ($r = 0.395$, $p = 0.019$), as well as scores of language fluency and visual spatial ability in ACE-R ($r = 0.374$, $p = 0.027$; $r = 0.363$, $p = 0.032$). A scatterplot was depicted to show the fit line and relationship between P2 amplitude and AVLT-20 min recall (**Figure 4**).

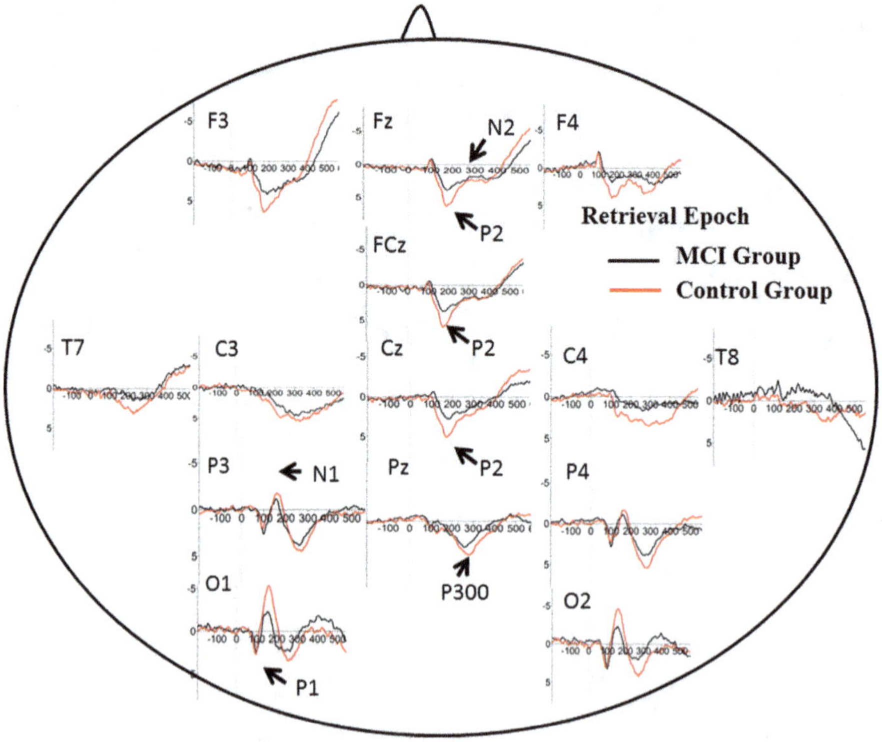

FIGURE 3 | Grand average ERP waveform in aMCI (black line) and normal control group (red line) during encoding period in WM task. Time was shown in milliseconds where stimulus onset was at 0, and potentials were shown in micro-voltage.

Standardized Low Resolution Tomography Analysis (sLORETA)

Based on the results showed above, we performed statistical non-parametric mapping (SnPM) during P2 and P300 time range (in the retrieval epoch) to show different activation in these specific temporal intervals. The statistical difference between groups for current density at the source is shown in **Table 4**. The brain areas that show activation differences at <0.05 level are shown in **Figure 5** (positive in yellow color, while negative in blue color with reference of MCI group). As shown in **Table 4**, the difference in P2 time range was maximum at BA 11 (medial frontal gyrus) of the right frontal cortex (Log of ratio of averages $= 0.846$, $p < 0.01$). Besides, BA 10 (superior frontal gyrus) also showed markedly activated in control group during P2 time range. However, the difference in cortex activation during P300 time range did not reach significant level.

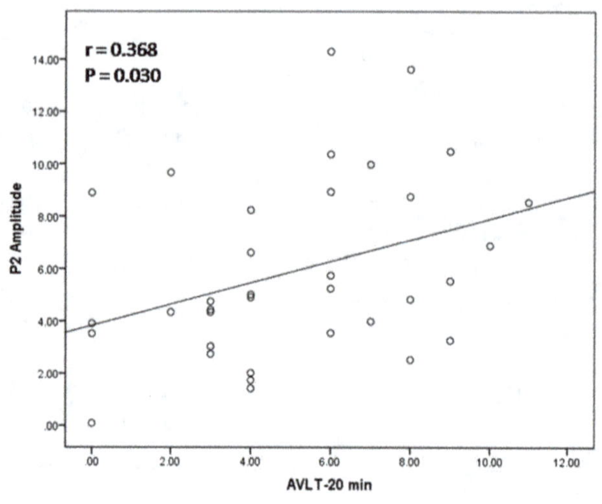

FIGURE 4 | Relation between P2 amplitude and score of auditory verbal learning test (recall after 20 min). The scatterplot and best fit line ($r = 0.368$ and $p = 0.030$) referred to Pearson's correlation analysis.

DISCUSSION

Working Memory Task Performance and ERPs

It is shown that in the MCI and AD patients, longer maintenance intervals hampered the task performance. Patients performed significantly worse than controls on the associative WM task (van Geldorp et al., 2015). In our study, the two groups had similar age, sex proportion and education level. Meanwhile, the interval between two stimuli was fixed and relatively short (Pinal et al., 2015b). Although aMCI patients did have poor cognitive ability in psychometric tests, the results showed similar WM task performance (reaction time and latency) in two groups. However, the brain activity measured as ERPs still uncovered difference

TABLE 4 | Comparison of aMCI and normal control group in sLORETA (voxels showing maximal difference).

MNI coordinates			Brodmann area	Brain region	Log of ratio of average	*p*-Value
X	*y*	*Z*				
P2 TIME-RANGE DURING RETRIEVAL (150–250 ms)						
25	45	−10	11	Frontal lobe, Medial Frontal Gyrus	0.845	<0.05
25	45	−5	11	Frontal lobe, Medial Frontal Gyrus	0.845	<0.05
20	45	−5	10	Frontal lobe, Superior Frontal Gyrus	0.832	<0.05
P300 TIME-RANGE DURING RETRIEVAL (250–450 ms)						
−5	55	−25	11	Frontal lobe, Rectal Gyrus	0.512	>0.1

MNI, Montreal Neurological Institute.

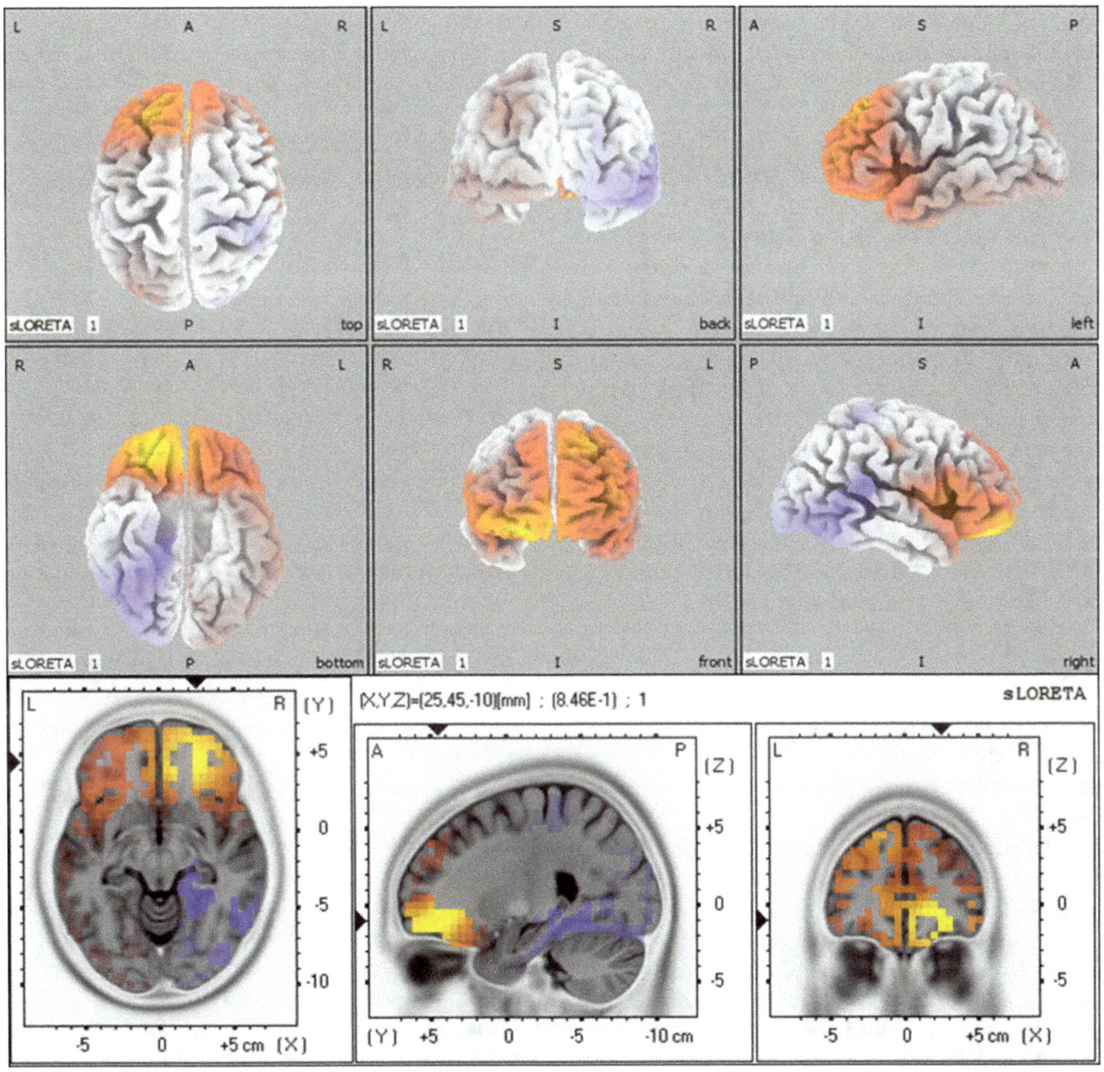

FIGURE 5 | The sLORETA images showing statistical differences between aMCI and control group (3D-view and slice-view) in the P2 time-range. The three slice-view images below located the maximal difference between aMCI group and control group (MNI coordinates *x*, *y*, *z* = 25, 45, −10). Positive difference was in yellow color with reference of MCI group.

under seemingly comparable WM performance. It suggested that brain activity deficit underlie behavioral change and the electrophysiological test provided opportunity of early detection and intervention.

Brain Activity and Neuropsychological Function

It is still unclear whether encoding or retrieval is impaired in MCI patients. In this exploratory study, the ERPs in encoding and retrieval epoch were separately analyzed. Some ERP components proved sensitive to probe stimulus. It is noted that the findings in ERPs made no sense until it could be related with real cognitive ability. Every ERP should be analyzed with the consideration of behavioral and cognitive ability.

P2: P2 has been related to various cognitive process: a semantic effect (Peressotti et al., 2012), top–down mechanism for rapid evaluation of stimulus significance (Paynter et al., 2009) or subjectively relevant stimuli (Schapkin et al., 2000; Potts and Tucker, 2001). Larger amplitude for P2 was observed in the control group than in MCI group. In WM model, retrieval requires phonological loop and central executive, which is generally defined as attention allocation efficiency (Germano and Kinsella, 2005; Wang et al., 2010). Previous studies concerning aging effects on P2 amplitude showed larger P2 amplitude in younger adults, suggesting deficit in the allocation of processing resources for the evaluation of stimulus significance. Consistently, positive correlation was found between the degree of improvement in WM capacity and the post-pre difference in P2 amplitudes after WM training (Li et al., 2015). However, the latency of P2 in the present study did not differ in two groups. It suggested little slowing in stimulus judgment during information encoding and retrieval in WM.

In DMS task, subjects had to search probe stimulus (a 2*3 letter matrix) for the sample, indicating involvement of attention allocation in the retrieval. Besides, the P2 amplitude found in retrieval epoch positively correlated with memory recall test (AVLT-20 min recall). These results supported the role of P2 in information retrieval, as well as regulation of attention allocation.

The P2 amplitude also showed correlation with visual-spatial score of ACE-R. The fact may give explanation that all subjects were not English native speakers and they largely recognize English letter via its appearance.

P300: P300 is widely studied in cognitive processes, and represented different psychological meaning under different tasks (Kirschner et al., 2015). Previous studies have found an age-related reduction in the amplitude of P300 component at parietal electrodes, suggesting lower amounts of processing resources available for allocation to stimulus categorization (McEvoy et al., 2001; Saliasi et al., 2013; Pinal et al., 2015a). However, the difference existed in encoding epoch, while our study showed difference of P300 amplitude in retrieval epoch when age was balanced between groups. Positive correlation was found between P300 amplitude and memory load, indicating its significance in modulating resources for stimulus classification and context updating (Pinal et al., 2014). As memory load was same in present two groups, difference in P300 suggested that aMCI patients could modulate fewer resources and thus evoked lower amplitude. Similar to P2, the latency of P300 in two groups did not differ from each other, suggesting relative spared processing speed in aMCI patients. The P300 amplitude also showed correlation with score of ACE-R, especially in language fluency and visual-spatial ability. It suggested that P300 might represent more general cognition ability, compared with P2.

N2: N2 (predominant in anterior part of brain) has been studied in correlation with visual information encoding (Nittono et al., 2007). Consistently, N2 waveform was obvious in anterior electrodes in the present study. Previous studies found positive association between N2 latency and task accuracy or N2 amplitude with memory load (Pinal et al., 2014, 2015a). Stimulus discrimination and classification may be reflected by N2 (Folstein and Van Petten, 2008), hence higher N2 amplitude happens when the stimulus includes more information load. There were no difference between aMCI and control group for N2 amplitude and latency. Low and fixed memory load (only one letter) in the present may give an explanation.

P1 and N1: It is generally accepted that these early ERP components usually represent perceptual processing of visual inputs (Vogel and Luck, 2000; Taylor, 2002). The present results indicate that the deficit in information retrieval does not affect perceptual processing of stimuli, which is also consist with DMS study in young and older subjects (Pinal et al., 2015a).

Medial Frontal Lobe in Working Memory

In the present study, MCI patients had less activated brain area in medial frontal area than control subject during P2 time range in WM retrieval. As MRI has high spatial resolution than ERPs, fMRI provides more precise activated location.

At retrieval, "retrieval-success network" was found in brain areas which is thought to be content-independent (Wagner et al., 2005; Huijbers et al., 2010). These areas found in fMRI studies include the posterior midline region consisting of the precuneus, retrosplenial cortex, and posterior cingulate, the medial prefrontal cortex as well as the hippocampus.

In a fMRI study with DMS task, correct decision at WM probe was linked to activation in the anterior and posterior midline brain structures (Bergmann et al., 2015). The result was generally consisted with our findings in sLORETA. As ERP provided higher time-resolution, frontal midline structures in 150–250 ms were less activated in aMCI group. Animal experiment provided evidence that shifting of attention set in the rat impaired with lesions of prefrontal cortex, and medial frontal cortex associated with impairment in initial acquisition and reversal learning.

As discussed above, P2 correlated with attention allocation in the retrieval. Locations found in sLORETA further verified its neuro-anatomical basis and functional significance.

One limitation of the present study is a bit fewer channel data (32-channel data) in sLORETA analysis. Though our findings in sLORETA was generally consistent with fMRI study, 64 or 128-channel EEG cap in further studies could provide more detailed and accurate information.

CONCLUSION

The aim of the present study was to explore brain activity changes in MCI patients during WM task. We tried to find clinically significant electrophysiological waveform for WM and its location in the cortex. The results revealed that brain activity during retrieval process of WM was impaired in aMCI patients, while encoding process spared. In retrieval process, the amplitude of P2 indicated deficient function of central executive in the WM model. Besides, medial and superior frontal gyrus markedly activated during P2 time range in the control group. The findings in the present study suggested WM retrieval deficit in aMCI patients, probably due to dysfunction of central executive (attention allocation) based on medial and superior frontal gyrus. It may provide new biomarker for early detection and intervention for aMCI.

AUTHOR CONTRIBUTIONS

All three authors cooperated and contributed to the design and plan of the present study. BL was in charge of ERP data acquisition, analysis and manuscript writing. HT was in charge of neuropsychological assessments and analysis. SC was in charge of clinical diagnosis and manuscript verifying.

ACKNOWLEDGMENTS

This work was supported by grants from the National Natural Science Foundation of China [grant numbers 81400888, 91332107].

REFERENCES

Aggarwal, N. T., Wilson, R. S., Beck, T. L., Bienias, J. L., and Bennett, D. A. (2005). Mild cognitive impairment in different functional domains and incident Alzheimer's disease. *J. Neurol. Neurosurg. Psychiatr.* 76, 1479–1484. doi: 10.1136/jnnp.2004.053561

Albert, M. S., Moss, M. B., Tanzi, R., and Jones, K. (2001). Preclinical prediction of AD using neuropsychological tests. *J. Int. Neuropsychol. Soc.* 7, 631–639. doi: 10.1017/S1355617701755105

Baddeley, A. (2012). Working memory: theories, models, and controversies. *Annu. Rev. Psychol.* 63, 1–29. doi: 10.1146/annurev-psych-120710-100422

Baddeley, A. D. (2001). Is working memory still working? *Am. Psychol.* 56, 851–864. doi: 10.1037/0003-066X.56.11.851

Barriga-Paulino, C. I., Rojas Benjumea, M. A., Rodriguez-Martinez, E. I., and Gomez Gonzalez, C. M. (2015). Fronto-temporo-occipital activity changes with age during a visual working memory developmental study in children, adolescents and adults. *Neurosci. Lett.* 599, 26–31. doi: 10.1016/j.neulet.2015.05.017

Bergmann, H. C., Daselaar, S. M., Beul, S. F., Rijpkema, M., Fernandez, G., and Kessels, R. P. (2015). Brain activation during associative short-term memory maintenance is not predictive for subsequent retrieval. *Front. Hum. Neurosci.* 9:479. doi: 10.3389/fnhum.2015.00479

Ding, D., Zhao, Q., Guo, Q., Meng, H., Wang, B., Luo, J., et al. (2015). Prevalence of mild cognitive impairment in an urban community in China: a cross-sectional analysis of the Shanghai aging study. *Alzheimers Dement.* 11, 300–309.e2. doi: 10.1016/j.jalz.2013.11.002

Fang, R., Wang, G., Huang, Y., Zhuang, J. P., Tang, H. D., Wang, Y., et al. (2014). Validation of the Chinese version of Addenbrooke's cognitive examination-revised for screening mild Alzheimer's disease and mild cognitive impairment. *Dement. Geriatr. Cogn. Disord.* 37, 223–231. doi: 10.1159/000353541

Folstein, J. R., and Van Petten, C. (2008). Influence of cognitive control and mismatch on the N2 component of the ERP: a review. *Psychophysiology* 45, 152–170. doi: 10.1111/j.1469-8986.2007.00602.x

Galashan, D., Fehr, T., and Herrmann, M. (2015). Differences between target and non-target probe processing-combined evidence from fMRI, EEG and fMRI-constrained source analysis. *Neuroimage* 111, 289–299. doi: 10.1016/j.neuroimage.2015.02.044

Gauthier, S., Reisberg, B., Zaudig, M., Petersen, R. C., Ritchie, K., Broich, K., et al. (2006). International psychogeriatric association expert conference on mild cognitive I. Mild cognitive impairment. *Lancet* 367, 1262–1270. doi: 10.1016/S0140-6736(06)68542-5

Germano, C., and Kinsella, G. J. (2005). Working memory and learning in early Alzheimer's disease. *Neuropsychol. Rev.* 15, 1–10. doi: 10.1007/s11065-005-3583-7

Grober, E., and Kawas, C. (1997). Learning and retention in preclinical and early Alzheimer's disease. *Psychol. Aging* 12, 183–188. doi: 10.1037/0882-7974.12.1.183

Huijbers, W., Pennartz, C. M., and Daselaar, S. M. (2010). Dissociating the "retrieval success" regions of the brain: effects of retrieval delay. *Neuropsychologia* 48, 491–497. doi: 10.1016/j.neuropsychologia.2009.10.006

Jia, J., Zhou, A., Wei, C., Jia, X., Wang, F., Li, F., et al. (2014). The prevalence of mild cognitive impairment and its etiological subtypes in elderly Chinese. *Alzheimers Dement.* 10, 439–447. doi: 10.1016/j.jalz.2013.09.008

Katzman, R., Zhang, M. Y., Ouang Ya, Q., Wang, Z. Y., Liu, W. T., Yu, E., et al. (1988). A Chinese version of the mini-mental state examination; impact of illiteracy in a Shanghai dementia survey. *J. Clin. Epidemiol.* 41, 971–978. doi: 10.1016/0895-4356(88)90034-0

Kirschner, A., Cruse, D., Chennu, S., Owen, A. M., and Hampshire, A. (2015). A P300-based cognitive assessment battery. *Brain Behav.* 5, e00336. doi: 10.1002/brb3.336

Li, W., Guo, Z., Jones, J. A., Huang, X., Chen, X., Liu, P., et al. (2015). Training of working memory impacts neural processing of vocal pitch regulation. *Sci. Rep.* 5:16562. doi: 10.1038/srep16562

McEvoy, L. K., Pellouchoud, E., Smith, M. E., and Gevins, A. (2001). Neurophysiological signals of working memory in normal aging. *Brain Res. Cogn. Brain Res.* 11, 363–376. doi: 10.1016/S0926-6410(01)00009-X

Missonnier, P., Deiber, M. P., Gold, G., Herrmann, F. R., Millet, P., Michon, A., et al. (2007). Working memory load-related electroencephalographic parameters can differentiate progressive from stable mild cognitive impairment. *Neuroscience* 150, 346–356. doi: 10.1016/j.neuroscience.2007.09.009

Missonnier, P., Gold, G., Fazio-Costa, L., Michel, J. P., Mulligan, R., Michon, A., et al. (2005). Early event-related potential changes during working memory activation predict rapid decline in mild cognitive impairment. *J. Gerontol. A Biol. Sci. Med. Sci.* 60, 660–666. doi: 10.1093/gerona/60.5.660

Nittono, H., Shibuya, Y., and Hori, T. (2007). Anterior N2 predicts subsequent viewing time and interest rating for novel drawings. *Psychophysiology* 44, 687–696. doi: 10.1111/j.1469-8986.2007.00539.x

Pandey, A. K., Kamarajan, C., Tang, Y., Chorlian, D. B., Roopesh, B. N., Manz, N., et al. (2012). Neurocognitive deficits in male alcoholics: an ERP/sLORETA analysis of the N2 component in an equal probability Go/NoGo task. *Biol. Psychol.* 89, 170–182. doi: 10.1016/j.biopsycho.2011.10.009

Pasquier, F., Grymonprez, L., Lebert, F., and Van der Linden, M. (2001). Memory impairment differs in frontotemporal dementia and Alzheimer's disease. *Neurocase* 7, 161–171. doi: 10.1093/neucas/7.2.161

Paynter, C. A., Reder, L. M., and Kieffaber, P. D. (2009). Knowing we know before we know: ERP correlates of initial feeling-of-knowing. *Neuropsychologia* 47, 796–803. doi: 10.1016/j.neuropsychologia.2008.12.009

Peressotti, F., Pesciarelli, F., Mulatti, C., and Dell'Acqua, R. (2012). Event-related potential evidence for two functionally dissociable sources of semantic effects in the attentional blink. *PLoS ONE* 7:e49099. doi: 10.1371/journal.pone.0049099

Petersen, R. C., Smith, G. E., Waring, S. C., Ivnik, R. J., Tangalos, E. G., and Kokmen, E. (1999). Mild cognitive impairment: clinical characterization and outcome. *Arch. Neurol.* 56, 303–308. doi: 10.1001/archneur.56.3.303

Pinal, D., Zurron, M., and Diaz, F. (2014). Effects of load and maintenance duration on the time course of information encoding and retrieval in working memory: from perceptual analysis to post-categorization processes. *Front. Hum. Neurosci.* 8:165. doi: 10.3389/fnhum.2014.00165

Pinal, D., Zurron, M., and Diaz, F. (2015a). Age-related changes in brain activity are specific for high order cognitive processes during successful encoding of information in working memory. *Front. Aging Neurosci.* 7:75. doi: 10.3389/fnagi.2015.00075

Pinal, D., Zurron, M., and Diaz, F. (2015b). An event related potentials study of the effects of age, load and maintenance duration on working memory recognition. *PLoS ONE* 10:e0143117. doi: 10.1371/journal.pone.0143117

Potts, G. F., and Tucker, D. M. (2001). Frontal evaluation and posterior representation in target detection. *Brain Res. Cogn. Brain Res.* 11, 147–156. doi: 10.1016/S0926-6410(00)00075-6

Ravaglia, G., Forti, P., Montesi, F., Lucicesare, A., Pisacane, N., Rietti, E., et al. (2008). Mild cognitive impairment: epidemiology and dementia risk in an elderly Italian population. *J. Am. Geriatr. Soc.* 56, 51–58. doi: 10.1111/j.1532-5415.2007.01503.x

Saliasi, E., Geerligs, L., Lorist, M. M., and Maurits, N. M. (2013). The relationship between P3 amplitude and working memory performance differs in young and older adults. *PLoS ONE* 8:e63701. doi: 10.1371/journal.pone.0063701

Schapkin, S. A., Gusev, A. N., and Kuhl, J. (2000). Categorization of unilaterally presented emotional words: an ERP analysis. *Acta Neurobiol. Exp. (Wars).* 60, 17–28.

Taylor, M. J. (2002). Non-spatial attentional effects on P1. *Clin. Neurophysiol.* 113, 1903–1908. doi: 10.1016/S1388-2457(02)00309-7

van Geldorp, B., Heringa, S. M., van den Berg, E., Olde Rikkert, M. G., Biessels, G. J., and Kessels, R. P. (2015). Working memory binding and episodic memory formation in aging, mild cognitive impairment, and Alzheimer's dementia. *J. Clin. Exp. Neuropsychol.* 37, 538–548. doi: 10.1080/13803395.2015.1037722

Vogel, E. K., and Luck, S. J. (2000). The visual N1 component as an index of a discrimination process. *Psychophysiology* 37, 190–203. doi: 10.1111/1469-8986.3720190

Wagner, A. D., Shannon, B. J., Kahn, I., and Buckner, R. L. (2005). Parietal lobe contributions to episodic memory retrieval. *Trends Cogn. Sci.* 9, 445–453. doi: 10.1016/j.tics.2005.07.001

Wang, Y., Song, Y., Qu, Z., and Ding, Y. (2010). Task difficulty modulates electrophysiological correlates of perceptual learning. *Int. J. Psychophysiol.* 75, 234–240. doi: 10.1016/j.ijpsycho.2009.11.006

Zhao, Q., Lv, Y., Zhou, Y., Hong, Z., and Guo, Q. (2012). Short-term delayed recall of auditory verbal learning test is equivalent to long-term delayed recall for identifying amnestic mild cognitive impairment. *PLoS ONE* 7:e51157. doi: 10.1371/journal.pone.0051157

7

Microglial Cell Dysregulation in Brain Aging and Neurodegeneration

Rommy von Bernhardi[1]*, *Laura Eugenín-von Bernhardi*[1] and *Jaime Eugenín*[2]*

[1] Department of Neurology, Faculty of Medicine, Pontificia Universidad Católica de Chile, Santiago, Chile, [2] Laboratory of Neural Systems, Department of Biology, Faculty of Chemistry and Biology, Universidad de Santiago de Chile (USACH), Santiago, Chile

Edited by:
Fei Yin,
University of Southern California, USA

Reviewed by:
Carsten Culmsee,
Philipps-University of Marburg, Germany
Jian Luo,
Palo Alto Veterans Institute for Research, Inc. (PAVIR), USA

***Correspondence:**
Rommy von Bernhardi,
Department of Neurology, Faculty of Medicine, Pontificia Universidad Católica de Chile, Marcoleta 391, Santiago 8330024, Chile
rvonb@med.puc.cl;
Jaime Eugenín,
Laboratory of Neural Systems, Department of Biology, Faculty of Chemistry and Biology, Universidad de Santiago de Chile (USACH), Avenida Libertador Bernardo O'Higgins 3363, Santiago, Chile
jaime.eugenin@usach.cl

Aging is the main risk factor for neurodegenerative diseases. In aging, microglia undergoes phenotypic changes compatible with their activation. Glial activation can lead to neuroinflammation, which is increasingly accepted as part of the pathogenesis of neurodegenerative diseases, including Alzheimer's disease (AD). We hypothesize that in aging, aberrant microglia activation leads to a deleterious environment and neurodegeneration. In aged mice, microglia exhibit an increased expression of cytokines and an exacerbated inflammatory response to pathological changes. Whereas LPS increases nitric oxide (NO) secretion in microglia from young mice, induction of reactive oxygen species (ROS) predominates in older mice. Furthermore, there is accumulation of DNA oxidative damage in mitochondria of microglia during aging, and also an increased intracellular ROS production. Increased ROS activates the redox-sensitive nuclear factor *kappa* B, which promotes more neuroinflammation, and can be translated in functional deficits, such as cognitive impairment. Mitochondria-derived ROS and cathepsin B, are also necessary for the microglial cell production of interleukin-1β, a key inflammatory cytokine. Interestingly, whereas the regulatory cytokine TGFβ1 is also increased in the aged brain, neuroinflammation persists. Assessing this apparent contradiction, we have reported that TGFβ1 induction and activation of Smad3 signaling after inflammatory stimulation are reduced in adult mice. Other protective functions, such as phagocytosis, although observed in aged animals, become not inducible by inflammatory stimuli and TGFβ1. Here, we discuss data suggesting that mitochondrial and endolysosomal dysfunction could at least partially mediate age-associated microglial cell changes, and, together with the impairment of the TGFβ1-Smad3 pathway, could result in the reduction of protective activation and the facilitation of cytotoxic activation of microglia, resulting in the promotion of neurodegenerative diseases.

Keywords: Alzheimer's disease, glia, mitochondria, neurodegenerative diseases, neuroinflammation, oxidative stress, reactive oxygen species, transforming growth factor-β

Introduction

Aging is a complex process of cumulative changes. A key hallmark is the progressive decline in physiological functions and behavioral capacity, which is observed at various levels of the organism, in particular at the central nervous system (CNS; Smith et al., 2005). These changes can lead to altered behavior, memory impairment, or loss of several control functions (Lipsitz and Goldberger, 1992; Lipsitz, 2002; Glenn et al., 2004). In addition, some responses of the immune system, in special related to adaptive immune system, also decline with age, increasing the susceptibility to infections and cancer. By contrast, other immune responses are exacerbated, facilitating the onset of autoimmune diseases (Yung and Julius, 2008) or the generation of a mild chronic neuroinflammation mediated by the dysregulation of the innate immune system, as will be discussed here. Therefore, aging can affect several tissues and processes, leading to highly complex functional changes.

Microglia undergoes several age-related changes that contribute to the generation of a chronic mild inflammatory environment, including an increased production of inflammatory cytokines and the production of reactive oxygen species (ROS). These changes have been linked to the appearance of cognitive deficits and the onset of chronic neurodegenerative diseases. Therefore, it has been proposed that aging of microglia could contribute to other age-associated brain changes and cognitive decline (Conde and Streit, 2006a,b; Streit, 2006; von Bernhardi, 2010; Aguzzi et al., 2013; Kettenmann et al., 2013).

Normal Brain Aging

Several structural and functional changes associated with normal brain aging have been reported. Brain mass decreases in the order of 2 to 3% per decade after the age of 50. Individuals that are 80 years or older, brain mass is reduced by 10% compared with that of young adults (Drachman, 2006). Magnetic resonance imaging (MRI) and voxel-based morphometry (VBM) show that age specially affects the volume of gray and white matter at prefrontal, parietal, and temporal areas (Ge et al., 2002; Sowell et al., 2003; Salat et al., 2004). Complex learning abilities, such as dual tasks (ea. memorizing a word list while walking), show a progressive decrease during aging (Lindenberger et al., 2000; Salat et al., 2005). Nevertheless, cognitive decline in aging is highly variable; many older people keep intact their cognitive abilities (Shock et al., 1984) until advanced ages.

At the cellular level, shortening of telomeres and activation of tumor suppressor genes, as well as accumulation of DNA damage, oxidative stress, and mild chronic inflammatory activity are characteristic of aging cells. Various tissues, including the brain show an imbalance between pro- and anti-inflammatory cytokine levels. In addition, potentially damaging mediators, such as cytokines, radical species (**Figure 1**), and eicosanoids among others, are produced in response to the exposure to physical, chemical or biological agents, such as ionic radiation, pollutants, pathogens, etc. (Dröge and Schipper, 2007; Vijg and Campisi, 2008). Both humans and mice show decreased levels of interleukin 10 (IL10; Ye and Johnson, 2001), and increased levels of tumor necrosis factor α (TNFα) and IL1β in the CNS (Lukiw, 2004; Streit et al., 2004a), and IL6 in plasma (Ye and Johnson, 2001; Godbout and Johnson, 2004). In addition, increased transforming growth factor β1 (TGFβ1) mRNA a key cytokine regulator, has been observed in the brain of aged mice and rats (Bye et al., 2001).

At the same time, several changes induced by an aged micro-environment, such as increased systemic inflammation, increased permeability of the blood-brain barrier (BBB), and degeneration of neurons and other brain cells, could contribute to the production of ROS. It has been proposed that BBB permeability increases in aged animals (Blau et al., 2012; Enciu et al., 2013), facilitating perhaps infiltration by monocytes releasing mitochondria-generated ROS. An age-related increase in the number of $CD11b^{+}$ $CD45^{high}$ cells, compatible with infiltrated monocytes, has been reported in the brain of aged rats (Blau et al., 2012). Likewise, expression levels of chemotactic molecules, such as interferon-inducible protein 10 (IIP10) and monocyte chemotactic protein-1 (MCP-1), are increased in the hippocampal region (Blau et al., 2012).

Glial Cells, Neuroinflammation and Oxidative Stress

Neuroinflammation is choreographed by microglia and astrocytes, and is defined by increased levels of a complex arrangement of mediators, including IL1β, TNFα and TGFβ, all of which are increased in aged individuals (McGeer and McGeer, 2001; von Bernhardi, 2007; von Bernhardi et al., 2010). Microglia are the brain resident macrophages (Hemmer et al., 2002; Ransohoff and Perry, 2009; Rivest, 2009) providing its first line of defense. In the brain of healthy adults, microglia are slender ramified cells that constantly survey brain parenchyma (Davalos et al., 2005; Nimmerjahn et al., 2005). When stimulated, microglia activate, enlarge their cell body (Nimmerjahn et al., 2005; Frank-Cannon et al., 2009) and change their functional properties (Liu et al., 2001; von Bernhardi and Eugenín, 2004; Lue et al., 2010). Microglia sense and act on a broad range of stimuli, including autoimmune injury, infection, ischemia, toxic insults and trauma (Streit, 2002; Kim and de Vellis, 2005; Schwab and McGeer, 2008; Lue et al., 2010; von Bernhardi et al., 2010). They recognize a broad spectrum of molecular targets, such as glycolipids, lipoproteins, nucleotides, peptides, (Nakamura, 2002; van Rossum and Hanisch, 2004; Pocock and Kettenmann, 2007), abnormally processed, modified or aggregated proteins (e.g., Aβ), inflammatory cytokines, and damaged neurons, which are the strongest inducers of microglia activation (Nakamura, 2002; Hanisch and Kettenmann, 2007; Ransohoff and Perry, 2009; Lue et al., 2010; Schuitemaker et al., 2012). Depending on the stimuli, microglia undergoes different activation patterns (Gordon, 2003; Martinez et al., 2008; Mosser and Edwards, 2008). They include (i) classical M1 activation, which can associate with cytotoxicity, (ii) alternative phagocytic/neuroprotective M2 activation (Gordon, 2003; Martinez et al., 2008) or (iii) regulatory activation (Mosser and Edwards, 2008). Thus, activated microglia show a continuum spectrum of activation patterns, resulting in the expression of different cytokines and cytokine receptors (Town et al., 2005).

Commitment to the M1 macrophage lineage (Satoh et al., 2010) is defined by the activation of a member of the interferon-regulatory factor (IRF) family. IRF5 activates genes encoding for inflammatory cytokines, such as TNFs, IL6, IL12 and IL23, and tumor suppressors (Ouyang et al., 2007; Krausgruber et al., 2011). M2 polarization is controlled by IRF4

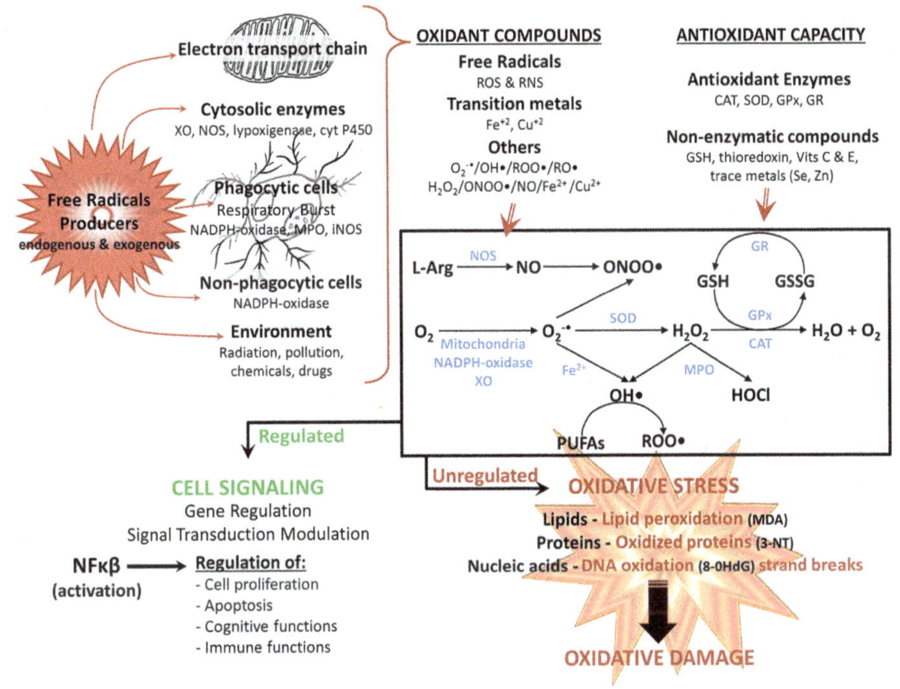

FIGURE 1 | Reactive species participate in normal cellular function or in pathological mechanisms depending on their overproduction. Reactive oxygen species (**ROS**) and reactive nitrogen species (**RNS**), are produced through several mechanisms by the cell: the electron transport chain in mitochondria, various cytosolic and membrane enzymes (i.e., xanthine oxidase (**XO**), nitric oxide synthase (**NOS**), NADPH oxidase complex, etc.), as well as exogenously provided by the environment. At the same time, cells have several antioxidant defense mechanisms for detoxifying ROS and RNS, including enzymes (i.e., superoxide dismutase (**SOD**), catalase (**CAT**), glutathione peroxidase (**GPx**), glutathione reductase (**GR**) and nonenzymatic antioxidants (i.e., reduced glutathione (**GSH**), vitamins **E** and **C**. The main generation pathways of ROS and RNS are also shown: the reduction of O_2 occurs by diverse mechanisms (i.e., mitochondria, XO, NADPH-oxidase complex) leading to formation of superoxide anion (**$O_2^{\bullet-}$**); which is easily transformed to hydrogen peroxide (**H_2O_2**) either nonenzymatically or by SOD. H_2O_2 is converted to H_2O by CAT, or by GPx, which together with the GR regenerate GSH. In addition, under stress conditions and high concentration of transition metal (i.e., iron ions—**Fe**), O_2 •- can generate hydroxyl radical **(OH•)**, which in turn can react with polyunsaturated fatty acids (**PUFAs**) and generate peroxyl radical (**ROO•**). Finally, O_2 •- can react with nitric oxide (**NO**; depending on NOS), producing the highly reactive peroxinitrite (**ONOO•**) anion, whereas H_2O_2 is converted to hypochlorous acid (**HOCl**) by myeloperoxidase (**MPO**). The balance between oxidants compounds and antioxidant defense determines the end result. Optimal physiologic levels leads to beneficial effects, with ROS and RNS acting as second messengers in intracellular signaling cascades (modulation of gene regulation and signal transduction pathways, mainly by activation of NFκB), regulating several physiological functions (i.e., cognitive and immune functions). However, when overproduction of ROS/RNS is higher than the antioxidant system, the equilibrium status favors oxidant vs. antioxidant reactions, leading to **oxidative stress**, in which ROS/RNS have harmful effects, because of their reaction with various macromolecules (lipids, proteins and nucleic acids), contributing to cellular and tissue oxidative damage, and the development of age-related impairments. **Oxidation products**: 3-NT, 3-nitrotyrosine; 8-OHdG, 8-hydroxy-2-deoxyguanosine; malondialdehyde (**MDA**); alkoxyl radical (**RO•**).

(Satoh et al., 2010; Krausgruber et al., 2011). Cyclic AMP-response element binding protein (CREB)–mediated induction of transcription factor C/EBPβ upregulates M2-specific genes (Ruffell et al., 2009), whereas activation of transcription factor nuclear factor *kappa*-light-chain-enhancer of activated B cells (NFκB)-p50 is associated with the inhibition of M1-activation genes (Porta et al., 2009). Secretion of IL4, IL10 and TGFβ by M2-activated macrophages, promote humoral immune responses and down-regulate M1-mediated responses, inhibiting several inflammatory functions (Town et al., 2005). Originally, it was thought that M2 activation resulted in protective functions. However, there is evidence that M2 cytokines such as IL4, IL5, IL9, and IL13 also result in the induction of some chronic inflammatory processes (Wynn, 2003). As for regulatory macrophages; they appear to arise at later stages of adaptive immune responses, being their primary role limiting inflammatory activation (Mosser, 2003). Regulatory macrophages appear to be generated through several signaling pathways, involving extracellular signal-regulated kinases/mitogen-activated protein kinases (ERK/MAPK; Lucas et al., 2005; Mosser and Edwards, 2008).

Microglia are activated in nearly all CNS diseases (Kreutzberg, 1996; Hanisch and Kettenmann, 2007; Neumann et al., 2009), producing and secreting a broad spectrum of inflammatory mediators, such as eicosanoids, cytokines (Nakamura, 2002; Kim and de Vellis, 2005; Tichauer et al., 2007), chemokines, ROS, nitric oxide (NO·), small metabolites, proteases (ea. α-antichymotrypsin and α-antitrypsin), and inflammatory markers (ea. serum amyloid P and C-reactive protein; Li et al., 2007; Tichauer et al., 2007; Neumann et al., 2009; Lue et al., 2010).

Those inflammatory mediators regulate innate immune defense and have profound effects on neuronal properties, modifying synaptic function (Selkoe, 2002; Di Filippo et al., 2008). In addition, microglia can also induce bystander damage of neurons, especially under conditions of strong or long lasting stimulation, and depending on the environmental context (Li et al., 2007; von Bernhardi, 2007). In fact, cytotoxic activation of microglia is associated with neuronal loss and decline of cognitive and neurobehavioral function (Cagnin et al., 2001; Kim and de Vellis, 2005; Block et al., 2007). Nevertheless, microglia also secretes trophic factors and modulator cytokines, being active partners in neuroprotection.

Neuroinflammation establishes a complex interaction with oxidizing agents through redox sensors present in enzymes, receptors, and transcription factors. Those factors affect neuron-glia crosstalk and neuronal function (Liu et al., 2012), resulting later in neurodegenerative changes (Raj et al., 2014). Signal transduction of various cytokines, themselves critical mediators of oxidative stress, neuroinflammation, and even neurodegenerative changes, are modified by the redox status (Mrak and Griffin, 2005; Kierdorf et al., 2010). Oxidative stress, a result of the equilibrium between production and detoxification of radical species (**Figure 1**), further increases inflammatory cytokines, creating a vicious cycle (Rosales-Corral et al., 2010), and affects the maintenance of cellular homeostasis and cell survival (Satoh and Lipton, 2007).

Mitochondria were often thought to be the main responsible for ROS overproduction and oxidative stress. However, NADPH oxidase (NOX) enzymes participation is also an important ROS-generating system (Bordt and Polster, 2014). Activation of the phagocyte NADPH oxidase (NOX2) in microglia, plays a role in neuroinflammation, but appears also to contribute to neuronal death under pathologic conditions (Qin et al., 2013; Jiang et al., 2015). Moreover, ROS production can also depend on other NOX isoforms, which are detected also in astrocytes and neurons (Nayernia et al., 2014). Whereas ROS derived from normal NADPH oxidase function is required for processes such as neuronal signaling, memory, and central homeostasis (Jiang et al., 2015), overproduction of ROS contributes to excessive oxidative stress, resulting in neuronal dysfunction and neurotoxicity (Zhang et al., 2014). ROS regulates several signal transduction pathways, including for some trophic factors and hormones. NFκB is a transcription factor activated by ROS and inflammatory mediators that participates both in protective and deleterious responses, depending on the context of stimulation that will result in the co-activation of various signaling pathways. It activates genes regulating cellular survival, growth, differentiation, inflammation, and cell death. Under non-stimulated conditions, NFκB is kept inactive by IκB (inhibitor of κB) in the cytoplasmic compartment. High concentrations of ROS inactivate NFκB through oxidation of its p50 subunit, inhibiting its DNA binding. In contrast to the inhibitory effect of high ROS levels, moderate levels of ROS lead to the sequential phosphorylation, polyubiquitination and degradation of IκB, allowing the activation of NFκB (**Figures 1, 2**). Once activated, and depending on the context, NFκB plays a pro-survival role by inhibiting c-Jun N-terminal kinases/stress-activated protein kinase (JNK) and caspase cell death pathways and upregulating transcriptional activation of anti-apoptotic proteins and genes involved in decreasing mitochondrial ROS (mtROS), especially those coding for manganese superoxide dismutase (MnSOD; Patten et al., 2010). TNFα also activates NFκB associated with neuroprotection against β-amyloid (Aβ) neurotoxicity *in vitro* (Barger et al., 1995), and NFκB activates anti-apoptotic responses and protects neurons from excitotoxicity and ischemic brain injury (Pennypacker et al., 2001; Bhakar et al., 2002; Mattson, 2005).

On the other hand, NFκB activation can also be detrimental. NFκB has a key role in the initiation and amplification of inflammation through its response to inflammatory stimuli mediated by TNFα or IL1, leading to the induction of several cytokines and chemokines. Activation of NFκB and MAPK pathways are conspicuous in oxidative stress- (Chen et al., 2009; Chongthammakun et al., 2009) and Aβ-induced (Song et al., 2004) neuronal cell death. In addition to NFκB, other transcription factors are activated by inflammatory conditions, such as peroxisome proliferator-activated receptor gamma (PPARγ) and signal transducer and activator of transcription (STAT-1) and have also been implicated in Alzheimer's disease (AD; Sastre et al., 2006; Cho et al., 2007).

The brain is particularly vulnerable to oxidative stress. Vulnerability depends on its: (i) high oxygen metabolic rate (consumes approximately 20% of the total consumption of oxygen of a mammal), (ii) high dependence on oxidative metabolism for obtaining energy, (iii) high content of iron, an endogenous catalyzer for the generation of ROS and reactive nitrogen species (RNS), (iv) lower content of antioxidant enzymes compared with other organs (Floyd and Hensley, 2002; Mattson et al., 2002); and (v) low ability to eliminate mutations not removed by cell replacement as consequence of the post-mitotic nature of neurons. Aged, or injured brains of any sort, show oxidative modifications in nucleic acids, proteins, lipids, and sugars (**Figure 1**). Several of those oxidative damage and changes result in a loss of function (Lovell et al., 2001; Halliwell, 2006).

Age-Related Changes of Microglia

Microglial cell changes have been documented in aging. However, many of those changes are also observed in neurodegenerative conditions. Thus, it is still unclear whether these changes are reactive to the underlying pathophysiology. Although there is an agreement on the fact that degenerative diseases are not the natural continuous progression of age-related decline, both aging and neurodegenerative disease appear to be highly multifactorial conditions that also share many relevant factors. Aging is a mayor risk factor for the development of many neurodegenerative diseases. Furthermore, neuroinflammation and oxidative stress (both reportedly associated with non-pathological aging in humans and animal models) are common features for several disease phenotypes. Studies in cell cultures and animal models suggest the existence of altered activation states and cellular senescence in the aged brain. Not only aging

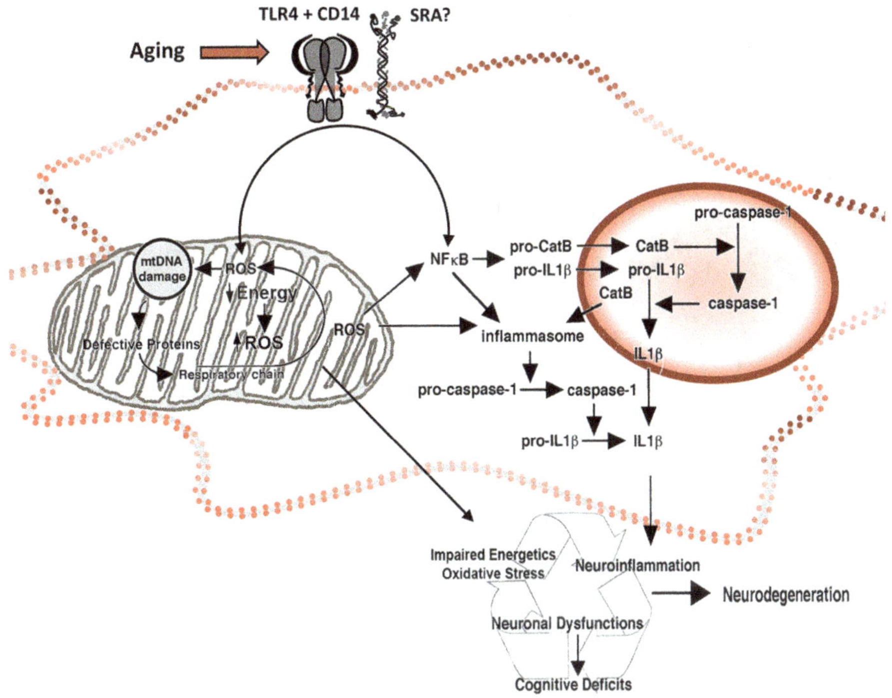

FIGURE 2 | Reactive oxygen species and inflammation in the aged microglia. Representation of the participation of mitochondria and lysosomes in the increased production of ROS and inflammatory cytokines by aged microglia. Increased intracellular ROS activate redox-sensitive NFκB through a pathway mediated by mitochondrial ROS (associated with decreased energetic production and increased release of ROS by the electron transport chain) and a ROS-independent pathway, potentiating neuroinflammation. The activation of NFκB induces production of pro-CatB and pro-IL1β, and the activation of inflammasome in the cytoplasm. Pro-CatB is processed into CatB in the lysosome, which in turn, mediates the activation of pro-caspase-1 to caspase 1 and increases the processing of pro-IL1β, releasing increased amounts of IL1β both in the phagolysosome and the cytoplasm, as well as potentially potentiate apoptosis. Changes on the expression of pattern recognition receptors, like TLR4 CD14 and SRA, result in changes on neuroinflammatory activation and oxidative stress by activating NFκB and the release of ROS.

appears to be a key risk factor for neurodegenerative as well as other chronic diseases (Mosher and Wyss-Coray, 2014; Cho et al., 2015), but the presence of those diseases potentiate also the appearance of aging and senescence related markers (Baron et al., 2014; Mosher and Wyss-Coray, 2014; Bachstetter et al., 2015).

There is high heterogeneity of microglia in various neurodegenerative diseases and those phenotypes share common characteristics with aging (Bachstetter et al., 2015) as well as the pattern of microglia gene expression is shared by aging and neurodegenerative conditions (Holtman et al., 2015). Moreover, many of the changes described in aged microglia represent changes that occur during aging; meaning that, they do not appear when reaching a certain age threshold, but they change through life, as the individual ages. Analysis of transcriptome data from postmortem studies of frontal cortex from 381 healthy individuals with ages spanning from young teenagers to people older than 80 years of age, show that microglia gene markers assemble into a transcriptional module in a gene co-expression network (Wehrspaun et al., 2015), whose expression pattern show a negative correlation with age. Genes that encode microglia surface receptors for neuron and/or microglia crosstalk are especially affected. In addition, they found that microglia are controlled by brain-expressed transcription factors, including *RUNX1*, *IRF8*, *PU.1*, and *TAL1* (Kierdorf and Prinz, 2013), which are master regulators for the age-dependent microglia module. As the authors highlighted, identification of age-dependent gene modules in adulthood are relevant for understanding critical periods for susceptibility to late-onset diseases (Wehrspaun et al., 2015).

Senescent microglia display morphological changes (**Figure 3**), with fewer and shorter processes, increased soma volume, and formation of spheroid swellings, which is referred as "dystrophic microglia" (Streit et al., 2004b; Conde and Streit, 2006a,b; Streit, 2006; Flanary et al., 2007). Microglia co-localize with neurodegenerating neurons, and show clumping, with loss of their homogeneous tissue distribution, and accumulation of phagocytic inclusions (Hart et al., 2012; Tremblay et al., 2012; Hefendehl et al., 2014). Live imaging shows that the dynamic response of microglia to injury changes with age. Young microglia increase their motility and extend ramifications rapidly when exposed to ATP, an injury-associated signal, or to a focal tissue injury. In contrast, aged microglia are less dynamic and ramified and further reduce their dynamism when exposed to ATP. On the other hand, disaggregation of aged microglia from the site of injury becomes slow, indicating

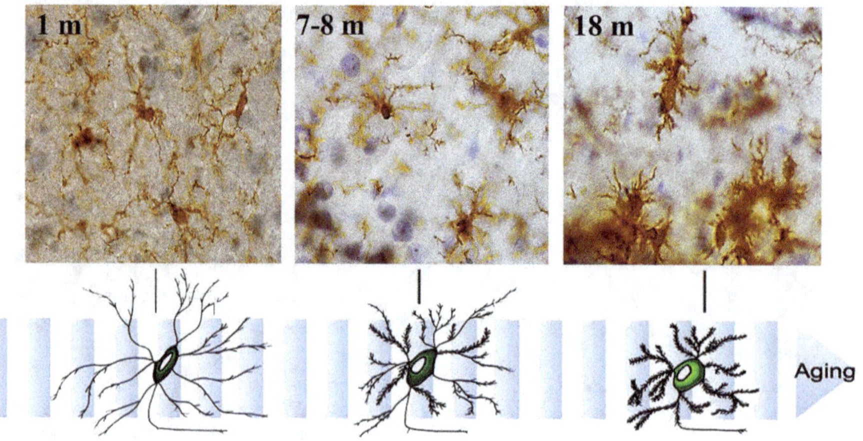

FIGURE 3 | Aging-related morphological changes of microglia. Microglial cell morphology changes with aging. Immunohistochemistry for Iba-1 (a constitutive identity marker for monocyte-macrophage cells) and counterstaining with hematoxylin of hippocampal sections from animals of different ages (1- to 18-month old). Microglia obtained from young mice have a small cell body and very long and slender ramifications. As mice age, microglia gradually show bigger cell bodies and progressively shorter and thicker cell processes.

that aged microglia tend to show sustained responses (Damani et al., 2011). Both in aging (Flanary and Streit, 2004) and in AD (Flanary et al., 2007), microglia show telomere shortening and decreased telomerase activity, which are speculated to be one of the factors underlying the diminution of some functional activities, such as clearance (phagocytosis plus effective removal of the compounds) and basal proliferation (Harry, 2013). Reduced microglia replication could also result in a depletion of healthy microglia, favoring the participation of more senescent and dysfunctional cells (Mosher and Wyss-Coray, 2014).

Activated microglia are the primary cellular source of both inflammatory molecules and oxidative products (**Figure 4**). (Pawate et al., 2004; Qin et al., 2005b; Hayashi et al., 2008). Microglia from aged brains show increased basal production of IL6 and enhanced lypopolysaccharide (LPS)-induced IL6 and IL1β, compared with microglia from young mice brains in culture (Ye and Johnson, 1999; Sierra et al., 2007). They appear to be activated also under normal physiological conditions. In aging, mild stimulatory events or minor injuries, otherwise easily solved, could induce damage and initiate a disease process. TGFβ1 is a strong regulator of neuroinflammation and cytotoxicity and its signaling pathway could be part of the switch mechanism from protective to deleterious activation of microglia. Its downstream canonical signaling involves the Smad pathway, which transduce extracellular signals from ligands acting as transcription factors (Derynck and Zhang, 2003), as well as a complex Smad independent signaling (Weiss and Attisano, 2013). TGFβ1 secreted by hippocampal neurons and astrocytes regulates microglial cell activation, attenuating the release of inflammatory cytokines and reactive species (Chen et al., 2002; Mittaud et al., 2002; Herrera-Molina and von Bernhardi, 2005; Herrera-Molina et al., 2012), protecting neuronal cells *in vitro* (Hu et al., 1995; Lieb et al., 2003; Herrera-Molina and von Bernhardi, 2005) and promoting microglia-mediated Aβ phagocytosis and degradation (Wyss-Coray et al., 2001). These regulatory effects of TGFβ1 are mediated by Smad3-dependent mechanisms (Flores and von Bernhardi, 2012; Tichauer and von Bernhardi, 2012), as well as the reported inhibition of lipopolysaccharide (LPS)-induced macrophage and microglial activation (Werner et al., 2000; Le et al., 2004). TGFβ1 Smad3 pathway also participates in the inhibition of the production of radical species induced by inflammatory stimuli and in the induction of amyloid-β (Aβ) phagocytosis *in vitro* (Tichauer and von Bernhardi, 2012).

TGFβ1 levels are elevated in aged individual (Blobe et al., 2000; Tichauer et al., 2014). However, recent reports show that induction of the Smad3 pathway by inflammatory conditions is decreased in normal aging (Tichauer et al., 2014). Interestingly, this signaling pathway is impaired in AD patients and mouse models for AD, resulting in Aβ accumulation, Aβ-induced neurodegeneration, and neurofibrillary tangle formation (Tesseur et al., 2006; Ueberham et al., 2006). Evidence gathered over the last two decades indicate that TGFβ signaling impairment often lead to neuroinflammation, neuronal dysfunction and neurodegenerative changes, and could be involved in the pathogenesis of neurodegenerative diseases (Tesseur and Wyss-Coray, 2006). Given the complex signaling pathway activated by TGFβ, which in addition to the Smad pathway also activates Smad-independent signaling, including ERK/MAPK, P38 MAPK, JNK, and PI3K (Derynck and Zhang, 2003; Weiss and Attisano, 2013), a decreased activation of Smad3 in an environment presenting elevated levels of TGFβ, as observed in aging, could result in an increased activation of MAPKs and PI3K, which are signaling pathways also involved in inflammatory activation. Such an imbalance on the signaling activated by TGFβ could explain, at least partially, the maintenance of increased levels of microglial cell activation, oxidative stress and mild neuroinflammation, although TGFβ1,

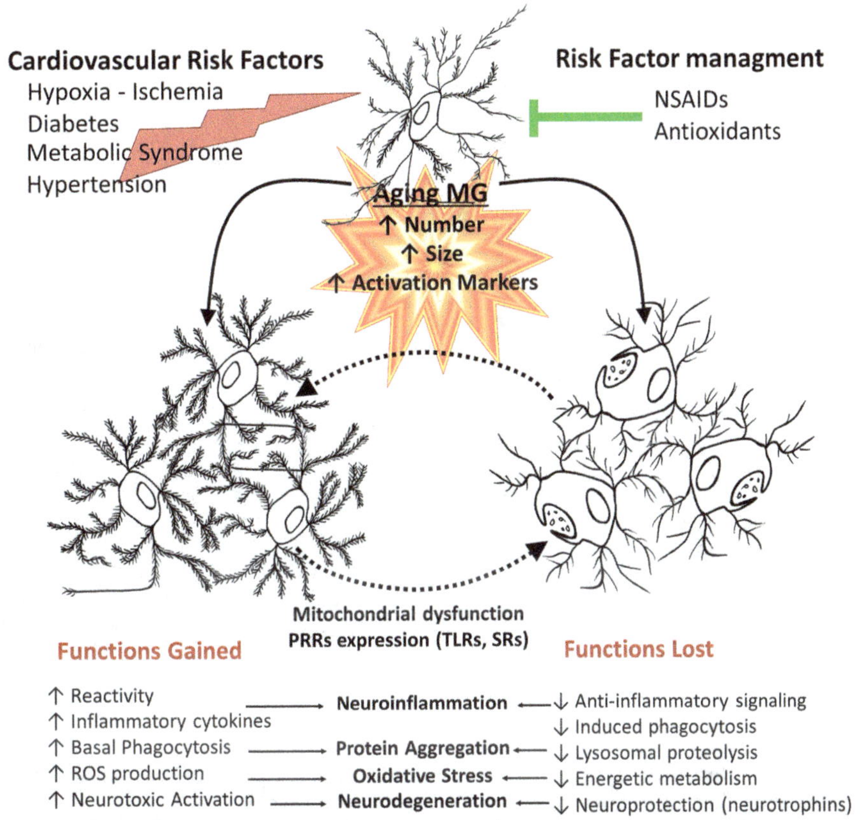

FIGURE 4 | Age-related changes of microglial cell function. In aged brains, there is an increased number, size and activation of microglia. This is affected by additional systemic pathophysiological changes associated with other age related changes, environmental factors and disease processes, such as cardiovascular risk factors and metabolic syndrome or injuries. Deleterious processes further promote an inflammatory environment, increasing cytotoxic microglial cell activation, whereas risk factor management and pharmacological interventions can promote a healthy aging. Aged microglia changes depend both on gained and lost functions. They have increased basal phagocytic activity, although a reduced capacity to induce phagocytosis when stimulated, together with reduced lysosomal activity, resulting in a decreased clearance activity. Microglia also shows an increased production of inflammatory cytokines and reactive species. Those changes result in a shift of balance towards decreased protective functions and an increased neurotoxicity.

one of the main regulatory cytokines decreasing inflammatory activation, is increased in aged mice (Tichauer et al., 2014). Those results indicate that TGFβ1-Smad3 signaling could be a therapeutic target for AD treatment.

Another alternative is that stimuli that normally would trigger a protective response, in conditions of age-related impairment of normal homeostatic mechanisms result in a persistent activation, which is associated, for example, to a robust induction of oxidative stress (**Figures 4, 5**; von Bernhardi, 2007; Herrup, 2010), or to the upregulation of NFκB. In fact, NFκB response is age-dependent, and it is another candidate for age-dependent changes due to its role in the regulation of immunity, inflammation, and cell death (Adler et al., 2007). Blockade of NFκB in aged mice has been reported to reverse the gene expression program and cell morphology, "rejuvenating" old mice (Adler et al., 2008). TNFα signaling involves NFκB, resulting in a beneficial or detrimental response depending on the age and the type of stimuli. Stimulation of 24 month-old rat neurons with TNFα plus Aβ is toxic, whereas those same stimuli are protective for 10 month-old neurons (Patel and Brewer, 2008). The down-regulation of TNFs receptors TNFR1 and TNFR2 signaling observed in aging results in defective NFκB activation and fails to provide a neuroprotective response against Aβ toxicity by TNFα (Patel and Brewer, 2008). NFκB accumulates in the nuclei of old neurons; an effect that is also produced by blocking TNFR2. An alternative explanation for the failure of NFκB to activate protective pathways could depend on high concentrations of ROS (Parihar and Brewer, 2007), and the oxidized redox state of aged cells (Parihar et al., 2008). The redox state of NFκB could be a control mechanism regulating its availability (Sulciner et al., 1996). It is unclear whether the over-production of ROS, through a vicious cycle in the aging mitochondria, may activate redox-sensitive NFkB, thereby provoking excessive inflammation in the aged brain (Hayashi et al., 2008; Nakanishi and Wu, 2009; **Figure 2**).

When exposed to endotoxins like LPS, microglia derived from adult mice secrete high amounts of ROS, whereas young animals microglia predominately produce NO·, with little ROS (Tichauer et al., 2014). Aged microglia become more inflammatory

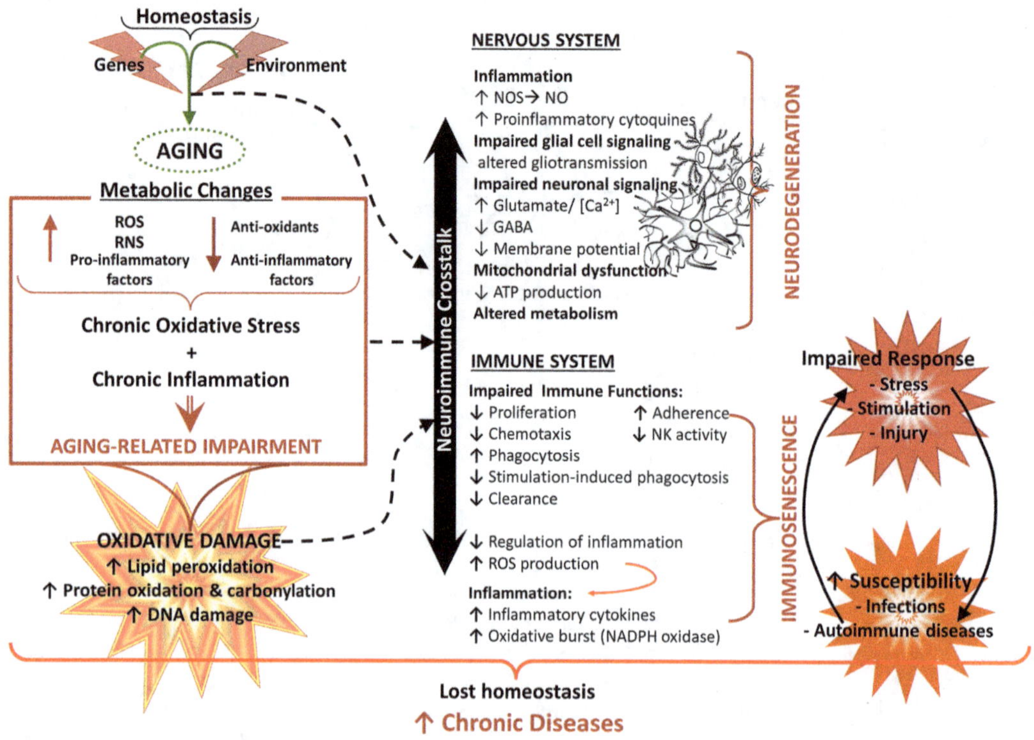

FIGURE 5 | Aging of the nervous and immune system and the neuroimmune crosstalk. Healthy aging of the nervous and immune systems depend both on genetic and environmental (lifestyle) factors. Aging is associated with a state of low grade chronic oxidative stress and inflammation (with production of reactive mediators and inflammatory compounds and a decreased antioxidant and anti-inflammatory capacity), which appear to be the cause of an important part of age-related deterioration of the nervous and the immune systems, as well as of the neuroimmune communication. Because of their complex functions, the central nervous system (CNS) and the immune system are especially vulnerable to oxidative damage (i.e., lipid peroxidation, protein oxidation, DNA damage), which contributes to oxidative stress and inflammation. Age-related changes in the immune function, known as immunosenescence, results in increased susceptibility to infections and cancer, inflammation and autoimmune diseases. In the CNS, oxidative stress has a negative impact on function, leading to mitochondrial dysfunction and impaired energetic metabolism, altered neuronal and glial signaling. There may be disruption of the cycle glutamate-glutamine and increased levels of neuronal calcium, which are involved in mechanisms of neuronal damage leading to loss of function, excitotoxicity and apoptosis. In addition, dysfunction of the neuron-glia crosstalk leads to a chronic neuroinflammation, which promotes a prolonged activation of microglia and further induction of dysfunction and degenerative changes. All these alterations contribute to functional decline and the development of neurodegenerative diseases. **NO**, nitric oxide; **NOS**, nitric oxide synthase; **RNS**, reactive nitrogen species; **ROS**, reactive oxygen species.

than their younger counterparts upon systemic inflammatory stimulation; thus exacerbating neurodegenerative changes (Combrinck et al., 2002; Cunningham et al., 2005; Godbout et al., 2005; Sierra et al., 2007). Systemic inflammation also causes aged microglia to become more responsive than young microglia, increasing production of inflammatory cytokines (IL1β, IL6 and TNFα). The resulting exacerbated response to inflammatory challenges appears to depend on the priming of microglia by previous activation experience. Primed microglia undergoes a phenotypic shift towards a sensitized state, responding to a secondary "triggering" stimulus more rapidly and robustly than non-primed cells (Harry, 2013). Therefore, the exacerbated response to stimuli of aged microglia can contribute to neuronal damage (**Figure 5**) and the onset of chronic diseases (Perry et al., 2003, 2007; Perry, 2004).

Age-related changes on cell response involve changes on microglia receptors (**Figures 2, 4**). Aged microglia show upregulation of Toll-like receptors (TLRs), and TLR4 co-receptor CD14 (Letiembre et al., 2007), as well as age-related changes in signal transduction of TLR4. There are changes in the expression profile of scavenger receptors (SRs; Yamamoto et al., 2002; Hickman et al., 2008). TLRs, CD14, and SRs are pattern recognition receptors (PRRs), key participants of the host defense response and the phagocytosis of pathogen-associated molecules pattern (PAMPs) and damage-associated molecules pattern (DAMPs), being crucial for the innate immune response The activation of these receptors by diverse ligands is associated with activation of microglial cell (Godoy et al., 2012; Murgas et al., 2012, 2014), production of inflammatory mediators, and uptake of pathogens and macromolecules, including Aβ (Alarcón et al., 2005). Thus, changes on their expression pattern affect cell activation (Cornejo and Von Bernhardi, 2013). In addition, aged microglia also express some surface antigens that are not normally expressed by their young counterparts, including the major histocompatibility complex II (MHCII), associated with antigen presentation, and ED1, the rodent equivalent of CD68, associated with phagocytosis. Regardless of the increased CD68, aged microglia are not better phagocytes than young microglia (Floden and Combs, 2011). In fact, aged microglia appear to have a decreased ability to phagocytose Aβ compared with microglia from young mice (Floden and Combs, 2011). We observed that although basal phagocytosis by microglia obtained from 1-year old mice is slightly increased compared with young mice, phagocytosis fails to be induced by TGFβ (Tichauer et al., 2014) or LPS (Cornejo et al., 2014), and is not coupled to an effective clearance machinery (**Figure 5**). Moreover, in addition to phagocytosis, protein homeostasis is impaired at several levels, including chaperone-mediated protein folding and stability, protein trafficking, protein degradation and autophagy. A major consequence of these impairments is the aggregation of abnormal proteins, which is an important neuropathological finding in several neurodegenerative diseases, such as Parkinson's disease (PD) and AD (Taylor and Dillin, 2011). Taken together, age-related changes in receptors expression could account for alterations observed in microglial cell function, providing insight on cell phenotypes that could play a role in the pathophysiological changes leading to neurodegenerative diseases.

Autophagy capacity can regulate mitochondrial integrity, ROS production, and subsequent NLR family, pyrin containing 3 (NLRP3) inflammasome activation (Nakahira et al., 2011; Zhou et al., 2011; Salminen et al., 2012). NLRP3 activation is negatively regulated by autophagy, because damaged mitochondria producing high amounts of ROS are removed by autophagy. In fact, inhibition of autophagy triggers accumulation of damaged mitochondria (Zhou et al., 2011), which produce more ROS.

Mitochondrial DNA (mtDNA), which encodes components of the mitochondria electron transfer complexes, is highly susceptible to ROS-mediated damage, due to its close proximity to the ROS generated by the respiratory chain and to its decreased number of protective histones and DNA-binding proteins. Aging-related accumulation of mtDNA damage results in a reduced expression of mitochondria electron transfer complexes, in especial complexes I and IV, because they contain a relatively large number of mtDNA-encoded subunits. The reduced activity of complex I further facilitates the generation of ROS (Lin et al., 2002), establishing a vicious cycle (Kang et al., 2007; **Figure 2**). Most cells have protective mechanisms, depending on enzymatic breakdown or scavenging of ROS (**Figure 1**). However, antioxidant systems appear to be less functional in the brain, which can lead to persistent increased levels of ROS and RNS reacting with the various target molecules (Halliwell, 2006).

Functional decline of lysosomes and mitochondria in microglia produces an exacerbated generation of ROS and inflammatory mediators, which could further promote microglia aging (Hayashi et al., 2008). Accumulation of mitochondrial DNA oxidative damage in microglia during aging, increases ROS production. The increased intracellular ROS, in turn, activates the redox-sensitive nuclear factor *kappa* B, inducing neuroinflammation (Nakanishi and Wu, 2009), which in turn also promotes oxidative stress. Mitochondria-derived ROS and cathepsin B, are also involved in the microglial production of interleukin-1β (**Figure 2**).

During aging, autophagy efficiency declines and becomes dysfunctional, resulting in the accumulation of waste materials within cells (Salminen et al., 2012). On the other hand, induction of phagocytosis on LPS-primed microglia can cause lysosomal damage. The release of cathepsin B (CatB), a lysosomal cysteine protease, into the cytoplasm triggers the activation of the NLRP3, leading to the production and secretion of IL1β (**Figure 2**) and IL18 (Halle et al., 2008; Hornung et al., 2008). Interestingly, a NLRP3-deficient AD mice model show improvement of their spatial memory deficits, a reduced expression of brain caspase-1 and IL1β, and enhanced Aβ clearance (Heneka et al., 2013). In addition of Aβ, cholesterol crystals is also a major causative factor of age-related diseases such as atherosclerosis, and also shows activation of the inflammasome in a CatB-dependent manner (Duewell et al., 2010; Masters et al., 2010).

Aged Microglia-Related Neuronal Impairment and Neurodegenerative Diseases

Age-dependent changes gradually have a toll on brain homeostasis and function (Herrup, 2010; von Bernhardi et al., 2010), changing glial cell reactivity (von Bernhardi, 2007). Cytotoxic activation of microglia, increased production of inflammatory cytokines, and ROS combined with impaired ability to regulate increased oxidative stress in the aging brain (Conde and Streit, 2006b; von Bernhardi et al., 2010). Those changes appear to be causative factors for neurodegenerative processes, (**Figure 5**; Block et al., 2007) and the associated decline in motor and cognitive functions (Forster et al., 1996; Navarro et al., 2002).

Chronic inflammation induces deficits in long-term potentiation (LTP), the major neuronal substrate for learning and memory, in middle-aged but not in young rats (Liu et al., 2012). Similarly, *in vivo* microinjection of fibrillary Aβ in the cortex of aged rhesus monkeys showed neurodegeneration, tau phosphorylation, and microglial cell proliferation, but not in young monkeys, suggesting that Aβ neurotoxicity is a pathological response of the aging brain (Geula et al., 1998). In this context, microglia upregulated production of IL1β, is possibly implicated in age-associated cognitive impairments (Rachal Pugh et al., 2001; Maher et al., 2006). As mentioned above, aged microglia actively participate in the genesis of neuronal damage in neurodegenerative diseases, through production of inflammatory mediators and ROS (Block et al., 2007), but also because of the impairment of their neuroprotective functions (**Figure 5**). Thus, microglia contribute to the death of dopaminergic neurons in PD, forebrain neurons in AD, and motor neurons in amyotrophic lateral sclerosis (ALS; Boillée et al., 2006; Mount et al., 2007). Similarly, TNFα promotes PD progression (McCoy et al., 2006), whereas the absence of TNFR1 protects against AD- and PD-like disease in mice (Sriram et al., 2002; He et al., 2007).

Neurodegenerative diseases often have increased generation of RNS and ROS as an early event (Perry et al., 2002; Shi and Gibson, 2007), which can contribute to neuronal cell injury via various redox reactions (**Figure 1**). Deficiency in antioxidant enzymes, such as superoxide dismutase (SOD), increases disease associated phenomena (Li et al., 2004a), increasing tau phosphorylation (Melov et al., 2007), and amyloid and tau aggregation (Li et al., 2004a), and accelerates behavioral impairment (Esposito et al., 2006). Thus, oxidative damage in the brain of AD patients and animal models is more abundant than that observed in age-matched control individuals. Conversely, increased expression of antioxidant enzymes attenuates AD phenotype (Dumont et al., 2009).

There are additional mechanisms for reactive species-related impairment, NO· target cysteine residues of proteins to form S-nitrosothiols (SNOs). The interaction with proteins that are targets of S-nitrosylation represents NO· signal transduction (Hess et al., 2005). S-nitrosylation switches the on-off functions of receptors, GTPases, and transcription factors, and can affect mitochondrial function. NO· reversibly inhibits complexes I and IV (Clementi et al., 1998), further increasing release of ROS by mitochondria, further promoting dysfunction of mitochondrial dynamics (Bossy-Wetzel and Lipton, 2003; Barsoum et al., 2006). Moreover, S-nitrosylation modulates GTPase activity of the mitochondrial fission protein dynamin-related protein 1 (Drp1), favoring altered mitochondrial dynamics, synaptic damage, and eventually neuronal death (Cho et al., 2009). Other examples relevant for aging and neurodegeneration are: (i) the S-nitrosylation of protein-disulfide isomerase (PDI, an enzyme relevant for the maturation and transport of unfolded secretory proteins), which abolishes PDI-mediated inhibition of neurodegenerative changes triggered by endoplasmic reticulum (ER) stress, misfolded proteins, or proteasome inhibition (Uehara et al., 2006); and (ii) the S-nitrosylation of ApoE, resulting in changes of its interaction with low-density lipoprotein (LDL) receptors (Abrams et al., 2011).

Microglia and Alzheimer's Disease

Neurodegenerative diseases, including AD, involve several converging disease mechanisms, generating a functional interplay between neurons and glial cells (**Figure 5**). The AD brain is characterized by the presence of senile plaques, constituted by aggregated Aβ, and neurofibrillary tangles (NFTs), formed by hyper-phosphorylated tau, as well by synapse and neuronal loss (Uylings and de Brabander, 2002), and glial cell activation (Kim and de Vellis, 2005; Jellinger, 2006; Heneka and O'banion, 2007; von Bernhardi, 2007; von Bernhardi et al., 2010). Interestingly, Alzheimer, on his original descriptions, already stated that these lesions were markers of an upstream process rather than the disease cause (Davis and Chisholm, 1999). The fact that brain innate immune response could be involved in the genesis of neurodegenerative diseases (Nguyen et al., 2002; Björkqvist et al., 2009; von Bernhardi et al., 2010), lead to re-consider the role of Aβ and propose glia to be a leading factor in the pathology of AD (von Bernhardi, 2007). The hippocampus, one of the regions affected early by neurodegeneration in AD, is one of the most densely populated by microglia together with the *Substantia nigra*. However, most scientists who adhere to the "amyloid cascade hypothesis" of AD, view Aβ as the cause of AD and neuroinflammation just as a consequence of glia activation (Akiyama et al., 2000; Heneka and O'banion, 2007; Hirsch and Hunot, 2009).

Microglia are intimately associated with Aβ plaques in AD, but not with the diffuse Aβ plaques of the normal aged brain (Itagaki et al., 1989; von Bernhardi et al., 2001; von Bernhardi, 2007; Hashioka et al., 2008; Heurtaux et al., 2010). The trigger for microglia activation is unclear, but the invasion of plaques by active microglia has been reported in AD transgenic mice models, when Aβ is injected into the brain or in *in vitro* experiments (von Bernhardi et al., 2001; Alarcón et al., 2005; Reed-Geaghan et al., 2009; Njie et al., 2012; Thanopoulou et al., 2010). Their activation by Aβ (Simard et al., 2006; Hashioka et al., 2008; Koenigsknecht-Talboo et al., 2008) results in cell transformation (Husemann et al., 2001). Microglia aging is associated with several mechanisms underlying the formation and accumulation of Aβ aggregates. Microglia clearance (phagocytosis plus degradation) of Aβ is reduced leading to its initial accumulation (Floden and Combs, 2011; Zhao et al., 2014), as well as its capacity to migrate (Sheng et al., 1998; Damani et al., 2011) and shift among inflammatory activation patterns towards a more phagocytic stage (Sierra et al., 2007; Streit et al., 2009; Schuitemaker et al., 2012). Similar results have been reported on AD patients (Mawuenyega et al., 2010). There is an age-related impairment of phagocytosis (Harry et al., 2000; Zhao et al., 2014) and clearance. Clearance by both microglia and astrocytes appears to depend on peroxisome proliferator-activated receptor-γ (PPARγ) and apolipoprotein E (apoE) levels, which promote the proteolytic clearance of soluble forms of Aβ (Mandrekar-Colucci et al., 2012). In addition, human genetic studies indicate that coding variants of TREM2, a regulator of microglia activation and phagocytosis, are suggestive of microglia immune senescence (Guerreiro et al., 2013), and results in a substantial risk for AD. Plaque-associated reactive microglia in these animals show enhanced staining for TNFα and IL-1β (Benzing et al., 1999). Neuroinflammation as well as other stressors promote production and release of Aβ (Lee et al., 2007; Mosher and Wyss-Coray, 2014) as well as its amyloidogenicity, favoring its aggregation. However, acute increased levels of various inflammatory factors, including IL1β and IL6 are associated with activation of glial cells and reduced amyloid pathology (Chakrabarty et al., 2010; Jiang et al., 2015), although chronic neuroinflammation fails promoting amyloid removal. Promotion of Aβ production and aggregation has been also observed secondary to microglia-related ROS through a stress response or depending on oxidative modifications of the peptide (Giasson et al., 2002).

Importantly, Aβ is also clearly indicated as a source of oxidative stress (Varadarajan et al., 2000), as Aβ activates microglia to produce extracellular superoxide radical ($O_2{\cdot}^-$; Qin et al., 2002; Bamberger et al., 2003), and can be a potent inducer of NFκB via the induction of intracellular ROS (Lee et al., 2005; Valerio et al., 2006) as well as through the TNFR1 signaling, which results in neuronal apoptosis (Li et al., 2004b; Valerio et al., 2006).

In addition to the role of oxidative stress in neuron dysfunction and degeneration, secondary to Aβ neurotoxicity, excitotoxicity, aggregation of proteins, and impaired calcium metabolism (Kuchibhotla et al., 2008; Lopez et al., 2008; Santos et al., 2010a,b), ROS appears to be a common mediator unifying the spectrum of cellular mechanisms leading to AD (**Figure 6**). Oxidative damage of the brain of AD patients and animal models include lipid peroxidation (Praticò et al., 1998; Butterfield and Lauderback, 2002; Butterfield, 2002; Butterfield et al., 2002), and oxidation of proteins and nucleic acids (Nunomura et al., 2001, 2004). RNA and DNA oxidation could impair protein synthesis, DNA repair, and transcription, and could eventually lead to cell death (**Figure 1**; Ding et al., 2006). Oxidation of mtDNA is 10-fold more abundant than that of nDNA. Increased mtDNA oxidation could lead to the reported mitochondrial abnormalities, which may contribute to the increase of O2·- leakage, ultimately resulting into elevated oxidative stress (Swerdlow, 2007; Swerdlow et al., 2010).

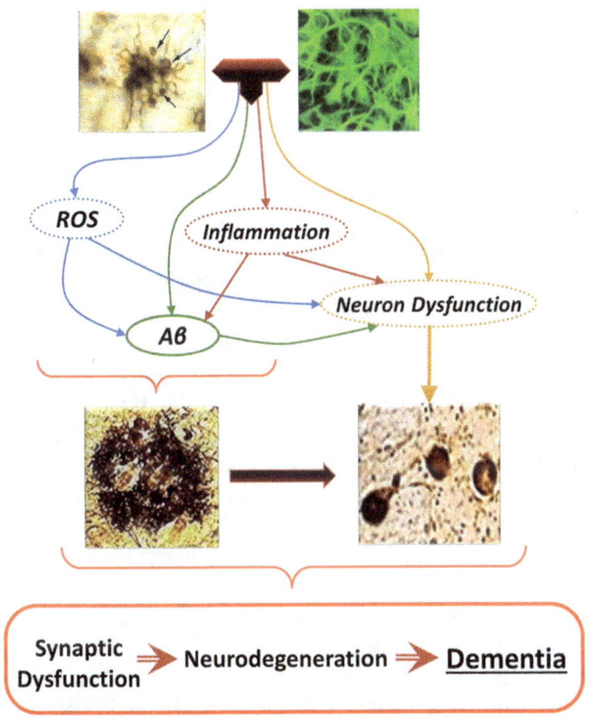

FIGURE 6 | The "Glial Cell Dysregulation Hypothesis" of Alzheimer's disease (AD). The glial cell dysregulation hypothesis proposes that AD has its cause on changes on the activation of microglia and on impaired regulation, which become increasingly cytotoxic decreasing their defensive functions. Impaired activation results in oxidative stress, persistent neuroinflammation and neuronal dysfunction, all of which can also induce production and aggregation of Aβ, and additional neuronal dysfunction. Inflammatory activation, secondary to aging and to various forms of stimuli or injury through life, can result in glial cell dysregulation. Dysregulated activation of glia, through the abnormal release of cytokines, reactive species, and other mediators, contributes to the increased expression of Aβ as well to functional and degenerative changes of neurons, perpetuating abnormal activation of glia, synaptic dysfunction and cell damage.

Glia actively promote neuronal dysfunction and neurodegeneration (von Bernhardi, 2007) through oxidative stress mechanisms by: (i) modifying intracellular proteins and lipids (Lovell et al., 2001; Halliwell, 2006; Zhu et al., 2007); (ii) inducing mitochondrial dysfunction, which increases production of ROS, and activates caspases, activating cell death pathway (Baloyannis, 2006; Lin and Beal, 2006a,b) and ATP depletion (Baloyannis, 2006); (iii) facilitating formation of ubiquitinated aggregates of misfolded proteins (Oddo, 2008) as consequence of the impairment of energy-dependent ubiquitin–proteasome pathway and abnormal phosphorylation of cytoskeleton components (Arnaud et al., 2006); (iv) inhibiting glial cell excitatory amino-acid transporter 2 (EAAT2) activity (Tian et al., 2010) inducing release of glutamate by astrocytes (Lauderback et al., 2001). Overactive glutamate receptors increase intracellular free calcium, causing mitochondrial toxicity (Mahad et al., 2008; Kawamata and Manfredi, 2010) and affect several calcium-dependent enzymes leading to dysfunction and initiation of apoptosis (Mattson and Chan, 2003); and (v) activating microglia (**Figure 4**) and astrocytes to produce and release inflammatory cytokines (von Bernhardi, 2007; Agostinho et al., 2010; Lee et al., 2010; von Bernhardi et al., 2010) and other reactive mediators (NO·, ROS; Zhu et al., 2007; von Bernhardi, 2007; Block, 2008; Agostinho et al., 2010; von Bernhardi et al., 2010). These factors activate signaling pathways of cytokines as well as of eicosanoids produced by cyclooxygenase-2 (COX-2; Wang et al., 2004; Trepanier and Milgram, 2010). Aging and AD also present changes in enzymes involved in glutathione (GSH) metabolism (**Figure 1**; comprehensive view on glutathione peroxidase (GPx), in Toppo et al. (2009). glutathione S-transferase (GST) activity is decreased in the AD amygdale, hippocampus, parietal lobe, and nucleus basalis of Meynert (Lovell et al., 1998). Decreased glutathione S-transferase omega-1 (GSTO1; Li et al., 2003), can be involved in the activation of IL1β (Laliberte et al., 2003), a fundamental component in the early inflammatory response of AD (Grimaldi et al., 2000; Griffin and Mrak, 2002).

Recapitulating, we consider that neurodegenerative changes in AD are consequence of "mis-activated", dysfunctional microglia, proposing the "glia dysregulation hypothesis" (**Figure 6**; von Bernhardi, 2007). The innate immune response, normally protective, becomes abnormally activated, contributing to cytotoxicity (**Figure 5**; Nguyen et al., 2002; Wyss-Coray and Mucke, 2002; Saud et al., 2005; von Bernhardi, 2007). Normally activated microglia are important as the scavenger cells of the CNS. However, if they fail responding to their normal regulatory feedback and/or they show an impaired ability to clear Aβ (Paresce et al., 1997; von Bernhardi, 2007), glial cells could become predominantly cytotoxic. The distinction is relevant when developing therapeutic approaches. The aim of therapy should be oriented to potentiate a protective pattern of microglial cell function rather than functionally inhibiting microglia as it is most often proposed now.

Treatment Strategies for Neurodegenerative Diseases

Modulation of Microglial Cell Activation

Microglia are important actors for maintenance, repair and defense, although dysregulated microglia have deleterious effects. An effective microglia/neuroinflammation based therapy should target regulation of microglial cell response towards a beneficial pattern of activation, rather than their elimination. Because microglial function, as well as the deleterious effect of oxidative damage are associated with the activation of NADPH oxidase and the production of ROS that will act on both intracellular and extracellular targets (Block et al., 2006, 2007), this enzyme complex appears as a relevant therapeutic target. Originally linked only to respiratory burst in phagocytes, over the last decade it has been reported that NADPH oxidase homologues on diverse cells including neurons also play roles in normal function. Several peptides and small molecules, have been reported to inhibit NADPH oxidase, with potential neuroprotective effect over the last decade (Choi et al., 2005; Qin et al., 2005a). Because inhibition of NADPH oxidase activation targets the major generator of high amounts of ROS by microglia, its inhibition would reduce several inflammatory factors, including eicosanoids like PGE_2 (Wang et al., 2004). The challenge is to develop tools targeting NADPH oxidase isoforms responsible for overproduction of ROS by phagocytes like microglia. The efficacy as neuroprotector of the NADPH oxidase inhibitor diphenyleneiodonium has been reported in both LPS- and 1-methyl-4-phenyl-1,2,3,6-tetrahydropyridine-treated mice (Wang et al., 2015). Diphenyleneiodonium attenuates progressive dopaminergic degeneration, with high efficacy in protecting the remaining neuronal population and restoring motor function even at late stages of disease progression in PD mouse models. Neuroprotection is associated with inhibition of microglial cell activation, decreased α-synuclein aggregation, and reduction of inflammatory mediators (Wang et al., 2015).

Also some inflammatory cytokines have been considered as possible therapeutic targets for AD (Greig et al., 2004; Heneka and O'banion, 2007; Lee et al., 2010). However, a side effect on therapies blocking inflammatory cytokines is the immune suppression caused by these drugs that leaves the patient prone to suffer grave infections. Systemic administration of the anti-inflammatory antibiotic minocycline, which inhibits microglia activation (Kohman et al., 2013a) affects strongly microglia, but also astrocytes, perivascular, meningeal, and infiltrating macrophages. It has been reported that minocycline restores LTP deficits, while normalizing the level of IL1β. These beneficial effects indicate that neuroinflammation could contribute to the deficits in synaptic plasticity, learning and memory observed during normal aging. However, minocycline use reveals the complexity of the effects of microglia function in neurodegenerative disease models. Minocycline show different effects on microglial cell activation and cognitive function along different phases of the life spans of animal models (Kohman et al., 2013a) suggesting that although inhibition of microglia can be beneficial at one stage of disease progression, it becomes detrimental at others.

Activation of Antioxidant Pathways

Reduction of ROS and oxidative stress could be also achieved through the activation of antioxidant pathways. In addition to the relatively weak antioxidant defenses of the brain, brain aging also determines loss of the endogenous mechanisms of free radical scavenging. Among cellular antioxidant defenses, heat shock proteins have been regarded as cytoprotector for oxidative damage-dependent mechanisms in neurodegenerative diseases. Among the stress proteins, the redox-regulated heme-oxygenase 1 (HO-1) gene, and its activation represents a protective system potentially active against brain oxidative injury. HO-1 polymorphisms have been associated with increased AD susceptibility, and dysregulation of the HO system has been associated with brain aging and the pathogenesis of AD (Markesbery, 1997; Pappolla et al., 1998). AD patients' brains present microglia recruitment by neurons with tau abnormalities. Those cell clusters correlate with increased levels of NRF2 and HO-1, suggesting an attempt of the diseased brain to limit microgliosis. Microglial cells HO-1 could be especially relevant for the regulation of neurotoxic mediators, being responsible of the antinflammatory effect of compounds such as schizandrin C (Park et al., 2013) and several other compounds (Foresti et al., 2013). Lastres-Becker et al. recently showed that fractalkine activated AKT in microglia, upregulating the transcription factor NRF2, and its target genes including HO-1. Fractalkine regulates microglial cell activation in neurodegenerative diseases. In a mouse model of tauopathy, they confirmed that NRF2- and fractalkine receptor-KO mice did not express HO-1 in microglia and showed they played a crucial role in the attenuation of neuroinflammation. Those observations suggest that NRF2-dependent induction of HO-1 could limit over-activation of microglia (Lastres-Becker et al., 2014). *In vitro* studies report a decreased HO-1 expression in HIV-infected macrophages. HO-1 deficiency correlates with increased glutamate and neurotoxicity, whereas HO-1 siRNA knockdown or its enzymatic inhibition in HIV-infected macrophages increased supernatant glutamate and neurotoxicity. In contrast, induction of HO-1 by dimethyl fumarate (DMF) decreased glutamate and neurotoxicity. Furthermore, increased IFNγ, as observed in CNS HIV infection, reduced HO-1 expression in cultured human astrocytes and macrophages (Gill et al., 2014). There are reports that activation of HO-1 is strongly protective against oxidative damage and cell death in neurons. Thus, modulation of HO-1 should represent a potential pharmaceutical strategy for the treatment of neurodegenerative disorders (Racchi et al., 2008; Schipper and Song, 2015).

Mitochondrial Antioxidants

Mitochondria have key roles in the production of ROS and in apoptosis signaling. Several compounds targeting mitochondria are currently being tested in clinical trials for treatment of neurodegenerative diseases. Mitochondrial antioxidants appear to be especially interesting at preclinical level (Szeto et al., 2014). Coenzyme Q10 (CoQ10), a carrier of the electron transport chain of oxidative phosphorylation, has been shown to be neuroprotective by attenuating mitochondrial dysfunction and aging (Shetty et al., 2014). However, the fact that these oral antioxidants cross poorly the BBB, has slowed down their therapeutical use; directing new research towards more soluble, shorter chain CoQ10 derivatives, such as idebenone [6-(10-hydroxydecyl-2,3-dimethoxy-5-methyl-1,4-benzoquinone], decylubiquinone (dUb), and MitoQ10. MitoQ10 has the advantage of being accumulated within mitochondria, where it is activated into ubiquinol, which can reduce mitochondrial oxidative damage (Lu et al., 2008). Other class of mitochondrial antioxidants are Szeto-Schiller (SS) peptides (Szeto, 2014), which localize in mitochondria at a broad condition of mitochondrial membrane potential. *In vivo* experiments revealed that SS peptides are protective, increasing survival and motor performance, and decreasing cell death (Moreira et al., 2010). In PD animal models, SS peptides also protect dopaminergic neurons against MPTP neurotoxicity (Moreira et al., 2010).

Therapeutic effects of the regulation of NADPH oxidase and antioxidant treatment will not be restricted exclusively to microglia. However, the development of drugs for specific isoforms and the fact that neuroinflammation is mostly driven by microglia and astrocytes, will have an enormous impact on the cytotoxic activation of glial cells, by reducing both ROS, inflammatory cytokines and endogenous inflammatory mediators.

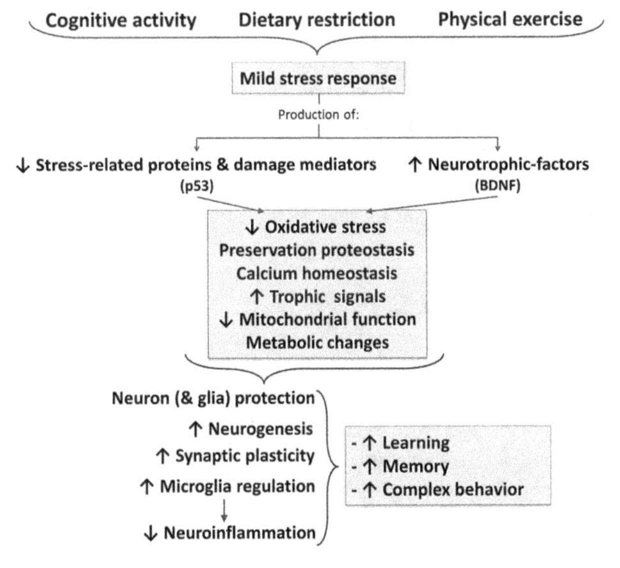

FIGURE 7 | Life style changes as a strategy for aging well. Cognitive activity, dietary caloric restriction and moderate physical exercise induce mild stress responses which results in a decreased production of stress proteins and reduction of oxidative stress. In additions, there is an increased production of neurotrophic factors, among which brain-derived neurotrophic factor (BDNF) appears to be one of the most important, but also participate growth hormone (GH) and insulin growth factor 1 (IGF1). Decreased stress signal and increased trophic signal acts on mitochondrial function, improving energetic metabolism and reducing oxidative stress to a protective level. Stress signals and ROS, below a certain threshold concentration, induce survival signals capable of restoring cellular homeostasis but, at higher or continued levels, can contribute to aging and degenerative changes.

Life-Style Changes Prevent Microglia dysrEgulation and Cytotoxic Activation

Accumulating evidence show that exercise, dietary restriction, cognitive intervention (enriched environment) as well as other mild stressors can play a role in reducing microglial activation and priming during aging (**Figure 7**). Moderate exercising is capable of even reducing the exaggerated neuroinflammation in response to infection-type of stimuli in aged animals, with its increased cytokine production and cognitive deficit (Barrientos et al., 2011), and age-related microglial sensitization (Barrientos et al., 2011; Kohman et al., 2013b), suggesting that exercise could be an effective intervention to prevent microglial cell aging. Furthermore, In adult APP/PS1 mice, exercise increase neurobehavioral performance, which is associated with increased numbers of certain populations of cholinergic and serotoninergic neurons, and reduced Aβ levels and microglia activation (Ke et al., 2011). Beneficial effects of exercise and cognitive intervention could, at least in part, result from its induction of brain-derived neurotrophic factor (BDFN; Barrientos et al., 2011; Polito et al., 2014). Although most of reports are related to the effect of BDNF on neuron function and survival, there are reports on its effect on inhibiting activation of microglia (Garofalo et al., 2015). Dietary restriction also appears to attenuate age-related activation of microglia, resulting in beneficial effects on neurodegeneration and cognitive decline (Morgan et al., 2007). It has anti-inflammatory and anti-apoptotic effects (Loncarevic-Vasiljkovic et al., 2012), and has been shown to elicit many health promoting benefits, delaying immunosenescence and attenuating neurodegeneration in animal models of AD and PD. However, the mechanisms involved in the effect of dietary restriction on microglial cell activation are poorly understood. Exposure to dietary restriction attenuates LPS-induced fever, and LPS-induced microglial activation in some specific brain regions, including the arcuate and ventromedial nuclei of the hypothalamus and the subfornical organ. Activation of microglia in the hypothalamic nuclei was positively correlated with body temperature (Radler et al., 2014). Dietary restriction suppresses LPS-induced secretion of inflammatory cytokines, and shifts hypothalamic signaling pathways to an anti-inflammatory bias (Radler et al., 2015).

Interestingly, both exercise and dietary restriction have been recently shown to promote mitochondrial biogenesis and expression of mitochondrial transcription factor A (TFAM) in the rat brain (Picca et al., 2012; Zhang et al., 2012). Collectively, exercise, cognitive activity, and dietary restriction could be effective ways to slowdown brain aging by preventing microglia aging through secretion of growth factor and regulatory cytokines. Although those effects are not restricted to microglia, the fact that microglia are the major drivers of neuroinflammation, determines that interventions affecting them can have an enormous impact on the brain homeostatic response.

Concluding Remarks

Aging is a major risk factor for the great majority of neurodegenerative diseases. Age dependent changes, including increased glial cell activation, neuroinflammation, oxidative stress, impaired mitochondrial function, and impaired protein processing, could lead to the dysregulation of microglial cell functions resulting, among several alterations in cytotoxicity and accumulation of Aβ, generating the hallmark histopathology of AD. Whereas each of these age-dependent changes are discreet in the normal aging process, their combined effect, together with the genetic background and environmental conditions could initiate the vicious circle of cytotoxic activation (von Bernhardi, 2007). Participation of oxidative stress could be both a trigger and a consequence of Aβ accumulation, mitochondrial impairment, cytotoxic activation of microglia, proteasome dysfunction and protein misfolding, contributing to the potentiation of the other disease mechanisms. Additionally, oxidative stress, cytotoxicity and Aβ aggregation further decrease proteasome activity, creating a vicious circle leading to more Aβ and tau aggregation.

Microglia, in a close crosstalk with astrocytes, neurons and other brain cells, serve crucial functions as the scavenger system of the CNS, providing beneficial functions as tissue repair in the CNS. However, chronic, dysregulated activation of microglia appears to lead to deleterious effects inducing malfunction and damage of brain cells. What drives this dysregulation is not fully understood, but age-related impairment of regulatory mechanisms, as observed for TGBβ transduction signaling (Tichauer et al., 2014) are a promising hypothesis for understanding cytotoxic activation in aged individuals (von Bernhardi et al., 2011). Nonetheless, despite the undeniable potential of activated microglia to become deleterious, microglia have a profound immune-modulatory and reparative potential in the CNS. Thus, instead of abolishing microglia activation as it is most often proposed, strategies to potentiate those beneficial functions while inhibiting cytotoxic activation should be developed. Such strategy may well constitute the way to treat neurodegenerative disorders, but demands a better understanding of the protective and modulatory pathways of immune activation. Additional research is needed for the identification of new pathways that may decrease the impact of microglial cell dysfunction, in order of breaking the vicious circle leading to neurotoxicity.

Further research is necessary to develop effective pharmacological interventions against brain aging. Most of the proposed targets, antioxidants, anti-inflammatory drugs affecting cytokines, and microglia inhibitors, deeply affect physiological cell signaling and functions, including pro-survival signaling pathways, resulting in unacceptable side effects. In that perspective, multi-target pharmacological approaches aimed to reestablish normal regulation of microglia in the aged brain may be future research avenue for slowing senescence-related impairment. Furthermore, non-pharmacological strategies, like exercise, life style changes and dietary restriction, could promote a healthy aging through their effects on promoting microglial physiological functions, while reducing inflammation and ROS production.

Acknowledgments

Support by grants FONDECYT 1131025 (RvB) and 1130874 (JE) is acknowledged.

References

Abrams, A. J., Farooq, A., and Wang, G. (2011). S-nitrosylation of ApoE in Alzheimer's disease. *Biochemistry* 50, 3405–3407. doi: 10.1021/bi200266v

Adler, A. S., Kawahara, T. L., Segal, E., and Chang, H. Y. (2008). Reversal of aging by NFkappaB blockade. *Cell Cycle* 7, 556–559. doi: 10.4161/cc.7.5.5490

Adler, A. S., Sinha, S., Kawahara, T. L., Zhang, J. Y., Segal, E., and Chang, H. Y. (2007). Motif module map reveals enforcement of aging by continual NF-kappaB activity. *Genes Dev.* 21, 3244–3257. doi: 10.1101/gad.1588507

Agostinho, P., Cunha, R. A., and Oliveira, C. (2010). Neuroinflammation, oxidative stress and the pathogenesis of Alzheimer's disease. *Curr. Pharm. Des.* 16, 2766–2778. doi: 10.2174/138161210793176572

Aguzzi, A., Barres, B. A., and Bennett, M. L. (2013). Microglia: scapegoat, saboteur, or something else? *Science* 339, 156–161. doi: 10.1126/science.1227901

Akiyama, H., Barger, S., Barnum, S., Bradt, B., Bauer, J., Cole, G. M., et al. (2000). Inflammation and Alzheimer's disease. *Neurobiol. Aging* 21, 383–421. doi: 10.1016/S0197-4580(00)00124-X

Alarcón, R., Fuenzalida, C., Santibáñez, M., and Von Bernhardi, R. (2005). Expression of scavenger receptors in glial cells. Comparing the adhesion of astrocytes and microglia from neonatal rats to surface-bound beta-amyloid. *J. Biol. Chem.* 280, 30406–30415. doi: 10.1074/jbc.m414686200

Arnaud, L., Robakis, N. K., and Figueiredo-Pereira, M. E. (2006). It may take inflammation, phosphorylation and ubiquitination to 'tangle' in Alzheimer's disease. *Neurodegener. Dis.* 3, 313–319. doi: 10.1159/000095638

Bachstetter, A. D., Van Eldik, L. J., Schmitt, F. A., Neltner, J. H., Ighodaro, E. T., Webster, S. J., et al. (2015). Disease-related microglia heterogeneity in the hippocampus of Alzheimer's disease, dementia with Lewy bodies and hippocampal sclerosis of aging. *Acta Neuropathol. Commun.* 3:32. doi: 10.1186/s40478-015-0209-z

Baloyannis, S. J. (2006). Mitochondrial alterations in Alzheimer's disease. *J. Alzheimers Dis.* 9, 119–126.

Bamberger, M. E., Harris, M. E., McDonald, D. R., Husemann, J., and Landreth, G. E. (2003). A cell surface receptor complex for fibrillar beta-amyloid mediates microglial activation. *J. Neurosci.* 23, 2665–2674.

Barger, S. W., Hörster, D., Furukawa, K., Goodman, Y., Krieglstein, J., and Mattson, M. P. (1995). Tumor necrosis factors alpha and beta protect neurons against amyloid beta-peptide toxicity: evidence for involvement of a kappa B-binding factor and attenuation of peroxide and Ca2+ accumulation. *Proc. Natl. Acad. Sci. U S A* 92, 9328–9332. doi: 10.1073/pnas.92.20.9328

Baron, R., Babcock, A. A., Nemirovsky, A., Finsen, B., and Monsonego, A. (2014). Accelerated microglial pathology is associated with Abeta plaques in mouse models of Alzheimer's disease. *Aging Cell* 13, 584–595. doi: 10.1111/acel.12210

Barrientos, R. M., Frank, M. G., Crysdale, N. Y., Chapman, T. R., Ahrendsen, J. T., Day, H. E., et al. (2011). Little exercise, big effects: reversing aging and infection-induced memory deficits and underlying processes. *J. Neurosci.* 31, 11578–11586. doi: 10.1523/JNEUROSCI.2266-11.2011

Barsoum, M. J., Yuan, H., Gerencser, A. A., Liot, G., Kushnareva, Y., Graber, S., et al. (2006). Nitric oxide-induced mitochondrial fission is regulated by dynamin-related GTPases in neurons. *EMBO J.* 25, 3900–3911. doi: 10.1038/sj.emboj.7601253

Benzing, W. C., Wujek, J. R., Ward, E. K., Shaffer, D., Ashe, K. H., Younkin, S. G., et al. (1999). Evidence for glial-mediated inflammation in aged APP(SW) transgenic mice. *Neurobiol. Aging* 20, 581–589. doi: 10.1016/s0197-4580(99)00065-2

Bhakar, A. L., Tannis, L. L., Zeindler, C., Russo, M. P., Jobin, C., Park, D. S., et al. (2002). Constitutive nuclear factor-kappa B activity is required for central neuron survival. *J. Neurosci.* 22, 8466–8475.

Björkqvist, M., Wild, E. J., and Tabrizi, S. J. (2009). Harnessing immune alterations in neurodegenerative diseases. *Neuron* 64, 21–24. doi: 10.1016/j.neuron.2009.09.034

Blau, C. W., Cowley, T. R., O'sullivan, J., Grehan, B., Browne, T. C., Kelly, L., et al. (2012). The age-related deficit in LTP is associated with changes in perfusion and blood-brain barrier permeability. *Neurobiol. Aging* 33, 1005.e1023–1005.e1035. doi: 10.1016/j.neurobiolaging.2011.09.035

Blobe, G. C., Schiemann, W. P., and Lodish, H. F. (2000). Role of transforming growth factor beta in human disease. *N. Engl. J. Med.* 342, 1350–1358. doi: 10.1056/NEJM200005043421807

Block, M. L. (2008). NADPH oxidase as a therapeutic target in Alzheimer's disease. *BMC Neurosci.* 9(Suppl. 2):S8. doi: 10.1186/1471-2202-9-s2-s8

Block, M. L., Li, G., Qin, L., Wu, X., Pei, Z., Wang, T., et al. (2006). Potent regulation of microglia-derived oxidative stress and dopaminergic neuron survival: substance P vs. dynorphin. *FASEB J.* 20, 251–258. doi: 10.1096/fj.05-4553com

Block, M. L., Zecca, L., and Hong, J. S. (2007). Microglia-mediated neurotoxicity: uncovering the molecular mechanisms. *Nat. Rev. Neurosci.* 8, 57–69. doi: 10.1038/nrn2038

Boillée, S., Yamanaka, K., Lobsiger, C. S., Copeland, N. G., Jenkins, N. A., Kassiotis, G., et al. (2006). Onset and progression in inherited ALS determined by motor neurons and microglia. *Science* 312, 1389–1392. doi: 10.1126/science.1123511

Bordt, E. A., and Polster, B. M. (2014). NADPH oxidase- and mitochondria-derived reactive oxygen species in proinflammatory microglial activation: a bipartisan affair? *Free Radic. Biol. Med.* 76, 34–46. doi: 10.1016/j.freeradbiomed.2014.07.033

Bossy-Wetzel, E., and Lipton, S. A. (2003). Nitric oxide signaling regulates mitochondrial number and function. *Cell Death Differ.* 10, 757–760. doi: 10.1038/sj.cdd.4401244

Butterfield, D. A. (2002). Amyloid beta-peptide (1–42)-induced oxidative stress and neurotoxicity: implications for neurodegeneration in Alzheimer's disease brain. A review. *Free Radic. Res.* 36, 1307–1313. doi: 10.1080/1071576021000049890

Butterfield, D. A., Castegna, A., Lauderback, C. M., and Drake, J. (2002). Evidence that amyloid beta-peptide-induced lipid peroxidation and its sequelae in Alzheimer's disease brain contribute to neuronal death. *Neurobiol. Aging* 23, 655–664. doi: 10.1016/s0197-4580(01)00340-2

Butterfield, D. A., and Lauderback, C. M. (2002). Lipid peroxidation and protein oxidation in Alzheimer's disease brain: potential causes and consequences involving amyloid beta-peptide-associated free radical oxidative stress. *Free Radic. Biol. Med.* 32, 1050–1060. doi: 10.1016/s0891-5849(02)00794-3

Bye, N., Zieba, M., Wreford, N. G., and Nichols, N. R. (2001). Resistance of the dentate gyrus to induced apoptosis during ageing is associated with increases in transforming growth factor-beta1 messenger RNA. *Neuroscience* 105, 853–862. doi: 10.1016/s0306-4522(01)00236-6

Cagnin, A., Brooks, D. J., Kennedy, A. M., Gunn, R. N., Myers, R., Turkheimer, F. E., et al. (2001). *In vivo* measurement of activated microglia in dementia. *Lancet* 358, 461–467. doi: 10.1016/s0140-6736(01)05625-2

Chakrabarty, P., Jansen-West, K., Beccard, A., Ceballos-Diaz, C., Levites, Y., Verbeeck, C., et al. (2010). Massive gliosis induced by interleukin-6 suppresses Abeta deposition in vivo: evidence against inflammation as a driving force for amyloid deposition. *FASEB J.* 24, 548–559. doi: 10.1096/fj.09-141754

Chen, L., Liu, L., Yin, J., Luo, Y., and Huang, S. (2009). Hydrogen peroxide-induced neuronal apoptosis is associated with inhibition of protein phosphatase 2A and 5, leading to activation of MAPK pathway. *Int. J. Biochem. Cell. Biol.* 41, 1284–1295. doi: 10.1016/j.biocel.2008.10.029

Chen, S., Luo, D., Streit, W. J., and Harrison, J. K. (2002). TGF-beta1 upregulates CX3CR1 expression and inhibits fractalkine-stimulated signaling in rat microglia. *J. Neuroimmunol.* 133, 46–55. doi: 10.1016/s0165-5728(02)00354-5

Cho, S. H., Chen, J. A., Sayed, F., Ward, M. E., Gao, F., Nguyen, T. A., et al. (2015). SIRT1 deficiency in microglia contributes to cognitive decline in aging and neurodegeneration via epigenetic regulation of IL-1beta. *J. Neurosci.* 35, 807–818. doi: 10.1523/jneurosci.2939-14.2015

Cho, H. J., Kim, S. K., Jin, S. M., Hwang, E. M., Kim, Y. S., Huh, K., et al. (2007). IFN-gamma-induced BACE1 expression is mediated by activation of JAK2 and ERK1/2 signaling pathways and direct binding of STAT1 to BACE1 promoter in astrocytes. *Glia* 55, 253–262. doi: 10.1002/glia.20451

Cho, D. H., Nakamura, T., Fang, J., Cieplak, P., Godzik, A., Gu, Z., et al. (2009). S-nitrosylation of Drp1 mediates beta-amyloid-related mitochondrial fission and neuronal injury. *Science* 324, 102–105. doi: 10.1126/science.1171091

Choi, S. H., Lee, D. Y., Chung, E. S., Hong, Y. B., Kim, S. U., and Jin, B. K. (2005). Inhibition of thrombin-induced microglial activation and NADPH oxidase by minocycline protects dopaminergic neurons in the substantia nigra in vivo. *J. Neurochem.* 95, 1755–1765. doi: 10.1111/j.1471-4159.2005.03503.x

Chongthammakun, V., Sanvarinda, Y., and Chongthammakun, S. (2009). Reactive oxygen species production and MAPK activation are implicated in tetrahydrobiopterin-induced SH-SY5Y cell death. *Neurosci. Lett.* 449, 178–182. doi: 10.1016/j.neulet.2008.10.106

Clementi, E., Brown, G. C., Feelisch, M., and Moncada, S. (1998). Persistent inhibition of cell respiration by nitric oxide: crucial role of S-nitrosylation of mitochondrial complex I and protective action of glutathione. *Proc. Natl. Acad. Sci. U S A* 95, 7631–7636. doi: 10.1073/pnas.95.13.7631

Combrinck, M. I., Perry, V. H., and Cunningham, C. (2002). Peripheral infection evokes exaggerated sickness behaviour in pre-clinical murine prion disease. *Neuroscience* 112, 7–11. doi: 10.1016/s0306-4522(02)00030-1

Conde, J. R., and Streit, W. J. (2006a). Effect of aging on the microglial response to peripheral nerve injury. *Neurobiol. Aging* 27, 1451–1461. doi: 10.1016/j.neurobiolaging.2005.07.012

Conde, J. R., and Streit, W. J. (2006b). Microglia in the aging brain. *J. Neuropathol. Exp. Neurol.* 65, 199–203. doi: 10.1097/01.jnen.0000202887.22082.63

Cornejo, F., and Von Bernhardi, R. (2013). Role of scavenger receptors in glia-mediated neuroinflammatory response associated with Alzheimer's disease. *Mediators Inflamm.* 2013:895651. doi: 10.1155/2013/895651

Cornejo, F. A., Vruwink, M., Metz, C., Ramírez, G., and Von Bernhardi, R. (2014). "Role of scavenger receptor class A in glial cell activation in Alzheimer's disease," in *Social Neuroscience Abstract 44th Annual Meeting*, Washington, DC.

Cunningham, C., Wilcockson, D. C., Campion, S., Lunnon, K., and Perry, V. H. (2005). Central and systemic endotoxin challenges exacerbate the local inflammatory response and increase neuronal death during chronic neurodegeneration. *J. Neurosci.* 25, 9275–9284. doi: 10.1523/jneurosci.2614-05.2005

Damani, M. R., Zhao, L., Fontainhas, A. M., Amaral, J., Fariss, R. N., and Wong, W. T. (2011). Age-related alterations in the dynamic behavior of microglia. *Aging Cell* 10, 263–276. doi: 10.1111/j.1474-9726.2010.00660.x

Davalos, D., Grutzendler, J., Yang, G., Kim, J. V., Zuo, Y., Jung, S., et al. (2005). ATP mediates rapid microglial response to local brain injury in vivo. *Nat. Neurosci.* 8, 752–758. doi: 10.1038/nn1472

Davis, J. N. 2nd, and Chisholm, J. C. (1999). Alois Alzheimer and the amyloid debate. *Nature* 400:810. doi: 10.1038/23571

Derynck, R., and Zhang, Y. E. (2003). Smad-dependent and Smad-independent pathways in TGF-beta family signalling. *Nature* 425, 577–584. doi: 10.1038/nature02006

Di Filippo, M., Sarchielli, P., Picconi, B., and Calabresi, P. (2008). Neuroinflammation and synaptic plasticity: theoretical basis for a novel, immune-centred, therapeutic approach to neurological disorders. *Trends Pharmacol. Sci.* 29, 402–412. doi: 10.1016/j.tips.2008.06.005

Ding, Q., Markesbery, W. R., Cecarini, V., and Keller, J. N. (2006). Decreased RNA and increased RNA oxidation, in ribosomes from early Alzheimer's disease. *Neurochem. Res.* 31, 705–710. doi: 10.1007/s11064-006-9071-5

Drachman, D. A. (2006). Aging of the brain, entropy and Alzheimer disease. *Neurology* 67, 1340–1352. doi: 10.1212/01.wnl.0000240127.89601.83

Dröge, W., and Schipper, H. M. (2007). Oxidative stress and aberrant signaling in aging and cognitive decline. *Aging Cell* 6, 361–370. doi: 10.1111/j.1474-9726.2007.00294.x

Duewell, P., Kono, H., Rayner, K. J., Sirois, C. M., Vladimer, G., Bauernfeind, F. G., et al. (2010). NLRP3 inflammasomes are required for atherogenesis and activated by cholesterol crystals. *Nature* 464, 1357–1361. doi: 10.1038/nature08938

Dumont, M., Wille, E., Stack, C., Calingasan, N. Y., Beal, M. F., and Lin, M. T. (2009). Reduction of oxidative stress, amyloid deposition and memory deficit by manganese superoxide dismutase overexpression in a transgenic mouse model of Alzheimer's disease. *FASEB J.* 23, 2459–2466. doi: 10.1096/fj.09-132928

Enciu, A. M., Gherghiceanu, M., and Popescu, B. O. (2013). Triggers and effectors of oxidative stress at blood-brain barrier level: relevance for brain ageing and neurodegeneration. *Oxid. Med. Cell. Longev.* 2013:297512. doi: 10.1155/2013/297512

Esposito, L., Raber, J., Kekonius, L., Yan, F., Yu, G. Q., Bien-Ly, N., et al. (2006). Reduction in mitochondrial superoxide dismutase modulates Alzheimer's disease-like pathology and accelerates the onset of behavioral changes in human amyloid precursor protein transgenic mice. *J. Neurosci.* 26, 5167–5179. doi: 10.1523/jneurosci.0482-06.2006

Flanary, B. E., Sammons, N. W., Nguyen, C., Walker, D., and Streit, W. J. (2007). Evidence that aging and amyloid promote microglial cell senescence. *Rejuvenation Res.* 10, 61–74. doi: 10.1089/rej.2006.9096

Flanary, B. E., and Streit, W. J. (2004). Progressive telomere shortening occurs in cultured rat microglia, but not astrocytes. *Glia* 45, 75–88. doi: 10.1002/glia.10301

Floden, A. M., and Combs, C. K. (2011). Microglia demonstrate age-dependent interaction with amyloid-beta fibrils. *J. Alzheimers Dis.* 25, 279–293. doi: 10.3233/JAD-2011-101014

Flores, B., and von Bernhardi, R. (2012). Transforming growth factor beta1 modulates amyloid beta-induced glial activation through the Smad3-dependent induction of MAPK phosphatase-1. *J. Alzheimers Dis.* 32, 417–429. doi: 10.3233/JAD-2012-120721

Floyd, R. A., and Hensley, K. (2002). Oxidative stress in brain aging. Implications for therapeutics of neurodegenerative diseases. *Neurobiol. Aging* 23, 795–807. doi: 10.1016/s0197-4580(02)00019-2

Foresti, R., Bains, S. K., Pitchumony, T. S., de Castro Brás, L. E., Drago, F., Dubois-Randé, J. L., et al. (2013). Small molecule activators of the Nrf2-HO-1 antioxidant axis modulate heme metabolism and inflammation in BV2 microglia cells. *Pharmacol. Res.* 76, 132–148. doi: 10.1016/j.phrs.2013.07.010

Forster, M. J., Dubey, A., Dawson, K. M., Stutts, W. A., Lal, H., and Sohal, R. S. (1996). Age-related losses of cognitive function and motor skills in mice are associated with oxidative protein damage in the brain. *Proc. Natl. Acad. Sci. U S A* 93, 4765–4769. doi: 10.1073/pnas.93.10.4765

Frank-Cannon, T. C., Alto, L. T., Mcalpine, F. E., and Tansey, M. G. (2009). Does neuroinflammation fan the flame in neurodegenerative diseases? *Mol. Neurodegener.* 4:47. doi: 10.1186/1750-1326-4-47

Garofalo, S., D'Alessandro, G., Chece, G., Brau, F., Maggi, L., Rosa, A., et al. (2015). Enriched environment reduces glioma growth through immune and non-immune mechanisms in mice. *Nat. Commun.* 6:6623. doi: 10.1038/ncomms7623

Ge, Y., Grossman, R. I., Babb, J. S., Rabin, M. L., Mannon, L. J., and Kolson, D. L. (2002). Age-related total gray matter and white matter changes in normal adult brain. Part I: volumetric MR imaging analysis. *AJNR Am. J. Neuroradiol.* 23, 1327–1333.

Geula, C., Wu, C. K., Saroff, D., Lorenzo, A., Yuan, M., and Yankner, B. A. (1998). Aging renders the brain vulnerable to amyloid beta-protein neurotoxicity. *Nat. Med.* 4, 827–831. doi: 10.1038/nm0798-827

Giasson, B. I., Ischiropoulos, H., Lee, V. M., and Trojanowski, J. Q. (2002). The relationship between oxidative/nitrative stress and pathological inclusions in Alzheimer's and Parkinson's diseases. *Free Radic. Biol. Med.* 32, 1264–1275. doi: 10.1016/s0891-5849(02)00804-3

Gill, A. J., Kovacsics, C. E., Cross, S. A., Vance, P. J., Kolson, L. L., Jordan-Sciutto, K. L., et al. (2014). Heme oxygenase-1 deficiency accompanies neuropathogenesis of HIV-associated neurocognitive disorders. *J. Clin. Invest.* 124, 4459–4472. doi: 10.1172/jci72279

Glenn, C. F., Chow, D. K., David, L., Cooke, C. A., Gami, M. S., Iser, W. B., et al. (2004). Behavioral deficits during early stages of aging in Caenorhabditis elegans result from locomotory deficits possibly linked to muscle frailty. *J. Gerontol. A Biol. Sci. Med. Sci.* 59, 1251–1260. doi: 10.1093/gerona/59.12.1251

Godbout, J. P., Chen, J., Abraham, J., Richwine, A. F., Berg, B. M., Kelley, K. W., et al. (2005). Exaggerated neuroinflammation and sickness behavior in aged mice following activation of the peripheral innate immune system. *FASEB J.* 19, 1329–1331. doi: 10.1096/fj.05-3776fje

Godbout, J. P., and Johnson, R. W. (2004). Interleukin-6 in the aging brain. *J. Neuroimmunol.* 147, 141–144. doi: 10.1016/j.jneuroim.2003.10.031

Godoy, B., Murgas, P., Tichauer, J., and Von Bernhardi, R. (2012). Scavenger receptor class A ligands induce secretion of IL1beta and exert a modulatory effect on the inflammatory activation of astrocytes in culture. *J. Neuroimmunol.* 251, 6–13. doi: 10.1016/j.jneuroim.2012.06.004

Gordon, S. (2003). Alternative activation of macrophages. *Nat. Rev. Immunol.* 3, 23–35. doi: 10.1038/nri978

Greig, N. H., Mattson, M. P., Perry, T., Chan, S. L., Giordano, T., Sambamurti, K., et al. (2004). New therapeutic strategies and drug candidates for neurodegenerative diseases: p53 and TNF-alpha inhibitors and GLP-1 receptor agonists. *Ann. N Y Acad. Sci.* 1035, 290–315. doi: 10.1196/annals.1332.018

Griffin, W. S., and Mrak, R. E. (2002). Interleukin-1 in the genesis and progression of and risk for development of neuronal degeneration in Alzheimer's disease. *J. Leukoc. Biol.* 72, 233–238.

Grimaldi, L. M., Casadei, V. M., Ferri, C., Veglia, F., Licastro, F., Annoni, G., et al. (2000). Association of early-onset Alzheimer's disease with an interleukin-1alpha gene polymorphism. *Ann. Neurol.* 47, 361–365. doi: 10.1002/1531-8249(200003)47:3<361::aid-ana12>3.0.co;2-n

Guerreiro, R., Wojtas, A., Bras, J., Carrasquillo, M., Rogaeva, E., Majounie, E., et al. (2013). TREM2 variants in Alzheimer's disease. *N. Engl. J. Med.* 368, 117–127. doi: 10.1056/NEJMoa1211851

Halle, A., Hornung, V., Petzold, G. C., Stewart, C. R., Monks, B. G., Reinheckel, T., et al. (2008). The NALP3 inflammasome is involved in the innate immune response to amyloid-beta. *Nat. Immunol.* 9, 857–865. doi: 10.1038/ni.1636

Halliwell, B. (2006). Oxidative stress and neurodegeneration: where are we now? *J. Neurochem.* 97, 1634–1658. doi: 10.1111/j.1471-4159.2006.03907.x

Hanisch, U. K., and Kettenmann, H. (2007). Microglia: active sensor and versatile effector cells in the normal and pathologic brain. *Nat. Neurosci.* 10, 1387–1394. doi: 10.1038/nn1997

Harry, G. J. (2013). Microglia during development and aging. *Pharmacol. Ther.* 139, 313–326. doi: 10.1016/j.pharmthera.2013.04.013

Harry, G. J., Lefebvre d'Hellencourt, C., Bruccoleri, A., and Schmechel, D. (2000). Age-dependent cytokine responses: trimethyltin hippocampal injury in wild-type, APOE knockout and APOE4 mice. *Brain Behav. Immun.* 14, 288–304. doi: 10.1006/brbi.2000.0606

Hart, A. D., Wyttenbach, A., Perry, V. H., and Teeling, J. L. (2012). Age related changes in microglial phenotype vary between CNS regions: grey versus white matter differences. *Brain Behav. Immun.* 26, 754–765. doi: 10.1016/j.bbi.2011.11.006

Hashioka, S., Miklossy, J., Schwab, C., Klegeris, A., and Mcgeer, P. L. (2008). Adhesion of exogenous human microglia and THP-1 cells to amyloid plaques of postmortem Alzheimer's disease brain. *J. Alzheimers Dis.* 14, 345–352.

Hayashi, Y., Yoshida, M., Yamato, M., Ide, T., Wu, Z., Ochi-Shindou, M., et al. (2008). Reverse of age-dependent memory impairment and mitochondrial DNA damage in microglia by an overexpression of human mitochondrial transcription factor a in mice. *J. Neurosci.* 28, 8624–8634. doi: 10.1523/jneurosci.1957-08.2008

He, P., Zhong, Z., Lindholm, K., Berning, L., Lee, W., Lemere, C., et al. (2007). Deletion of tumor necrosis factor death receptor inhibits amyloid beta generation and prevents learning and memory deficits in Alzheimer's mice. *J. Cell Biol.* 178, 829–841. doi: 10.1083/jcb.200705042

Hefendehl, J. K., Neher, J. J., Sühs, R. B., Kohsaka, S., Skodras, A., and Jucker, M. (2014). Homeostatic and injury-induced microglia behavior in the aging brain. *Aging Cell* 13, 60–69. doi: 10.1111/acel.12149

Hemmer, B., Archelos, J. J., and Hartung, H. P. (2002). New concepts in the immunopathogenesis of multiple sclerosis. *Nat. Rev. Neurosci.* 3, 291–301. doi: 10.1038/nrn784

Heneka, M. T., Kummer, M. P., Stutz, A., Delekate, A., Schwartz, S., Vieira-Saecker, A., et al. (2013). NLRP3 is activated in Alzheimer's disease and contributes to pathology in APP/PS1 mice. *Nature* 493, 674–678. doi: 10.1038/nature11729

Heneka, M. T., and O'banion, M. K. (2007). Inflammatory processes in Alzheimer's disease. *J. Neuroimmunol.* 184, 69–91. doi: 10.1016/j.jneuroim.2006.11.017

Herrera-Molina, R., Flores, B., Orellana, J. A., and von Bernhardi, R. (2012). Modulation of interferon-gamma-induced glial cell activation by transforming growth factor beta1: a role for STAT1 and MAPK pathways. *J. Neurochem.* 123, 113–123. doi: 10.1111/j.1471-4159.2012.07887.x

Herrera-Molina, R., and von Bernhardi, R. (2005). Transforming growth factor-beta 1 produced by hippocampal cells modulates microglial reactivity in culture. *Neurobiol. Dis.* 19, 229–236. doi: 10.1016/j.nbd.2005.01.003

Herrup, K. (2010). Reimagining Alzheimer's disease--an age-based hypothesis. *J. Neurosci.* 30, 16755–16762. doi: 10.1523/jneurosci.4521-10.2010

Hess, D. T., Matsumoto, A., Kim, S. O., Marshall, H. E., and Stamler, J. S. (2005). Protein S-nitrosylation: purview and parameters. *Nat. Rev. Mol. Cell Biol.* 6, 150–166. doi: 10.1038/nrm1569

Heurtaux, T., Michelucci, A., Losciuto, S., Gallotti, C., Felten, P., Dorban, G., et al. (2010). Microglial activation depends on beta-amyloid conformation: role of the formylpeptide receptor 2. *J. Neurochem.* 114, 576–586. doi: 10.1111/j.1471-4159.2010.06783.x

Hickman, S. E., Allison, E. K., and El Khoury, J. (2008). Microglial dysfunction and defective β-amyloid clearance pathways in aging Alzheimer's disease mice. *J. Neurosci.* 28, 8354–8360. doi: 10.1523/JNEUROSCI.0616-08.2008

Hirsch, E. C., and Hunot, S. (2009). Neuroinflammation in Parkinson's disease: a target for neuroprotection? *Lancet Neurol.* 8, 382–397. doi: 10.1016/s1474-4422(09)70062-6

Holtman, I. R., Raj, D. D., Miller, J. A., Schaafsma, W., Yin, Z., Brouwer, N., et al. (2015). Induction of a common microglia gene expression signature by aging and neurodegenerative conditions: a co-expression meta-analysis. *Acta Neuropathol. Commun.* 3:31. doi: 10.1186/s40478-015-0203-5

Hornung, V., Bauernfeind, F., Halle, A., Samstad, E. O., Kono, H., Rock, K. L., et al. (2008). Silica crystals and aluminum salts activate the NALP3 inflammasome through phagosomal destabilization. *Nat. Immunol.* 9, 847–856. doi: 10.1038/ni.1631

Hu, S., Sheng, W. S., Peterson, P. K., and Chao, C. C. (1995). Cytokine modulation of murine microglial cell superoxide production. *Glia* 13, 45–50. doi: 10.1002/glia.440130106

Husemann, J., Loike, J. D., Kodama, T., and Silverstein, S. C. (2001). Scavenger receptor class B type I (SR-BI) mediates adhesion of neonatal murine microglia to fibrillar beta-amyloid. *J. Neuroimmunol.* 114, 142–150. doi: 10.1016/s0165-5728(01)00239-9

Itagaki, S., McGeer, P. L., Akiyama, H., Zhu, S., and Selkoe, D. (1989). Relationship of microglia and astrocytes to amyloid deposits of Alzheimer disease. *J. Neuroimmunol.* 24, 173–182. doi: 10.1016/0165-5728(89)90115-x

Jellinger, K. A. (2006). Alzheimer 100--highlights in the history of Alzheimer research. *J. Neural Transm.* 113, 1603–1623. doi: 10.1007/s00702-006-0578-3

Jiang, L., Chen, S. H., Chu, C. H., Wang, S. J., Oyarzabal, E., Wilson, B., et al. (2015). A novel role of microglial NADPH oxidase in mediating extra-synaptic function of norepinephrine in regulating brain immune homeostasis. *Glia* 63, 1057–1072. doi: 10.1002/glia.22801

Kang, D., Kim, S. H., and Hamasaki, N. (2007). Mitochondrial transcription factor A (TFAM): roles in maintenance of mtDNA and cellular functions. *Mitochondrion* 7, 39–44. doi: 10.1016/j.mito.2006.11.017

Kawamata, H., and Manfredi, G. (2010). Mitochondrial dysfunction and intracellular calcium dysregulation in ALS. *Mech. Ageing Dev.* 131, 517–526. doi: 10.1016/j.mad.2010.05.003

Ke, H. C., Huang, H. J., Liang, K. C., and Hsieh-Li, H. M. (2011). Selective improvement of cognitive function in adult and aged APP/PS1 transgenic mice by continuous non-shock treadmill exercise. *Brain Res.* 1403, 1–11. doi: 10.1016/j.brainres.2011.05.056

Kettenmann, H., Kirchhoff, F., and Verkhratsky, A. (2013). Microglia: new roles for the synaptic stripper. *Neuron* 77, 10–18. doi: 10.1016/j.neuron.2012.12.023

Kierdorf, K., and Prinz, M. (2013). Factors regulating microglia activation. *Front. Cell. Neurosci.* 7:44. doi: 10.3389/fncel.2013.00044

Kierdorf, K., Wang, Y., and Neumann, H. (2010). Immune-mediated CNS damage. *Results Probl. Cell Differ.* 51, 173–196. doi: 10.1007/400_2008_15

Kim, S. U., and de Vellis, J. (2005). Microglia in health and disease. *J. Neurosci. Res.* 81, 302–313. doi: 10.1002/jnr.20562

Koenigsknecht-Talboo, J., Meyer-Luehmann, M., Parsadanian, M., Garcia-Alloza, M., Finn, M. B., Hyman, B. T., et al. (2008). Rapid microglial response around amyloid pathology after systemic anti-Abeta antibody administration in PDAPP mice. *J. Neurosci.* 28, 14156–14164. doi: 10.1523/jneurosci.4147-08.2008

Kohman, R. A., Bhattacharya, T. K., Kilby, C., Bucko, P., and Rhodes, J. S. (2013a). Effects of minocycline on spatial learning, hippocampal neurogenesis and microglia in aged and adult mice. *Behav. Brain Res.* 242, 17–24. doi: 10.1016/j.bbr.2012.12.032

Kohman, R. A., Bhattacharya, T. K., Wojcik, E., and Rhodes, J. S. (2013b). Exercise reduces activation of microglia isolated from hippocampus and brain of aged mice. *J. Neuroinflammation* 10:114. doi: 10.1186/1742-2094-10-114

Krausgruber, T., Blazek, K., Smallie, T., Alzabin, S., Lockstone, H., Sahgal, N., et al. (2011). IRF5 promotes inflammatory macrophage polarization and TH1-TH17 responses. *Nat. Immunol.* 12, 231–238. doi: 10.1038/ni.1990

Kreutzberg, G. W. (1996). Microglia: a sensor for pathological events in the CNS. *Trends Neurosci.* 19, 312–318. doi: 10.1016/0166-2236(96)10049-7

Kuchibhotla, K. V., Goldman, S. T., Lattarulo, C. R., Wu, H. Y., Hyman, B. T., and Bacskai, B. J. (2008). Abeta plaques lead to aberrant regulation of calcium homeostasis in vivo resulting in structural and functional disruption of neuronal networks. *Neuron* 59, 214–225. doi: 10.1016/j.neuron.2008.06.008

Laliberte, R. E., Perregaux, D. G., Hoth, L. R., Rosner, P. J., Jordan, C. K., Peese, K. M., et al. (2003). Glutathione s-transferase omega 1-1 is a target of cytokine release inhibitory drugs and may be responsible for their effect on interleukin-1beta posttranslational processing. *J. Biol. Chem.* 278, 16567–16578. doi: 10.1074/jbc.m211596200

Lastres-Becker, I., Innamorato, N. G., Jaworski, T., Rábano, A., Kügler, S., Van Leuven, F., et al. (2014). Fractalkine activates NRF2/NFE2L2 and heme oxygenase 1 to restrain tauopathy-induced microgliosis. *Brain* 137, 78–91. doi: 10.1093/brain/awt323

Lauderback, C. M., Hackett, J. M., Huang, F. F., Keller, J. N., Szweda, L. I., Markesbery, W. R., et al. (2001). The glial glutamate transporter, GLT-1, is oxidatively modified by 4-hydroxy-2-nonenal in the Alzheimer's disease brain: the role of Abeta1-42. *J. Neurochem.* 78, 413–416. doi: 10.1046/j.1471-4159.2001.00451.x

Le, Y., Iribarren, P., Gong, W., Cui, Y., Zhang, X., and Wang, J. M. (2004). TGF-beta1 disrupts endotoxin signaling in microglial cells through Smad3 and MAPK pathways. *J. Immunol.* 173, 962–968. doi: 10.4049/jimmunol.173.2.962

Lee, Y. J., Han, S. B., Nam, S. Y., Oh, K. W., and Hong, J. T. (2010). Inflammation and Alzheimer's disease. *Arch. Pharm. Res.* 33, 1539–1556. doi: 10.1007/s12272-010-1006-7

Lee, J. Y., Kweon, H. S., Cho, E., Byun, H. R., Kim, D. H., Kim, Y. H., et al. (2007). Upregulation of tPA/plasminogen proteolytic system in the periphery of amyloid deposits in the Tg2576 mouse model of Alzheimer's disease. *Neurosci. Lett.* 423, 82–87. doi: 10.1016/j.neulet.2007.06.037

Lee, J. M., Li, J., Johnson, D. A., Stein, T. D., Kraft, A. D., Calkins, M. J., et al. (2005). Nrf2, a multi-organ protector? *FASEB J.* 19, 1061–1066. doi: 10.1096/fj.04-2591hyp

Letiembre, M., Hao, W., Liu, Y., Walter, S., Mihaljevic, I., Rivest, S., et al. (2007). Innate immune receptor expression in normal brain aging. *Neuroscience* 146, 248–254. doi: 10.1016/j.neuroscience.2007.01.004

Li, F., Calingasan, N. Y., Yu, F., Mauck, W. M., Toidze, M., Almeida, C. G., et al. (2004a). Increased plaque burden in brains of APP mutant MnSOD heterozygous knockout mice. *J. Neurochem.* 89, 1308–1312. doi: 10.1111/j.1471-4159.2004.02455.x

Li, J., Stein, T. D., and Johnson, J. A. (2004b). Genetic dissection of systemic autoimmune disease in Nrf2-deficient mice. *Physiol. Genomics* 18, 261–272. doi: 10.1152/physiolgenomics.00209.2003

Li, L., Lu, J., Tay, S. S., Moochhala, S. M., and He, B. P. (2007). The function of microglia, either neuroprotection or neurotoxicity, is determined by the equilibrium among factors released from activated microglia in vitro. *Brain Res.* 1159, 8–17. doi: 10.1016/j.brainres.2007.04.066

Li, Y. J., Oliveira, S. A., Xu, P., Martin, E. R., Stenger, J. E., Scherzer, C. R., et al. (2003). Glutathione S-transferase omega-1 modifies age-at-onset of Alzheimer disease and Parkinson disease. *Hum. Mol. Genet.* 12, 3259–3267. doi: 10.1093/hmg/ddg357

Lieb, K., Engels, S., and Fiebich, B. L. (2003). Inhibition of LPS-induced iNOS and NO synthesis in primary rat microglial cells. *Neurochem. Int.* 42, 131–137. doi: 10.1016/s0197-0186(02)00076-1

Lin, M. T., and Beal, M. F. (2006a). Alzheimer's APP mangles mitochondria. *Nat. Med.* 12, 1241–1243. doi: 10.1038/nm1106-1241

Lin, M. T., and Beal, M. F. (2006b). Mitochondrial dysfunction and oxidative stress in neurodegenerative diseases. *Nature* 443, 787–795. doi: 10.1038/nature05292

Lin, M. T., Simon, D. K., Ahn, C. H., Kim, L. M., and Beal, M. F. (2002). High aggregate burden of somatic mtDNA point mutations in aging and Alzheimer's disease brain. *Hum. Mol. Genet.* 11, 133–145. doi: 10.1093/hmg/11.2.133

Lindenberger, U., Marsiske, M., and Baltes, P. B. (2000). Memorizing while walking: increase in dual-task costs from young adulthood to old age. *Psychol. Aging* 15, 417–436. doi: 10.1037//0882-7974.15.3.417

Lipsitz, L. A. (2002). Dynamics of stability: the physiologic basis of functional health and frailty. *J. Gerontol. A Biol. Sci. Med. Sci.* 57, B115–B125. doi: 10.1093/gerona/57.3.b115

Lipsitz, L. A., and Goldberger, A. L. (1992). Loss of 'complexity' and aging. Potential applications of fractals and chaos theory to senescence. *JAMA* 267, 1806–1809. doi: 10.1001/jama.1992.03480130122036

Liu, B., Wang, K., Gao, H. M., Mandavilli, B., Wang, J. Y., and Hong, J. S. (2001). Molecular consequences of activated microglia in the brain: overactivation induces apoptosis. *J. Neurochem.* 77, 182–189. doi: 10.1046/j.1471-4159.2001.00216.x

Liu, X., Wu, Z., Hayashi, Y., and Nakanishi, H. (2012). Age-dependent neuroinflammatory responses and deficits in long-term potentiation in the hippocampus during systemic inflammation. *Neuroscience* 216, 133–142. doi: 10.1016/j.neuroscience.2012.04.050

Loncarevic-Vasiljkovic, N., Pesic, V., Todorovic, S., Popic, J., Smiljanic, K., Milanovic, D., et al. (2012). Caloric restriction suppresses microglial activation and prevents neuroapoptosis following cortical injury in rats. *PLoS One* 7:e37215. doi: 10.1371/journal.pone.0037215

Lopez, J. R., Lyckman, A., Oddo, S., Laferla, F. M., Querfurth, H. W., and Shtifman, A. (2008). Increased intraneuronal resting [Ca2+] in adult Alzheimer's disease mice. *J. Neurochem.* 105, 262–271. doi: 10.1111/j.1471-4159.2007.05135.x

Lovell, M. A., Xie, C., and Markesbery, W. R. (1998). Decreased glutathione transferase activity in brain and ventricular fluid in Alzheimer's disease. *Neurology* 51, 1562–1566. doi: 10.1212/wnl.51.6.1562

Lovell, M. A., Xie, C., and Markesbery, W. R. (2001). Acrolein is increased in Alzheimer's disease brain and is toxic to primary hippocampal cultures. *Neurobiol. Aging* 22, 187–194. doi: 10.1016/s0197-4580(00)00235-9

Lu, C., Zhang, D., Whiteman, M., and Armstrong, J. S. (2008). Is antioxidant potential of the mitochondrial targeted ubiquinone derivative MitoQ conserved in cells lacking mtDNA? *Antioxid. Redox Signal.* 10, 651–660. doi: 10.1089/ars.2007.1865

Lucas, M., Zhang, X., Prasanna, V., and Mosser, D. M. (2005). ERK activation following macrophage FcgammaR ligation leads to chromatin modifications at the IL-10 locus. *J. Immunol.* 175, 469–477. doi: 10.4049/jimmunol.175.1.469

Lue, L. F., Kuo, Y. M., Beach, T., and Walker, D. G. (2010). Microglia activation and anti-inflammatory regulation in Alzheimer's disease. *Mol. Neurobiol.* 41, 115–128. doi: 10.1007/s12035-010-8106-8

Lukiw, W. J. (2004). Gene expression profiling in fetal, aged and Alzheimer hippocampus: a continuum of stress-related signaling. *Neurochem. Res.* 29, 1287–1297. doi: 10.1023/b:nere.0000023615.89699.63

Mahad, D., Ziabreva, I., Lassmann, H., and Turnbull, D. (2008). Mitochondrial defects in acute multiple sclerosis lesions. *Brain* 131, 1722–1735. doi: 10.1093/brain/awn105

Maher, F. O., Clarke, R. M., Kelly, A., Nally, R. E., and Lynch, M. A. (2006). Interaction between interferon gamma and insulin-like growth factor-1 in hippocampus impacts on the ability of rats to sustain long-term potentiation. *J. Neurochem.* 96, 1560–1571. doi: 10.1111/j.1471-4159.2006.03664.x

Mandrekar-Colucci, S., Karlo, J. C., and Landreth, G. E. (2012). Mechanisms underlying the rapid peroxisome proliferator-activated receptor-gamma-mediated amyloid clearance and reversal of cognitive deficits in a murine model of Alzheimer's disease. *J. Neurosci.* 32, 10117–10128. doi: 10.1523/JNEUROSCI.5268-11.2012

Markesbery, W. R. (1997). Oxidative stress hypothesis in Alzheimer's disease. *Free Radic. Biol. Med.* 23, 134–147. doi: 10.1016/s0891-5849(96)00629-6

Martinez, F. O., Sica, A., Mantovani, A., and Locati, M. (2008). Macrophage activation and polarization. *Front. Biosci.* 13, 453–461. doi: 10.2741/2692

Masters, S. L., Dunne, A., Subramanian, S. L., Hull, R. L., Tannahill, G. M., Sharp, F. A., et al. (2010). Activation of the NLRP3 inflammasome by islet amyloid polypeptide provides a mechanism for enhanced IL-1beta in type 2 diabetes. *Nat. Immunol.* 11, 897–904. doi: 10.1038/ni.1935

Mattson, M. P. (2005). NF-kappaB in the survival and plasticity of neurons. *Neurochem. Res.* 30, 883–893. doi: 10.1007/s11064-005-6961-x

Mattson, M. P., and Chan, S. L. (2003). Neuronal and glial calcium signaling in Alzheimer's disease. *Cell Calcium* 34, 385–397. doi: 10.1016/s0143-4160(03)00128-3

Mattson, M. P., Chan, S. L., and Duan, W. (2002). Modification of brain aging and neurodegenerative disorders by genes, diet and behavior. *Physiol. Rev.* 82, 637–672. doi: 10.1152/physrev.00004.2002

Mawuenyega, K. G., Sigurdson, W., Ovod, V., Munsell, L., Kasten, T., Morris, J. C., et al. (2010). Decreased clearance of CNS beta-amyloid in Alzheimer's disease. *Science* 330:1774. doi: 10.1126/science.1197623

McCoy, M. K., Martinez, T. N., Ruhn, K. A., Szymkowski, D. E., Smith, C. G., Botterman, B. R., et al. (2006). Blocking soluble tumor necrosis factor signaling with dominant-negative tumor necrosis factor inhibitor attenuates loss of dopaminergic neurons in models of Parkinson's disease. *J. Neurosci.* 26, 9365–9375. doi: 10.1523/jneurosci.1504-06.2006

McGeer, P. L., and McGeer, E. G. (2001). Inflammation, autotoxicity and Alzheimer disease. *Neurobiol. Aging* 22, 799–809. doi: 10.1016/s0197-4580(01)00289-5

Melov, S., Adlard, P. A., Morten, K., Johnson, F., Golden, T. R., Hinerfeld, D., et al. (2007). Mitochondrial oxidative stress causes hyperphosphorylation of tau. *PLoS One* 2:e536. doi: 10.1371/journal.pone.0000536

Mittaud, P., Labourdette, G., Zingg, H., and Guenot-Di Scala, D. (2002). Neurons modulate oxytocin receptor expression in rat cultured astrocytes: involvement of TGF-beta and membrane components. *Glia* 37, 169–177. doi: 10.1002/glia.10029

Moreira, P. I., Zhu, X., Wang, X., Lee, H. G., Nunomura, A., Petersen, R. B., et al. (2010). Mitochondria: a therapeutic target in neurodegeneration. *Biochim. Biophys. Acta* 1802, 212–220. doi: 10.1016/j.bbadis.2009.10.007

Morgan, T. E., Wong, A. M., and Finch, C. E. (2007). Anti-inflammatory mechanisms of dietary restriction in slowing aging processes. *Interdiscip. Top. Gerontol.* 35, 83–97. doi: 10.1159/000096557

Mosher, K. I., and Wyss-Coray, T. (2014). Microglial dysfunction in brain aging and Alzheimer's disease. *Biochem. Pharmacol.* 88, 594–604. doi: 10.1016/j.bcp.2014.01.008

Mosser, D. M. (2003). The many faces of macrophage activation. *J. Leukoc. Biol.* 73, 209–212. doi: 10.1189/jlb.0602325

Mosser, D. M., and Edwards, J. P. (2008). Exploring the full spectrum of macrophage activation. *Nat. Rev. Immunol.* 8, 958–969. doi: 10.1038/nri2448

Mount, M. P., Lira, A., Grimes, D., Smith, P. D., Faucher, S., Slack, R., et al. (2007). Involvement of interferon-gamma in microglial-mediated loss of dopaminergic neurons. *J. Neurosci.* 27, 3328–3337. doi: 10.1523/jneurosci.5321-06.2007

Mrak, R. E., and Griffin, W. S. (2005). Glia and their cytokines in progression of neurodegeneration. *Neurobiol. Aging* 26, 349–354. doi: 10.1016/j.neurobiolaging.2004.05.010

Murgas, P., Cornejo, F. A., Merino, G., and Von Bernhardi, R. (2014). SR-A regulates the inflammatory activation of astrocytes. *Neurotox. Res.* 25, 68–80. doi: 10.1007/s12640-013-9432-1

Murgas, P., Godoy, B., and Von Bernhardi, R. (2012). Abeta potentiates inflammatory activation of glial cells induced by scavenger receptor ligands and inflammatory mediators in culture. *Neurotox. Res.* 22, 69–78. doi: 10.1007/s12640-011-9306-3

Nakahira, K., Haspel, J. A., Rathinam, V. A., Lee, S. J., Dolinay, T., Lam, H. C., et al. (2011). Autophagy proteins regulate innate immune responses by inhibiting the release of mitochondrial DNA mediated by the NALP3 inflammasome. *Nat. Immunol.* 12, 222–230. doi: 10.1038/ni.1980

Nakamura, Y. (2002). Regulating factors for microglial activation. *Biol. Pharm. Bull.* 25, 945–953. doi: 10.1248/bpb.25.945

Nakanishi, H., and Wu, Z. (2009). Microglia-aging: roles of microglial lysosome- and mitochondria-derived reactive oxygen species in brain aging. *Behav. Brain Res.* 201, 1–7. doi: 10.1016/j.bbr.2009.02.001

Navarro, A., Sánchez Del Pino, M. J., Gómez, C., Peralta, J. L., and Boveris, A. (2002). Behavioral dysfunction, brain oxidative stress and impaired mitochondrial electron transfer in aging mice. *Am. J. Physiol. Regul. Integr. Comp. Physiol.* 282, R985–R992. doi: 10.1152/ajpregu.00537.2001

Nayernia, Z., Jaquet, V., and Krause, K. H. (2014). New insights on NOX enzymes in the central nervous system. *Antioxid. Redox Signal.* 20, 2815–2837. doi: 10.1089/ars.2013.5703

Neumann, H., Kotter, M. R., and Franklin, R. J. (2009). Debris clearance by microglia: an essential link between degeneration and regeneration. *Brain* 132, 288–295. doi: 10.1093/brain/awn109

Nguyen, M. D., Julien, J. P., and Rivest, S. (2002). Innate immunity: the missing link in neuroprotection and neurodegeneration? *Nat. Rev. Neurosci.* 3, 216–227. doi: 10.1038/nrn752

Nimmerjahn, A., Kirchhoff, F., and Helmchen, F. (2005). Resting microglial cells are highly dynamic surveillants of brain parenchyma in vivo. *Science* 308, 1314–1318. doi: 10.1126/science.1110647

Njie, E. G., Boelen, E., Stassen, F. R., Steinbusch, H. W., Borchelt, D. R., and Streit, W. J. (2012). Ex vivo cultures of microglia from young and aged rodent brain reveal age-related changes in microglial function. *Neurobiol. Aging* 195, e1–e12. doi: 10.1016/j.neurobiolaging.2010.05.008

Nunomura, A., Chiba, S., Lippa, C. F., Cras, P., Kalaria, R. N., Takeda, A., et al. (2004). Neuronal RNA oxidation is a prominent feature of familial Alzheimer's disease. *Neurobiol. Dis.* 17, 108–113. doi: 10.1016/j.nbd.2004.06.003

Nunomura, A., Perry, G., Aliev, G., Hirai, K., Takeda, A., Balraj, E. K., et al. (2001). Oxidative damage is the earliest event in Alzheimer disease. *J. Neuropathol. Exp. Neurol.* 60, 759–767.

Oddo, S. (2008). The ubiquitin-proteasome system in Alzheimer's disease. *J. Cell. Mol. Med.* 12, 363–373. doi: 10.1111/j.1582-4934.2008.00276.x

Ouyang, X., Negishi, H., Takeda, R., Fujita, Y., Taniguchi, T., and Honda, K. (2007). Cooperation between MyD88 and TRIF pathways in TLR synergy via IRF5 activation. *Biochem. Biophys. Res. Commun.* 354, 1045–1051. doi: 10.1016/j.bbrc.2007.01.090

Pappolla, M. A., Chyan, Y. J., Omar, R. A., Hsiao, K., Perry, G., Smith, M. A., et al. (1998). Evidence of oxidative stress and in vivo neurotoxicity of beta-amyloid in a transgenic mouse model of Alzheimer's disease: a chronic oxidative paradigm for testing antioxidant therapies in vivo. *Am. J. Pathol.* 152, 871–877.

Paresce, D. M., Chung, H., and Maxfield, F. R. (1997). Slow degradation of aggregates of the Alzheimer's disease amyloid beta-protein by microglial cells. *J. Biol. Chem.* 272, 29390–29397. doi: 10.1074/jbc.272.46.29390

Parihar, M. S., and Brewer, G. J. (2007). Simultaneous age-related depolarization of mitochondrial membrane potential and increased mitochondrial reactive oxygen species production correlate with age-related glutamate excitotoxicity in rat hippocampal neurons. *J. Neurosci. Res.* 85, 1018–1032. doi: 10.1002/jnr.21218

Parihar, M. S., Kunz, E. A., and Brewer, G. J. (2008). Age-related decreases in NAD(P)H and glutathione cause redox declines before ATP loss during glutamate treatment of hippocampal neurons. *J. Neurosci. Res.* 86, 2339–2352. doi: 10.1002/jnr.21679

Park, S. Y., Park, S. J., Park, T. G., Rajasekar, S., Lee, S. J., and Choi, Y. W. (2013). Schizandrin C exerts anti-neuroinflammatory effects by upregulating phase II detoxifying/antioxidant enzymes in microglia. *Int. Immunopharmacol.* 17, 415–426. doi: 10.1016/j.intimp.2013.06.032

Patel, J. R., and Brewer, G. J. (2008). Age-related differences in NFkappaB translocation and Bcl-2/Bax ratio caused by TNFalpha and Abeta42 promote survival in middle-age neurons and death in old neurons. *Exp. Neurol.* 213, 93–100. doi: 10.1016/j.expneurol.2008.05.007

Patten, D. A., Germain, M., Kelly, M. A., and Slack, R. S. (2010). Reactive oxygen species: stuck in the middle of neurodegeneration. *J. Alzheimers Dis.* 20, S357–S367. doi: 10.3233/JAD-2010-100498

Pawate, S., Shen, Q., Fan, F., and Bhat, N. R. (2004). Redox regulation of glial inflammatory response to lipopolysaccharide and interferongamma. *J. Neurosci. Res.* 77, 540–551. doi: 10.1002/jnr.20180

Pennypacker, K. R., Kassed, C. A., Eidizadeh, S., Saporta, S., Sanberg, P. R., and Willing, A. E. (2001). NF-kappaB p50 is increased in neurons surviving hippocampal injury. *Exp. Neurol.* 172, 307–319. doi: 10.1006/exnr.2001.7817

Perry, V. H. (2004). The influence of systemic inflammation on inflammation in the brain: implications for chronic neurodegenerative disease. *Brain Behav. Immun.* 18, 407–413. doi: 10.1016/j.bbi.2004.01.004

Perry, G., Cash, A. D., and Smith, M. A. (2002). Alzheimer disease and oxidative stress. *J. Biomed. Biotechnol.* 2, 120–123. doi: 10.1155/S1110724302203010

Perry, V. H., Cunningham, C., and Holmes, C. (2007). Systemic infections and inflammation affect chronic neurodegeneration. *Nat. Rev. Immunol.* 7, 161–167. doi: 10.1038/nri2015

Perry, V. H., Newman, T. A., and Cunningham, C. (2003). The impact of systemic infection on the progression of neurodegenerative disease. *Nat. Rev. Neurosci.* 4, 103–112. doi: 10.1038/nrn1032

Picca, A., Fracasso, F., Pesce, V., Cantatore, P., Joseph, A. M., Leeuwenburgh, C., et al. (2012). Age- and calorie restriction-related changes in rat brain mitochondrial DNA and TFAM binding. *Age (Dordr)* 35, 1607–1620. doi: 10.1007/s11357-012-9465-z

Pocock, J. M., and Kettenmann, H. (2007). Neurotransmitter receptors on microglia. *Trends Neurosci.* 30, 527–535. doi: 10.1016/j.tins.2007.07.007

Polito, L., Chierchia, A., Tunesi, M., Bouybayoune, I., Kehoe, P. G., Albani, D., et al. (2014). Environmental enrichment lessens cognitive decline in APP23 mice without affecting brain sirtuin expression. *J. Alzheimers Dis.* 42, 851–864. doi: 10.3233/JAD-131430

Porta, C., Rimoldi, M., Raes, G., Brys, L., Ghezzi, P., Di Liberto, D., et al. (2009). Tolerance and M2 (alternative) macrophage polarization are related processes orchestrated by p50 nuclear factor kappaB. *Proc. Natl. Acad. Sci. U S A* 106, 14978–14983. doi: 10.1073/pnas.0809784106

Praticò, D., MY Lee, V., Trojanowski, J. Q., Rokach, J., and Fitzgerald, G. A. (1998). Increased F2-isoprostanes in Alzheimer's disease: evidence for enhanced lipid peroxidation in vivo. *FASEB J.* 12, 1777–1783.

Qin, L., Block, M. L., Liu, Y., Bienstock, R. J., Pei, Z., Zhang, W., et al. (2005a). Microglial NADPH oxidase is a novel target for femtomolar neuroprotection against oxidative stress. *FASEB J.* 19, 550–557. doi: 10.1096/fj.04-2857com

Qin, L., Li, G., Qian, X., Liu, Y., Wu, X., Liu, B., et al. (2005b). Interactive role of the toll-like receptor 4 and reactive oxygen species in LPS-induced microglia activation. *Glia* 52, 78–84. doi: 10.1002/glia.20225

Qin, L., Liu, Y., Cooper, C., Liu, B., Wilson, B., and Hong, J. S. (2002). Microglia enhance beta-amyloid peptide-induced toxicity in cortical and mesencephalic neurons by producing reactive oxygen species. *J. Neurochem.* 83, 973–983. doi: 10.1046/j.1471-4159.2002.01210.x

Qin, L., Liu, Y., Hong, J. S., and Crews, F. T. (2013). NADPH oxidase and aging drive microglial activation, oxidative stress and dopaminergic neurodegeneration following systemic LPS administration. *Glia* 61, 855–868. doi: 10.1002/glia.22479

Racchi, M., Uberti, D., Govoni, S., Memo, M., Lanni, C., Vasto, S., et al. (2008). Alzheimer's disease: new diagnostic and therapeutic tools. *Immun. Ageing* 5:7. doi: 10.1186/1742-4933-5-7

Rachal Pugh, C., Fleshner, M., Watkins, L. R., Maier, S. F., and Rudy, J. W. (2001). The immune system and memory consolidation: a role for the cytokine IL-1β. *Neurosci. Biobehav. Rev.* 25, 29–41. doi: 10.1016/s0149-7634(00)00048-8

Radler, M. E., Hale, M. W., and Kent, S. (2014). Calorie restriction attenuates lipopolysaccharide (LPS)-induced microglial activation in discrete regions of the hypothalamus and the subfornical organ. *Brain Behav. Immun.* 38, 13–24. doi: 10.1016/j.bbi.2013.11.014

Radler, M. E., Wright, B. J., Walker, F. R., Hale, M. W., and Kent, S. (2015). Calorie restriction increases lipopolysaccharide-induced neuropeptide Y immunolabeling and reduces microglial cell area in the arcuate hypothalamic nucleus. *Neuroscience* 285, 236–247. doi: 10.1016/j.neuroscience.2014.11.014

Raj, D. D., Jaarsma, D., Holtman, I. R., Olah, M., Ferreira, F. M., Schaafsma, W., et al. (2014). Priming of microglia in a DNA-repair deficient model of accelerated aging. *Neurobiol. Aging* 35, 2147–2160. doi: 10.1016/j.neurobiolaging.2014.03.025

Ransohoff, R. M., and Perry, V. H. (2009). Microglial physiology: unique stimuli, specialized responses. *Annu. Rev. Immunol.* 27, 119–145. doi: 10.1146/annurev.immunol.021908.132528

Reed-Geaghan, E. G., Savage, J. C., Hise, A. G., and Landreth, G. E. (2009). CD14 and toll-like receptors 2 and 4 are required for fibrillar Abeta-stimulated microglial activation. *J. Neurosci.* 29, 11982–11992. doi: 10.1523/JNEUROSCI.3158-09.2009

Rivest, S. (2009). Regulation of innate immune responses in the brain. *Nat. Rev. Immunol.* 9, 429–439. doi: 10.1038/nri2565

Rosales-Corral, S., Reiter, R. J., Tan, D. X., Ortiz, G. G., and Lopez-Armas, G. (2010). Functional aspects of redox control during neuroinflammation. *Antioxid. Redox Signal.* 13, 193–247. doi: 10.1089/ars.2009.2629

Ruffell, D., Mourkioti, F., Gambardella, A., Kirstetter, P., Lopez, R. G., Rosenthal, N., et al. (2009). A CREB-C/EBPbeta cascade induces M2 macrophage-specific gene expression and promotes muscle injury repair. *Proc. Natl. Acad. Sci. U S A* 106, 17475–17480. doi: 10.1073/pnas.0908641106

Salat, D. H., Buckner, R. L., Snyder, A. Z., Greve, D. N., Desikan, R. S., Busa, E., et al. (2004). Thinning of the cerebral cortex in aging. *Cereb. Cortex* 14, 721–730. doi: 10.1093/cercor/bhh032

Salat, D. H., Tuch, D. S., Hevelone, N. D., Fischl, B., Corkin, S., Rosas, H. D., et al. (2005). Age-related changes in prefrontal white matter measured by diffusion tensor imaging. *Ann. N Y Acad. Sci.* 1064, 37–49. doi: 10.1196/annals.1340.009

Salminen, A., Ojala, J., Kaarniranta, K., and Kauppinen, A. (2012). Mitochondrial dysfunction and oxidative stress activate inflammasomes: impact on the aging process and age-related diseases. *Cell. Mol. Life Sci.* 69, 2999–3013. doi: 10.1007/s00018-012-0962-0

Santos, R. X., Correia, S. C., Wang, X., Perry, G., Smith, M. A., Moreira, P. I., et al. (2010a). Alzheimer's disease: diverse aspects of mitochondrial malfunctioning. *Int. J. Clin. Exp. Pathol.* 3, 570–581.

Santos, R. X., Correia, S. C., Wang, X., Perry, G., Smith, M. A., Moreira, P. I., et al. (2010b). A synergistic dysfunction of mitochondrial fission/fusion dynamics and mitophagy in Alzheimer's disease. *J. Alzheimers Dis.* 20(Suppl. 2), S401–S412. doi: 10.3233/JAD-2010-100666

Sastre, M., Klockgether, T., and Heneka, M. T. (2006). Contribution of inflammatory processes to Alzheimer's disease: molecular mechanisms. *Int. J. Dev. Neurosci.* 24, 167–176. doi: 10.1016/j.ijdevneu.2005.11.014

Satoh, T., and Lipton, S. A. (2007). Redox regulation of neuronal survival mediated by electrophilic compounds. *Trends Neurosci.* 30, 37–45. doi: 10.1016/j.tins.2006.11.004

Satoh, T., Takeuchi, O., Vandenbon, A., Yasuda, K., Tanaka, Y., Kumagai, Y., et al. (2010). The Jmjd3-Irf4 axis regulates M2 macrophage polarization and host responses against helminth infection. *Nat. Immunol.* 11, 936–944. doi: 10.1038/ni.1920

Saud, K., Herrera-Molina, R., and Von Bernhardi, R. (2005). Pro- and anti-inflammatory cytokines regulate the ERK pathway: implication of the timing for the activation of microglial cells. *Neurotox. Res.* 8, 277–287. doi: 10.1007/bf03033981

Schipper, H. M., and Song, W. (2015). A Heme Oxygenase-1 Transducer model of degenerative and developmental brain disorders. *Int. J. Mol. Sci.* 16, 5400–5419. doi: 10.3390/ijms16035400

Schuitemaker, A., van der Doef, T. F., Boellaard, R., van der Flier, W. M., Yaqub, M., Windhorst, A. D., et al. (2012). Microglial activation in healthy aging. *Neurobiol. Aging* 33, 1067–1072. doi: 10.1016/j.neurobiolaging.2010.09.016

Schwab, C., and McGeer, P. L. (2008). Inflammatory aspects of Alzheimer disease and other neurodegenerative disorders. *J. Alzheimers Dis.* 13, 359–369.

Selkoe, D. J. (2002). Alzheimer's disease is a synaptic failure. *Science* 298, 789–791. doi: 10.1126/science.1074069

Sheng, J. G., Mrak, R. E., and Griffin, W. S. (1998). Enlarged and phagocytic, but not primed, interleukin-1 alpha-immunoreactive microglia increase with age in normal human brain. *Acta Neuropathol.* 95, 229–234. doi: 10.1007/s004010050792

Shetty, R. A., Ikonne, U. S., Forster, M. J., and Sumien, N. (2014). Coenzyme Q10 and alpha-tocopherol reversed age-associated functional impairments in mice. *Exp. Gerontol.* 58, 208–218. doi: 10.1016/j.exger.2014.08.007

Shi, Q., and Gibson, G. E. (2007). Oxidative stress and transcriptional regulation in Alzheimer disease. *Alzheimer Dis. Assoc. Disord.* 21, 276–291. doi: 10.1097/wad.0b013e31815721c3

Shock, N., Greulich, R., Costa, P., Andres, R., Lakatta, E., Arenberg, D., et al. (1984). *Normal Human Aging: The Baltimore Longitudinal Study of Aging.* Baltimore: US Department of Health and Human Services.

Sierra, A., Gottfried-Blackmore, A. C., McEwen, B. S., and Bulloch, K. (2007). Microglia derived from aging mice exhibit an altered inflammatory profile. *Glia* 55, 412–424. doi: 10.1002/glia.20468

Simard, A. R., Soulet, D., Gowing, G., Julien, J. P., and Rivest, S. (2006). Bone marrow-derived microglia play a critical role in restricting senile plaque formation in Alzheimer's disease. *Neuron* 49, 489–502. doi: 10.1016/j.neuron.2006.01.022

Smith, R. G., Betancourt, L., and Sun, Y. (2005). Molecular endocrinology and physiology of the aging central nervous system. *Endocr. Rev.* 26, 203–250. doi: 10.1210/er.2002-0017

Song, Y. S., Park, H. J., Kim, S. Y., Lee, S. H., Yoo, H. S., Lee, H. S., et al. (2004). Protective role of Bcl-2 on beta-amyloid-induced cell death of differentiated PC12 cells: reduction of NF-kappaB and p38 MAP kinase activation. *Neurosci. Res.* 49, 69–80. doi: 10.1016/j.neures.2004.01.010

Sowell, E. R., Peterson, B. S., Thompson, P. M., Welcome, S. E., Henkenius, A. L., and Toga, A. W. (2003). Mapping cortical change across the human life span. *Nat. Neurosci.* 6, 309–315. doi: 10.1038/nn1008

Sriram, K., Matheson, J. M., Benkovic, S. A., Miller, D. B., Luster, M. I., and O'Callaghan, J. P. (2002). Mice deficient in TNF receptors are protected against dopaminergic neurotoxicity: implications for Parkinson's disease. *FASEB J.* 16, 1474–1476. doi: 10.1096/fj.02-0216fje

Streit, W. J. (2002). Microglia as neuroprotective, immunocompetent cells of the CNS. *Glia* 40, 133–139. doi: 10.1002/glia.10154

Streit, W. J. (2006). Microglial senescence: does the brain's immune system have an expiration date? *Trends Neurosci.* 29, 506–510. doi: 10.1016/j.tins.2006.07.001

Streit, W. J., Braak, H., Xue, Q. S., and Bechmann, I. (2009). Dystrophic (senescent) rather than activated microglial cells are associated with tau pathology and likely precede neurodegeneration in Alzheimer's disease. *Acta Neuropathol.* 118, 475–485. doi: 10.1007/s00401-009-0556-6

Streit, W. J., Mrak, R. E., and Griffin, W. S. (2004a). Microglia and neuroinflammation: a pathological perspective. *J. Neuroinflammation* 1:14. doi: 10.1186/1742-2094-1-14

Streit, W. J., Sammons, N. W., Kuhns, A. J., and Sparks, D. L. (2004b). Dystrophic microglia in the aging human brain. *Glia* 45, 208–212. doi: 10.1002/glia.10319

Sulciner, D. J., Irani, K., Yu, Z. X., Ferrans, V. J., Goldschmidt-Clermont, P., and Finkel, T. (1996). rac1 regulates a cytokine-stimulated, redox-dependent pathway necessary for NF-kappaB activation. *Mol. Cell. Biol.* 16, 7115–7121.

Swerdlow, R. H. (2007). Is aging part of Alzheimer's disease, or is Alzheimer's disease part of aging? *Neurobiol. Aging* 28, 1465–1480. doi: 10.1016/j.neurobiolaging.2006.06.021

Swerdlow, R. H., Burns, J. M., and Khan, S. M. (2010). The Alzheimer's disease mitochondrial cascade hypothesis. *J. Alzheimers Dis.* 20(Suppl. 2), S265–S279. doi: 10.3233/JAD-2010-100339

Szeto, H. H. (2014). First-in-class cardiolipin-protective compound as a therapeutic agent to restore mitochondrial bioenergetics. *Br. J. Pharmacol.* 171, 2029–2050. doi: 10.1111/bph.12461

Szeto, H. H., James, L. P., and Atkinson, A. J. (2014). Mitochondrial pharmacology: its future is now. *Clin. Pharmacol. Ther.* 96, 629–633. doi: 10.1038/clpt.2014.177

Taylor, R. C., and Dillin, A. (2011). Aging as an event of proteostasis collapse. *Cold Spring Harb. Perspect. Biol.* 3:a004440. doi: 10.1101/cshperspect.a004440

Tesseur, I., and Wyss-Coray, T. (2006). A role for TGF-beta signaling in neurodegeneration: evidence from genetically engineered models. *Curr. Alzheimer Res.* 3, 505–513. doi: 10.2174/156720506779025297

Tesseur, I., Zou, K., Esposito, L., Bard, F., Berber, E., Can, J. V., et al. (2006). Deficiency in neuronal TGF-beta signaling promotes neurodegeneration and Alzheimer's pathology. *J. Clin. Invest.* 116, 3060–3069. doi: 10.1172/jci27341

Thanopoulou, K., Fragkouli, A., Stylianopoulou, F., and Georgopoulos, S. (2010). Scavenger receptor class B type I (SR-BI) regulates perivascular macrophages and modifies amyloid pathology in an Alzheimer mouse model. *Proc. Natl. Acad. Sci. U S A* 107, 20816–20821. doi: 10.1073/pnas.1005888107

Tian, G., Kong, Q., Lai, L., Ray-Chaudhury, A., and Lin, C. L. (2010). Increased expression of cholesterol 24S-hydroxylase results in disruption of glial glutamate transporter EAAT2 association with lipid rafts: a potential role in Alzheimer's disease. *J. Neurochem.* 113, 978–989. doi: 10.1111/j.1471-4159.2010.06661.x

Tichauer, J. E., Flores, B., Soler, B., Eugenín-von Bernhardi, L., Ramírez, G., and von Bernhardi, R. (2014). Age-dependent changes on TGFbeta1 Smad3 pathway modify the pattern of microglial cell activation. *Brain Behav. Immun.* 37, 187–196. doi: 10.1016/j.bbi.2013.12.018

Tichauer, J., Saud, K., and von Bernhardi, R. (2007). Modulation by astrocytes of microglial cell-mediated neuroinflammation: effect on the activation of microglial signaling pathways. *Neuroimmunomodulation* 14, 168–174. doi: 10.1159/000110642

Tichauer, J. E., and von Bernhardi, R. (2012). Transforming growth factor-beta stimulates beta amyloid uptake by microglia through Smad3-dependent mechanisms. *J. Neurosci. Res.* 90, 1970–1980. doi: 10.1002/jnr.23082

Toppo, S., Flohé, L., Ursini, F., Vanin, S., and Maiorino, M. (2009). Catalytic mechanisms and specificities of glutathione peroxidases: variations of a basic scheme. *Biochim. Biophys. Acta* 1790, 1486–1500. doi: 10.1016/j.bbagen.2009.04.007

Town, T., Nikolic, V., and Tan, J. (2005). The microglial "activation" continuum: from innate to adaptive responses. *J. Neuroinflammation* 2:24. doi: 10.1186/1742-2094-2-24

Tremblay, M. E., Zettel, M. L., Ison, J. R., Allen, P. D., and Majewska, A. K. (2012). Effects of aging and sensory loss on glial cells in mouse visual and auditory cortices. *Glia* 60, 541–558. doi: 10.1002/glia.22287

Trepanier, C. H., and Milgram, N. W. (2010). Neuroinflammation in Alzheimer's disease: are NSAIDs and selective COX-2 inhibitors the next line of therapy? *J. Alzheimers Dis.* 21, 1089–1099. doi: 10.3233/JAD-2010-090667

Ueberham, U., Ueberham, E., Gruschka, H., and Arendt, T. (2006). Altered subcellular location of phosphorylated Smads in Alzheimer's disease. *Eur. J. Neurosci.* 24, 2327–2334. doi: 10.1111/j.1460-9568.2006.05109.x

Uehara, T., Nakamura, T., Yao, D., Shi, Z. Q., Gu, Z., Ma, Y., et al. (2006). S-nitrosylated protein-disulphide isomerase links protein misfolding to neurodegeneration. *Nature* 441, 513–517. doi: 10.1038/nature04782

Uylings, H. B., and de Brabander, J. M. (2002). Neuronal changes in normal human aging and Alzheimer's disease. *Brain Cogn.* 49, 268–276. doi: 10.1006/brcg.2001.1500

Valerio, A., Boroni, F., Benarese, M., Sarnico, I., Ghisi, V., Bresciani, L. G., et al. (2006). NF-kappaB pathway: a target for preventing beta-amyloid (Abeta)-induced neuronal damage and Abeta42 production. *Eur. J. Neurosci.* 23, 1711–1720. doi: 10.1111/j.1460-9568.2006.04722.x

van Rossum, D., and Hanisch, U. K. (2004). Microglia. *Metab. Brain Dis.* 19, 393–411. doi: 10.1023/B:MEBR.0000043984.73063.d8

Varadarajan, S., Yatin, S., Aksenova, M., and Butterfield, D. A. (2000). Review: Alzheimer's amyloid beta-peptide-associated free radical oxidative stress and neurotoxicity. *J. Struct. Biol.* 130, 184–208. doi: 10.1006/jsbi.2000.4274

Vijg, J., and Campisi, J. (2008). Puzzles, promises and a cure for ageing. *Nature* 454, 1065–1071. doi: 10.1038/nature07216

von Bernhardi, R. (2007). Glial cell dysregulation: a new perspective on Alzheimer disease. *Neurotox. Res.* 12, 215–232. doi: 10.1007/bf03033906

von Bernhardi, R. (2010). Immunotherapy in Alzheimer's disease: where do we stand? Where should we go? *J. Alzheimers Dis.* 19, 405–421. doi: 10.3233/JAD-2010-1248

von Bernhardi, R., and Eugenín, J. (2004). Microglial reactivity to beta-amyloid is modulated by astrocytes and proinflammatory factors. *Brain Res.* 1025, 186–193. doi: 10.1016/j.brainres.2004.07.084

von Bernhardi, R., Ramírez, G., Matile, H., and Döbeli, H. (2001). Immobilized amyloid precursor protein constructs: a tool for the in vitro screening of glial cell reactivity. *Eur. J. Neurosci.* 14, 946–956. doi: 10.1046/j.0953-816x.2001.01715.x

von Bernhardi, R., Tichauer, J. E., and Eugenín, J. (2010). Aging-dependent changes of microglial cells and their relevance for neurodegenerative disorders. *J. Neurochem.* 112, 1099–1114. doi: 10.1111/j.1471-4159.2009.06537.x

von Bernhardi, R., Tichauer, J., and Eugenín-von Bernhardi, L. (2011). Proliferating culture of aged microglia for the study of neurodegenerative diseases. *J. Neurosci. Methods* 202, 65–69. doi: 10.1016/j.jneumeth.2011.08.027

Wang, Q., Qian, L., Chen, S. H., Chu, C. H., Wilson, B., Oyarzabal, E., et al. (2015). Post-treatment with an ultra-low dose of NADPH oxidase inhibitor diphenyleneiodonium attenuates disease progression in multiple Parkinson's disease models. *Brain* 138, 1247–1262. doi: 10.1093/brain/awv034

Wang, T., Qin, L., Liu, B., Liu, Y., Wilson, B., Eling, T. E., et al. (2004). Role of reactive oxygen species in LPS-induced production of prostaglandin E2 in microglia. *J. Neurochem.* 88, 939–947. doi: 10.1046/j.1471-4159.2003.02242.x

Wehrspaun, C. C., Haerty, W., and Ponting, C. P. (2015). Microglia recapitulate a hematopoietic master regulator network in the aging human frontal cortex. *Neurobiol. Aging* 36, 2443.e9–2443.e20. doi: 10.1016/j.neurobiolaging.2015.04.008

Weiss, A., and Attisano, L. (2013). The TGFbeta superfamily signaling pathway. *Wiley Interdiscip. Rev. Dev. Biol.* 2, 47–63. doi: 10.1002/wdev.86

Werner, F., Jain, M. K., Feinberg, M. W., Sibinga, N. E., Pellacani, A., Wiesel, P., et al. (2000). Transforming growth factor-beta 1 inhibition of macrophage activation is mediated via Smad3. *J. Biol. Chem.* 275, 36653–36658. doi: 10.1074/jbc.m004536200

Wynn, T. A. (2003). IL-13 effector functions. *Annu. Rev. Immunol.* 21, 425–456. doi: 10.1146/annurev.immunol.21.120601.141142

Wyss-Coray, T., Lin, C., Yan, F., Yu, G. Q., Rohde, M., McConlogue, L., et al. (2001). TGF-β1 promotes microglial amyloid-beta clearance and reduces plaque burden in transgenic mice. *Nat. Med.* 7, 612–618. doi: 10.1038/87945

Wyss-Coray, T., and Mucke, L. (2002). Inflammation in neurodegenerative disease–a double-edged sword. *Neuron* 35, 419–432. doi: 10.1016/s0896-6273(02)00794-8

Yamamoto, K., Shimokawa, T., Yi, H., Isobe, K., Kojima, T., Loskutoff, D. J., et al. (2002). Aging accelerates endotoxin-induced thrombosis : increased responses of plasminogen activator inhibitor-1 and lipopolysaccharide signaling with aging. *Am. J. Pathol.* 161, 1805–1814. doi: 10.1016/s0002-9440(10)64457-4

Ye, S. M., and Johnson, R. W. (1999). Increased interleukin-6 expression by microglia from brain of aged mice. *J. Neuroimmunol.* 93, 139–148. doi: 10.1016/s0165-5728(98)00217-3

Ye, S. M., and Johnson, R. W. (2001). An age-related decline in interleukin-10 may contribute to the increased expression of interleukin-6 in brain of aged mice. *Neuroimmunomodulation* 9, 183–192. doi: 10.1159/000049025

Yung, R. L., and Julius, A. (2008). Epigenetics, aging and autoimmunity. *Autoimmunity* 41, 329–335. doi: 10.1080/08916930802024889

Zhang, J., Malik, A., Choi, H. B., Ko, R. W., Dissing-Olesen, L., and MacVicar, B. A. (2014). Microglial CR3 activation triggers long-term synaptic depression in the hippocampus via NADPH oxidase. *Neuron* 82, 195–207. doi: 10.1016/j.neuron.2014.01.043

Zhang, Q., Wu, Y., Zhang, P., Sha, H., Jia, J., Hu, Y., et al. (2012). Exercise induces mitochondrial biogenesis after brain ischemia in rats. *Neuroscience* 205, 10–17. doi: 10.1016/j.neuroscience.2011.12.053

Zhao, W., Zhang, J., Davis, E. G., and Rebeck, G. W. (2014). Aging reduces glial uptake and promotes extracellular accumulation of Abeta from a lentiviral vector. *Front. Aging Neurosci.* 6:210. doi: 10.3389/fnagi.2014.00210

Zhou, R., Yazdi, A. S., Menu, P., and Tschopp, J. (2011). A role for mitochondria in NLRP3 inflammasome activation. *Nature* 469, 221–225. doi: 10.1038/nature09663

Zhu, X., Su, B., Wang, X., Smith, M. A., and Perry, G. (2007). Causes of oxidative stress in Alzheimer disease. *Cell. Mol. Life Sci.* 64, 2202–2210. doi: 10.1007/s00018-007-7218-4

8

Common Effects of Amnestic Mild Cognitive Impairment on Resting-State Connectivity Across Four Independent Studies

Angela Tam[1,2,3], Christian Dansereau[3,4], AmanPreet Badhwar[3,4], Pierre Orban[2,3], Sylvie Belleville[3,4], Howard Chertkow[1], Alain Dagher[1], Alexandru Hanganu[3,5,6], Oury Monchi[3,4,5,6], Pedro Rosa-Neto[1,2], Amir Shmuel[1], Seqian Wang[1,2], John Breitner[1,2] and Pierre Bellec[3,4]* for the Alzheimer's Disease Neuroimaging Initiative†*

[1] McGill University, Montreal, QC, Canada, [2] Douglas Mental Health University Institute, Research Centre, Montreal, QC, Canada, [3] Centre de Recherche de L'institut Universitaire de Gériatrie de Montréal, Montreal, QC, Canada, [4] Université de Montréal, Montreal, QC, Canada, [5] University of Calgary, Calgary, AB, Canada, [6] Hotchkiss Brain Institute, Calgary, AB, Canada

Edited by:
Junfeng Sun,
Shanghai Jiao Tong University, China

Reviewed by:
Donald G. McLaren,
University of Wisconsin-Madison, USA
Rui Li,
Chinese Academy of Sciences, China

***Correspondence:**
Angela Tam
angela.tam@mail.mcgill.ca;
Pierre Bellec
pierre.bellec@criugm.qc.ca

†Data used in preparing this article were obtained from the Alzheimer's Disease Neuroimaging Initiative (ADNI) database (adni.loni.usc.edu). As such, the investigators within the ADNI contributed to the design and implementation of ADNI and/or provided data but most of them did not participate in this analysis or writing this report. A complete list of ADNI investigators can be found at: http://adni.loni.usc.edu/wp-content/uploads/how_to_apply/ADNI_Acknowledgement_List.pdf.

Resting-state functional connectivity is a promising biomarker for Alzheimer's disease. However, previous resting-state functional magnetic resonance imaging studies in Alzheimer's disease and amnestic mild cognitive impairment (aMCI) have shown limited reproducibility as they have had small sample sizes and substantial variation in study protocol. We sought to identify functional brain networks and connections that could consistently discriminate normal aging from aMCI despite variations in scanner manufacturer, imaging protocol, and diagnostic procedure. We therefore combined four datasets collected independently, including 112 healthy controls and 143 patients with aMCI. We systematically tested multiple brain connections for associations with aMCI using a weighted average routinely used in meta-analyses. The largest effects involved the superior medial frontal cortex (including the anterior cingulate), dorsomedial prefrontal cortex, striatum, and middle temporal lobe. Compared with controls, patients with aMCI exhibited significantly decreased connectivity between default mode network nodes and between regions of the cortico-striatal-thalamic loop. Despite the heterogeneity of methods among the four datasets, we identified common aMCI-related connectivity changes with small to medium effect sizes and sample size estimates recommending a minimum of 140 to upwards of 600 total subjects to achieve adequate statistical power in the context of a multisite study with 5–10 scanning sites and about 10 subjects per group and per site. If our findings can be replicated and associated with other established biomarkers of Alzheimer's disease (e.g., amyloid and tau quantification), then these functional connections may be promising candidate biomarkers for Alzheimer's disease.

Keywords: fMRI, mild cognitive impairment, connectome, resting-state, default mode network, meta-analysis

INTRODUCTION

Resting-state connectivity in functional magnetic resonance imaging (fMRI) captures the spatial coherence of spontaneous fluctuations in blood oxygenation. Resting-state fMRI is a promising technique that may be useful as an early biomarker for Alzheimer's disease (AD), a neurodegenerative process that develops over decades before patients suffer from dementia. The possibility that disturbed resting-state connectivity may be an early marker for AD is supported by studies of mild cognitive impairment (MCI), a disorder characterized by objective cognitive deficits without dementia, i.e., without impairment in activities of daily living, and more specifically by studies of amnestic MCI (aMCI), the most common subtype of MCI characterized by memory deficits (Petersen et al., 2001). These studies showed altered functional connectivity in MCI compared with cognitively normal elderly (CN; Sorg et al., 2007; Bai et al., 2009; Liang et al., 2012; Wu et al., 2014), but they relied on small sample sizes ($n = \sim 40$) and differed in many aspects of their protocols, e.g., recruitment and image acquisition procedures. If resting-state fMRI is to serve as a useful biomarker of AD, or any pathology, for clinical practice or research, we must determine if changes in functional connectivity differences between groups of subjects are robust to such variation in study protocols. Therefore, we sought to identify brain connections that showed consistent MCI-related changes across multiple independent studies. If such connections exist, they may be used as targets to be examined alongside other established AD biomarkers (e.g., amyloid and tau measures) in order to validate resting-state fMRI's potential as a biomarker for AD.

Resting-state connectivity studies have consistently found decreased connectivity between nodes within the default mode network (DMN) in patients with AD or MCI compared with CN (Sorg et al., 2007; Bai et al., 2009; Zhang et al., 2010; Koch et al., 2012; Liang et al., 2012). Less consistent are reports of alterations in the executive attentional, frontoparietal, and anterior temporal networks (Sorg et al., 2007; Zhang et al., 2010; Gour et al., 2011; Agosta et al., 2012; Liang et al., 2012; Wu et al., 2014) due to the literature's bias toward investigating the DMN. Further inconsistencies can be found in some studies that have reported increased connectivity between the middle temporal lobe and other DMN areas in MCI (Qi et al., 2010), while others have reported decreased connectivity between these same regions (Bai et al., 2009) and others have reported no significant differences between MCI and CN (Koch et al., 2012).

One obvious explanation for such inconsistency may be these studies' small sample sizes resulting in low statistical power (Kelly et al., 2012). Beyond this, however, there are other methodological differences that may compromise the comparison of results across independent studies. For example, the criteria for recruiting subjects with MCI, e.g., Petersen (2004) vs. NIA-AA recommendations (Albert et al., 2011) may differ among studies. Different study samples may also reflect different socio-cultural characteristics of recruiting sites, e.g., ethnicity, language, diet, socioeconomic status. The fMRI measurements themselves can also be affected by differences in details of the image acquisition such as scanner make and model (Friedman et al., 2006), sequence parameters such as repetition time, flip angle, or acquisition volume (Friedman and Glover, 2006), experimental design such as eyes-open/eyes-closed (Yan et al., 2009) or experiment duration (van Dijk et al., 2010), and scanning environment such as sound attenuation measures (Elliott et al., 1999), room temperature (Vanhoutte et al., 2006), or head-motion restraint techniques (Edward et al., 2000).

To identify robust changes in resting-state connectivity between aMCI and CN, we implemented a meta-analysis of four independent resting-state fMRI datasets (ADNI2 and three small single-site studies) using a weighted average implemented by Willer et al. (2010). Rather than relying on a priori target regions or connections, we leveraged the large sample size to perform a systematic search of brain connections affected by aMCI, an approach termed a "connectome-wide association study" (Shehzad et al., 2014). In addition, we relied on functionally-defined brain parcellations using an automated clustering procedure and we explored the impact of the number of brain clusters (called resolution) on observed differences (Bellec et al., 2015).

METHODS

Participants

We combined data from four independent studies: the Alzheimer's Disease Neuroimaging Initiative 2 (ADNI2) sample, two samples from the Centre de recherche de l'institut universitaire de gériatrie de Montréal (CRIUGMa and CRIUGMb), and a sample from the Montreal Neurological Institute (MNI; Wu et al., 2014). All participants gave their written informed consent to engage in these studies, which were approved by the research ethics board of the respective institutions, and included consent for data sharing with collaborators as well as secondary analysis. Ethical approval was also obtained at the site of secondary analysis (CRIUGM).

The ADNI2 data used in the preparation of this article were obtained from the Alzheimer's Disease Neuroimaging Initiative (ADNI) database (adni.loni.usc.edu). ADNI was launched in 2003 by the National Institute on Aging, the National Institute of Biomedical Imaging and Bioengineering, the Food and Drug Administration, private pharmaceutical companies and non-profit organizations, as a \$60 million, 5-year public-private partnership representing efforts of co-investigators from numerous academic institutions and private corporations. ADNI was followed by ADNI-GO and ADNI-2 that included newer techniques. Subjects included in this study were recruited by ADNI-2 from all 13 sites that acquired resting-state fMRI on Philips scanners across North America. For up-to-date information, see www.adni-info.org.

The combined sample included 112 CN and 143 aMCI prior to quality control. After quality control, 99 CN and 129 aMCI remained. In the CN group, the mean age was 72.0 (*s.d.* $= 7.0$) years, and 37% were men. Mean age of the aMCI subjects was 72.3 (*s.d.* $= 7.6$) years, and 50% were men. An independent samples t-test did not reveal any significant difference in age between the groups ($t = 0.759, p = 0.448$). A chi-squared test revealed a trend toward a significant difference in gender distribution between the groups ($\chi^2 = 3.627, p = 0.057$). Note that both age and gender were entered as confounding variables in the statistical analysis below. See **Table 1** for sample size and demographic information from the individual studies after passing quality control (for information about the original cohorts before quality control, see Supplementary Table 1).

All subjects underwent cognitive testing (e.g., memory, language, and executive function; see **Table 2** for a list of specific tests used in each study). Exclusion criteria common to all studies included: Contraindications to MRI, presence or history of axis I psychiatric disorders (e.g., depression, bipolar disorder, schizophrenia), presence or history of neurologic disease with potential impact on cognition (e.g., Parkinson's disease), and presence or history of substance abuse. CN subjects could not meet criteria for MCI or dementia. Those with aMCI had memory complaints, objective cognitive loss (based on neuropsychological testing), but had intact functional abilities and did not meet criteria for dementia. In ADNI2, the diagnosis of aMCI was made based on an education adjusted abnormal score on the Logical Memory II subscale (Delayed Paragraph Recall, Paragraph A only) from the Wechsler Memory Scale and a Clinical Dementia Rating (CDR) of 0.5. In both CRIUGMa and CRIUGMb, the diagnosis of aMCI was made based on scores equal to or >1.5 standard deviations below the mean adjusted for age and education on memory tests. At the MNI, the diagnosis of aMCI relied on the Petersen criteria (2004). At both CRIUGMb and MNI, aMCI diagnoses were made with input from a neurologist. See the Supplementary Methods (Datasheet 1 in Supplementary Material) for greater details for each study.

Imaging Data Acquisition

All resting-state fMRI and structural scans were acquired on 3T scanners. We performed analyses on the first usable scan (typically the baseline scan) from ADNI2 and applied clinical diagnoses from the same study time point as the first usable scan for each participant in that dataset. See **Table 3** for acquisition parameters for each sample.

Computational Environment

All experiments were performed using the NeuroImaging Analysis Kit (NIAK[1]; Bellec et al., 2011) version 0.12.18, under CentOS version 6.3 with Octave[2] version 3.8.1 and the Minc toolkit[3] version 0.3.18. Analyses were executed in parallel on the "Guillimin" supercomputer[4], using the pipeline system for Octave and Matlab (Bellec et al., 2012), version 1.0.2. The scripts used for processing can be found on Github[5].

Pre-processing

Each fMRI dataset was corrected for slice timing; a rigid-body motion was then estimated for each time frame, both within and between runs, as well as between one fMRI run and the T1 scan for each subject (Collins and Evans, 1997). The T1 scan was itself non-linearly co-registered to the Montreal Neurological Institute (MNI) ICBM152 stereotaxic symmetric template (Fonov et al., 2011), using the CIVET pipeline (Ad-Dab'bagh et al., 2006). The rigid-body, fMRI-to-T1 and T1-to-stereotaxic transformations were all combined to resample the fMRI in MNI space at a 3 mm isotropic resolution. To minimize artifacts due to excessive motion, all time frames showing a displacement >0.5 mm were removed (Power et al., 2012). A minimum of 50 unscrubbed volumes per run was required for further analysis (13 CN and 14 aMCI were rejected from the original cohort of 112 CN and 143 aMCI). Neither the rate of rejection nor the frame displacement values (before and after scrubbing) varied significantly among the

[1]http://simexp.github.io/niak/.
[2]https://www.gnu.org/software/octave/.
[3]http://www.bic.mni.mcgill.ca/ServicesSoftware/ServicesSoftwareMincToolKit.
[4]http://www.calculquebec.ca/en/resources/compute-servers/guillimin.
[5]https://github.com/SIMEXP/mcinet.

TABLE 1 | Demographic information in all studies after quality control.

		ADNI2	CRIUGMa	CRIUGMb	MNI	Combined sample
CN	**N**	**49**	**18**	**17**	**15**	**99**
	Mean age (*s.d.*)	74.4 (6.8)	71.2 (8.0)	70.4 (4.6)	67.0 (5.7)	72.0 (7.0)
	Number male (%)	21 (43%)	7 (39%)	2 (12%)	7 (47%)	37 (37%)
	Mean years of education (*s.d.*)[a]	16.9 (2.2)	14.9 (2.3)	15.1 (2.8)	15.0 (3.1)	16.0 (2.6)
	MMSE mean (range)	28.7 (25–30)	28.8 (27–30)	n/a	29.0 (27–30)	n/a
	MoCA mean (range)	n/a	27.8 (22–30)	28.4 (26–30)	n/a	n/a
aMCI	**N**	**82**	**8**	**21**	**18**	**129**
	Mean age (*s.d.*)	71.2 (7.3)	79.9 (6.1)	74.8 (7.0)	71.2 (8.1)	72.3 (7.6)
	Number male (%)	43 (52%)	3 (38%)	12 (57%)	7 (39%)	65 (50%)
	Mean years of education (*s.d.*)[a]	16.2 (2.6)	13.7 (3.8)	14.8 (4.2)	13.1 (3.1)	15.5 (3.2)
	MMSE mean (range)	28.1 (24–30)*	26.1 (22–29)*	n/a	26.1 (22–30)*	n/a
	MoCA mean (range)	n/a	23.3 (20–29)*	24.6 (16–29)*	n/a	n/a

MMSE, Mini-mental state examination; MoCA, Montreal Cognitive Assessment.
**Significant difference between aMCI and CN (within study) for independent samples t-test at $p \leq 0.05$.*
[a]Missing values for education for subjects in ADNI2 (1 CN, 1 aMCI), CRIUGMb (2 aMCI), and MNI (3 CN, 6 aMCI).

TABLE 2 | Neuropsychological tests that were used in each study.

Test	ADNI2	CRIUGMa	CRIUGMb	MNI
Mini-mental state examination (MMSE)	x	x		x
Montreal Cognitive Assessment (MoCA)	x	x	x	
Clinical Dementia Rating (CDR)	x		x	
ADAS-Cog	x			
Everyday Cognition (ECog)	x			
Trail making	x (Trails A and B)	x (Trails A and B)	x (Trails A and B)	x (DKEFS)
Boston naming test	x	x	x	x
Digit span		x	x	x
Color-word interference (DKEFS)		x	x	x
Rey auditory verbal learning test	x	x		x
Verbal fluency	x	x	x (MEC)	x (DKEFS)
Clock drawing	x	x		
Visual object and space perception battery		x		
Brixton spatial anticipation test			x	
Hooper visual organization test			x	
Rey complex figure		x	x	x
Aggie figures learning test				x
16-Item free and cued recall (RL/RI-16)			x	
Pyramid and palm trees test		x		
Weschler memory scale—logical memory subtest	x	x	x	

MEC, Montréal évaluation de la communication; DKEFS, Delis–Kaplan Executive Function System.

four samples or between CN and aMCI. The following nuisance covariates were regressed out from fMRI time series: slow time drifts (basis of discrete cosines with a 0.01 Hz high-pass cut-off), average signals in conservative masks of the white matter and the lateral ventricles as well as the first 3–10 principal components (median numbers for ADNI2, CRIUGMa, CRIUGMb, and MNI were 9, 6, 7, and 7, respectively, and accounting for 95% variance) of the six rigid-body motion parameters and their squares (Lund et al., 2006; Giove et al., 2009). The fMRI volumes were finally spatially smoothed with a 6 mm isotropic Gaussian blurring kernel. A more detailed description of the pipeline can be found on the NIAK website[6] and Github[7].

Bootstrap Analysis of Stable Clusters (BASC)

We applied a BASC to identify clusters that consistently exhibited similar spontaneous BOLD fluctuations in individual subjects, and were spatially stable across subjects. We first applied a region-growing algorithm to reduce each fMRI dataset into a time × space array, with 957 regions (Bellec et al., 2006). BASC replicates a hierarchical Ward clustering 1000 times and computes the probability that a pair of regions fall in the same cluster, a measure called stability. The region × region stability matrix is fed into a clustering procedure to derive consensus clusters, which are composed of regions with a high average probability of being assigned to the same cluster across all replications. At the individual level, the clustering was applied to the similarity of regional time series, which was replicated using a circular block bootstrap. Consensus clustering was applied to the average individual stability matrix to identify group clusters. The group clustering was replicated via bootstrapping of subjects in the group. A consensus clustering was finally applied on the group stability matrix to generate group consensus clusters.

The cluster procedure was carried out at a specific number of clusters (called resolution). Using a "multiscale stepwise selection" (MSTEPS) method (Bellec, 2013), we determined a subset of resolutions that provided an accurate summary of the group stability matrices generated over a fine grid of resolutions: 4, 6, 12, 22, 33, 65, 111, and 208.

Derivation of Functional Connectomes

For each resolution K, and each pair of distinct clusters, the between-clusters connectivity was measured by the Fisher transform of the Pearson's correlation between the average time series of the clusters. The within-cluster connectivity was the Fisher transform of the average correlation between time series inside the cluster. An individual connectome was thus a $K \times K$ matrix. See **Figures 1A,B** for an illustration of a parcellation and associated connectome.

Statistical Testing

To test for differences between aMCI and CN at a given resolution, we used a general linear model (GLM) for each connection between two clusters. The GLM included an intercept, the age and sex of participants, and the average frame

[6]http://niak.simexp-lab.org/pipe_preprocessing.html.
[7]https://github.com/SIMEXP/mcinet/tree/master/preprocess.

TABLE 3 | Structural and functional scan acquisition parameters.

	ADNI2[a]	CRIUGMa	CRIUGMb	MNI
Scanner manufacturer	**Philips**	**Siemens**	**Siemens**	**Siemens**
STRUCTURAL				
No. channels	8	32	32	32
No. slices	170	176	176	176
Slice thickness (mm)	1.2	1	1	1
In-plane resolution (mm × mm)	1 × 1	1 × 1	1 ×1	1 × 1
Matrix size	256 × 256	240 × 256	256 × 256	256 × 256
FOV (mm^2)	256	240/256	256	256
TR (s)	6.8	2.3	2.53	2.3
TE (ms)	3.09	2.91	1.64	2.98
TI (s)	n/a	0.9	1.2	0.9
FA (°)	9	9	7	9
Slice gap	0	0	0	0
Imaging plane	Sagittal	Sagittal	Sagittal	Sagittal
NEX	1	1	1	1
FUNCTIONAL				
No. runs	1	1	3	3
No. channels	8	32	32	32
No. volumes	140	240	150	160
No. slices	48	33	42	38
Slice thickness (mm)	3.3	4	3.4	3.6
In-plane resolution (mm × mm)	3.3 × 3.3	3 × 3	3.4 × 3.4	3.6 × 3.6
Matrix size	64 × 64	64 × 64	64 × 64	64 × 64
FOV (mm^2)	212	192	218	230
TR (s)	3	2	2.6	2
TE (ms)	30	30	30	30
FA (°)	80	90	90	90
Slice gap	0	0	0	0
Imaging plane	Axial	Axial	Axial	Axial
NEX	1	1	1	1
Total scan time (min:s)	7:00	8:00	19:30	16:00

[a]*http://adni.loni.usc.edu/wp-content/uploads/2011/04/ADNI_3T_Philips_2.6.pdf.*

displacement of the runs involved in the analysis. The contrast of interest (aMCI–CN) was represented by a dummy covariate coding the difference in average connectivity between the two groups. All covariates except the intercept were corrected to a zero mean (**Figure 1C**). The GLM was estimated independently for each scanning protocol. In addition to distinguishing between CRIUGMa, CRIUGMb, MNI, and ADNI2, ADNI2 was subdivided into five sub-studies based on the use of different Philips scanner models (i.e., Achieva, Gemini, Ingenia, Ingenuity, and Intera). We dropped all subjects scanned with Ingenuity (2 CN, 1 aMCI) due to the elimination of all aMCI subjects within that site by the scrubbing procedure and its small sample size. We therefore estimated seven independent GLMs for each protocol (ADNI2-Achieva, ADNI2-Gemini, ADNI2-Ingenia, ADNI2-Intera, CRIUGMa, CRIUGMb, MNI). The estimated effects were combined across all protocols through inverse variance based weighted averaging (Willer et al., 2010; **Figure 1D**).

Resolutions containing fewer than 50 clusters have been suggested to have higher sensitivity based on prior independent work (Bellec et al., 2015). The GLM was first applied at an a priori resolution of $K = 33$, which was the lowest number of clusters for which the DMN could be clearly decomposed into subnetworks (Supplementary Figure 1, visit Figshare for 3D volumes of brain parcellations[8] and see Supplementary Table 2 for a list of the 33 clusters and their numerical IDs). The false-discovery rate (FDR) across connections was controlled at $q^{FDR} \leq 0.1$ (Benjamini and Hochberg, 1995). In addition to the analysis at resolution 33, we assessed the impact of that parameter by replicating the GLM analysis at the seven resolutions selected by MSTEPS (Supplementary Figure 2). We implemented an omnibus test (family-wise error rate $\alpha \leq 0.05$) to assess the overall presence of significant differences between groups, pooling FDR results across all resolutions (Bellec et al., 2015). If the omnibus test across resolutions was not significant, then no test would be deemed significant. Since this omnibus test was significant, we used the FDR threshold of $q \leq 0.1$ to explore single resolutions.

RESULTS

Functional Connectivity Differences Between aMCI and CN

The omnibus test pooling significant differences in connectivity between aMCI and CN across all resolutions was significant at $\alpha \leq 0.05$ ($p \leq 0.0056$). In line with prior observations on independent datasets (Bellec et al., 2015), resolutions containing fewer than 50 clusters were associated with a higher rate of discovery (**Figure 2**). At resolution 33, significant group differences between aMCI and CN were seen across the whole brain (**Figure 3A**). Four brain clusters were associated with 47% of all significant changes found across the connectome: the superior medial frontal cortex (including anterior cingulate), dorsomedial prefrontal cortex, striatum, and middle temporal lobe (**Figures 3B,C**, Supplementary Table 3). Supplementary Table 3 contains a list of parcels that account for all non-redundant significant connectivity differences between aMCI and CN. For example, the first-ranked seed (superior medial frontal cortex) was associated with 13.4% of connections that differ between the groups. The second-ranked seed (dorsomedial prefrontal cortex) was associated with an additional 12.7% of connectivity differences that did not overlap with or were not previously accounted for by the first seed. Note that if a given parcel was associated with a significant effect with another region that ranked in the table, then that parcel may not be listed in the table (i.e., this table is not a comprehensive list of parcels that show significant effects, as a given parcel may involve a region in the table at a higher rank which already accounted for its effects). Given that the top four clusters explained nearly half of the findings, they were further characterized in seed-based connectivity analyses, which revealed that aMCI showed decreased connectivity between DMN nodes and between areas of the cortico-striatal-thalamic loop (**Figure 4**). More specifically, in aMCI compared to CN, the superior medial frontal cortex displayed significantly reduced connectivity with

[8]http://dx.doi.org/10.6084/m9.figshare.1480461.

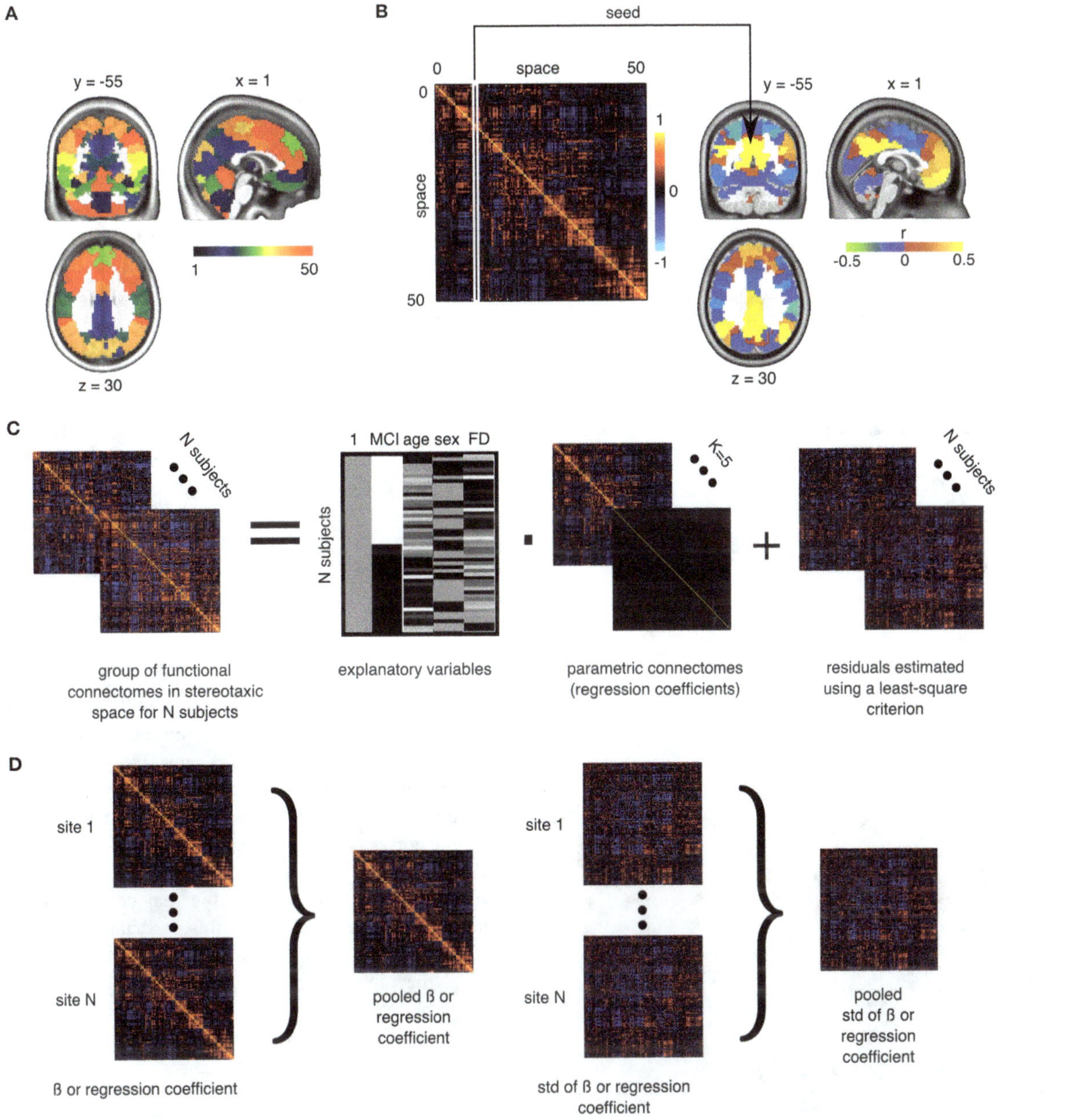

FIGURE 1 | Application of general linear models to connectomes. (A) The brain is functionally parcellated into K (e.g., 50) clusters generated through a clustering algorithm. **(B)** The connectome is a $K \times K$ matrix measuring functional connectivity between and within clusters. **(C)** A general linear model is used to test the association between phenotypes and connectomes, independently at each connection, at the group level. **(D)** In a multisite situation, independent site-specific effects are estimated and then pooled through weighted averaging (Willer et al., 2010).

the ventromedial prefrontal cortex, striatum, thalamus, temporal lobes, hippocampus, inferior parietal lobes, and precuneus (**Figure 4A**). aMCI showed reduced connectivity between the dorsomedial prefrontal cortex with temporal lobe regions, ventral frontal areas, thalamus, striatum, and the cuneus (**Figure 4B**). The striatum in aMCI also exhibited decreased connectivity with the sensorimotor cortex, thalamus, and frontal and parietal regions (**Figure 4C**). Lastly, in aMCI, the middle temporal lobe displayed significantly decreased connectivity with the posterior cingulate, precuneus, inferior parietal lobes, hippocampus, and frontal areas (**Figure 4D**).

Sample-Specific Effects

The statistical model we used to combine GLM analyses across sites was based on a weighted average. The possibility thus existed that an effect would be significant in the pooled analysis because it was driven by a very strong effect in a single sample, instead of being consistent across all samples. When we examined

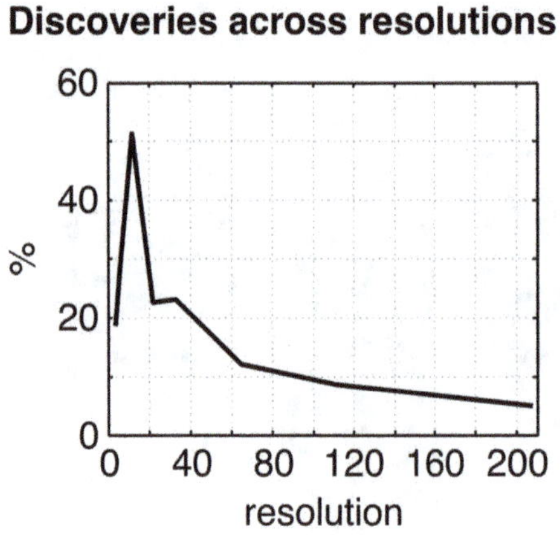

FIGURE 2 | Plot of the percentage of connections identified as significant by the statistical comparison between aMCI and CN across the connectome ($q^{FDR} \leq 0.1$), as a function of the resolutions selected by MSTEPS.

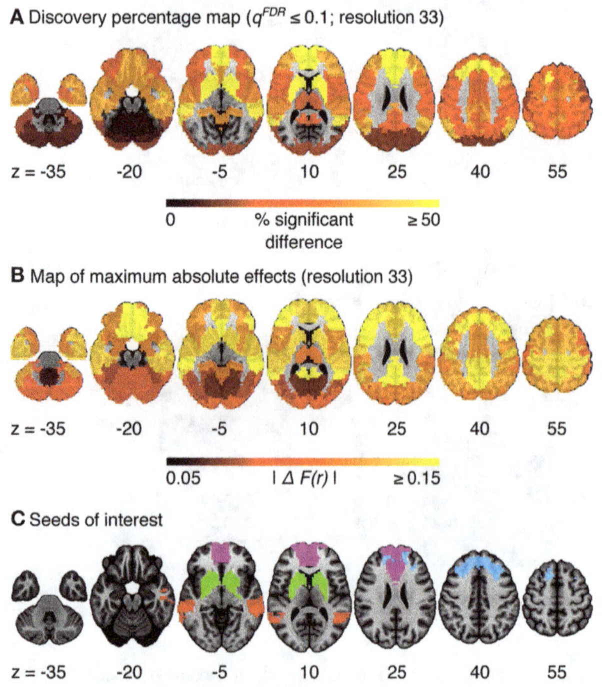

FIGURE 3 | (A) Map of the percentage of connections associated with a given cluster and identified as significant by the statistical comparison between aMCI and CN, at a resolution of 33 clusters ($q^{FDR} \leq 0.1$). **(B)** Maximum absolute difference in average connectivity between aMCI and CN, across all connections associated with a cluster, at resolution 33. ΔF(r) signifies the difference in Fisher-transformed correlation values between the groups. **(C)** Four clusters of interest (superior medial frontal cortex, dorsomedial prefrontal cortex, striatum, middle temporal lobe) were selected out of 33 for further characterization.

effects in each sample independently, we detected no findings or very few significant findings. We then explored the whole brain connectivity of the top four seed regions (superior medial frontal cortex, dorsomedial prefrontal cortex, striatum, and middle temporal lobe) within each sample. The majority of effects found at each sample did not appear to be consistent or reproducible across studies as the comparison between aMCI and CN varied substantially among the seven samples (**Figure 5**, Supplementary Figures 3–5). We assessed the extent at which findings among the seven samples were similar by calculating correlation coefficients across the spatial maps for the average connectivity values in CN, the average connectivity values in aMCI, and differences in connectivity values between aMCI and CN among the samples. We found that the difference maps, contrasting aMCI and CN, were weakly correlated on average across studies and protocols (mean $r = 0.06$, min $r = -0.64$, max $r = 0.69$). The average connectivity maps among studies in both CN and aMCI were generally highly correlated with each other (for CN, mean $r = 0.68$, min $r = -0.16$, max $r = 0.95$; for aMCI, mean $r = 0.67$, min $r = -0.10$, max $r = 0.97$). These results were expected given the small sample sizes of most independent samples (Kelly et al., 2012), but still sobering as the majority of the literature on aMCI and fMRI has used small sample sizes.

However, despite the large observed variations in the spatial distribution of aMCI vs. CN contrasts, there were still clear consistent trends across studies and protocols. We indeed found that aMCI-related connectivity changes that surpassed the FDR threshold in the pooled analysis showed similar trends in the vast majority of samples across seeds and connections, where the independent aMCI samples consistently exhibited decreased connectivity compared to the CN samples (**Figures 5**, **6**, Supplementary Figures 3–5). For example, the pooled analysis revealed that, compared to CN, aMCI exhibited significantly reduced connectivity between the superior medial frontal cortex cortex (the region in which connectivity was most affected by aMCI) and the middle temporal lobes. This change appeared to be common to the majority of the independent samples (**Figures 5**, **6A**). For this particular seed, the change in connectivity was mainly due to regions with positive correlations in CN having smaller correlation values closer to zero in aMCI in the individual samples (**Figures 5**, **6A**). For sample-specific effects in other seeds and connections, please see Supplementary Figures 3–9.

Effect Sizes and Sample Size Estimates

We measured the effect sizes of the difference between groups at each significant connection by calculating Cohen's *d*, via a weighted average of the effect sizes per individual sample. We found small to medium effect sizes, ranging from $d = 0.10$–0.48, with an average effect size of $d = 0.32$. Note that these effect sizes are potentially inflated since we have focussed on significant results only. We also calculated the sample sizes required to achieve 80% power, based on the effect sizes estimated by Cohen's *d*, the assumption of balanced groups, Gaussian distributions, bilateral tests, and $\alpha = 0.05$, for each connection. We found that the estimated sample sizes ranged from 140 to upwards of 600 total subjects, which further suggests that findings from small samples, similar to the seven samples we included when assessed independently, are not expected to be reliable. As noted above, as we used the same sample to estimate the location of effects and

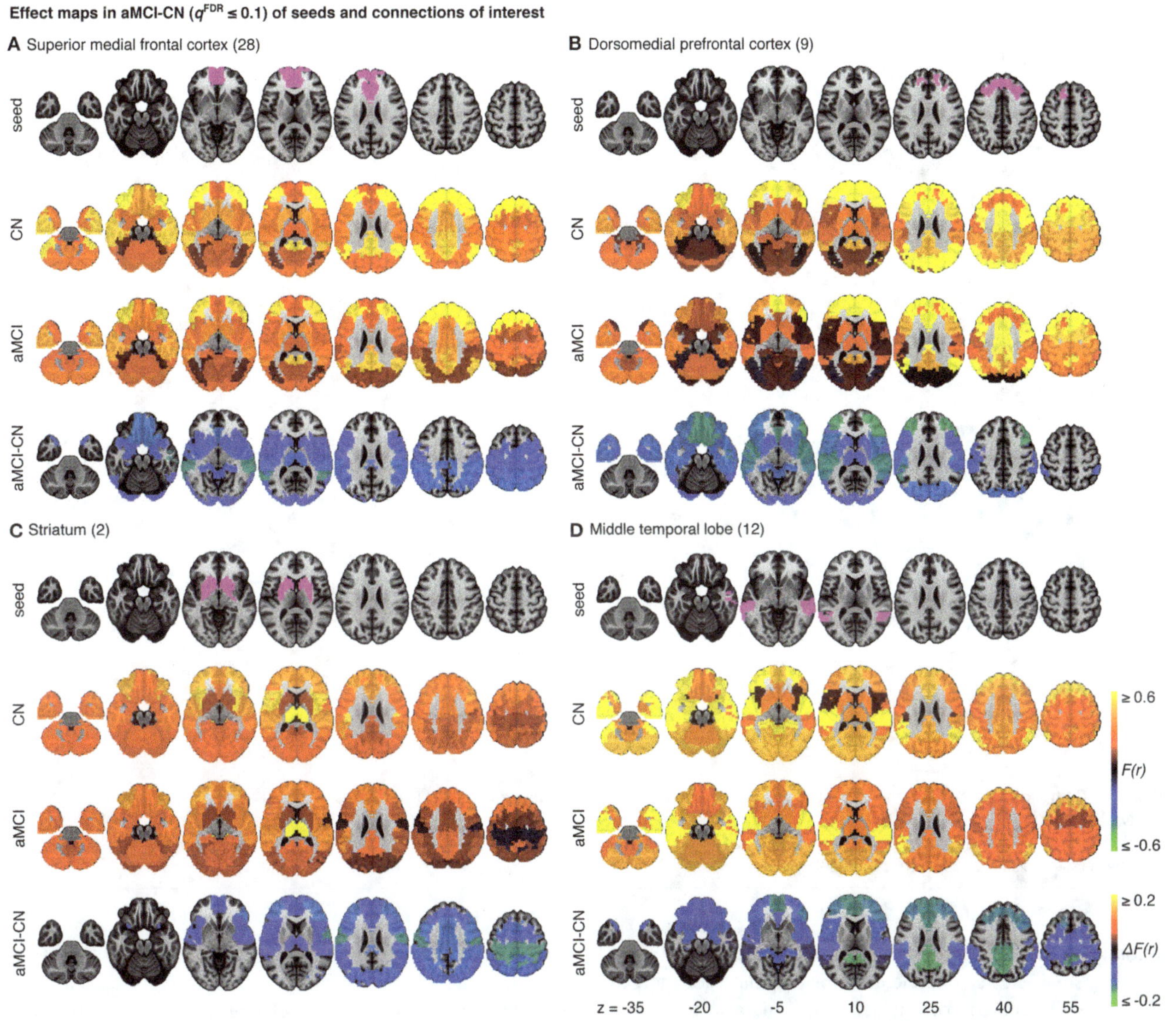

FIGURE 4 | Effect maps for a selection of four seeds that show effects related to aMCI at resolution 33. Effect maps reveal the spatial distribution of the changes in functional connectivity for **(A)** the superior medial frontal cortex, **(B)** the dorsomedial prefrontal cortex, **(C)** striatum, and **(D)** the middle temporal lobe. All connections shown in the maps of difference in average connectivity between aMCI and CN are significant at $q^{FDR} \leq 0.1$. For each panel, the top line maps the spatial location of the seed region in magenta, the second and third lines show the connectivity (Fisher-transformed correlation values, $F(r)$) between the designated seed region and the rest of the brain in CN and aMCI, respectively, and the fourth line shows a difference map between aMCI and CN [difference in Fisher-transformed correlation values, $\Delta F(r)$]. The numbers in parentheses refer to the numerical IDs of the clusters in the 3D parcellation volume, as listed in Supplementary Table 2.

their size, these sample size estimates are possibly optimistic, i.e., deflated compared to a replication on an independent sample. See **Figure 6** and Supplementary Figures 6–9 for Cohen's *d* and sample size estimates for each significant connection that was reported in **Figure 4**.

Effect of Resolution on the GLM

The percentage of discoveries in significant differences between aMCI and CN across the connectomes varied markedly as a function of resolution, as selected by the MSTEPS procedure. Higher resolutions were associated with fewer discoveries, especially beyond resolution 65 (Supplementary Figure 10A). By contrast, the maximal amplitude of differences in average connectivity associated with a particular cluster did not decrease substantially, and sometimes increased, when the resolution increased (Supplementary Figure 10B). The decrease in percentage of discovery thus likely reflected a cost associated with an increased number of multiple comparisons in the FDR procedure, rather than a loss in signal quality. Regarding the clusters that were selected for our seed-based analyses (the superior medial frontal cortex, dorsomedial prefrontal cortex, striatum, and middle temporal lobe), the associated effect maps (without statistical threshold) were highly consistent across different resolutions (Supplementary Figures 11, 12), with the

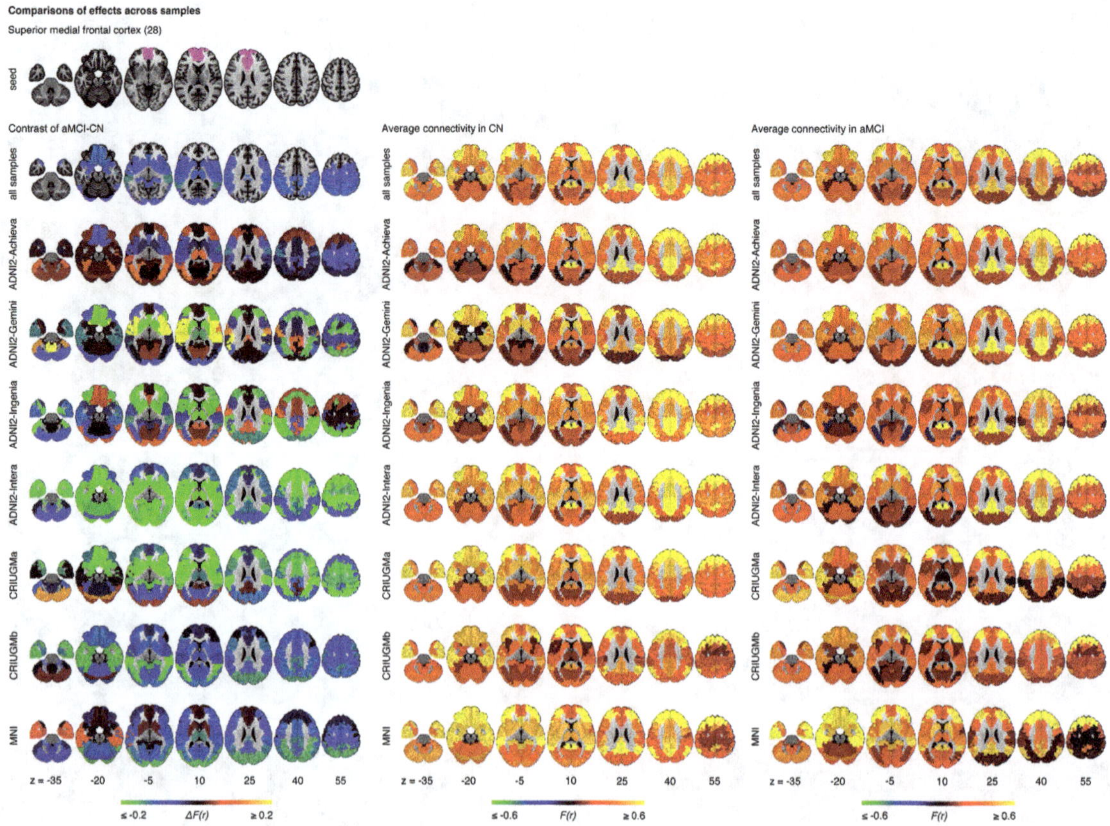

FIGURE 5 | Comparisons of effects in the superior medial frontal cortex across samples. This figure illustrates functional connectivity changes between aMCI and CN, average connectivity in CN, and average connectivity in aMCI in each site (ADNI2-Achieva, ADNI2-Gemini, ADNI2-Ingenia, ADNI2-Intera, CRIUGMa, CRIUGMb, MNI) independently of other sites and when samples are pooled together (all samples). The number in parentheses refers to the numerical ID of the seed in the 3D parcellation volume, as listed in Supplementary Table 2.

potential exception of very low resolutions where, for example, a relatively small cluster like the anterior cingulate got merged with a large distributed cortical network. This also replicated a prior study on the effect of multiresolution parcellations on GLM analysis (Bellec et al., 2015). Lastly, signal-to-noise ratio did not have a significant impact on the results (Supplementary Figure 13).

DISCUSSION

We report resting-state functional connectivity differences in the superior medial frontal cortex, dorsomedial prefrontal cortex, striatum, and middle temporal lobe between aMCI and CN subjects when multiple studies were combined together. Despite protocol differences, we found that aMCI exhibited reduced connectivity within areas of the DMN and cortico-striatal-thalamic loop compared to CN. Previous studies suggested these altered patterns of functional connectivity in MCI may result from the coevolution of multiple AD-associated biological processes, namely structural degeneration (Pievani et al., 2010; Coupé et al., 2012), neurofibrillary and amyloid pathologies (Small et al., 2006), and cerebrovascular dysfunction (Villeneuve and Jagust, 2015).

The superior medial frontal cortex and middle temporal lobes, both of which are DMN nodes, were among the seed regions with the greatest amount of aMCI-related connectivity changes with other brain areas. Decreased connectivity in aMCI patients was found between these two nodes and other DMN regions, including the posterior cingulate, precuneus, inferior parietal lobes, ventromedial prefrontal cortex, and hippocampus. Our findings support previous studies that used small single-site samples and reported reduced DMN connectivity in MCI and AD patients (Sorg et al., 2007; Bai et al., 2009; Agosta et al., 2012; Koch et al., 2012). Alterations in the DMN may reflect increased amyloid burden in aMCI patients as it has been shown that amyloid plaques impair default mode connectivity (Hedden et al., 2009; Sheline et al., 2010b; Mormino et al., 2011).

We found reduced connectivity within the frontal lobes, notably between ventral and dorsal areas. Decreased functional connectivity between the ventral and dorsal frontal regions could reflect degeneration in gray matter and in white matter tracts connecting these areas. Longitudinal studies have shown greater prefrontal cortex atrophy in MCI over time, as well as in those transitioning to AD, compared to CN (McDonald et al., 2009; Carmichael et al., 2013). Cortico-cortical white matter bundles, e.g., superior longitudinal fasciculus, have also

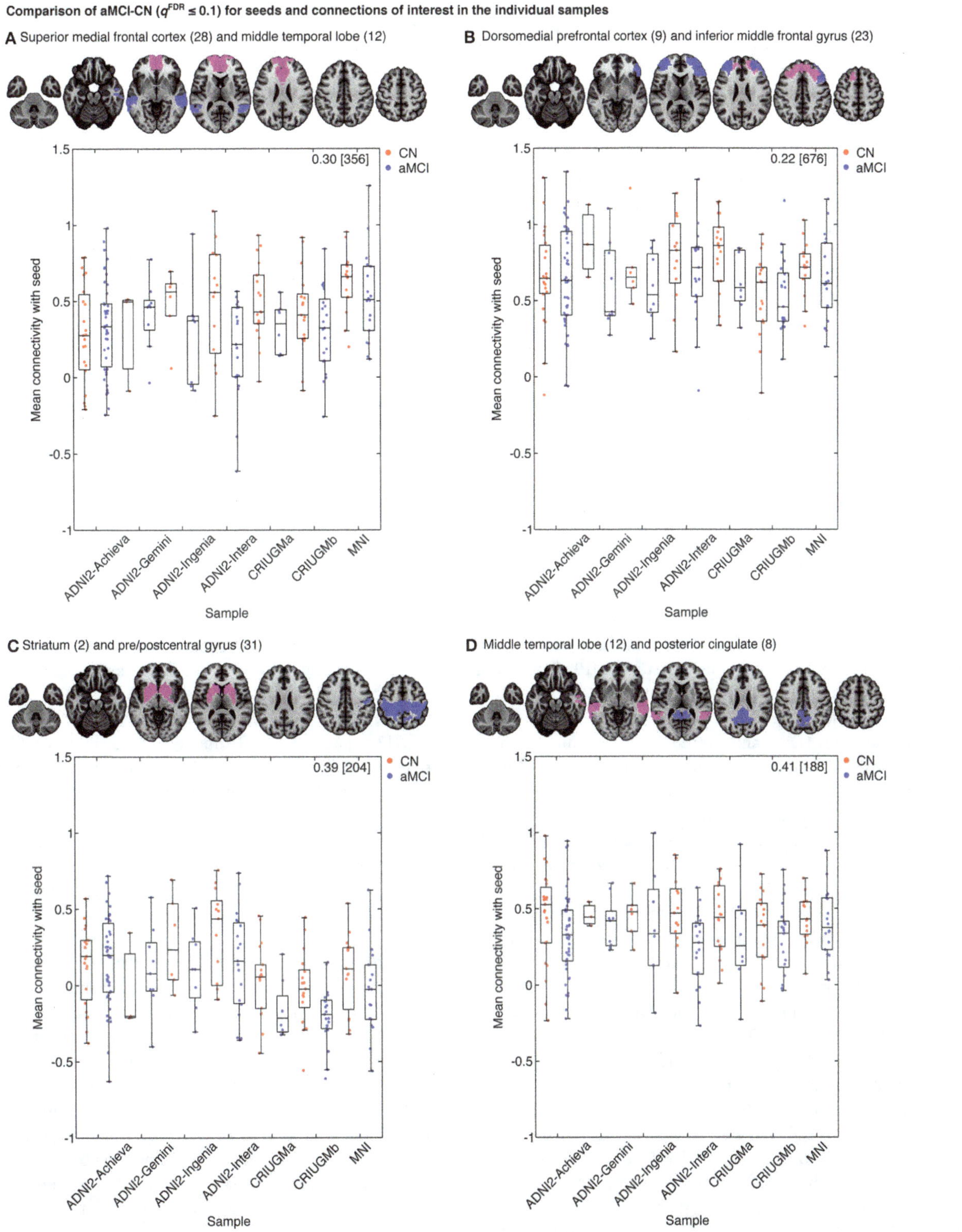

FIGURE 6 | Mean connectivity between (A) the superior medial frontal cortex and middle temporal lobe, (B) the dorsomedial prefrontal cortex and middle frontal gyrus, (C) the striatum and pre/postcentral gyrus, and (D) middle temporal lobe and posterior cingulate in CN and aMCI in the independent samples. Each map displays the seed (pink) and a selected cluster (blue) whose connectivity with the seed significantly differed between CN and aMCI in the pooled analysis. The box-whisker plots display the mean connectivity (Fisher-transformed correlation values) between the seed and the selected parcel, overlaid

(Continued)

FIGURE 6 | Continued
over individual data points, in the CN and MCI groups in the ADNI2-Achieva, ADNI2-Gemini, ADNI2-Ingenia, ADNI2-Intera, CRIUGMa, CRIUGMb, and MNI samples. We also report the Cohen's *d* (a weighted average of the effect sizes per sample) followed by a sample size estimate (for 80% power, balanced groups, bilateral tests, Gaussian distributions, and $\alpha = 0.05$) in square brackets in the top-right corner of each plot. The numbers in parentheses in the titles refer to the numerical IDs of the seeds in the 3D parcellation volume, as listed in Supplementary Table 2. For box-whisker plots for all significant clusters with each of these seeds, see Supplementary Figures 6–9.

been demonstrated to degenerate in patients with MCI and AD (Pievani et al., 2010). Additionally, functional connectivity changes may reflect the regional effect of increased amyloid burden (Sheline et al., 2010b), and PIB-PET work has shown the frontal lobe to be one of the first regions in which amyloid accumulates in autosomal dominant AD mutation carriers (Bateman et al., 2012). Our results may also be due to neurofibrillary pathology as it typically appears in the prefrontal cortex during MCI (Bossers et al., 2010). Lastly, cerebral hypoperfusion in the frontal lobe of MCI (Chao et al., 2009) may have contributed to our results.

We also observed functional disconnection between the temporal and frontal lobes in aMCI. Effects in the temporal lobes were expected given that the temporal lobe is a region known to suffer from significant AD pathology in preclinical phases (Guillozet et al., 2003). Structural connectivity may also explain the functional connectivity changes between the frontal and temporal regions, since degeneration of white matter tracts between these areas, e.g., the uncinate fasciculus, occurs with the progression from MCI to AD and correlates with episodic memory impairment in MCI (Pievani et al., 2010; Rémy et al., 2015). Furthermore, examining the integrity of the arcuate fasciculus, a major language tract that connects the frontal and temporal lobes (Dick and Tremblay, 2012), might reveal a biological basis for language impairments such as word-finding difficulties in MCI and AD, (Nutter-Upham et al., 2008). Brain areas that subserve language function could be important targets to investigate given recent evidence that multilingualism, like other forms of cognitive reserve, may help delay the onset of AD (Chertkow et al., 2010).

Unexpectedly, we also found significant effects in the striatum, which showed reduced connectivity in aMCI with the sensorimotor cortex, frontal and parietal regions, and thalamus. While not initially expected, these findings may reflect earlier observations that regions within the cortico-striatal-thalamic loops are vulnerable to AD pathology. For example, previous work demonstrated the presence of substantial amyloid burden in the striatum in both autosomal dominant and sporadic forms of AD (Braak and Braak, 1990; Villemagne et al., 2009), and the striatum may be the first region in which amyloid deposition occurs in autosomal dominant AD (Klunk et al., 2007; Bateman et al., 2012). Furthermore, significant neurodegeneration is known to occur with AD in the striatum and thalamus (de Jong et al., 2008; Madsen et al., 2010), so our results might reflect the brain's capacity for functional plasticity in response to amyloid or neurodegeneration in these regions. Motor cortex hyperexcitability has also been shown in AD, and this suggests that inhibitory circuits leading to the motor cortex may be affected in the disease (Ferreri et al., 2011). Patients with AD also demonstrate changes in swallowing which have been associated with altered cortical activity (Humbert et al., 2010). Our results may support these observations. Additionally, our findings may represent a biological basis for the cognitive and motor symptoms of MCI (Aggarwal et al., 2006) since the striatum and the rest of the basal ganglia have been implicated in stimulus-response associative learning and memory and motor skill acquisition and execution (Packard and Knowlton, 2002; Doyon et al., 2009). Future research should examine the potential relationship between connectivity in the cortico-striatal-thalamic loops and motor function in aMCI and AD.

Our findings contrasted with previous, smaller single-site studies that have variously reported decreased and increased connectivity. The reports of increased connectivity (Bai et al., 2009; Qi et al., 2010; Gour et al., 2011) may have reflected unique attributes of particular protocols or the choices made with respect to pre-processing steps, for example using global signal regression (Saad et al., 2012). Given that our sample size estimates suggest the use of hundreds of subjects to obtain adequate statistical power, it is not surprising that discrepancies between our results and previous findings generated from smaller, likely underpowered, studies exist. Even when we examined the samples in our study (ADNI2-Achieva, ADNI2-Gemini, ADNI2-Ingenia, ADNI2-Intera, CRIUGMa, CRIUGMb, MNI) independently of each other, we found inconsistent effects among the samples. It is only by combining the studies together in a meta-analysis that we were able to find some common differences in functional connectomes between patients with aMCI and CN. This finding underscores the need for multisite studies with large sample sizes in order to generate reproducible results, as previously suggested in the field of autism research (Haar et al., 2014).

Among our study's limitations is that it was not possible to model each of the 13 ADNI2 sites independently because the sites tended to be small and unbalanced in the numbers of patients and controls. We therefore chose to model each scanner model within ADNI2 separately based on the recommendation of a reviewer. A previous version of the analysis (published as a preprint[9]) had not modeled the different scanner models in ADNI2 and instead treated ADNI2 as a single site. This previous analysis yielded fewer significant findings, but the results were still mostly consistent with what is reported here. Our results suggest that modeling scanner models may have a positive impact on fMRI association studies, but further experiments would be required to confirm that this trend is reproducible. We must also note that the METAL averaging is only representative of the specific samples that were averaged, especially using only

[9]http://dx.doi.org/10.1101/019646.

Philips and Siemens scanners, and it is unclear how our findings may replicate in other studies that would employ a different combination of protocols, say using GE scanners. In particular, our sample size estimates have to be interpreted with caution. They may first be under-estimated, because they were not derived from pre-specified locations, but rather associated with the connections showing the largest effects in our particular sample. These sample sizes were also derived from a meta-analysis combining particular types of studies. We only had 3T scanners from two manufacturers, Siemens and Philips. For the Siemens studies, all were from the same model. For the Philips studies, the scanning protocol was identical at every site, and only the scanner model varied across scanners. Finally, a fairly large number of patients and controls (generally more than 10 subjects per group) was scanned for each variant of the scanning protocol. The sample size estimate may turn out quite differently for a single site study or on the contrary for a study with a very large number of sites and with only a few subjects per site.

Our study is also limited by its cross-sectional nature, which precludes inference that the functional changes we found would necessarily predict progression toward Alzheimer's dementia. Furthermore, aMCI has many underlying causes aside from AD. It is possible that some subjects in our cohort had cognitive impairments due to Lewy Body dementia, for example. However, all samples in the current study had inclusion criteria that enriched for subjects that had aMCI likely due to AD and excluded aMCI subjects with other co-morbidities, such as depression or Parkinson's disease. Also, we did not account for structural atrophy, despite a bias for increased detection in functional differences due to differences in underlying structure (Dukart and Bertolino, 2014). However, aMCI-related gray matter changes likely co-localize to some extent with functional changes, and the aim of our work was to map out functional changes rather than study their interaction with atrophy. We did not account for other variables, such as APOE genotype (Sheline et al., 2010a), amyloid deposition (Sheline et al., 2010b), presence of neurofibrillary tangles (Maruyama et al., 2013), and cerebrovascular mechanisms (Villeneuve and Jagust, 2015). At least some of these could potentially have explained the observed aMCI-related functional connectivity changes as part of an underlying disease mechanism. Large-scale multimodal studies, incorporating genomics, proteomics, and multimodal imaging will be needed to identify the interactions between these and other physiological facets of the pathology. Despite combining several samples together, we still only achieved relatively limited power, given that sample size estimates required at least 140 to over 600 total subjects to consistently identify effects between groups. Lastly, because of the explorative approach used in our study, the resulting estimates of effect sizes may have been inflated and discussion of possible pathological mechanisms for our findings was speculative. However, our discoveries may be used as follow-up targets in future work. Upcoming research should not only attempt to verify our findings by using these regions and their associated connections with hypothesis-driven approaches (e.g., seed-based correlation analyses), but also to extend them to cohorts that include Alzheimer's dementia and other clinical populations (e.g., CN with significant amyloid deposition) and to longitudinal studies that characterize individuals' progression to dementia. Finally, future studies should aim to determine whether our findings are associated with established biomarkers of AD (e.g., amyloid and tau quantification) in order to probe the potential of these functional connections as biomarkers.

Overall, our results supported previous findings of DMN connectivity changes in AD and MCI (Greicius et al., 2004; Sorg et al., 2007), given that three of the identified seeds (superior medial frontal cortex, dorsomedial prefrontal cortex, middle temporal lobe) are part of this network. It is noteworthy, however, that our strongest observed effects reported here were not in the same DMN regions typically described in earlier resting-state studies of MCI and AD, viz, posterior cingulate/precuneus (Sheline et al., 2010b; Zhang et al., 2010). Unexpected changes were also found in the striatum, and this may reflect the advantages of "mining" the whole-brain connectome to search for new biomarkers of mild cognitive impairment and possibly the early progression of the pathophysiologic substrate of Alzheimer's disease. If confirmed, our results could suggest the utility of these regions in resting-state fMRI as a biomarker endpoint in clinical trials.

ACKNOWLEDGMENTS

We thank Sven Joubert, Isabelle Rouleau, and Sophie Benoit for their contribution in collection of the CRIUGMa dataset. We thank Tom Nichols for his comments and suggestions. Collection of the CRIUGMb dataset was supported by the Alzheimer's Society of Canada. Collection of the MNI dataset was supported by Industry Canada/Montreal Neurological Institute Centre of excellence in commercialization and research. This work was supported by CIHR (133359) and NSERC (436141-2013). Data collection and sharing for this project was funded by the Alzheimer's Disease Neuroimaging Initiative (ADNI; National Institutes of Health Grant U01 AG024904) and DOD ADNI (Department of Defense award number W81XWH-12-2-0012). ADNI is funded by the National Institute on Aging, the National Institute of Biomedical Imaging and Bioengineering, and through generous contributions from the following: Alzheimer's Association; Alzheimer's Drug Discovery Foundation; Araclon Biotech; BioClinica, Inc.; Biogen Idec Inc.; Bristol-Myers Squibb Company; Eisai Inc.; Elan Pharmaceuticals, Inc.; Eli Lilly and Company; EuroImmun; F. Hoffmann-La Roche Ltd., and its affiliated company Genentech, Inc.; Fujirebio; GE Healthcare; IXICO Ltd.; Janssen Alzheimer Immunotherapy Research & Development, LLC.; Johnson & Johnson Pharmaceutical Research & Development LLC.; Medpace, Inc.; Merck & Co., Inc.; Meso Scale Diagnostics, LLC.; NeuroRx Research; Neurotrack Technologies; Novartis Pharmaceuticals Corporation; Pfizer Inc.; Piramal Imaging; Servier; Synarc Inc.; and Takeda Pharmaceutical Company. The Canadian Institutes of Health Research is providing funds to support ADNI clinical sites in Canada. Private sector contributions are facilitated by the Foundation for the National Institutes of Health (www.fnih.org). The grantee organization is the Northern California Institute for Research and Education, and the study is coordinated by the Alzheimer's Disease Cooperative Study at the University of California, San Diego. ADNI data are disseminated by the Laboratory for Neuro Imaging at the University of Southern California.

REFERENCES

Ad-Dab'bagh, Y., Einarson, D., Lyttelton, O., Muehlboeck, J. S., Mok, K., Ivanov, O., et al. (2006). "The CIVET image-processing environment: a fully automated comprehensive pipeline for anatomical neuroimaging research," in *Proceedings of the 12th Annual Meeting of the Organization for Human Brain Mapping* (Florence), 2266.

Aggarwal, N. T., Wilson, R. S., Beck, T. L., Bienias, J. L., and Bennett, D. A. (2006). Motor dysfunction in mild cognitive impairment and the risk of incident Alzheimer disease. *Arch. Neurol.* 63, 1763–1769. doi: 10.1001/archneur.63.12.1763

Agosta, F., Pievani, M., Geroldi, C., Copetti, M., Frisoni, G. B., and Filippi, M. (2012). Resting state fMRI in Alzheimer's disease: beyond the default mode network. *Neurobiol. Aging* 33, 1564–1578. doi: 10.1016/j.neurobiolaging.2011.06.007

Albert, M. S., DeKosky, S. T., Dickson, D., Dubois, B., Feldman, H. H., Fox, N. C., et al. (2011). The diagnosis of mild cognitive impairment due to Alzheimer's disease: recommendations from the National Institute on Aging-Alzheimer's Association workgroups on diagnostic guidelines for Alzheimer's disease. *Alzheimers. Dement.* 7, 270–279. doi: 10.1016/j.jalz.2011.03.008

Bai, F., Watson, D. R., Yu, H., Shi, Y., Yuan, Y., and Zhang, Z. (2009). Abnormal resting-state functional connectivity of posterior cingulate cortex in amnestic type mild cognitive impairment. *Brain Res.* 1302, 167–174. doi: 10.1016/j.brainres.2009.09.028

Bateman, R. J., Xiong, C., Benzinger, T. L. S., Fagan, A., Goate, A., Fox, N. C., et al. (2012). Clinical and biomarker changes in dominantly inherited Alzheimer's disease. *N. Engl. J. Med.* 367, 795–804. doi: 10.1056/NEJMoa1202753

Bellec, P. (2013). "Mining the hierarchy of resting-state brain networks: selection of representative clusters in a multiscale structure," in International Workshop on *Pattern Recognition in Neuroimaging* (Philadelphia, PA), 54–57. doi: 10.1109/prni.2013.23

Bellec, P., Benhajali, Y., Carbonell, F., Dansereau, C., Albouy, G., Pelland, M., et al. (2015). Impact of the resolution of brain parcels on connectome-wide association studies in fMRI. *NeuroImage* 123, 212–228. doi: 10.1016/j.neuroimage.2015.07.071

Bellec, P., Carbonell, F. M., Perlbarg, V., Lepage, C., Lyttelton, O., Fonov, V., et al. (2011). "A neuroimaging analysis kit for Matlab and Octave," in *Proceedings of the 17th International Conference on Functional Mapping of the Human Brain.* (Québec City, QC).

Bellec, P., Lavoie-Courchesne, S., Dickinson, P., Lerch, J. P., Zijdenbos, A. P., and Evans, A. (2012). The pipeline system for Octave and Matlab (PSOM): a lightweight scripting framework and execution engine for scientific workflows. *Front. Neuroinform.* 6:7. doi: 10.3389/fninf.2012.00007

Bellec, P., Perlbarg, V., Jbabdi, S., Pélégrini-Issac, M., Anton, J.-L., Doyon, J., et al. (2006). Identification of large-scale networks in the brain using fMRI. *Neuroimage* 29, 1231–1243. doi: 10.1016/j.neuroimage.2005.08.044

Benjamini, Y., and Hochberg, Y. (1995). Controlling the false discovery rate: a practical and powerful approach to multiple testing. *J. R. Stat. Soc. B* 57, 289–300. doi: 10.2307/2346101

Bossers, K., Wirz, K. T. S., Meerhoff, G. F., Essing, A. H. W., van Dongen, J. W., Houba, P., et al. (2010). Concerted changes in transcripts in the prefrontal cortex precede neuropathology in Alzheimer's disease. *Brain* 133, 3699–3723. doi: 10.1093/brain/awq258

Braak, H., and Braak, E. (1990). Alzheimer's disease: striatal amyloid deposits and neurofibrillary changes. *J. Neuropathol. Exp. Neurol.* 49, 215. doi: 10.1097/00005072-199005000-00003

Carmichael, O., McLaren, D. G., Tommet, D., Mungas, D., Jones, R. N., for the Alzheimer's Disease Neuroimaging Initiative (2013). Coevolution of brain structures in amnestic mild cognitive impairment. *NeuroImage* 66, 449–456. doi: 10.1016/j.neuroimage.2012.10.029

Chao, L. L., Pa, J., Duarte, A., Schuff, N., Weiner, M. W., Kramer, J. H., et al. (2009). Patterns of cerebral hypoperfusion in amnestic and dysexecutive MCI. Alzheimer Dis. Assoc. Disord. 23, 245–252. doi: 10.1097/WAD.0b013e318199ff46

Chertkow, H., Whitehead, V., Phillips, N., Wolfson, C., Atherton, J., and Bergman, H. (2010). Multilingualism (but not always bilingualism) delays the onset of alzheimer disease: evidence from a bilingual community. Alzheimer Dis. Assoc. Disord. 24, 118–125. doi: 10.1097/WAD.0b013e3181ca1221

Collins, D. L., and Evans, A. C. (1997). Animal: validation and applications of nonlinear registration-based segmentation. *Int. J. Patt. Recogn. Artif. Intell.* 11, 1271–1294. doi: 10.1142/S0218001497000597

Coupé, P., Eskildsen, S. F., Manjón, J. V., Fonov, V. S., Collins, D. L., for the Alzheimer's Disease Neuroimaging Initiative (2012). Simultaneous segmentation and grading of anatomical structures for patient"s classification: application to Alzheimer"s disease. *NeuroImage* 59, 3736–3747. doi: 10.1016/j.neuroimage.2011.10.080

de Jong, L. W., van der Hiele, K., Veer, I. M., Houwing, J. J., Westendorp, R. G. J., Bollen, E. L. E. M., et al. (2008). Strongly reduced volumes of putamen and thalamus in Alzheimer's disease: an MRI study. *Brain* 131, 3277–3285. doi: 10.1093/brain/awn278

Dick, A. S., and Tremblay, P. (2012). Beyond the arcuate fasciculus: consensus and controversy in the connectional anatomy of language. *Brain* 135, 3529–3550. doi: 10.1093/brain/aws222

Doyon, J., Bellec, P., Amsel, R., Penhune, V., Monchi, O., Carrier, J., et al. (2009). Contributions of the basal ganglia and functionally related brain structures to motor learning. *Behav. Brain Res.* 199, 61–75. doi: 10.1016/j.bbr.2008.11.012

Dukart, J., and Bertolino, A. (2014). When structure affects function – the need for partial volume effect correction in functional and resting state magnetic resonance imaging studies. *PLoS ONE* 9:e114227. doi: 10.1371/journal.pone.0114227

Edward, V., Windischberger, C., Cunnington, R., Erdler, M., Lanzenberger, R., Mayer, D., et al. (2000). Quantification of fMRI artifact reduction by a novel plaster cast head holder. *Hum. Brain Mapp.* 11, 207–213. doi: 10.1002/1097-0193(200011)11:3<207::AID-HBM60>3.0.CO;2-J

Elliott, M. R., Bowtell, R. W., and Morris, P. G. (1999). The effect of scanner sound in visual, motor, and auditory functional MRI. *Magn. Reson. Med.* 41, 1230–1235.

Ferreri, F., Pasqualetti, P., Määttä, S., Ponzo, D., Guerra, A., Bressi, F., et al. (2011). Motor cortex excitability in Alzheimer's disease: a transcranial magnetic stimulation follow-up study. *Neurosci. Lett.* 492, 94–98. doi: 10.1016/j.neulet.2011.01.064

Fonov, V., Evans, A., Botteron, K., Almli, C. R., McKinstry, R. C., and Collins, D. L. (2011). Unbiased average age-appropriate atlases for pediatric studies. *NeuroImage* 54, 313–327. doi: 10.1016/j.neuroimage.2010.07.033

Friedman, L., and Glover, G. H. (2006). Report on a multicenter fMRI quality assurance protocol. *J. Magn. Reson. Imaging* 23, 827–839. doi: 10.1002/jmri.20583

Friedman, L., Glover, G. H., and Fbirn Consortium (2006). Reducing interscanner variability of activation in a multicenter fMRI study: controlling for signal-to-fluctuation-noise-ratio (SFNR) differences. *NeuroImage* 33, 471–481. doi: 10.1016/j.neuroimage.2006.07.012

Giove, F., Gili, T., Iacovella, V., Macaluso, E., and Maraviglia, B. (2009). Images-based suppression of unwanted global signals in resting-state functional connectivity studies. *Magn. Reson. Imaging* 27, 1058–1064. doi: 10.1016/j.mri.2009.06.004

Gour, N., Ranjeva, J.-P., Ceccaldi, M., Confort-Gouny, S., Barbeau, E., Soulier, E., et al. (2011). Basal functional connectivity within the anterior temporal network is associated with performance on declarative memory tasks. *NeuroImage* 58, 687–697. doi: 10.1016/j.neuroimage.2011.05.090

Greicius, M. D., Srivastava, G., Reiss, A. L., and Menon, V. (2004). Default-mode network activity distinguishes Alzheimer's disease from healthy aging:

evidence from functional MRI. *Proc. Natl. Acad. Sci. U.S.A.* 101, 4637–4642. doi: 10.1073/pnas.0308627101

Guillozet, A. L., Weintraub, S., Mash, D. C., and Mesulam, M. M. (2003). Neurofibrillary tangles, amyloid, and memory in aging and mild cognitive impairment. *Arch. Neurol.* 60, 729–736. doi: 10.1001/archneur.60.5.729

Haar, S., Berman, S., Behrmann, M., and Dinstein, I. (2014). Anatomical Abnormalities in Autism? *Cereb. Cortex.* doi: 10.1093/cercor/bhu242. [Epub ahead of print].

Hedden, T., van Dijk, K. R. A., Becker, J. A., Sperling, R. A., Johnson, K. A., and Buckner, R. L. (2009). Disruption of functional connectivity in clinically normal older adults harboring amyloid burden. *J. Neurosci.* 29, 12686–12694. doi: 10.1523/JNEUROSCI.3189-09.2009

Humbert, I. A., McLaren, D. G., Kosmatka, K., Fitzgerald, M., Johnson, S., Porcaro, E., et al. (2010). Early deficits in cortical control of swallowing in Alzheimer's disease. *J. Alzheimers Dis.* 19, 1185–1197. doi: 10.3233/JAD-2010-1316

Kelly, C., Biswal, B. B., Craddock, R. C., Castellanos, F. X., and Milham, M. P. (2012). Characterizing variation in the functional connectome: promise and pitfalls. *Trends Cogn. Sci.* 16, 181–188. doi: 10.1016/j.tics.2012.02.001

Klunk, W. E., Price, J. C., Mathis, C. A., Tsopelas, N. D., Lopresti, B. J., Ziolko, S. K., et al. (2007). Amyloid deposition begins in the striatum of presenilin-1 mutation carriers from two unrelated pedigrees. *J. Neurosci.* 27, 6174–6184. doi: 10.1523/JNEUROSCI.0730-07.2007

Koch, W., Teipel, S., Mueller, S., Benninghoff, J., Wagner, M., Bokde, A. L. W., et al. (2012). Diagnostic power of default mode network resting state fMRI in the detection of Alzheimer's disease. *Neurobiol. Aging* 33, 466–478. doi: 10.1016/j.neurobiolaging.2010.04.013

Liang, P., Wang, Z., Yang, Y., and Li, K. (2012). Three subsystems of the inferior parietal cortex are differently affected in mild cognitive impairment. *J. Alzheimers Dis.* 30, 475–487. doi: 10.3233/JAD-2012-111721

Lund, T. E., Madsen, K. H., Sidaros, K., Luo, W.-L., and Nichols, T. E. (2006). Non-white noise in fMRI: does modelling have an impact? *Neuroimage* 29, 54–66. doi: 10.1016/j.neuroimage.2005.07.005

Madsen, S. K., Ho, A. J., Hua, X., Saharan, P. S., Toga, A. W., Jack, C. R., et al. (2010). 3D maps localize caudate nucleus atrophy in 400 Alzheimer's disease, mild cognitive impairment, and healthy elderly subjects. *Neurobiol. Aging* 31, 1312–1325. doi: 10.1016/j.neurobiolaging.2010.05.002

Maruyama, M., Shimada, H., Suhara, T., Shinotoh, H., Ji, B., Maeda, J., et al. (2013). Imaging of tau pathology in a tauopathy mouse model and in alzheimer patients compared to normal controls. *Neuron* 79, 1094–1108. doi: 10.1016/j.neuron.2013.07.037

McDonald, C. R., McEvoy, L. K., Gharapetian, L., Fennema-Notestine, C., Hagler, D. J., Holland, D., et al. (2009). Regional rates of neocortical atrophy from normal aging to early Alzheimer disease. *Neurology* 73, 457–465. doi: 10.1212/WNL.0b013e3181b16431

Mormino, E. C., Smiljic, A., Hayenga, A. O., Onami, S. H., Greicius, M. D., Rabinovici, G. D., et al. (2011). Relationships between β-amyloid and functional connectivity in different components of the default mode network in aging. *Cereb. Cortex* 21, 2399–2407. doi: 10.1093/cercor/bhr025

Nutter-Upham, K. E., Saykin, A. J., Rabin, L. A., Roth, R. M., Wishart, H. A., Pare, N., et al. (2008). Verbal fluency performance in amnestic MCI and older adults with cognitive complaints. *Arch. Clin. Neuropsychol.* 23, 229–241. doi: 10.1016/j.acn.2008.01.005

Packard, M. G., and Knowlton, B. J. (2002). Learning and memory functions of the Basal Ganglia. *Annu. Rev. Neurosci.* 25, 563–593. doi: 10.1146/annurev.neuro.25.112701.142937

Petersen, R. C. (2004). Mild cognitive impairment as a diagnostic entity. *J. Intern. Med.* 256, 183–194. doi: 10.1111/j.1365-2796.2004.01388.x

Petersen, R. C., Doody, R., Kurz, A., Mohs, R. C., Morris, J. C., Rabins, P. V., et al. (2001). Current concepts in mild cognitive impairment. *Arch. Neurol.* 58, 1985–1992. doi: 10.1001/archneur.58.12.1985

Pievani, M., Agosta, F., Pagani, E., Canu, E., Sala, S., Absinta, M., et al. (2010). Assessment of white matter tract damage in mild cognitive impairment and Alzheimer's disease. *Hum. Brain Mapp.* 31, 1862–1875. doi: 10.1002/hbm.20978

Power, J. D., Barnes, K. A., Snyder, A. Z., Schlaggar, B. L., and Petersen, S. E. (2012). Spurious but systematic correlations in functional connectivity MRI networks arise from subject motion. *Neuroimage* 59, 2142–2154. doi: 10.1016/j.neuroimage.2011.10.018

Qi, Z., Wu, X., Wang, Z., Zhang, N., Dong, H., Yao, L., et al. (2010). Impairment and compensation coexist in amnestic MCI default mode network. *Neuroimage* 50, 48–55. doi: 10.1016/j.neuroimage.2009.12.025

Rémy, F., Vayssière, N., Saint-Aubert, L., Barbeau, E., and Pariente, J. (2015). White matter disruption at the prodromal stage of Alzheimer's disease: relationships with hippocampal atrophy and episodic memory performance. *Neuroimage Clin.* 7, 482–492. doi: 10.1016/j.nicl.2015.01.014

Saad, Z. S., Gotts, S. J., Murphy, K., Chen, G., Jo, H. J., Martin, A., et al. (2012). Trouble at rest: how correlation patterns and group differences become distorted after global signal regression. *Brain Connect.* 2, 25–32. doi: 10.1089/brain.2012.0080

Shehzad, Z., Kelly, C., Reiss, P. T., Cameron Craddock, R., Emerson, J. W., McMahon, K., et al. (2014). A multivariate distance-based analytic framework for connectome-wide association studies. *NeuroImage* 93(Pt 1), 74–94. doi: 10.1016/j.neuroimage.2014.02.024

Sheline, Y. I., Morris, J. C., Snyder, A. Z., Price, J. L., Yan, Z., D'Angelo, G., et al. (2010a). APOE4 allele disrupts resting state fMRI connectivity in the absence of amyloid plaques or decreased CSF A 42. *J. Neurosci.* 30, 17035–17040. doi: 10.1523/JNEUROSCI.3987-10.2010

Sheline, Y. I., Raichle, M. E., Snyder, A. Z., Morris, J. C., Head, D., Wang, S., et al. (2010b). Amyloid plaques disrupt resting state default mode network connectivity in cognitively normal elderly. *Biol. Psychiatry* 67, 584–587. doi: 10.1016/j.biopsych.2009.08.024

Small, G. W., Kepe, V., Ercoli, L. M., Siddarth, P., Bookheimer, S. Y., Miller, K. J., et al. (2006). PET of brain amyloid and tau in mild cognitive impairment. *N. Engl. J. Med.* 355, 2652–2663. doi: 10.1056/NEJMoa054625

Sorg, C., Riedl, V., Mühlau, M., Calhoun, V. D., Eichele, T., Läer, L., et al. (2007). Selective changes of resting-state networks in individuals at risk for Alzheimer's disease. *Proc. Natl. Acad. Sci. U.S.A.* 104, 18760–18765. doi: 10.1073/pnas.0708803104

van Dijk, K. R. A., Hedden, T., Venkataraman, A., Evans, K. C., Lazar, S. W., and Buckner, R. L. (2010). Intrinsic functional connectivity as a tool for human connectomics: theory, properties, and optimization. *J. Neurophysiol.* 103, 297–321. doi: 10.1152/jn.00783.2009

Vanhoutte, G., Verhoye, M., and van der Linden, A. (2006). Changing body temperature affects the T2* signal in the rat brain and reveals hypothalamic activity. *Magn. Reson. Med.* 55, 1006–1012. doi: 10.1002/mrm.20861

Villemagne, V. L., Ataka, S., Mizuno, T., Brooks, W. S., Wada, Y., Kondo, M., et al. (2009). High striatal amyloid beta-peptide deposition across different autosomal Alzheimer disease mutation types. *Arch. Neurol.* 66, 1537–1544. doi: 10.1001/archneurol.2009.285

Villeneuve, S., and Jagust, W. J. (2015). Imaging vascular disease and amyloid in the aging brain: implications for treatment. *J. Prev. Alzheimers Dis.* 2, 64–70. doi: 10.14283/jpad.2015.47

Willer, C. J., Li, Y., and Abecasis, G. R. (2010). METAL: fast and efficient meta-analysis of genomewide association scans. *Bioinformatics* 26, 2190–2191. doi: 10.1093/bioinformatics/btq340

Wu, L., Soder, R. B., Schoemaker, D., Carbonnell, F., Sziklas, V., Rowley, J., et al. (2014). Resting state executive control network adaptations in amnestic mild cognitive impairment. *J. Alzheimers Dis.* 40, 993–1004. doi: 10.3233/JAD-131574

Yan, C.-G., Liu, D., He, Y., Zou, Q., Zhu, C., Zuo, X., et al. (2009). Spontaneous Brain activity in the default mode network is sensitive to different resting-state conditions with limited cognitive load. *PLoS ONE* 4:e5743. doi: 10.1371/journal.pone.0005743

Zhang, H.-Y., Wang, S.-J., Liu, B., Ma, Z.-L., Yang, M., Zhang, Z., et al. (2010). Resting brain connectivity: changes during the progress of Alzheimer disease. *Radiology* 256, 598–606. doi: 10.1148/radiol.10091701

9

Interaction of Basal Forebrain Cholinergic Neurons with the Glucocorticoid System in Stress Regulation and Cognitive Impairment

*Saswati Paul[1], Won Kyung Jeon[2], Jennifer L. Bizon[3] and Jung-Soo Han[1]**

[1] Department of Biological Sciences, Konkuk University, Seoul, South Korea, [2] Herbal Medicine Research Division, Korea Institute of Oriental Medicine, Daejeon, South Korea, [3] Department of Neuroscience, College of Medicine, Evelyn F. and William L. McKnight Brain Institute, University of Florida, Gainesville, FL, USA

Edited by:
Enrique Cadenas, University of Southern California, USA

Reviewed by:
Junming Wang, University of Mississippi Medical Center, USA
Anna Maria Colangelo, University of Milano-Bicocca, Italy

***Correspondence:**
Jung-Soo Han, Department of Biological Sciences, Konkuk University, 120 Neungdong-ro, Gwangjin-gu, Seoul 143-701, South Korea
jshan06@konkuk.ac.kr

A substantial number of studies on basal forebrain (BF) cholinergic neurons (BFCN) have provided compelling evidence for their role in the etiology of stress, cognitive aging, Alzheimer's disease (AD), and other neurodegenerative diseases. BFCN project to a broad range of cortical sites and limbic structures, including the hippocampus, and are involved in stress and cognition. In particular, the hippocampus, the primary target tissue of the glucocorticoid stress hormones, is associated with cognitive function in tandem with hypothalamic-pituitary-adrenal (HPA) axis modulation. The present review summarizes glucocorticoid and HPA axis research to date in an effort to establish the manner in which stress affects the release of acetylcholine (ACh), glucocorticoids, and their receptor in the context of cognitive processes. We attempt to provide the molecular interactive link between the glucocorticoids and cholinergic system that contributes to BFCN degeneration in stress-induced acceleration of cognitive decline in aging and AD. We also discuss the importance of animal models in facilitating such studies for pharmacological use, to which could help decipher disease states and propose leads for pharmacological intervention.

Keywords: cholinergic neuron, stress, aging, basal forebrain, hippocampus, glucocorticoid, glucocorticoid receptor

Introduction

Since its inception, the cholinergic hypothesis has generated considerable interest. It has been used to decipher the different orchestrating functions and dysfunctions in the nervous system associated with Alzheimer's disease (AD) and other neurodegenerative diseases. This hypothesis has been used to further understand cognitive impairment and neurodegenerative diseases by evaluating and tracing brain functions in normal and aging brains (Gallagher and Colombo, 1995; Contestabile, 2011). The main components of the cholinergic pathway are: (1) the neurotransmitter acetylcholine (ACh); (2) acetylcholinesterase (AChE), which breaks down ACh; (3) choline acetyltransferase, an enzyme that synthesizes ACh; and (4) ACh receptors, specifically the nicotinic ACh receptor, and the muscarinic ACh receptor (mAChR). Evidence from previous research on normal aging (Drachman et al., 1982),

AD (Whitehouse et al., 1982), and anti-cholinergic (Newhouse et al., 1988, 1994) and pro-cholinergic drug administration (Davis and Mohs, 1982) supports the major role of the cholinergic system in aged-related cognitive decline. Extensive research has established the relationship between cognitive impairment and the cholinergic system in the basal forebrain (BF; Baxter and Chiba, 1999). The involvement of the cholinergic system in regulating stress is also evident from studies that acute/inescapable stress enhanced release of ACh and induced expression of genes that regulate ACh availability in the hippocampus and prefrontal cortex (Mark et al., 1996; Kaufer et al., 1998). Cognitive processes are influenced by the acute and chronic stress-induced release of glucocorticoids, stress hormones that influence the function of the prefrontal cortex and hippocampus (Popoli et al., 2011). Stress and stress hormone plays a well-established role in mental health and impaired cognition. It is correlated with hippocampal volume and age-related cognitive decline (Lupien et al., 1994, 2009), suggesting that sustained stress, via glucocorticoid hypersecretion, leads to hippocampal damage (Uno et al., 1989). Prolonged overproduction of glucocorticoids can be detrimental to brain structure, whereas insufficient glucocorticoid signaling can lead to stress-related pathological conditions (Raison and Miller, 2003). This emphasizes the need for the careful regulation of glucocorticoid exposure. Impairment of the hypothalamic-pituitary-adrenal (HPA) axis in response to stress is also associated with cognitive dysfunction in aged animals (Issa et al., 1990; Bizon et al., 2001). In addition, HPA activity was blunt in elderly compared to young adult participants (Hatzinger et al., 2011). Therefore, new therapeutic approaches acting on the HPA axis and its receptor signaling should take into account.

Activation of the septo-hippocampal cholinergic system is considered as an important aspect in the adaptive response to stress and is influenced by neuronal and hormonal stimuli. This septo-hippocampal activation seems to initialize following activation of the pituitary-adrenocortical axis (Gilad et al., 1985; Gilad, 1987) and may then affect glucocorticoid secretion via the HPA axis (Herman et al., 1996). The HPA axis plays an important role in the adaptation to stress by modulating hippocampal activity. Thus, the hippocampus, along with cholinergic innervation from the BF, is involved in regulating the HPA axis stress response. Activation of the HPA axis mediates responses that enable an organism to maintain its homeostasis. Hence, neurodegeneration of cholinergic neurons, a pathological characteristic in AD and aging, makes the elderly vulnerable to stress, resulting in cognitive impairment.

The extent to which the cholinergic system is involved in stress, cognition, and neurological disorders has been reported in several significant research reports. Therefore, we attempt to develop a supporting background for our recent studies in rats (aged or with cholinergic lesions) on HPA axis dysfunction in response to stress and altered glucocorticoid receptor (GR) signaling in the hippocampus. We also describe the interactive link between the glucocorticoid and cholinergic systems in aging and stress.

Overview of the Basal Forebrain Cholinergic System

An anatomical simplified overview of BF cholinergic neurons is summarized in **Figure 1**, including cells located in the medial septum (MS), the vertical limb of the diagonal band of Broca (VDB), and the nucleus basalis of Meynert–extending to the substantia innominata in the rodent brain. These structures send cholinergic projections to a broad range of neocortical sites as well as structures in the limbic system, including the hippocampus (Mesulam et al., 1983; Gallagher and Colombo, 1995). Thus, the septo-hippocampal pathway, which arises from the medial septal nucleus and nucleus of the diagonal band, is the main structure of the central cholinergic system and the main source of cholinergic innervation to the hippocampal formation. A topographical model of the septo-hippocampal pathway has been constructed based on various lesion, tracing, and immunocytochemical methods in the septal and hippocampal regions (Lewis et al., 1967; Dutar et al., 1995). The MS is connected to the hippocampus, via the fimbria and dorsal fornix, and to the medial cortex (Lewis and Shute, 1967; Teles-Grilo Ruivo and Mellor, 2013). The cornu ammonis (CA) 1 pyramidal and dentate granule (DG) cell layers in the dorsal hippocampus receive afferent inputs from the VDB, and these cell layers in the ventral hippocampus receive inputs from the both MS and VDB (McKinney et al., 1983; Nyakas et al., 1987).

Cholinergic Hypothesis in Disease Etiology

The cholinergic hypothesis has been implicated in the etiology of AD, various types of dementia, and aging, and is rooted in degeneration of BF cholinergic neurons causing cognitive deficit (Bartus et al., 1982; Bartus, 2000; Sarter et al., 2003). This theory, however, remains controversial. Although enhancement of cholinergic function by cholinergic agents (e.g., AChE inhibitors) in AD and age-related cognitive deficit supported the hypothesis, other research subsequently pinpointed the involvement of other factors, such as dopamine projections to the frontal cortex, amyloid deposition, and increased glucocorticoid levels (Dumas and Newhouse, 2011). More specifically, hypersecretion of glucocorticoid, or A-beta-altered HPA axis function, have been implicated in hippocampal impairment in AD (Hibberd et al., 2000; Brureau et al., 2013) Additionally, elevated glucocorticoid levels and impaired GR signaling are associated with HPA dysfunction, resulting in cognitive decline in elderly subjects (Issa et al., 1990; Lupien et al., 1994; Bizon et al., 2001; Mizoguchi et al., 2009). Therefore, a possible pathophysiological link between glucocorticoids and the age-dependent decline in BF cholinergic function, especially in the CA1, CA3, and DG regions of hippocampus, has also been established (Hörtnagl et al., 1993). Craig et al. postulated a new cholinergic hypothesis version for AD, where loss of MS cholinergic input to the hippocampus induces hippocampal vulnerability, resulting in greater cognitive impairment in response to subsequent insults, such as stress or injury (Craig et al., 2011).

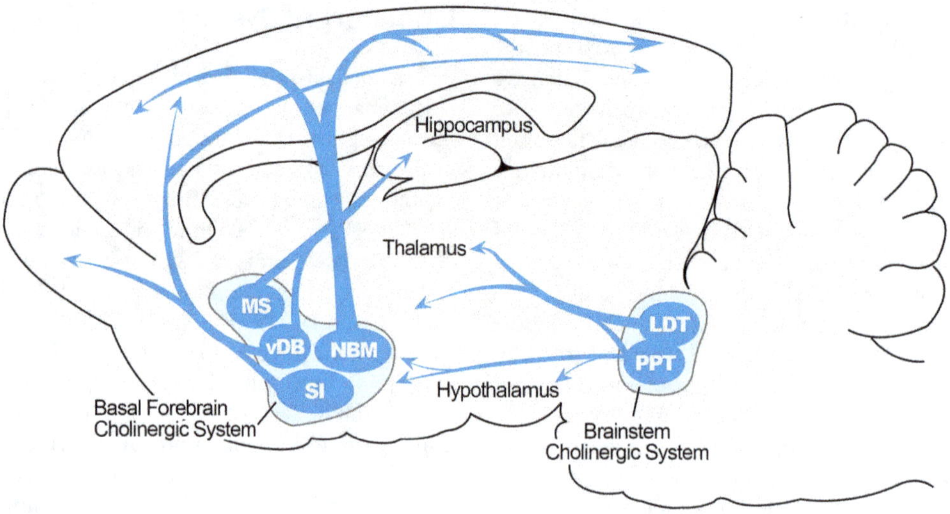

FIGURE 1 | Illustrated overview of the basal forebrain cholinergic pathway. Cholinergic projections include the medial septum (MS), vertical limbs of the diagonal band of Broca (vDB), nucleus basalis of Meynert (NBM), and substantia innominate (SI) projecting to the hippocampus, thalamus, olfactory bulb, and cortical region. Cholinergic pontomesencephalon neurons include laterodorsal tegmental (LDT) and pedunculopontine tegmental nuclei (PPT) projecting to hindbrain, thalamus, hypothalamus, and basal forebrain.

Implication of Lesion Studies in Evaluating Cholinergic Innervation

Application of the cholinergic hypothesis to animal model offers the ability to evaluate functional network and molecular pathway to understand neurocognitive diseases. Selection of animal (even among rodents) is important, as they differ in cholinergic tone, receptor activation, and relevance to human basal cholinergic activity (Van der Zee and Keijser, 2011). The adoption of the rodent as an animal model may compliment studies in primates due to effectiveness and cost-efficiency. Moreover, features such as short lifespans are an important factor to be considered in the study of late-onset or aging diseases (Gallagher et al., 2011). One major pathological hallmark of neurodegenerative disease that cause cognitive decline, is the dramatic loss of BF cholinergic projection neurons with reduced cholinergic innervation to the hippocampus and neocortex (Davies and Maloney, 1976; Whitehouse et al., 1981; Arendt et al., 1983; Mesulam, 2004). Additionally, the relative loss of cholinergic neurons and the decrease of the ACh synthesizing enzyme, choline acetyltransferase in the brain of AD patients is associated with cognitive impairment (Bartus, 2000). In animal studies, neurotoxin-induced BF lesions cause similar cognitive impairments (Olton, 1990). However, lesioning cholinergic BF neurons is challenging because they are intertwined with non-cholinergic neurons and there is a risk of damaging adjacent structures.

Although BF lesions using conventional lesion methods (e.g., electrolytic) produce varying manifestations of cognitive impairment, the development of methods that selectively interrupt the BF region has been attempted (Easton et al., 2012; Baxter and Bucci, 2013). An initial approach innovatively used 192IgG-saporin, a neurotoxin with a specific affinity for cholinergic neuron cell surface receptors (Wiley et al., 1991; Baxter and Bucci, 2013). A myriad of studies picked the hippocampal and septo-hippocampal regions of the BF as lesion sites to evaluate the cholinergic interventions observed in aging and cognition. Studies with selective BF neurotoxic lesion concluded this region was associated with cognitive function characterized by attention (Muir et al., 1993; Baxter et al., 1997, 1999; Bucci et al., 1998; Chiba et al., 1999; Chudasama et al., 2004), and learning and memory (Hepler et al., 1985; Hagan et al., 1988; Berger-Sweeney et al., 1994; Baxter et al., 1995; Janisiewicz et al., 2004). Furthermore, a significant correlation between cognitive impairment and decline in cholinergic markers for the septo-hippocampal projection in aged rats (Gallagher et al., 1990; Smith and Booze, 1995) supports the involvement of BF cholinergic neurons in cognition. More recently, animals with a saporin-induced partial loss of septo-hippocampal cholinergic neurons exhibited cognitive deficit (Brayda-Bruno et al., 2013). Other lesion studies extended the importance of the BF cholinergic system in the process of functional recovery from brain injury in young rats (Conner et al., 2005), which is intriguing in that animals with BF lesions may show deficits in cognitive function. Selective lesion of cholinergic inputs to the hippocampus has also been used to evaluate the effects of cholinergic receptors in regulating hippocampal ACh release (Thorne and Potter, 1995).

Though lesion studies have generated substantial controversy, the advent of this approach has generated new empirical tests and compelling information on the potential function of cholinergic and non-cholinergic neurons emanating from the BF. Additionally, this has unveiled the possible role played by loss of these neurons in stress, aging, and other neurocognitive diseases. More essentially, animal models are indispensable for recreating specific human pathogenic events, and invaluable for drug screening and therapeutic intervention assessment.

HPA Axis and Glucocorticoids in Stress Regulation and Aging

The HPA axis is an integral component in promoting resilience to stress. Most salient age-related changes in the stress response are thought to occur in the HPA axis. The HPA system is classically controlled by a range of afferent signals responsible for the coordinated release of various signaling markers. The hypothalamus is at the top of the hierarchy in the control of the central HPA axis. When the brain perceives a stressor, activation of the paraventricular nucleus of the hypothalamus triggers the release of corticotropin-releasing hormone. Corticotropin-releasing hormone stimulates pituitary adrenocorticotropic hormone (ACTH) release and activates the adrenal gland, which secretes glucocorticoids (cortisol in humans and corticosterone in rodents). Glucocorticoids released from the adrenal gland interact with the HPA axis by binding to specific GRs in the brain, forming a closed-loop feedback system and subsequently coping with stress (Sapolsky et al., 1986; Mizuno and Kimura, 1997; Srinivasan et al., 2013). Thus, glucocorticoids are the end product of the HPA axis and regulate a wide array of actions influencing neuronal function and metabolism (**Figure 2**).

Two types of steroid hormone receptors have been identified in tandem in the brain: the mineralocorticoid receptor (MR) and the GR. Expression of MR is considerably more restricted in the brain compared to the ubiquitous expression of GR, and both mediate classical genomic and non-genomic glucocorticoid actions by acting as nuclear transcriptional activators and repressors (Reul and de Kloet, 1985; Joëls, 2008; van der Laan and Meijer, 2008; Groeneweg et al., 2011). Moreover, the secretion of glucocorticoids and their binding to receptors leads to auto-regulatory decreases in receptor availability and *vice versa* (Sapolsky et al., 1984; Reul et al., 1987a,b). Actions of GR described above extends the role of GR beyond mediating glucocorticoid feedback following stress, whereas MR participates in basal HPA tone (Reul et al., 1987a; De Kloet et al., 1998) and the genomic action in adaptation and homeostasis after stress exposure (de Kloet, 2008). After GR binding, these activated receptors are translocated to the nucleus where they bind to the glucocorticoid responsive elements (GRE) and affect the transcriptional activity of target genes (Funder, 1997). Stress causes a down-regulation of GR through the increase of circulating glucocorticoids, eventually decreasing sensitivity to nuclear transcriptional activities. Glucocorticoid-GR can also activate transcription by binding directly as a homodimer to the GRE DNA sequence present in the promotors of target genes (e.g., *serum- and glucocorticoid-induced protein kinase, mitogen-activated protein kinase phosphatase-1*, etc) that has been reported to regulate cognitive function (Lee et al., 2007; Vyas and Maatouk, 2013; Cestari et al., 2014).

HPA activity tends to increase with age due to inefficiencies of glucocorticoid negative-feedback inhibition, resulting in elevated plasma levels of ACTH and glucocorticoids (Mizoguchi et al., 2009; Aguilera, 2011). A decrease in glucocorticoid negative-feedback inhibition is associated with the loss of GR and altered GR signaling in the forebrain (Issa et al., 1990; Bizon et al., 2001; Lund et al., 2004; Lee et al., 2012). Increased levels of glucocorticoids appear to threaten hippocampal neurons and direct the loss of dendrite complexity in the hippocampus (Hibberd et al., 2000). Inappropriate HPA axis regulation in aging is reviewed by Aguilera (2011) who stresses its adverse effect in stress-related brain disorders.

A link between HPA deregulation and disruption of GR has been observed in AD and other neurodegenerative diseases (Brureau et al., 2013; Vyas and Maatouk, 2013). Interestingly, though extra-hypothalamic GR sites receive attention for this glucocorticoid-mediated HPA inhibitory feedback; the hippocampus receives the utmost attention with regards to these effects (McEwen et al., 1968, 1969; Sapolsky et al., 1984, 1986; Herman et al., 1989). The influence of glucocorticoids on the HPA axis markedly depends on the available GR in individual

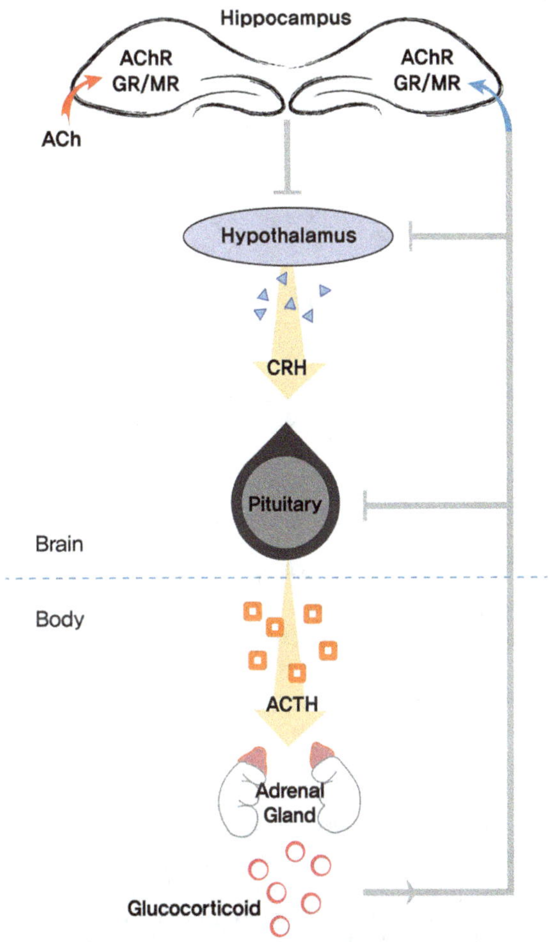

FIGURE 2 | Schematic diagram showing the role of the hippocampus in modulating the HPA (hypothalamic pituitary adrenocortical) axis. Stress triggers the release of glucocorticoids, which exerts feedback to the hippocampus, hypothalamus, and pituitary. Acetylcholine (ACh) is also involved in mediating neuroendocrine, emotional, and physiological responses in tandem with the HPA axis. AChR, acetylcholine receptors; GR, glucocorticoid receptor; MR, mineralocorticoid receptor; CRH, corticotropin-releasing hormone; ACTH, adrenocorticotropic hormone.

tissues (Simons, 2008). Abundant expression of GR in the forebrain (McEwen et al., 1969; McEwen and Wallach, 1973), and increased activity of the HPA axis in the absence of forebrain inhibition on HPA axis by damage of the forebrain (Jacobson and Sapolsky, 1991; van Haarst et al., 1996), contributes to the sequelae associated with GR malfunction. Taken together, forebrain GR expression is critical for HPA axis regulation in response to stress (Furay et al., 2008) and further adduces the role of GR in stress.

Cholinergic Neuron in Stress Regulation via HPA Axis and Cognitive Function

A further increase in ACh release was observed in the hippocampus after acute stress (Finkelstein et al., 1985; Gilad et al., 1985; Imperato et al., 1989). Corticosterone administration, mimicking the increase in the plasma corticosterone concentration produced by stress, induced hippocampal ACh (Imperato et al., 1989). These studies support the involvement of glucocorticoids in the cholinergic innervation of the hippocampus, and the activation of the HPA axis in the process. Stress-induced responses activated the septo-hippocampal cholinergic pathway within minutes (Gilad, 1987), which then induced ACh-mediated neuroendocrine, emotional, and physiological responses by stimulating the HPA axis (Newman et al., 2001). This HPA axis activation led to the release of corticosterone, a stress neurohormone (Nyakas et al., 1987; Calogero et al., 1988, 1990). Increased release of hippocampal ACh and glucocorticoids in response to stress was observed in young rats, but not in aged rats (Mizuno and Kimura, 1997). However, contradictory results have been reported. Proteomic analyses of the hippocampus of rats exposed to stress showed a decrease in a precursor protein of hippocampal cholinergic neurostimulating peptide (HCNP) leading to a loss of ACh production (Kim and Kim, 2007). HCNP stimulate the enzyme activity of choline acetyltransferase in neurons. It is also reported that expression levels of HCNP precursor protein mRNA were decreased in the hippocampus of AD patients (Maki et al., 2002). These reports indicate a possible intricate interplay between the level of glucocorticoids, ACh, and hippocampal cholinergic protein expression effecting septo-hippocampal cholinergic pathways.

Interestingly, a parallel increase in both plasma corticosterone and hippocampal ACh level has been validated as a consequence of elevated platform exposure, a relatively mild stress (Degroot et al., 2004). The interaction of glucocorticoid with ACh in the brain is well reviewed (Mora et al., 2012). Moreover, regulation of the HPA axis by glucocorticoid feedback and cholinergic brain function modulating stress responses depends on the intensity and predictability of stressful stimuli (Pitman et al., 1988; Martí and Armario, 1997; Morris and Rao, 2014).

Although ACh mediates its effects via both types of ACh receptors, mAChR are more involved in cognitive impairment and are densely present in the hippocampus (Dutar et al., 1995; Colgin et al., 2003; Drever et al., 2011). An excessive loss of mAChR in the hippocampus of Alzheimer's patients, and severely impaired muscarinic signaling associated with age-related cognitive decline (Bartus et al., 1982; Zhang et al., 2007), reveal the connection between the muscarinic-dependent cholinergic system and cognitive impairment. Scopolamine-induced mAChR blockade resulted in cognitive deficit in healthy adult humans (Voss et al., 2010). Additionally, mAChR antagonists significantly elevated plasma corticosterone in stressed rats, suggesting an inhibitory effect of mAChR stimulation on pituitary-adrenal function (Kile and Turner, 1985). This result is indicative of a correlation between corticosterone levels, mAChR availability, and cognitive function.

Basal Forebrain Cholinergic Neurons, Hippocampal Glucocorticoids, and Glucocorticoid Receptor in Stress Regulation and Cognitive Aging

The hippocampus is a brain structure crucially involved in memory, the neuroendocrine regulation of stress hormones, and termination of the stress response via HPA axis glucocorticoid-mediated inhibition (Mizuno and Kimura, 1997; Kim and Diamond, 2002). Studies showing hippocampal damage due to prolonged exposure to glucocorticoids or chronic stress in primates (Uno et al., 1989; Sapolsky et al., 1990) have been triggered an assessment of the cumulative impact of such exposures on the hippocampus using other animals. A number of studies reported that chronic stress or glucocorticoids contributed hippocampal cell death in adult rats (Sapolsky et al., 1985; Dachir et al., 1997). The hippocampus contains a high density of GR and is a target of glucocorticoid actions. Cognitive deficits are associated with a loss of hippocampal neurons, in particular pyramidal cells, due to increased glucocorticoid exposure (McEwen et al., 1968; McEwen, 1999; Hibberd et al., 2000). However, others failed to find hippocampal neuronal loss in rats (Bodnoff et al., 1995; Sousa et al., 1998; Coburn-Litvak et al., 2004), tree shrews (Vollmann-Honsdorf et al., 1997; Fuchs et al., 2001), primates (Leverenz et al., 1999), and humans (Müller et al., 2001). The inconsistencies in literatures on glucocorticoid-related cell death may arise from species-specific differences in expression levels of GR and MR (Conrad, 2008).

In any case, impairments of hippocampal dependent memory and synaptic plasticity, and structural alterations have been observed in the animals with chronic stress or corticosterone treatment (Bodnoff et al., 1995; Fuchs et al., 2001; Finsterwald and Alberini, 2014). Down-regulation of GR in the hippocampus follows the chronic corticosterone treatment. (Tornello et al., 1982). And GR signaling was altered in stress-related psychopathologies (Finsterwald and Alberini, 2014). Thus this indicates a connection between GR availability and cognitive function. As GR are responsible for negative feedback control of the adaptive stress response (De Kloet et al., 1998), a reduction in hippocampal GR is associated with post-stress glucocorticoid hypersecretion (Sapolsky, 1996). Additionally, glucocorticoid treatments exacerbated the cholinergic neurotoxin ethycholine aziridinium (AF64A)-induced cholinergic lesions in the hippocampus, suggesting a pathophysiological link between glucocorticoids and age-dependent declines in cholinergic function or cholinergic degeneration in AD (Hörtnagl et al., 1993). Moreover, the essential coordinating role of GR in regulating glucocorticoid secretion through the HPA axis in response to stress in aging is well documented (Issa et al., 1990; Herman et al., 1996; Bizon et al., 2001; Murphy et al., 2002; Furay et al., 2008; Mizoguchi et al., 2009).

Glucocorticoid receptor, when functioning as a ligand-dependent transcription factor, controls transcription by directly binding to positive and negative GRE, regulating transcriptional increases (anti-inflammatory) or decreases (HPA axis negative feedback) or inhibiting transcriptional activity of other factors (on pro-inflammatory molecules) (Silverman and Sternberg, 2012). The GR-DNA binding phenomenon is gradually receiving recognition, and research on the anti-inflammatory effects of GR-DNA binding has been reported in *in vivo* and *in vitro* studies (Reichardt et al., 1998, 2001; Schäcke et al., 2002; Clark, 2007). Target disruption of GR genes and impaired GR-DNA binding has been correlated with cognitive deficits in mice (Oitzl et al., 1997, 2001), while intra-hippocampal GR blockade with a GR antagonist produced memory impairments (Nikzad et al., 2011). Diminished GR signaling and GR mRNA in the aged hippocampus is related to memory impairment and HPA axis dysregulation (Bizon et al., 2001; Murphy et al., 2002; Lee et al., 2012). Furthermore, a decrease in the nuclear uptake of corticosterone, decreased nuclear translocation, and DNA binding deficits were observed in the hippocampus of the aged rat (Sapolsky et al., 1983; Murphy et al., 2002; Lee et al., 2012). This highlights the need to understand glucocorticoids-genomic interactions, as this may illuminate the role of GR in cognitive processes. Reduced expression of GR mRNA in the hippocampus and medial prefrontal cortex was also observed with memory-impaired aged rats relative to young controls and memory-unimpaired aged rats, with no change in the basal levels of circulating glucocorticoids (Bizon et al., 2001). Another source of GR signaling interference in hippocampal cognition may be mediated by the regulation of other intruding nuclear transcriptional factors, such as activator protein and nuclear factor κB (NF-κB; Yang-Yen et al., 1990; McKay and Cidlowski, 1998; Lund et al., 2004). Recently, reduced expression of FKBP5, a key GR modulator, and smaller hippocampal volumes were observed in posttraumatic stress disorder, which was reversed after cognitive behavioral therapy (Levy-Gigi et al., 2013). Supporting the above facts, decreased nuclear GR mRNA and protein was observed in aged rats with cognitive impairment, suggesting defective GR transport might affect the transcriptional properties of hippocampal neurons with HPA axis dysfunction and could have age-related impact on cognitive decline and the loss of stress regulation (Bizon et al., 2001; Lee et al., 2012).

Although high levels of glucocorticoids are not associated with the loss of hippocampal neurons (Leverenz et al., 1999), some studies suggest interplay between the accumulative factor of stress and aging in the process of cell loss (Hibberd et al., 2000). On the other hand, Notarianni recently proposed a role for GR signaling in the initiation and development of AD, implicating over-activation of GR with hypercortisolemia in promoting amyloid beta (Aβ) production that leads to Aβ deposition and associated neuroinflammation (Notarianni, 2013).

Chronic neuroinflammation in the BF is also linked to loss of cholinergic neurons and is responsible for cognitive impairment associated with aging and AD (Willard et al., 1999). Significant loss of cholinergic neurons in the MS/diagonal band was also observed in aged animals with memory impairment (Baskerville et al., 2006). A direct correlation between glucocorticoid regulation of GR via the HPA axis and impaired GR function as a mechanism for inflammation is well reviewed (Silverman and Sternberg, 2012), emphasizing its importance in the prevention and management of chronic stress. Further, upregulation of pro-inflammatory cytokines occurs in the cortex and hippocampus of rats with post-surgery stress, resulting in post-operative cognitive dysfunction. This surgery-induced inflammation can be reduced by acetylcholinesterase inhibitors (Kalb et al., 2013), pointing to the involvement of the cholinergic system in cognitive impairment associated with neuroinflammation.

Interaction of ACh Receptor and GR in the Hippocampus

Cognitive impairment was observed in healthy human subjects treated with scopolamine, a selective mAChR antagonist (Voss et al., 2010). Rats treated with scopolamine showed spatial working memory impairment in an 8-arm radial maze task and alterations in ventral hippocampi ACh release (Mishima et al., 2000). In addition, impairment of recognition memory in BF cholinergic lesioned animals was aggravated by scopolamine, emphasizing the importance of mAChR in cognitive function (Steckler et al., 1995). Deficit in the transduction of cholinergic mAChR signals has been detected in the hippocampus of aged rats (Smith and Booze, 1995), the cortex of aged monkeys (Vannucchi and Goldman-Rakic, 1991), and in AD patients (Flynn et al., 1991). Additionally, impaired mAChR binding was found in the striatum and hippocampus of aged rats (Anson et al., 1992; Yamagami et al., 1992; Nieves-Martinez et al., 2012).

Loss of mAChR exacerbates cognitive decline and AD pathology, such as increased plaques/tangles and cerebrovascular deposition of Aβ in AD mice (Medeiros et al., 2011). Treatment with selective muscarinic agonists resulted in reduced production of Aβ in AD patients (Hock et al., 2003). A speculative pathway, due to loss of mAChR function in rats, induced by selective hippocampal cholinergic lesions with AF64A is predicted to influence effects in stimulating nicotinic receptors that may modulate the release of ACh (Thorne and Potter, 1995). In context, it is predicted that loss of mAChR function might exert stimulatory effects on nicotinic receptors, which are well described in cognitive functions (Levin, 2013). This highlights the importance of mAChR in BF cognitive function. Decreased expression of mAChR in the hippocampal CA1 region of aged epileptic animals (Cavarsan et al., 2011), and severely impaired muscarinic signaling in the hippocampus of cognitively impaired rats (Zhang et al., 2007), illustrates the involvement of the cholinergic system with cognition. More recently, decreases in ACh and mAChR were observed in cognitively impaired mice (Park et al., 2013). Additionally, impaired hippocampal ACh release and cognitive deficits in mAChR knockout mice (Tzavara et al., 2003) coupled with mAChR antagonist impairment of memory in aged rats (Quirion et al., 1995; Klinkenberg and Blokland, 2010) implies a role for mAChR in the cholinergic hypothesis of cognition.

Activation of septo-hippocampal cholinergic neurons is manifested by increased release of ACh and choline uptake. This choline uptake is reduced below control levels in the presence of chronic stress, followed by an up-regulation of muscarinic binding sites (Finkelstein et al., 1985). Suppression of glucocorticoid secretion enhances hippocampal cholinergic transmission in rats (Mizoguchi et al., 2008). Furthermore, enhanced memory consolidation by striatal corticosterone injection was blocked by administration of scopolamine (Sánchez-Resendis et al., 2012), confirming the interactive relationship between glucocorticoids and cholinergic receptor. Glucocorticoid modulation of mAChR in lung (Scherrer et al., 1997), smooth muscle (Emala et al., 1997), chronic obstructive pulmonary disease (Johnson, 2005), and several brain nuclei in rats (Torres et al., 1991) suggests a similar pattern in hippocampal cholinergic neurons.

Rats with selective removal of hippocampal cholinergic input showed HPA axis dysfunction and decreased hippocampal GR levels (Han et al., 2002; Helm et al., 2002, 2004; Lim et al., 2012). Subsequent studies also revealed altered GR-protein kinase A (PKA)-NF-κB signaling in the hippocampus with loss of cholinergic input (Lim et al., 2011, 2012). The study regarding interactive effects of stress with loss of BFCN on cognitive function reported chronic stress induced impairment of working memory in rats with loss of hippocampal cholinergic input (Craig et al., 2008). Recently, we examined whether chronic stress aggravated cognitive deficit induced by selective BF cholinergic lesions leading to alterations in GR-PKA-NF-κB signaling. Lesioned rats receiving chronic stress showed a severe impairment in spatial memory and increased NF-κB signaling activation, which was substantiated by increased hippocampal pro-inflammatory gene expression, such as inducible nitric oxide synthase and cyclooxygenase-2 (Lee et al., 2013). These data indicate that the interaction between GR and ACh receptors is associated with stress-induced cognitive dysfunction.

Conclusion

The present review summarizes the current research and shows the importance of glucocorticoids and their receptor in modulating cognition in stress, aging, and AD via the cholinergic system. This may pave a new way in understanding the progression of the aforementioned diseases. Therefore, this review facilitates the understanding of the following: (1) involvement of both GR and ACh receptors in modulating cognition, thus providing a palliative approach for pharmaceutical interventions as these receptors are discussed in many research papers as a route to therapeutic intervention; (2) an interactive platform to mark the holistic consequences of cognitive impairment converging from varied neurological deficits; and finally; (3) an interactive role of glucocorticoids in the development of cognitive dysfunction and vulnerability of the hippocampus to such exposure. The main objective of this review was not only to highlight the possible underlying association between the various pathways and neural circuits involved in cognitive impairment, but also to enable the mitigation of such stress-induced cognitive morbidity by developing more effective pharmacotherapeutic strategies to ameliorate such diseases.

Acknowledgments

This paper was written as part of Konkuk University's research support program for its faculty on sabbatical leave in 2014 and supported by a grant (K15310) from the Korea Institute of Oriental Medicine (KIOM).

References

Aguilera, G. (2011). HPA axis responsiveness to stress: implications for healthy aging. *Exp. Gerontol.* 46, 90–95. doi: 10.1016/j.exger.2010.08.023

Anson, R. M., Cutler, R., Joseph, J. A., Yamagami, K., and Roth, G. S. (1992). The effects of aging on muscarinic receptor/G-protein coupling in the rat hippocampus and striatum. *Brain Res.* 598, 302–306. doi: 10.1016/0006-8993(92)90197-h

Arendt, T., Bigl, V., Arendt, A., and Tennstedt, A. (1983). Loss of neurons in the nucleus basalis of Meynert in Alzheimer's disease, paralysis agitans and Korsakoff's disease. *Acta Neuropathol.* 61, 101–108. doi: 10.1007/bf00697388

Bartus, R. T. (2000). On neurodegenerative diseases, models and treatment strategies: lessons learned and lessons forgotten a generation following the cholinergic hypothesis. *Exp. Neurol.* 163, 495–529. doi: 10.1006/exnr.2000.7397

Bartus, R. T., Dean, R. L., Beer, B., and Lippa, A. S. (1982). The cholinergic hypothesis of geriatric memory dysfunction. *Science* 217, 408–414. doi: 10.1126/science.7046051

Baskerville, K. A., Kent, C., Nicolle, M. M., Gallagher, M., and Mckinney, M. (2006). Aging causes partial loss of basal forebrain but no loss of pontine reticular cholinergic neurons. *Neuroreport* 17, 1819–1823. doi: 10.1097/wnr.0b013e32800fef5a

Baxter, M. G., and Bucci, D. J. (2013). Selective immunotoxic lesions of basal forebrain cholinergic neurons: twenty years of research and new directions. *Behav. Neurosci.* 127, 611–618. doi: 10.1037/a0033781

Baxter, M. G., Bucci, D. J., Gorman, L. K., Wiley, R. G., and Gallagher, M. (1995). Selective immunotoxic lesions of basal forebrain cholinergic cells: effects on learning and memory in rats. *Behav. Neurosci.* 109, 714–722. doi: 10.1037/0735-7044.109.4.714

Baxter, M. G., and Chiba, A. A. (1999). Cognitive functions of the basal forebrain. *Curr. Opin. Neurobiol.* 9, 178–183. doi: 10.1016/s0959-4388(99)80024-5

Baxter, M. G., Gallagher, M., and Holland, P. C. (1999). Blocking can occur without losses in attention in rats with selective removal of hippocampal cholinergic input. *Behav. Neurosci.* 113, 881–890. doi: 10.1037//0735-7044.113.5.881

Baxter, M. G., Holland, P. C., and Gallagher, M. (1997). Disruption of decrements in conditioned stimulus processing by selective removal of hippocampal cholinergic input. *J. Neurosci.* 17, 5230–5236.

Berger-Sweeney, J., Heckers, S., Mesulam, M. M., Wiley, R. G., Lappi, D. A., and Sharma, M. (1994). Differential effects on spatial navigation of immunotoxin-induced cholinergic lesions of the medial septal area and nucleus basalis magnocellularis. *J. Neurosci.* 14, 4507–4519.

Bizon, J. L., Helm, K. A., Han, J. S., Chun, H. J., Pucilowska, J., Lund, P. K., et al. (2001). Hypothalamic-pituitary-adrenal axis function and corticosterone receptor expression in behaviourally characterized young and aged long-evans rats. *Eur. J. Neurosci.* 14, 1739–1751. doi: 10.1046/j.0953-816x.2001.01781.x

Bodnoff, S. R., Humphreys, A. G., Lehman, J. C., Diamond, D. M., Rose, G. M., and Meaney, M. J. (1995). Enduring effects of chronic corticosterone treatment on spatial learning, synaptic plasticity and hippocampal neuropathology in young and mid-aged rats. *J. Neurosci.* 15, 61–69.

Brayda-Bruno, L., Mons, N., Yee, B. K., Micheau, J., Abrous, D. N., Nogues, X., et al. (2013). Partial loss in septo-hippocampal cholinergic neurons alters memory-dependent measures of brain connectivity without overt memory deficits. *Neurobiol. Dis.* 54, 372–381. doi: 10.1016/j.nbd.2013.01.010

Brureau, A., Zussy, C., Delair, B., Ogier, C., Ixart, G., Maurice, T., et al. (2013). Deregulation of hypothalamic-pituitary-adrenal axis functions in an Alzheimer's disease rat model. *Neurobiol. Aging* 34, 1426–1439. doi: 10.1016/j.neurobiolaging.2012.11.015

Bucci, D. J., Holland, P. C., and Gallagher, M. (1998). Removal of cholinergic input to rat posterior parietal cortex disrupts incremental processing of conditioned stimuli. *J. Neurosci.* 18, 8038–8046.

Calogero, A. E., Bernardini, R., Gold, P. W., and Chrousos, G. P. (1988). Regulation of rat hypothalamic corticotropin-releasing hormone secretion *in vitro*: potential clinical implications. *Adv. Exp. Med. Biol.* 245, 167–181. doi: 10.1007/978-1-4899-2064-5_13

Calogero, A. E., Kamilaris, T. C., Johnson, E. O., Tartaglia, M. E., and Chrousos, G. (1990). Recovery of the rat hypothalamic-pituitary-adrenal axis after discontinuation of prolonged treatment with the synthetic glucocorticoid agonist dexamethasone. *Endocrinology* 127, 1574–1579. doi: 10.1210/endo-127-4-1574

Cavarsan, C. F., Avanzi, R. D., Queiroz, C. M., Xavier, G. F., Mello, L. E., and Covolan, L. (2011). m1 Acetylcholine receptor expression is decreased in Hippocampal CA1 region of aged epileptic animals. *Aging Dis.* 2, 301–307.

Cestari, V., Rossi-Arnaud, C., Saraulli, D., and Costanzi, M. (2014). The MAP(K) of fear: from memory consolidation to memory extinction. *Brain Res. Bull.* 105, 8–16. doi: 10.1016/j.brainresbull.2013.09.007

Chiba, A. A., Bushnell, P. J., Oshiro, W. M., and Gallagher, M. (1999). Selective removal of cholinergic neurons in the basal forebrain alters cued target detection. *Neuroreport* 10, 3119–3123. doi: 10.1097/00001756-199909290-00044

Chudasama, Y., Dalley, J. W., Nathwani, F., Bouger, P., and Robbins, T. W. (2004). Cholinergic modulation of visual attention and working memory: dissociable effects of basal forebrain 192-IgG-saporin lesions and intraprefrontal infusions of scopolamine. *Learn. Mem.* 11, 78–86. doi: 10.1101/lm.70904

Clark, A. R. (2007). Anti-inflammatory functions of glucocorticoid-induced genes. *Mol. Cell. Endocrinol.* 275, 79–97. doi: 10.1016/j.mce.2007.04.013

Coburn-Litvak, P. S., Tata, D. A., Gorby, H. E., Mccloskey, D. P., Richardson, G., and Anderson, B. J. (2004). Chronic corticosterone affects brain weight and mitochondrial, but not glial volume fraction in hippocampal area CA3. *Neuroscience* 124, 429–438. doi: 10.1016/j.neuroscience.2003.11.031

Colgin, L. L., Kubota, D., and Lynch, G. (2003). Cholinergic plasticity in the hippocampus. *Proc. Natl. Acad. Sci. U S A* 100, 2872–2877. doi: 10.1073/pnas.0530289100

Conner, J. M., Chiba, A. A., and Tuszynski, M. H. (2005). The basal forebrain cholinergic system is essential for cortical plasticity and functional recovery following brain injury. *Neuron* 46, 173–179. doi: 10.1016/j.neuron.2005.03.003

Conrad, C. D. (2008). Chronic stress-induced hippocampal vulnerability: the glucocorticoid vulnerability hypothesis. *Rev. Neurosci.* 19, 395–411. doi: 10.1515/revneuro.2008.19.6.395

Contestabile, A. (2011). The history of the cholinergic hypothesis. *Behav. Brain Res.* 221, 334–340. doi: 10.1016/j.bbr.2009.12.044

Craig, L. A., Hong, N. S., Kopp, J., and McDonald, R. J. (2008). Emergence of spatial impairment in rats following specific cholinergic depletion of the medial septum combined with chronic stress. *Eur. J. Neurosci.* 27, 2262–2271. doi: 10.1111/j.1460-9568.2008.06179.x

Craig, L. A., Hong, N. S., and McDonald, R. J. (2011). Revisiting the cholinergic hypothesis in the development of Alzheimer's disease. *Neurosci. Biobehav. Rev.* 35, 1397–1409. doi: 10.1016/j.neubiorev.2011.03.001

Dachir, S., Kadar, T., Robinzon, B., and Levy, A. (1997). Nimodipine's protection against corticosterone-induced morphological changes in the hippocampus of young rats. *Brain Res.* 748, 175–183. doi: 10.1016/s0006-8993(96)01296-6

Davies, P., and Maloney, A. J. (1976). Selective loss of central cholinergic neurons in Alzheimer's disease. *Lancet* 2:1403. doi: 10.1016/s0140-6736(76)91936-x

Davis, K. L., and Mohs, R. C. (1982). Enhancement of memory processes in Alzheimer's disease with multiple-dose intravenous physostigmine. *Am. J. Psychiatry* 139, 1421–1424. doi: 10.1176/ajp.139.11.1421

Degroot, A., Wade, M., Salhoff, C., Davis, R. J., Tzavara, E. T., and Nomikos, G. G. (2004). Exposure to an elevated platform increases plasma corticosterone and hippocampal acetylcholine in the rat: reversal by chlordiazepoxide. *Eur. J. Pharmacol.* 493, 103–109. doi: 10.1016/s0014-2999(04)00386-3

de Kloet, E. R. (2008). About stress hormones and resilience to psychopathology. *J. Neuroendocrinol.* 20, 885–892. doi: 10.1111/j.1365-2826.2008.01707.x

De Kloet, E. R., Vreugdenhil, E., Oitzl, M. S., and Joëls, M. (1998). Brain corticosteroid receptor balance in health and disease. *Endocr. Rev.* 19, 269–301. doi: 10.1210/er.19.3.269

Drachman, D. A., Glosser, G., Fleming, P., and Longenecker, G. (1982). Memory decline in the aged: treatment with lecithin and physostigmine. *Neurology* 32, 944–950. doi: 10.1212/wnl.32.9.944

Drever, B. D., Riedel, G., and Platt, B. (2011). The cholinergic system and hippocampal plasticity. *Behav. Brain Res.* 221, 505–514. doi: 10.1016/j.bbr.2010.11.037

Dumas, J. A., and Newhouse, P. A. (2011). The cholinergic hypothesis of cognitive aging revisited again: cholinergic functional compensation. *Pharmacol. Biochem. Behav.* 99, 254–261. doi: 10.1016/j.pbb.2011.02.022

Dutar, P., Bassant, M. H., Senut, M. C., and Lamour, Y. (1995). The septohippocampal pathway: structure and function of a central cholinergic system. *Physiol. Rev.* 75, 393–427.

Easton, A., Douchamps, V., Eacott, M., and Lever, C. (2012). A specific role for septohippocampal acetylcholine in memory? *Neuropsychologia* 50, 3156–3168. doi: 10.1016/j.neuropsychologia.2012.07.022

Emala, C. W., Clancy, J., and Hirshman, C. A. (1997). Glucocorticoid treatment decreases muscarinic receptor expression in canine airway smooth muscle. *Am. J. Physiol.* 272, L745–L751.

Finkelstein, Y., Koffler, B., Rabey, J. M., and Gilad, G. M. (1985). Dynamics of cholinergic synaptic mechanisms in rat hippocampus after stress. *Brain Res.* 343, 314–319. doi: 10.1016/0006-8993(85)90749-8

Finsterwald, C., and Alberini, C. M. (2014). Stress and glucocorticoid receptor-dependent mechanisms in long-term memory: from adaptive responses to psychopathologies. *Neurobiol. Learn. Mem.* 112, 17–29. doi: 10.1016/j.nlm.2013.09.017

Flynn, D. D., Weinstein, D. A., and Mash, D. C. (1991). Loss of high-affinity agonist binding to M1 muscarinic receptors in Alzheimer's disease: implications for the failure of cholinergic replacement therapies. *Ann. Neurol.* 29, 256–262. doi: 10.1002/ana.410290305

Fuchs, E., Flügge, G., Ohl, F., Lucassen, P., Vollmann-Honsdorf, G. K., and Michaelis, T. (2001). Psychosocial stress, glucocorticoids and structural alterations in the tree shrew hippocampus. *Physiol. Behav.* 73, 285–291. doi: 10.1016/s0031-9384(01)00497-8

Funder, J. W. (1997). Glucocorticoid and mineralocorticoid receptors: biology and clinical relevance. *Annu. Rev. Med.* 48, 231–240. doi: 10.1146/annurev.med.48.1.231

Furay, A. R., Bruestle, A. E., and Herman, J. P. (2008). The role of the forebrain glucocorticoid receptor in acute and chronic stress. *Endocrinology* 149, 5482–5490. doi: 10.1210/en.2008-0642

Gallagher, M., Burwell, R. D., Kodsi, M. H., McKinney, M., Southerland, S., Vella-Rountree, L., et al. (1990). Markers for biogenic amines in the aged rat brain: relationship to decline in spatial learning ability. *Neurobiol. Aging* 11, 507–514. doi: 10.1016/0197-4580(90)90111-c

Gallagher, M., and Colombo, P. J. (1995). Ageing: the cholinergic hypothesis of cognitive decline. *Curr. Opin. Neurobiol.* 5, 161–168. doi: 10.1016/0959-4388(95)80022-0

Gallagher, M., Stocker, A. M., and Koh, M. T. (2011). Mindspan: lessons from rat models of neurocognitive aging. *ILAR J.* 52, 32–40. doi: 10.1093/ilar.52.1.32

Gilad, G. M. (1987). The stress-induced response of the septo-hippocampal cholinergic system. A vectorial outcome of psychoneuroendocrinological interactions. *Psychoneuroendocrinology* 12, 167–184. doi: 10.1016/0306-4530(87)90002-3

Gilad, G. M., Mahon, B. D., Finkelstein, Y., Koffler, B., and Gilad, V. H. (1985). Stress-induced activation of the hippocampal cholinergic system and the pituitary-adrenocortical axis. *Brain Res.* 347, 404–408. doi: 10.1016/0006-8993(85)90209-4

Groeneweg, F. L., Karst, H., de Kloet, E. R., and Joëls, M. (2011). Rapid non-genomic effects of corticosteroids and their role in the central stress response. *J. Endocrinol.* 209, 153–167. doi: 10.1530/joe-10-0472

Hagan, J. J., Salamone, J. D., Simpson, J., Iversen, S. D., and Morris, R. G. (1988). Place navigation in rats is impaired by lesions of medial septum and diagonal band but not nucleus basalis magnocellularis. *Behav. Brain Res.* 27, 9–20. doi: 10.1016/0166-4328(88)90105-2

Han, J. S., Bizon, J. L., Chun, H. J., Maus, C. E., and Gallagher, M. (2002). Decreased glucocorticoid receptor mRNA and dysfunction of HPA axis in rats after removal of the cholinergic innervation to hippocampus. *Eur. J. Neurosci.* 16, 1399–1404. doi: 10.1046/j.1460-9568.2002.02191.x

Hatzinger, M., Brand, S., Herzig, N., and Holsboer-Trachsler, E. (2011). In healthy young and elderly adults, hypothalamic-pituitary-adrenocortical axis reactivity (HPA AR) varies with increasing pharmacological challenge and with age, but not with gender. *J. Psychiatr. Res.* 45, 1373–1380. doi: 10.1016/j.jpsychires.2011.05.006

Helm, K. A., Han, J. S., and Gallagher, M. (2002). Effects of cholinergic lesions produced by infusions of 192 IgG-saporin on glucocorticoid receptor mRNA expression in hippocampus and medial prefrontal cortex of the rat. *Neuroscience* 115, 765–774. doi: 10.1016/s0306-4522(02)00487-6

Helm, K. A., Ziegler, D. R., and Gallagher, M. (2004). Habituation to stress and dexamethasone suppression in rats with selective basal forebrain cholinergic lesions. *Hippocampus* 14, 628–635. doi: 10.1002/hipo.10203

Hepler, D. J., Olton, D. S., Wenk, G. L., and Coyle, J. T. (1985). Lesions in nucleus basalis magnocellularis and medial septal area of rats produce qualitatively similar memory impairments. *J. Neurosci.* 5, 866–873.

Herman, J. P., Prewitt, C. M., and Cullinan, W. E. (1996). Neuronal circuit regulation of the hypothalamo-pituitary-adrenocortical stress axis. *Crit. Rev. Neurobiol.* 10, 371–394. doi: 10.1615/critrevneurobiol.v10.i3-4.50

Herman, J. P., Schäfer, M. K., Young, E. A., Thompson, R., Douglass, J., Akil, H., et al. (1989). Evidence for hippocampal regulation of neuroendocrine neurons of the hypothalamo-pituitary-adrenocortical axis. *J. Neurosci.* 9, 3072–3082.

Hibberd, C., Yau, J. L., and Seckl, J. R. (2000). Glucocorticoids and the ageing hippocampus. *J. Anat.* 197(Pt. 4), 553–562. doi: 10.1046/j.1469-7580.2000.19740553.x

Hock, C., Maddalena, A., Raschig, A., Müller-Spahn, F., Eschweiler, G., Hager, K., et al. (2003). Treatment with the selective muscarinic m1 agonist talsaclidine decreases cerebrospinal fluid levels of A beta 42 in patients with Alzheimer's disease. *Amyloid* 10, 1–6. doi: 10.3109/13506120308995249

Hörtnagl, H., Berger, M. L., Havelec, L., and Hornykiewicz, O. (1993). Role of glucocorticoids in the cholinergic degeneration in rat hippocampus induced by ethylcholine aziridinium (AF64A). *J. Neurosci.* 13, 2939–2945.

Imperato, A., Puglisi-Allegra, S., Casolini, P., Zocchi, A., and Angelucci, L. (1989). Stress-induced enhancement of dopamine and acetylcholine release in limbic structures: role of corticosterone. *Eur. J. Pharmacol.* 165, 337–338. doi: 10.1016/0014-2999(89)90735-8

Issa, A. M., Rowe, W., Gauthier, S., and Meaney, M. J. (1990). Hypothalamic-pituitary-adrenal activity in aged, cognitively impaired and cognitively unimpaired rats. *J. Neurosci.* 10, 3247–3254.

Jacobson, L., and Sapolsky, R. (1991). The role of the hippocampus in feedback regulation of the hypothalamic-pituitary-adrenocortical axis. *Endocr. Rev.* 12, 118–134. doi: 10.1210/edrv-12-2-118

Janisiewicz, A. M., Jackson, O. 3rd, Firoz, E. F., and Baxter, M. G. (2004). Environment-spatial conditional learning in rats with selective lesions of medial septal cholinergic neurons. *Hippocampus* 14, 265–273. doi: 10.1002/hipo.10175

Joëls, M. (2008). Functional actions of corticosteroids in the hippocampus. *Eur. J. Pharmacol.* 583, 312–321. doi: 10.1016/j.ejphar.2007.11.064

Johnson, M. (2005). Corticosteroids: potential beta2-agonist and anticholinergic interactions in chronic obstructive pulmonary disease. *Proc. Am. Thorac. Soc.* 2, 320–325; discussion 340–341. doi: 10.1513/pats.200504-040sr

Kalb, A., von Haefen, C., Sifringer, M., Tegethoff, A., Paeschke, N., Kostova, M., et al. (2013). Acetylcholinesterase inhibitors reduce neuroinflammation and -degeneration in the cortex and hippocampus of a surgery stress rat model. *PLoS One* 8:e62679. doi: 10.1371/journal.pone.0062679

Kaufer, D., Friedman, A., Seidman, S., and Soreq, H. (1998). Acute stress facilitates long-lasting changes in cholinergic gene expression. *Nature* 393, 373–377. doi: 10.1038/30741

Kile, J. P., and Turner, B. B. (1985). Serotonergic and cholinergic interaction in the regulation of pituitary-adrenal function in rats. *Experientia* 41, 1123–1127. doi: 10.1007/bf01951690

Kim, J. J., and Diamond, D. M. (2002). The stressed hippocampus, synaptic plasticity and lost memories. *Nat. Rev. Neurosci.* 3, 453–462. doi: 10.1038/nrn849

Kim, H. G., and Kim, K. L. (2007). Decreased hippocampal cholinergic neurostimulating peptide precursor protein associated with stress exposure in rat brain by proteomic analysis. *J. Neurosci. Res.* 85, 2898–2908. doi: 10.1002/jnr.21407

Klinkenberg, I., and Blokland, A. (2010). The validity of scopolamine as a pharmacological model for cognitive impairment: a review of animal behavioral studies. *Neurosci. Biobehav. Rev.* 34, 1307–1350. doi: 10.1016/j.neubiorev.2010.04.001

Lee, S. Y., Hwang, Y. K., Yun, H. S., and Han, J. S. (2012). Decreased levels of nuclear glucocorticoid receptor protein in the hippocampus of aged long-evans rats with cognitive impairment. *Brain Res.* 1478, 48–54. doi: 10.1016/j.brainres.2012.08.035

Lee, S. Y., Kim, M. S., and Han, J. S. (2013). Activation of NF-kappa κB signaling in the hippocampus without cholinergic input was aggravated by chronic stress. *Soc. Neurosci.* Abstract.

Lee, C. T., Ma, Y. L., and Lee, E. H. (2007). Serum- and glucocorticoid-inducible kinase1 enhances contextual fear memory formation through down-regulation of the expression of Hes5. *J. Neurochem.* 100, 1531–1542. doi: 10.1111/j.1471-4159.2006.04284.x

Leverenz, J. B., Wilkinson, C. W., Wamble, M., Corbin, S., Grabber, J. E., Raskind, M. A., et al. (1999). Effect of chronic high-dose exogenous cortisol on hippocampal neuronal number in aged nonhuman primates. *J. Neurosci.* 19, 2356–2361.

Levin, E. D. (2013). Complex relationships of nicotinic receptor actions and cognitive functions. *Biochem. Pharmacol.* 86, 1145–1152. doi: 10.1016/j.bcp.2013.07.021

Levy-Gigi, E., Szabó, C., Kelemen, O., and Kéri, S. (2013). Association among clinical response, hippocampal volume and FKBP5 gene expression in individuals with posttraumatic stress disorder receiving cognitive behavioral therapy. *Biol. Psychiatry* 74, 793–800. doi: 10.1016/j.biopsych.2013.05.017

Lewis, P. R., and Shute, C. C. (1967). The cholinergic limbic system: projections to hippocampal formation, medial cortex, nuclei of the ascending cholinergic reticular system and the subfornical organ and supra-optic crest. *Brain* 90, 521–540. doi: 10.1093/brain/90.3.521

Lewis, P. R., Shute, C. C., and Silver, A. (1967). Confirmation from choline acetylase analyses of a massive cholinergic innervation to the rat hippocampus. *J. Physiol.* 191, 215–224. doi: 10.1113/jphysiol.1967.sp008246

Lim, C. S., Hwang, Y. K., Kim, D., Cho, S. H., Bañuelos, C., Bizon, J. L., et al. (2011). Increased interactions between PKA and NF-kappaB signaling in the hippocampus following loss of cholinergic input. *Neuroscience* 192, 485–493. doi: 10.1016/j.neuroscience.2011.05.074

Lim, C. S., Kim, Y. J., Hwang, Y. K., Bañuelos, C., Bizon, J. L., and Han, J. S. (2012). Decreased interactions in protein kinase A-Glucocorticoid receptor signaling in the hippocampus after selective removal of the basal forebrain cholinergic input. *Hippocampus* 22, 455–465. doi: 10.1002/hipo.20912

Lund, P. K., Hoyt, E. C., Bizon, J., Smith, D. R., Haberman, R., Helm, K., et al. (2004). Transcriptional mechanisms of hippocampal aging. *Exp. Gerontol.* 39, 1613–1622. doi: 10.1016/j.exger.2004.06.018

Lupien, S., Lecours, A. R., Lussier, I., Schwartz, G., Nair, N. P., and Meaney, M. J. (1994). Basal cortisol levels and cognitive deficits in human aging. *J. Neurosci.* 14, 2893–2903.

Lupien, S. J., Mcewen, B. S., Gunnar, M. R., and Heim, C. (2009). Effects of stress throughout the lifespan on the brain, behaviour and cognition. *Nat. Rev. Neurosci.* 10, 434–445. doi: 10.1038/nrn2639

Maki, M., Matsukawa, N., Yuasa, H., Otsuka, Y., Yamamoto, T., Akatsu, H., et al. (2002). Decreased expression of hippocampal cholinergic neurostimulating peptide precursor protein mRNA in the hippocampus in Alzheimer disease. *J. Neuropathol. Exp. Neurol.* 61, 176–185.

Mark, G. P., Rada, P. V., and Shors, T. J. (1996). Inescapable stress enhances extracellular acetylcholine in the rat hippocampus and prefrontal cortex but not the nucleus accumbens or amygdala. *Neuroscience* 74, 767–774. doi: 10.1016/0306-4522(96)00211-4

Martí, O., and Armario, A. (1997). Influence of regularity of exposure to chronic stress on the pattern of habituation of pituitary-adrenal hormones, prolactin and glucose. *Stress* 1, 179–189. doi: 10.3109/10253899709001107

McEwen, B. S. (1999). Stress and hippocampal plasticity. *Annu. Rev. Neurosci.* 22, 105–122. doi: 10.1146/annurev.neuro.22.1.105

McEwen, B. S., and Wallach, G. (1973). Corticosterone binding to hippocampus: nuclear and cytosol binding *in vitro*. *Brain Res.* 57, 373–386. doi: 10.1016/0006-8993(73)90143-1

McEwen, B. S., Weiss, J. M., and Schwartz, L. S. (1968). Selective retention of corticosterone by limbic structures in rat brain. *Nature* 220, 911–912. doi: 10.1038/220911a0

McEwen, B. S., Weiss, J. M., and Schwartz, L. S. (1969). Uptake of corticosterone by rat brain and its concentration by certain limbic structures. *Brain Res.* 16, 227–241. doi: 10.1016/0006-8993(69)90096-1

McKay, L. I., and Cidlowski, J. A. (1998). Cross-talk between nuclear factor-kappa B and the steroid hormone receptors: mechanisms of mutual antagonism. *Mol. Endocrinol.* 12, 45–56. doi: 10.1210/me.12.1.45

McKinney, M., Coyle, J. T., and Hedreen, J. C. (1983). Topographic analysis of the innervation of the rat neocortex and hippocampus by the basal forebrain cholinergic system. *J. Comp. Neurol.* 217, 103–121. doi: 10.1002/cne.902170109

Medeiros, R., Kitazawa, M., Caccamo, A., Baglietto-Vargas, D., Estrada-Hernandez, T., Cribbs, D. H., et al. (2011). Loss of muscarinic M1 receptor exacerbates Alzheimer's disease-like pathology and cognitive decline. *Am. J. Pathol.* 179, 980–991. doi: 10.1016/j.ajpath.2011.04.041

Mesulam, M. (2004). The cholinergic lesion of Alzheimer's disease: pivotal factor or side show? *Learn. Mem.* 11, 43–49. doi: 10.1101/lm.69204

Mesulam, M. M., Mufson, E. J., Wainer, B. H., and Levey, A. I. (1983). Central cholinergic pathways in the rat: an overview based on an alternative nomenclature (Ch1-Ch6). *Neuroscience* 10, 1185–1201. doi: 10.1016/0306-4522(83)90108-2

Mishima, K., Iwasaki, K., Tsukikawa, H., Matsumoto, Y., Egashira, N., Abe, K., et al. (2000). The scopolamine-induced impairment of spatial cognition parallels the acetylcholine release in the ventral hippocampus in rats. *Jpn. J. Pharmacol.* 84, 163–173. doi: 10.1254/jjp.84.163

Mizoguchi, K., Ikeda, R., Shoji, H., Tanaka, Y., Maruyama, W., and Tabira, T. (2009). Aging attenuates glucocorticoid negative feedback in rat brain. *Neuroscience* 159, 259–270. doi: 10.1016/j.neuroscience.2008.12.020

Mizoguchi, K., Shoji, H., Ikeda, R., Tanaka, Y., Maruyama, W., and Tabira, T. (2008). Suppression of glucocorticoid secretion enhances cholinergic transmission in rat hippocampus. *Brain Res. Bull.* 76, 612–615. doi: 10.1016/j.brainresbull.2008.03.003

Mizuno, T., and Kimura, F. (1997). Attenuated stress response of hippocampal acetylcholine release and adrenocortical secretion in aged rats. *Neurosci. Lett.* 222, 49–52. doi: 10.1016/s0304-3940(97)13340-7

Mora, F., Segovia, G., Del Arco, A., de Blas, M., and Garrido, P. (2012). Stress, neurotransmitters, corticosterone and body-brain integration. *Brain Res.* 1476, 71–85. doi: 10.1016/j.brainres.2011.12.049

Morris, M. C., and Rao, U. (2014). Cortisol response to psychosocial stress during a depressive episode and remission. *Stress* 17, 51–58. doi: 10.3109/10253890.2013.857398

Muir, J. L., Page, K. J., Sirinathsinghji, D. J., Robbins, T. W., and Everitt, B. J. (1993). Excitotoxic lesions of basal forebrain cholinergic neurons: effects on learning, memory and attention. *Behav. Brain Res.* 57, 123–131. doi: 10.1016/0166-4328(93)90128-d

Müller, M. B., Lucassen, P. J., Yassouridis, A., Hoogendijk, W. J., Holsboer, F., and Swaab, D. F. (2001). Neither major depression nor glucocorticoid treatment affects the cellular integrity of the human hippocampus. *Eur. J. Neurosci.* 14, 1603–1612. doi: 10.1046/j.0953-816x.2001.01784.x

Murphy, E. K., Spencer, R. L., Sipe, K. J., and Herman, J. P. (2002). Decrements in nuclear glucocorticoid receptor (GR) protein levels and DNA binding in aged rat hippocampus. *Endocrinology* 143, 1362–1370. doi: 10.1210/en.143.4.1362

Newhouse, P. A., Potter, A., Corwin, J., and Lenox, R. (1994). Age-related effects of the nicotinic antagonist mecamylamine on cognition and behavior. *Neuropsychopharmacology* 10, 93–107. doi: 10.1038/npp.1994.11

Newhouse, P. A., Sunderland, T., Tariot, P. N., Weingartner, H., Thompson, K., Mellow, A. M., et al. (1988). The effects of acute scopolamine in geriatric depression. *Arch. Gen. Psychiatry* 45, 906–912. doi: 10.1001/archpsyc.1988.01800340028004

Newman, M. B., Nazian, S. J., Sanberg, P. R., Diamond, D. M., and Shytle, R. D. (2001). Corticosterone-attenuating and anxiolytic properties of mecamylamine in the rat. *Prog. Neuropsychopharmacol. Biol. Psychiatry* 25, 609–620. doi: 10.1016/s0278-5846(00)00178-0

Nieves-Martinez, E., Haynes, K., Childers, S. R., Sonntag, W. E., and Nicolle, M. M. (2012). Muscarinic receptor/G-protein coupling is reduced in the dorsomedial striatum of cognitively impaired aged rats. *Behav. Brain Res.* 227, 258–264. doi: 10.1016/j.bbr.2011.10.048

Nikzad, S., Vafaei, A. A., Rashidy-Pour, A., and Haghighi, S. (2011). Systemic and intrahippocampal administrations of the glucocorticoid receptor antagonist RU38486 impairs fear memory reconsolidation in rats. *Stress* 14, 459–464. doi: 10.3109/10253890.2010.548171

Notarianni, E. (2013). Hypercortisolemia and glucocorticoid receptor-signaling insufficiency in Alzheimer's disease initiation and development. *Curr. Alzheimer Res.* 10, 714–731. doi: 10.2174/15672050113109990137

Nyakas, C., Luiten, P. G., Spencer, D. G., and Traber, J. (1987). Detailed projection patterns of septal and diagonal band efferents to the hippocampus in the rat with emphasis on innervation of CA1 and dentate gyrus. *Brain Res. Bull.* 18, 533–545. doi: 10.1016/0361-9230(87)90117-1

Oitzl, M. S., de Kloet, E. R., Joëls, M., Schmid, W., and Cole, T. J. (1997). Spatial learning deficits in mice with a targeted glucocorticoid receptor gene disruption. *Eur. J. Neurosci.* 9, 2284–2296. doi: 10.1111/j.1460-9568.1997.tb01646.x

Oitzl, M. S., Reichardt, H. M., Joëls, M., and de Kloet, E. R. (2001). Point mutation in the mouse glucocorticoid receptor preventing DNA binding impairs spatial memory. *Proc. Natl. Acad. Sci. U S A* 98, 12790–12795. doi: 10.1073/pnas.231313998

Olton, D. S. (1990). Dementia: animal models of the cognitive impairments following damage to the basal forebrain cholinergic system. *Brain Res. Bull.* 25, 499–502. doi: 10.1016/0361-9230(90)90242-r

Park, S. J., Shin, E. J., Min, S. S., An, J., Li, Z., Hee Chung, Y., et al. (2013). Inactivation of JAK2/STAT3 signaling axis and downregulation of M1 mAChR cause cognitive impairment in klotho mutant mice, a genetic model of aging. *Neuropsychopharmacology* 38, 1426–1437. doi: 10.1038/npp.2013.39

Pitman, D. L., Ottenweller, J. E., and Natelson, B. H. (1988). Plasma corticosterone levels during repeated presentation of two intensities of restraint stress: chronic stress and habituation. *Physiol. Behav.* 43, 47–55. doi: 10.1016/0031-9384(88)90097-2

Popoli, M., Yan, Z., McEwen, B. S., and Sanacora, G. (2011). The stressed synapse: the impact of stress and glucocorticoids on glutamate transmission. *Nat. Rev. Neurosci.* 13, 22–37. doi: 10.1038/nrn3138

Quirion, R., Wilson, A., Rowe, W., Aubert, I., Richard, J., Doods, H., et al. (1995). Facilitation of acetylcholine release and cognitive performance by an M(2)-muscarinic receptor antagonist in aged memory-impaired. *J. Neurosci.* 15, 1455–1462.

Raison, C. L., and Miller, A. H. (2003). When not enough is too much: the role of insufficient glucocorticoid signaling in the pathophysiology of stress-related disorders. *Am. J. Psychiatry* 160, 1554–1565. doi: 10.1176/appi.ajp.160.9.1554

Reichardt, H. M., Kaestner, K. H., Tuckermann, J., Kretz, O., Wessely, O., Bock, R., et al. (1998). DNA binding of the glucocorticoid receptor is not essential for survival. *Cell* 93, 531–541. doi: 10.1016/s0092-8674(00)81183-6

Reichardt, H. M., Tuckermann, J. P., Göttlicher, M., Vujic, M., Weih, F., Angel, P., et al. (2001). Repression of inflammatory responses in the absence of DNA binding by the glucocorticoid receptor. *EMBO J.* 20, 7168–7173. doi: 10.1093/emboj/20.24.7168

Reul, J. M., and de Kloet, E. R. (1985). Two receptor systems for corticosterone in rat brain: microdistribution and differential occupation. *Endocrinology* 117, 2505–2511. doi: 10.1210/endo-117-6-2505

Reul, J. M., van den Bosch, F. R., and de Kloet, E. R. (1987a). Differential response of type I and type II corticosteroid receptors to changes in plasma steroid level and circadian rhythmicity. *Neuroendocrinology* 45, 407–412. doi: 10.1159/000124766

Reul, J. M., van den Bosch, F. R., and de Kloet, E. R. (1987b). Relative occupation of type-I and type-II corticosteroid receptors in rat brain following stress and dexamethasone treatment: functional implications. *J. Endocrinol.* 115, 459–467. doi: 10.1677/joe.0.1150459

Sánchez-Resendis, O., Medina, A. C., Serafín, N., Prado-Alcalá, R. A., Roozendaal, B., and Quirarte, G. L. (2012). Glucocorticoid-cholinergic interactions in the dorsal striatum in memory consolidation of inhibitory avoidance training. *Front. Behav. Neurosci.* 6:33. doi: 10.3389/fnbeh.2012.00033

Sapolsky, R. M. (1996). Why stress is bad for your brain. *Science* 273, 749–750. doi: 10.1126/science.273.5276.749

Sapolsky, R. M., Krey, L. C., and McEwen, B. S. (1983). Corticosterone receptors decline in a site-specific manner in the aged rat brain. *Brain Res.* 289, 235–240. doi: 10.1016/0006-8993(83)90024-0

Sapolsky, R. M., Krey, L. C., and McEwen, B. S. (1984). Glucocorticoid-sensitive hippocampal neurons are involved in terminating the adrenocortical stress response. *Proc. Natl. Acad. Sci. U S A* 81, 6174–6177. doi: 10.1073/pnas.81.19.6174

Sapolsky, R. M., Krey, L. C., and McEwen, B. S. (1985). Prolonged glucocorticoid exposure reduces hippocampal neuron number: implications for aging. *J. Neurosci.* 5, 1222–1227.

Sapolsky, R. M., Krey, L. C., and McEwen, B. S. (1986). The neuroendocrinology of stress and aging: the glucocorticoid cascade hypothesis. *Endocr. Rev.* 7, 284–301. doi: 10.1210/edrv-7-3-284

Sapolsky, R. M., Uno, H., Rebert, C. S., and Finch, C. E. (1990). Hippocampal damage associated with prolonged glucocorticoid exposure in primates. *J. Neurosci.* 10, 2897–2902.

Sarter, M., Bruno, J. P., and Givens, B. (2003). Attentional functions of cortical cholinergic inputs: what does it mean for learning and memory? *Neurobiol. Learn. Mem.* 80, 245–256. doi: 10.1016/s1074-7427(03)00070-4

Schäcke, H., Döcke, W. D., and Asadullah, K. (2002). Mechanisms involved in the side effects of glucocorticoids. *Pharmacol. Ther.* 96, 23–43. doi: 10.1016/s0163-7258(02)00297-8

Scherrer, D., Lach, E., Landry, Y., and Gies, J. P. (1997). Glucocorticoid modulation of muscarinic and beta-adrenergic receptors in guinea pig lung. *Fundam. Clin. Pharmacol.* 11, 111–116. doi: 10.1111/j.1472-8206.1997.tb00176.x

Silverman, M. N., and Sternberg, E. M. (2012). Glucocorticoid regulation of inflammation and its functional correlates: from HPA axis to glucocorticoid receptor dysfunction. *Ann. N Y Acad. Sci.* 1261, 55–63. doi: 10.1111/j.1749-6632.2012.06633.x

Simons, S. S. Jr. (2008). What goes on behind closed doors: physiological versus pharmacological steroid hormone actions. *Bioessays* 30, 744–756. doi: 10.1002/bies.20792

Smith, M. L., and Booze, R. M. (1995). Cholinergic and GABAergic neurons in the nucleus basalis region of young and aged rats. *Neuroscience* 67, 679–688. doi: 10.1016/0306-4522(95)00076-u

Sousa, N., Madeira, M. D., and Paula-Barbosa, M. M. (1998). Effects of corticosterone treatment and rehabilitation on the hippocampal formation of neonatal and adult rats. An unbiased stereological study. *Brain Res.* 794, 199–210. doi: 10.1016/s0006-8993(98)00218-2

Srinivasan, S., Shariff, M., and Bartlett, S. E. (2013). The role of the glucocorticoids in developing resilience to stress and addiction. *Front. Psychiatry* 4:68. doi: 10.3389/fpsyt.2013.00068

Steckler, T., Keith, A. B., Wiley, R. G., and Sahgal, A. (1995). Cholinergic lesions by 192 IgG-saporin and short-term recognition memory: role of the septohippocampal projection. *Neuroscience* 66, 101–114. doi: 10.1016/0306-4522(94)00603-3

Teles-Grilo Ruivo, L. M., and Mellor, J. R. (2013). Cholinergic modulation of hippocampal network function. *Front. Synaptic Neurosci.* 5:2. doi: 10.3389/fnsyn.2013.00002

Thorne, B., and Potter, P. E. (1995). Lesion with the neurotoxin AF64A alters hippocampal cholinergic receptor function. *Brain Res. Bull.* 38, 121–127. doi: 10.1016/0361-9230(95)00076-q

Tornello, S., Orti, E., De Nicola, A. F., Rainbow, T. C., and McEwen, B. S. (1982). Regulation of glucocorticoid receptors in brain by corticosterone treatment of adrenalectomized rats. *Neuroendocrinology* 35, 411–417. doi: 10.1159/000123429

Torres, N., Fanelli, M., Alvarez, A. L., Santajuliana, D., Finkielman, S., and Pirola, C. J. (1991). Glucocorticoid-induced hypertension in rats: role of the central muscarinic cholinergic system. *J. Endocrinol.* 129, 269–274. doi: 10.1677/joe.0.1290269

Tzavara, E. T., Bymaster, F. P., Felder, C. C., Wade, M., Gomeza, J., Wess, J., et al. (2003). Dysregulated hippocampal acetylcholine neurotransmission and impaired cognition in M2, M4 and M2/M4 muscarinic receptor knockout mice. *Mol. Psychiatry* 8, 673–679. doi: 10.1038/sj.mp.4001270

Uno, H., Tarara, R., Else, J. G., Suleman, M. A., and Sapolsky, R. M. (1989). Hippocampal damage associated with prolonged and fatal stress in primates. *J. Neurosci.* 9, 1705–1711.

van der Laan, S., and Meijer, O. C. (2008). Pharmacology of glucocorticoids: beyond receptors. *Eur. J. Pharmacol.* 585, 483–491. doi: 10.1016/j.ejphar.2008.01.060

Van der Zee, E. A., and Keijser, J. N. (2011). Localization of pre- and postsynaptic cholinergic markers in rodent forebrain: a brief history and comparison of rat and mouse. *Behav. Brain Res.* 221, 356–366. doi: 10.1016/j.bbr.2010.11.051

van Haarst, A. D., Oitzl, M. S., Workel, J. O., and de Kloet, E. R. (1996). Chronic brain glucocorticoid receptor blockade enhances the rise in circadian and stress-induced pituitary-adrenal activity. *Endocrinology* 137, 4935–4943. doi: 10.1210/en.137.11.4935

Vannucchi, M. G., and Goldman-Rakic, P. S. (1991). Age-dependent decrease in the affinity of muscarinic M1 receptors in neocortex of rhesus monkeys. *Proc. Natl. Acad. Sci. U S A* 88, 11475–11479. doi: 10.1073/pnas.88.24.11475

Vollmann-Honsdorf, G. K., Flügge, G., and Fuchs, E. (1997). Chronic psychosocial stress does not affect the number of pyramidal neurons in tree shrew hippocampus. *Neurosci. Lett.* 233, 121–124. doi: 10.1016/s0304-3940(97)00647-2

Voss, B., Thienel, R., Reske, M., Habel, U., and Kircher, T. (2010). Cognitive performance and cholinergic transmission: influence of muscarinic and nicotinic receptor blockade. *Eur. Arch. Psychiatry Clin. Neurosci.* 260(Suppl. 2), S106–S110. doi: 10.1007/s00406-010-0160-8

Vyas, S., and Maatouk, L. (2013). Contribution of glucocorticoids and glucocorticoid receptors to the regulation of neurodegenerative processes. *CNS Neurol. Disord. Drug Targets* 12, 1175–1193. doi: 10.2174/187152731131200125

Whitehouse, P. J., Price, D. L., Clark, A. W., Coyle, J. T., and DeLong, M. R. (1981). Alzheimer disease: evidence for selective loss of cholinergic neurons in the nucleus basalis. *Ann. Neurol.* 10, 122–126. doi: 10.1002/ana.410100203

Whitehouse, P. J., Price, D. L., Struble, R. G., Clark, A. W., Coyle, J. T., and Delon, M. R. (1982). Alzheimer's disease and senile dementia: loss of neurons in the basal forebrain. *Science* 215, 1237–1239. doi: 10.1126/science.7058341

Wiley, R. G., Oeltmann, T. N., and Lappi, D. A. (1991). Immunolesioning: selective destruction of neurons using immunotoxin to rat NGF receptor. *Brain Res.* 562, 149–153. doi: 10.1016/0006-8993(91)91199-b

Willard, L. B., Hauss-Wegrzyniak, B., and Wenk, G. L. (1999). Pathological and biochemical consequences of acute and chronic neuroinflammation within the basal forebrain cholinergic system of rats. *Neuroscience* 88, 193–200. doi: 10.1016/s0306-4522(98)00216-4

Yamagami, K., Joseph, J. A., and Roth, G. S. (1992). Decrement of muscarinic receptor-stimulated low-KM GTPase in striatum and hippocampus from the aged rat. *Brain Res.* 576, 327–331. doi: 10.1016/0006-8993(92)90698-9

Yang-Yen, H. F., Chambard, J. C., Sun, Y. L., Smeal, T., Schmidt, T. J., Drouin, J., et al. (1990). Transcriptional interference between c-Jun and the glucocorticoid receptor: mutual inhibition of DNA binding due to direct protein-protein interaction. *Cell* 62, 1205–1215. doi: 10.1016/0092-8674(90)90396-v

Zhang, H. Y., Watson, M. L., Gallagher, M., and Nicolle, M. M. (2007). Muscarinic receptor-mediated GTP-Eu binding in the hippocampus and prefrontal cortex is correlated with spatial memory impairment in aged rats. *Neurobiol. Aging* 28, 619–626. doi: 10.1016/j.neurobiolaging.2006.02.016

10

Non-Monotonic Reorganization of Brain Networks with Alzheimer's Disease Progression

HyoungKyu Kim [1†], *Kwangsun Yoo* [1†], *Duk L. Na* [2,3], *Sang Won Seo* [2,3], *Jaeseung Jeong* [1*] *and Yong Jeong* [1*]

[1] *Department of Bio and Brain Engineering, Korea Advanced Institute of Science and Technology, Daejeon, South Korea,*
[2] *Department of Neurology, Samsung Medical Center, Sungkyunkwan University School of Medicine, Seoul, South Korea,*
[3] *Neuroscience Center, Samsung Medical Center, Seoul, South Korea*

Edited by:
Junfeng Sun,
Shanghai Jiao Tong University, China

Reviewed by:
Franziska Matthäus,
University of Heidelberg, Germany
Rong Fang,
Rui Jin Hospital North Affiliated to Shanghai Jiao Tong University School of Medicine, China

****Correspondence:***
Jaeseung Jeong,
Department of Bio and Brain Engineering, Korea Advanced Institute of Science and Technology, 291 Daehak-ro, Yuseong-gu, Daejeon 305-701, South Korea
jsjeong@kaist.ac.kr;
Yong Jeong,
Laboratory for Cognitive Neuroscience and NeuroImaging, Department of Bio and Brain Engineering, Korea Advanced Institute of Science and Technology, 291 Daehak-ro, Yuseong-gu, Daejeon 305-701, South Korea
yong@kaist.ac.kr

† *These authors have contributed equally to this work.*

Background: Identification of stage-specific changes in brain network of patients with Alzheimer's disease (AD) is critical for rationally designed therapeutics that delays the progression of the disease. However, pathological neural processes and their resulting changes in brain network topology with disease progression are not clearly known.

Methods: The current study was designed to investigate the alterations in network topology of resting state fMRI among patients in three different clinical dementia rating (CDR) groups (i.e., CDR = 0.5, 1, 2) and amnestic mild cognitive impairment (aMCI) and age-matched healthy subject groups. We constructed density networks from these 5 groups and analyzed their network properties using graph theoretical measures.

Results: The topological properties of AD brain networks differed in a non-monotonic, stage-specific manner. Interestingly, local and global efficiency and betweenness of the network were rather higher in the aMCI and AD (CDR 1) groups than those of prior stage groups. The number, location, and structure of rich-clubs changed dynamically as the disease progressed.

Conclusions: The alterations in network topology of the brain are quite dynamic with AD progression, and these dynamic changes in network patterns should be considered meticulously for efficient therapeutic interventions of AD.

Keywords: Alzheimer's disease, complex network, resting state fMRI, functional connectivity, graph theory

Introduction

Alzheimer's disease (AD) is the most common type of dementia, affecting about 5–10% of the population above the age of 65 (Sunderland et al., 2006). Clinical symptoms of AD are characterized by progressive amnesia, followed by a gradual decline in all cognitive functions, resulting in dementia (Sunderland et al., 2006). AD usually exhibits a typical clinical course reflecting the underlying progressing neuropathology (Bianchetti and Trabucchi, 2001; Storey et al., 2002). In the early stage, memory impairment is the prominent feature because the pathology initiates near the medial temporal cortex. In the moderate stage, language problems or visuospatial dysfunctions become conspicuous as the pathology propagates to the other temporal and parietal cortices (Förstl and Kurz, 1999; Bianchetti and Trabucchi, 2001). In the late stage of the illness, most cognitive functions are severely impaired, including frontal executive functions such as judgment, abstract, or logical reasoning, and planning (Braak and Braak, 1991; Fox et al., 2001). The mild cognitive impairment (MCI) is accompanied by mild memory deterioration but does not disrupt the activities of daily living. Although MCI is very heterogeneous and has multiple subtypes, it is considered to represent an intermediate stage between normal and dementia. MCI has been shown to be more likely to develop AD than cognitively normal (Boyle et al., 2006). Among MCI subtypes, Anmestic MCI (aMCI) is considered as a prodromal stage of AD, having a high-risk for progression to AD (Fischer et al., 2007). In addition, aMCI has been intensitvely investigated for early diagnosis of AD (Petersen, 2004).

Identification of clinical stages in Alzheimer's patients is crucial for the development of appropriate therapeutics that may delay the progression of the disease (Trojanowski et al., 2010). Several studies have attempted to determine the characteristics of each clinical stage of AD based on the distributions and patterns of the neuropathology (Braak and Braak, 1991), cognitive and behavioral performance (Folstein et al., 1975) and severity of clinical features such as the clinical dementia rating (CDR) (Hughes et al., 1982). For example, studies using structural MR imaging have shown that the regional patterns and rate of atrophy differ across AD stages (Scahill et al., 2002; Thompson et al., 2003). Atrophy in the medial temporal lobe commences prior to symptom onset, and is then followed by a reduction in gray matter in the limbic and other neocortices with relative sparing of primary sensory areas. These results are generally consistent with the tau accumulation and the corresponding clinical features (Scahill et al., 2002; Thompson et al., 2003).

In another aspect, there have been several studies supporting the hypothesis that AD is a "disconnection syndrome" (Delbeuck et al., 2003). According to this hypothesis, AD results from the disruption of neuronal connections due to synaptic loss and eventually neuronal death. This feature can be approached by adopting the concept of functional or structural connectivity. As the severity of the disease increases, the functional connectivity among brain regions is assumed to be gradually reduced. Indeed, prior neuroimaging studies have shown that AD patients show disrupted white matter integrity and functional connectivity among distant brain regions (Celone et al., 2006; Zhang et al., 2007). However, how different degrees of disruptions of connectivity in AD across clinical stages influence global information processing of the brain is not clearly understood yet (Wang et al., 2006; Zhou et al., 2008; Bai et al., 2011).

To address this question, the current study employed complex network analysis methods and investigated brain network properties from resting state fMRI in AD, aMCI, and healthy subjects (HS) (Strogatz, 2001; Bullmore and Sporns, 2009). Complex network analysis has shown that the brain has non-random network properties including small world and scale free features and exhibits hierarchical organization with modularity (Achard et al., 2006; Hagmann et al., 2008). Several fMRI and MEG studies have reported that AD and aMCI patients have reduced small-worldness characterized by a longer characteristic path length than that of HS (Stam et al., 2007, 2009; Kendi et al., 2008; Lo et al., 2010). However, we should note that some network properties in AD are not consistent across studies (for reviews, Xie and He, 2011; Tijms et al., 2013), for example, different studies have found increases (Kendi et al., 2008), decreases (Stam et al., 2009), or no significant changes in the clustering coefficient of the brain network in AD patients (Stam et al., 2007; Lo et al., 2010; Sanz-Arigita et al., 2010). Moreover, some studies have reported conflicting results regarding the characteristic path length; one study showed a decrease in the characteristic path length in AD brains (Sanz-Arigita et al., 2010), whereas another study reported no change (Supekar et al., 2008). This discrepancy regarding the change in the network topology of the AD brain might result from the heterogeneity of patient populations at different clinical stages of AD or the different strategy of generating network in the previous studies. To overcome this, we attempted to use the uniformly measured data sets and to raise the stability of network topology during the constructing networks. The parameters of realignment and segmentation of MR images were chosen based on the previous neuroimaging studies using SPM (Della-Maggiore et al., 2002; Maldjian et al., 2003). The density threshold values were also determined as to show the clear features of the brain network as the density value changes in a wide range. The threshold values for the same density network are in Supplementary Table 1.

To the best of our knowledge, there have been no previous studies using graph theoretical measures to investigate the consecutive changes in brain network topology with AD progression. Therefore, the current study investigated and compared topological properties of the brain networks in AD patients in three different CDR stages, patients with aMCI, and age-matched HS.

Materials and Methods

Participants

A total of 278 subjects (112 AD, 87 aMCI, and 79 HS) were recruited consecutively at the memory disorder clinic in the Department of Neurology at Samsung Medical Center in Seoul, South Korea between March 2008 and February 2009. Each participant underwent MR scans, clinical interviews, neurological examinations, and comprehensive neuropsychological assessments. Patients with aMCI met the criteria proposed by Petersen et al. (1999). We diagnosed aMCI based on criteria of −1.5 to −1 SD of SVLT score. Patients with AD fulfilled the criteria for probable AD proposed by the National Institute of Neurological and Communicative Disorders and Stroke and the AD and Related Disorders Associations (NINCDS-ADRDA) (McKhann et al., 1984). AD patients were subdivided into three groups according to their CDR (Morris, 1993), 36 with a CDR of 0.5, 55 with a CDR of 1, and 22 with a CDR of 2. The HS group was comprised of 79 subjects with no history of cognitive impairment or neurological or psychiatric illness, and the subjects exhibited normal performance during neuropsychological testing. During various phases, 126 subjects were excluded from the study, and data from 152 subjects was included in the analysis.

While reviewing their neuropsychological tests, we excluded 31 subjects (5 NL, 6 aMCI, 3 AD patients with a CDR score of 0.5, 10 AD patients with a CDR score of 1, and 7 AD patients with a CDR score of 2 whose clinical information was incomplete on at least one neuropsychological item. We then constructed an individual brain network according to the method described in the following Section Construction of a Brain Network Using Resting State fMRI, but with a threshold of 0.8. We excluded outliers with network degrees below [the first quartile −1.5 times the interquartile range] or above [the third quartile +1.5 times the interquartile range]. The networks with small degrees during the measurement were considered to be noisy data, and the networks with large degrees could be affected by artifacts. The number of outliers excluded in this step was 82. We then again checked group-wise average ages. To match the average age among groups, we additionally excluded 13 subjects in the HS group. Every participant or their caregivers in this study provided written informed consent. This study was approved by the Institutional Review Board of Samsung Medical Center, Seoul, South Korea.

Neuropsychological Assessments

Each participant underwent neuropsychological testing using the Seoul Neuropsychological Screening Battery (SNSB), a standardized neuropsychological battery that includes validated tests for a variety of cognitive functions such as attention, language, visuospatial function, verbal, and visual memory, frontal executive function, and CDR (Kang and Na, 2003). Among these evaluations, scorable tests included the Digit Span Backward, the Korean version of the Boston Naming Test (K-BNT) (Kim and Na, 1999), the Rey-Osterrieth Complex Figure Test (RCFT) (Lezak, 1983), the Seoul Verbal Learning Test (SVLT; three learning-free recall trials of 12 words, a 20 min delayed recall trial for these 12 items, and a recognition test), motor tests (Contrasting program, a Go/NoGo test), the phonemic and semantic Controlled Oral Word Association Test (COWAT), and the Stroop Test (Color reading of 112 items during 2 min).

Acquisition and Preprocessing of MRI

MR images were acquired using a 3 Tesla MR scanner (Philips Intera Achieva, Philips Healthcare, The Netherlands). T1-weighted anatomical MR images (TR = 9.9 ms; TE = 4.6 ms; flip angle = 8°; FOV [FH, AP, RL] = 240 × 240 × 180 mm^2; matrix = 480 × 480; 360 slices [sagittal]; voxel size = 0.5 × 0.5 × 0.5 mm^3) and T2*-weighted MR images (resting state fMRI) were obtained using a gradient echo planar imaging pulse sequence (TR = 3000 ms; TE = 35 ms; flip angle = 90°; FOV [RL, AP, FH] = 220 × 220 × 140 mm^2; matrix = 128 × 128; 35 slices [transverse]; voxel size [RL, AP, FH] = 1.72 × 1.72 × 4 mm^3).

Pre-processing steps for resting state fMRI included slice-timing correction, motion correction, co-registration, segmentation, spatial normalization into Montreal Neurological Institute (MNI) space, and smoothing as described previously (Yoo et al., 2013). Pre-processing was performed using Statistical Parametric Mapping software 8.0 (SPM, http://www.fil.ion.ucl.ac.uk/spm/) in MATLAB R2011a (7.12).

Construction of a Brain Network Using Resting State fMRI

We selected 90 brain regions as nodes to construct a brain network using an Automated Anatomical Labeling (AAL) parcellation scheme (Tzourio-Mazoyer et al., 2002). To determine the functional connectivity (i.e., the edges) between the nodes, we calculated mutual information for each pair of 90 fMRI time series extracted from each node. We then constructed a network with the same density for each individual and containing the same number of edges in every individual graph to facilitate comparison of network properties. This allows the comparison between groups with a controlled number of nodes and edges, because network properties with the same threshold change dramatically with their number of degrees.

$$\text{Mutual information} = \sum_y \sum_x p(x, y) log \left(\frac{p(x, y)}{p(x) p(y)} \right)$$

where *p(x,y)* is the joint probability distribution function of X and Y, *p(x)* and *p(y)* are the marginal probability distribution functions of X and Y, and X, Y are the serial values of fMRI from selected two regions in this study.

The various density values were tested to construct brain networks. Among them, we finally selected the lowest fixed density that provided a sufficiently sparse network with a lower bound of density, minimizing the number of isolated nodes. The threshold of each network was applied separately for fixed density, 7%. The density equals the number of edges divided by possible connections in the network,

$$\text{Density} = \frac{2E}{N(N-1)}$$

wherein the number of nodes N and edges E. This allows the controlled comparison of network structure and properties among different groups.

Graph Theoretical Analysis of the Brain Network

After constructing an individual brain network for each subject, graph theoretical analysis was performed to obtain the topological information of the network. We then compared the whole brain network properties among the five groups (HS, aMCI, CDR 0.5, CDR 1, and CDR 2, ANOVA, and *post-hoc*). We compared seven network parameters, including the characteristic path length, clustering coefficient, global efficiency, local efficiency, betweenness centrality, assortativity, and modularity. The characteristic path length is the average of the minimum number of edges that have to be passed through between nodes. The clustering coefficient of a node is the rate of existing edges between the nearest neighbors vs. possible connections. Global and local efficiency indicate the information transfer between nodes. Global efficiency is the average of the inverse of the shortest path lengths of individual nodes. The local efficiency of an individual node is the inverse of the shortest path length connecting all neighbors of that node. The betweenness centrality of a single node is the number of shortest paths between nodes that must pass through the selected node dividing by the number of all paths to normalize. Assortativity is the correlation between the degrees of connected nodes. A positive assortativity indicates that high-degree nodes tend to connect to each other. The modularity is the fraction of the edges that fall within the given groups minus the expected fraction if edges were distributed at random. This analysis was performed using the Brain connectivity toolbox (Rubinov and Sporns, 2010). We also investigated the network properties of each brain lobe (frontal, parietal, occipital, and temporal lobes and the subcortical area). To do this, we first calculated nodal values for each of the 90 AAL ROIs and then took the average of these values within each lobe or area. We compared these lobar or areal properties across the five groups with AD progression (ANOVA and *post-hoc*). In this lobar analysis, we supposed that tests for each lobe are independent, hence no correction was applied.

Correlation Analysis between Network Topology and Clinical Information

We tested whether network properties were correlated with clinical measures by two methods. First, we examined whether a significant correlation existed between network properties and clinical information within each of the five groups. Second, we performed the same correlation analysis including all subjects regardless of groups. We calculated the Pearson's correlation coefficient between the network properties and clinical measures and determined the significance of correlation based on the *p*-value ($p < 0.05$). For the correlation analysis, uncorrected *p*-value was used.

Rich-club organization

The rich-club in a complex network is a group of hubs having dense connections among themselves. The rich-club organization provides important information on the higher-order hierarchical backbone structure of networks (Colizza et al., 2006; McAuley et al., 2007). The rich-club phenomenon in networks is designed to measure when the hubs of a network tend to be more densely connected among themselves than nodes of a lower degree (Colizza et al., 2006). Networks having a relatively high rich-club coefficient show the rich-club effect and have many links between high degree nodes. The rich-club coefficient of a network is can be a measurement of the robustness. The networks are usually resilient with high rich-club coefficient, because the densely connected hubs can maintain the network structure easily. The rich-club coefficients of networks were also calculated in each group. We computed the rich-club coefficients $\Phi(k)$ of the networks over a range of degrees (k). For a degree (k), the edges and nodes with a smaller degree than k were removed from the network. In the remaining network, the rich-club coefficient $\Phi(k)$ is the ratio of the current edges and possible number of edges among remaining nodes,

$$\Phi\left(k\right) = \frac{2E_{>k}}{N_{>k}\left(N_{>k}-1\right)}$$

where N is the number of remaining nodes and E is the number of current edges. The rich-club coefficient $\Phi(k)$ can be normalized with a set of random networks of the same size and similar degree distribution. A normalized rich-club coefficient Φ_{norm} of >1 can be described as a rich-club organization in a network (Colizza et al., 2006). We calculated the rich-club curve comparing the rich-club coefficient between subject groups and 1000 random networks by rewiring edges with a similar degree distribution for each level of k,

$$\Phi_{norm}\left(k\right) = \frac{\Phi\left(k\right)}{\Phi_{random}\left(k\right)}$$

We also determined whether the permutation test from the 1000 random networks was statistically significant. We showed that $\Phi\left(k\right)$ was significantly greater than the distribution of $\Phi_{random}\left(k\right)$, with a $p < 0.05$.

Statistical Test

For the statistical tests, we used One-Way ANOVA for group difference of each property, and the Tukey's honest significant difference (HSD) test for *post-hoc* test in every comparison. The Tukey's HSD was optimal for One-Way ANOVA and similar procedures with equal sizes originally. As you already know, it has been confirmed to be conservative for One-Way ANOVA with the different sample sizes as well.

Results

The demographics and neuropsychological results of subjects in the current study are listed in **Table 1**. There were significant differences among groups, with the higher CDR group showing poorer performance in every cognitive domain.

We investigated changes in the topology of brain networks spanning from HS, to subjects with aMCI, to subjects in the AD spectrum. **Figure 1** shows the reorganization of the network from the HS to AD patients with a CDR of 2 (ANOVA and *post-hoc*) with respect to three parameters: global efficiency, local efficiency, and betweenness centrality. We found a non-monotonic change in the brain network as AD progressed; these 3 network properties are higher in aMCI and CDR 1 groups than other three groups. In common, these three network properties were significantly lower in the CDR 0.5 group compared with the aMCI group or the CDR 1 group ($p < 0.05$, uncorrected).In addition, we estimated the characteristic path length, clustering coefficient, modularity, and assortativity and found similar fluctuating patterns with AD progression (see Supplementary Figure 1).

We then determined whether the topology of the brain network correlated with the performance of particular cognitive functions. We performed a correlation analysis between network measures and neuropsychological test scores for each group separately (**Table 2** and Supplementary Table 2). We found significant correlations between network properties and neuropsychological test scores primarily in the aMCI group ($p < 0.05$, uncorrected). The aMCI group showed a negative correlation between the scores of the Digit Span Backward, Naming K-BNT, RCFT copy, Go/NoGo, and COWAT Semantic tests and network properties. The HS showed significant correlations between the Stroop Test scores and network measures (global efficiency, betweenness centrality, and characteristic path length). In addition, the CDR 0.5 group showed significant positive correlations between the COWAT Phonemic score and betweenness centrality and characteristic

TABLE 1 | Demographics and clinical information.

	HC	aMCI	AD CDR 0.5	AD CDR 1	AD CDR 2
Subjects	31 (26F)	50 (28F)	25 (15F)	36 (20F)	10 (6F)
Age	67.6 (±6.3)	70.4 (±7.6)	70.0 (±8.4)	72.6 (±7.7)	70.9 (±6.9)
Digit span backward	4.3 (±1.5)	3.5 (±1.0)	2.9 (±1.3)[aaa]	2.8 (±1.3)[aaa]	2.9 (±1.1)[a]
K-BNT	48.5 (±7.5)	40.6 (±9.3)[aa]	35.0 (±12.5)[aaa]	36.5 (±10.1)[aaa]	30.6 (±11.7)[aaab]
RCFT copy	32.2 (±5.0)	29.9 (±5.2)	23.8 (±11.4)[aab]	23.4 (±9.9)[aaabb]	21.4 (±10.9)[aab]
SVLT delayed	7.4 (±2.0)	2.5 (±2.4)[aaa]	1.0 (±1.9)[aaab]	0.6 (±1.1)[aaabbb]	0.4 (±1.3)[aaab]
RCFT delayed	15.0 (±3.9)	7.9 (±5.2)[aaa]	2.6 (±2.8)[aaabbb]	1.7 (±3.0)[aaabbb]	1.1 (±1.9)[aaabbb]
Contrasting program	19.9 (±0.2)	19.7 (±1.4)	18.4 (±4.5)	15.4 (±7.2)[aaabbb]	11.4 (±8.6)[aaabbbccc]
Go/NoGo test	19.6 (±1.1)	18.7 (±3.1)	16.1 (±5.3)	12.0 (±6.7)[aaabbbcc]	8.2 (±6.7)[aaabbbccc]
Stroop test color reading	87.7 (±23.3)	73.8 (±23.9)	48.8 (±29.5)[aaabbb]	39.5 (±25.1)[aaabbb]	20.6 (±16.0)[aaabbbc]
MMSE	28.6 (±1.9)	26.5 (±2.2)[a]	22.4 (±3.9)[aaabbb]	19.6 (±4.0)[aaabbbcc]	17.0 (±3.4)[aaabbbccc]
CDR sum of boxes (SNSB)	0.7 (±0.5)	1.3 (±0.8)	3.1 (±1.3)[aaabbb]	5.2 (±1.4)[aaabbbccc]	10.8 (±1.9)[aaabbbcccddd]
COWAT semantic	32.4 (±7.5)	24.4 (±7.5)[aaa]	21.4 (±6.9)[aaa]	18.2 (±6.9)[aaabbb]	12.9 (±5.3)[aaabbbc]
COWAT phonemic	28.1 (±10.8)	18.4 (±9.7)[aaa]	17.6 (±11.1)[aaa]	13.5 (±8.3)[aaa]	11.8 (±8.8)[aaa]

ANOVA and post-hoc analysis was performed.
Significantly different when compared to normal (a: $p < 0.05$, aa: $p < 0.01$, aaa: $p < 0.001$).
Compared to aMCI (b: $p < 0.05$, bb: $p < 0.01$, bbb: $p < 0.001$).
Compared to AD CDR 0.5 (c: $p < 0.05$, cc: $p < 0.01$, ccc: $p < 0.001$).
Compared to AD CDR 1 (ddd: $p < 0.001$).

path length. In contrast, no significant correlations were found between neuropsychological test performances and network measures in the CDR 1 and CDR 2 groups. All significant results were negative correlations (except those found in the CDR 0.5 group) and are shown in **Table 2** and Supplementary Table 2. In addition, we performed the same analysis for all subjects and found a significant negative correlation of the COWAT semantic score with network topologies (betweenness centrality, characteristic path length, and clustering coefficient, $p < 0.05$, uncorrected, Supplementary Table 3).

Next, we examined whether the changes in the network properties of each lobe were reflected in whole-brain topology as AD progresses. For each of the three network measures, global, and local efficiency and betweenness centrality, the bilateral temporal lobe and right subcortex showed a non-monotonic reorganization with AD progression (**Figure 2**). Particularly, the left frontal lobe exhibited this reorganization pattern for global efficiency and betweenness centrality, whereas the left subcortex exhibited this reorganization with respect to local efficiency and betweenness (**Figure 2**). In addition, the right frontal and parietal lobes displayed similar non-monotonic reorganization only for betweenness centrality.

We determined if there were significant changes in lobar network properties among AD groups. For global efficiency, the right parietal lobe showed significantly lower efficiency in the CDR 0.5 and CDR 2 groups compared to the HS group ($p < 0.05$), and the right temporal lobe showed an higher in the CDR 1 group compared with the CDR 0.5 group ($p < 0.05$). For local efficiency, the right parietal lobe showed lower efficiency in the aMCI compared to the HS group ($p < 0.05$), and the right temporal lobe was higher in the CDR 1 group compared to its preceding group, CDR 0.5 ($p < 0.05$). In left hemisphere, the temporal lobe was higher in the aMCI and CDR 1 groups compared to the HS and CDR 0.5 groups, respectively ($p < 0.05$). All significant results are shown in **Figure 2**. Other network properties, i.e., the characteristic path length, clustering coefficient, modularity, and assortativity, also exhibited a similar pattern of change with AD progression (see Supplementary Figure 2).

Lastly, we examined the rich-club organization of the brain networks with AD progression. **Figures 3A–D**) shows the rich-club coefficient, normalized rich-club coefficient, number of nodes, and number of edges as a function of degree threshold k from 1 to 15 for AD patients in different CDR stages and HS. For k-values larger than 9, the largest normalized rich-club coefficient was observed in the HS group, followed by the CDR 1 group. The remaining groups showed similar normalized rich-club coefficients within a range of 1–1.5. For k-values equal to 9, the aMCI and CDR 1 groups exhibited higher original and normalized rich-club coefficients and a greater number of links within the rich-club organization relative to the other AD stages.

We observed varying distribution patterns of rich-club nodes for the degree threshold $k = 9$ across AD stages (**Figure 3E**). For a k of 9, the numbers of nodes of the rich-clubs were 21, 28, 25, 22, and 25, and the numbers of edges were 68, 124, 70, 93, and 88 from the HS to the CDR 2 group. The original rich-club coefficients for $k = 9$ were 0.32, 0.33, 0.23, 0.4, and 0.29, and the normalized rich-club coefficients were 1.41, 1.42, 1.05, 1.76, and 1.30 from the HS to the CDR 2 group. The rich-club coefficients of the original and normalized values and the number of edges within the rich-club varied non-monotonically, similar to the change of the whole brain network properties as AD progresses. Within the rich-club core of the brain, frontal regions were not connected with posterior regions in the HS group. In contrast, in the aMCI group, the rich-club consisted of an increased number of frontal regions, and those were well-connected with the other

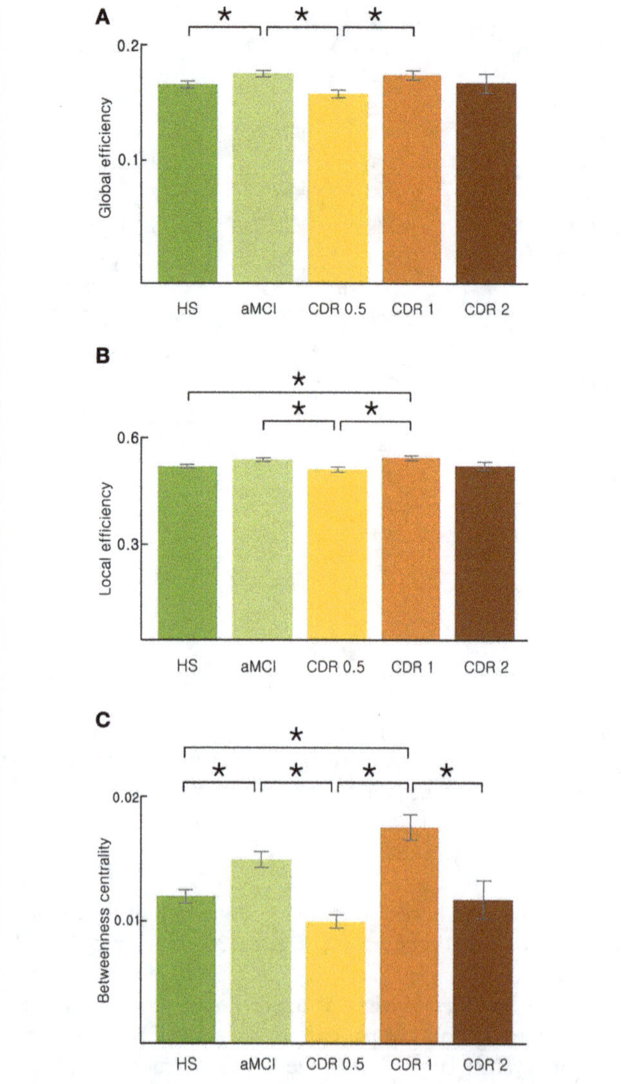

FIGURE 1 | Topological properties of the AD brain networks with the disease progression. (A) Global efficiency, **(B)** local efficiency, and **(C)** betweenness centrality changed stage-specifically in a non-monotonic manner. Significance is represented by an asterisk ($p < 0.05$, ANOVA and *post-hoc*).

posterior (parietal and occipital) regions. Interestingly, these frontal regions and their connectivity gradually decreased and disappeared in the CDR 1 group before increasing again in the CDR 2 group.

Discussion

We investigated changes in network properties from HS to subjects with prodromal and intermediate stages of AD by comparing topological measures of the brain network and determining their relationship with behavioral and clinical test scores. The current study first examined the whole process of alterations in brain networks from the time before AD onset to a severe AD stage. To properly examine and compare the topological reorganization of the brain network, it was necessary to construct networks with similar size. In the current study, we constructed a brain network with the same density (sparsity), avoiding the use of a specific threshold value. Because the density network contains the same number of edges, we were able to compare brain networks of the same size among groups.

We demonstrated the ongoing reorganization process of the brain network with AD progression. However, we did not observe a correlation between any network measure and clinical deterioration, e.g., CDR. Unexpectedly, this reorganization occurred stage-specifically in a non-monotonic manner (**Figure 1** and Supplementary Figure 1). It has been proposed that the progression of AD follows a sigmoidal curve (Jack and Holtzman, 2013). However, the smooth progressive change in each parameter is rather presumptive and mainly based on interpolation or extrapolation of limited evidence. Given the five stages of AD progression, we revealed that network topological properties, including network efficiency and betweenness centrality, were higher in the aMCI and CDR 1 groups compared to other AD groups or HS. First, the brain network in the aMCI group exhibited significantly higher efficiency compared to that of the previous stage, the HS group. Higher network efficiency and betweenness centrality would result from the presence of additional hub regions. In addition, the results from the correlation analysis between neuropsychological test scores and network properties support a stage-specific non-monotonicity. We found that correlations between neuropsychological scores

TABLE 2 | Correlation between network properties and clinical information within each group ($p < 0.05$, uncorrected, $p/R^2/r$).

		Global efficiency	Local efficiency	Betweenness centrality
HS	Stroop test color-reading correct	0.035/0.145/−0.381	–	0.025/0.162/−0.402
aMCI	Digit span backward	–	–	0.028/0.096/−0.310
	Naming K-BNT	–	0.021/0.106/−0.325	0.022/0.104/−0.323
	RCFT copy	–	0.028/0.096/−0.310	–
	Go/NoGo	–	0.010/0.131/−0.361	0.025/0.100/−0.317
	COWAT semantic	0.029/0.096/−0.310	0.010/0.131/−0.361	0.010/0.132/−0.363
AD CDR 0.5	COWAT phonemic	–	–	0.031/0.187/0.433

HS, healthy subject; aMCI, amnestic mild cognitive impairment; AD, Alzheimer's disease; CDR, clinical dementia rating.
R^2: goodness of fit by coefficient of determination; r: Person's correlation coefficient.

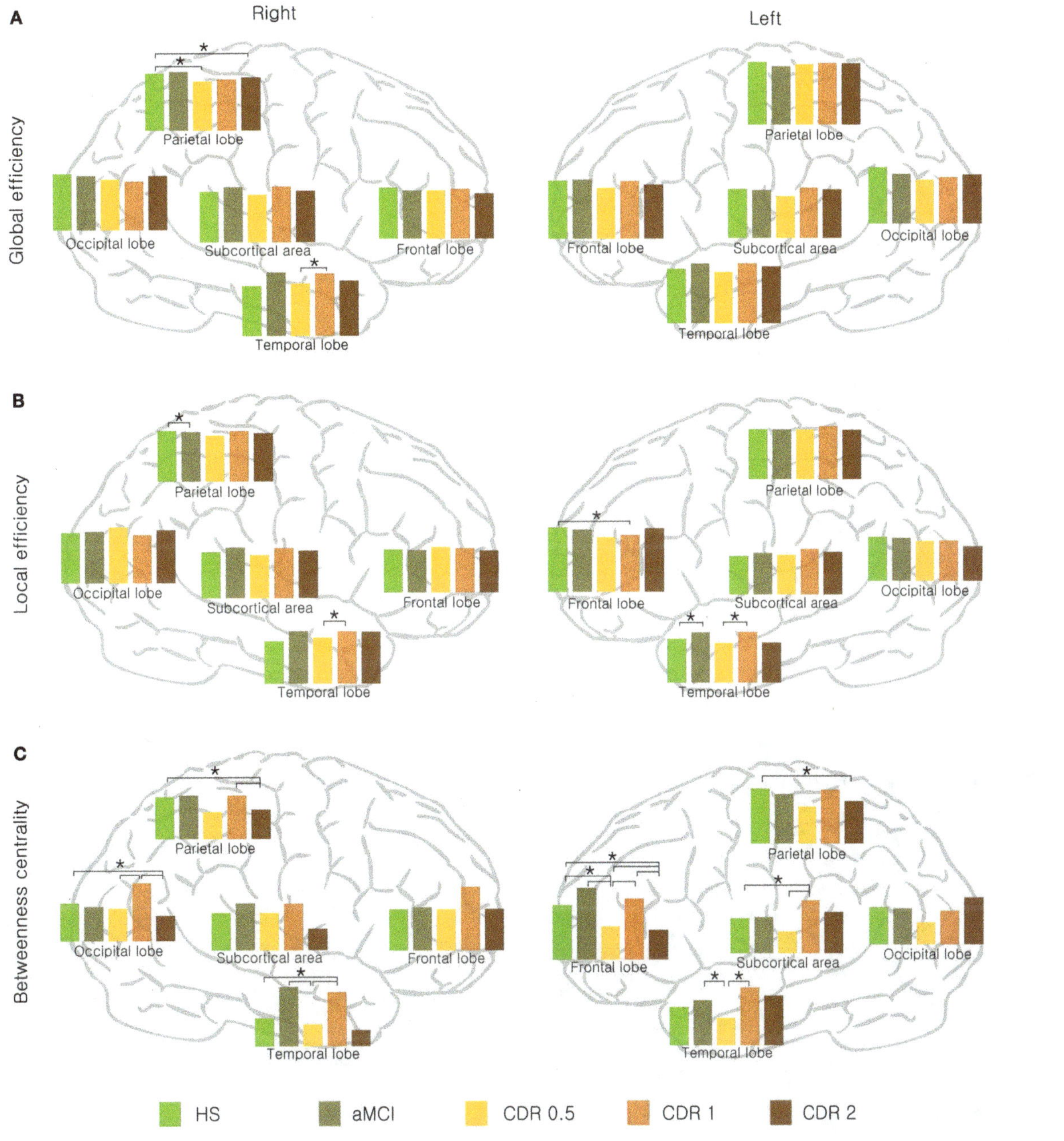

FIGURE 2 | Lobar network properties with AD progression. (A) Global efficiency, **(B)** local efficiency, and **(C)** betweenness centrality changed stage-specifically in a non-monotonic manner. Significance is represented by an asterisk ($p < 0.05$, ANOVA and *post-hoc*).

and network properties were distinguishable among each group of AD progression (**Table 2**, and Supplementary Tables 2, 3). The speculation for this finding is described in Supplementary Material.

It is interesting and unusual that an advanced disease stage has higher network efficiency than a previous stage. We speculate that this finding is in line with previous studies reporting hyperactivation in the hippocampus and other memory-related areas during cognitive and memory-related tasks in MCI patients (Dickerson et al., 2005; Hämäläinen et al., 2007) compared to HS and AD patients. In addition to the task-induced activation, increased resting state connectivity in aMCI patients compared to HS has also been reported (Sohn et al., 2014). Another study demonstrated that MCI patients exhibiting faster cognitive decline have greater hippocampal activation (Miller et al., 2008). Given that the resting state connectivity and the brain activation show a positive correlation with each other (Mennes et al., 2011), our result of increased brain network efficiency in aMCI patients is consistent with the aforementioned studies. The reorganization process of the rich-club core with AD progression is speculated

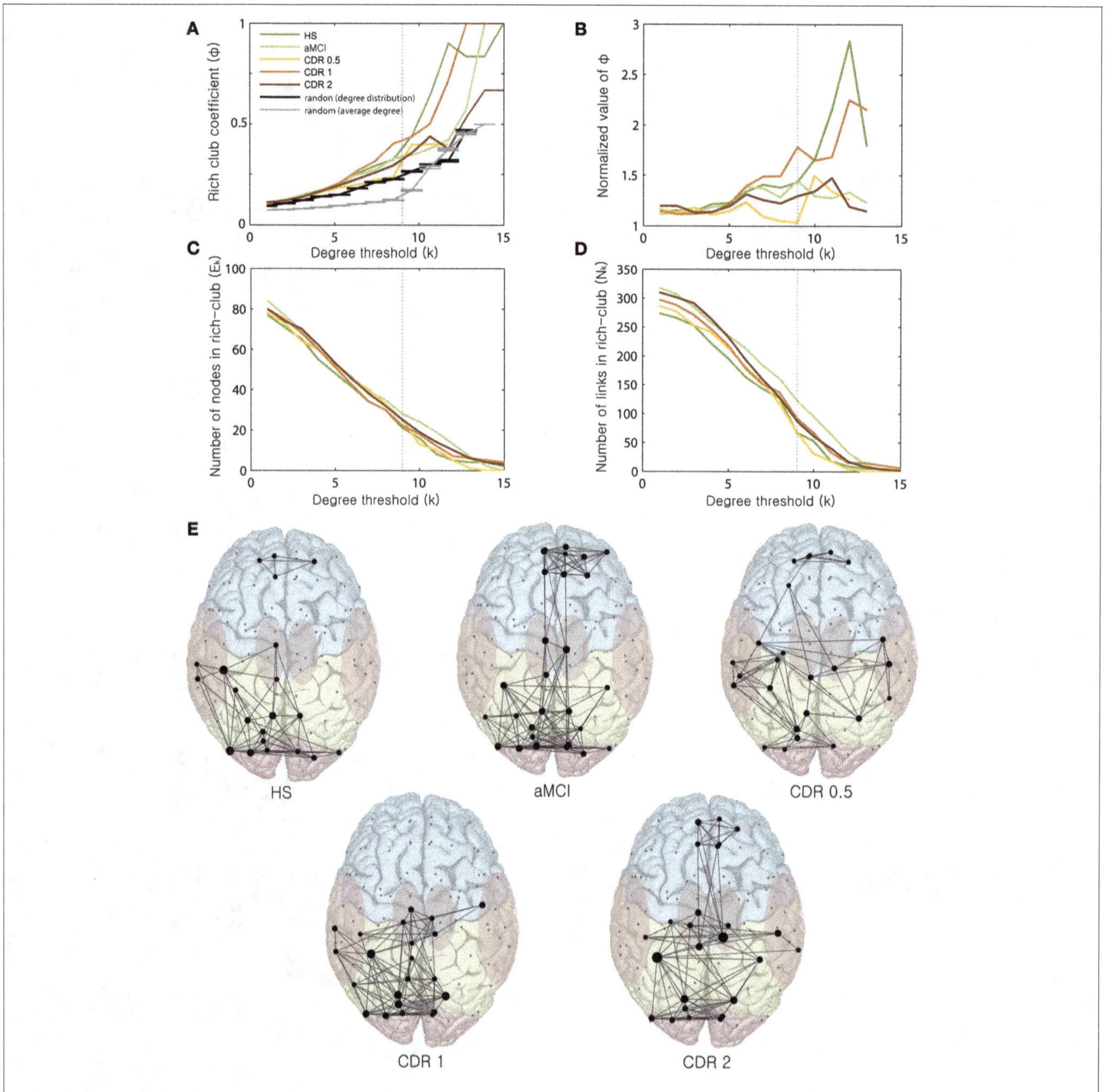

FIGURE 3 | Changes in rich-club organization as a function of k. Changes of the **(A)** rich-club coefficient, **(B)** normalized rich-club coefficient, **(C)** number of nodes within the rich-club, and **(D)** number of links within the rich-club are displayed with varying k-values ranging from 0 to 15. **(E)** Rich-club organization with AD progression. Representative networks for each stage are shown for $k = 9$.

in detail with other possibilities and scenarios of non-monotonic changes in AD brain networks in Supplementary Material.

We should be cautious in interpreting the results, because there are several limitations and ambiguous outcomes from these analyses. Moreover, we should note that these results appear to contrast with those of other previous studies. Based on this discrepancy, it is likely uncertain whether the non-monotonic changes in network parameters are generated by disease progression or not. We also mention that the mechanisms underlying the connections between network parameters and disease progression are not clear, because the parameters tended to be non-monotonic. Another recent study showed increasing path length and decreasing small-worldness of the density network with AD progression (Sun et al., 2014). This can be seen as opposite contrasting result with our study, although that study used different group stratification and different measurements of network construction compared with this study. We chose mutual information as a measure of functional connectivity, whereas the most common measure is the Pearson's correlation coefficient. The Pearson's correlation provides information about the linear relationship between regions but does not detect non-linear interactions among regions. Therefore, as an alternative approach that accounts for non-linear interactions, we used mutual information to construct the information transmission network of the brain. However, the path length used in the current study showed a mildly significant increase with the disease progression, whereas Sun et al. showed some regional betweenness centrality changes in non-monotonic values with disease progression. This discrepancy in the results between the studies using similar data and methods suggest that other elements may influence these network properties and indicate our limited understanding of the innate causal relationship between network parameters and AD. Based on these potential explanations for the observed non-monotonic network parameter changes in the current study, the possibility that our conclusions are incorrect or produced from other influences may not be excluded.

Rich-club organization also plays an unclear role in these results. Differences in rich-club network structure were observed not only between the groups exhibiting significantly different network parameters but also between groups exhibiting similar values. This makes our results difficult to interpret because the innate cause of rich-club structure changes remains still unclear. We should admit that the *post-hoc* analysis did not produce significant results in the analysis of lobar parameters. Because of the insufficient number of subjects in some groups, it is likely assumed that the lobar parameters are independent of each other. The *post-hoc* tests were calculated only for group dependency. This limitation suggests that we should interpret our major finding of the non-monotonic changes in the lobar parameters with extreme caution. In addition, we noted that HS, aMCI and AD severity in each CDR category were continuous variables in this analysis; however, since this study was a cross-sectional study, a longitudinal analysis is required to investigate the changes in each patient over time. The diagnoses of AD and aMCI were based on clinical criteria without any pathological or amyloid imaging data. Thus, dementia of other origins may have been included in these diagnoses, particularly aMCI. The large number of excluded subjects due to age-matching and abnormal correlation values between regions is another limitation of this study.

The change of brain network by AD progression and the innate principles are not fully uncovered. The diverse and even opposed results are reported through attempting various methods and measurements. This can be a good time to investigate this issue more seriously to find the causal relationship between brain network and disease progress of AD.

Acknowledgments

This research was supported by Basic Science Research Program through the National Research Foundation of Korea (NRF) funded by the Ministry of Education (NRF-2012R1A1A2044776), the Brain Research Program through the National Research Foundation of Korea (NRF) funded by the Ministry of Science, ICT and Future Planning (NRF-2010-0018843), the Basic Science Program through the National Research Foundation of Korea (NRF) funded by the Ministry of Education (NRF-2006-2005399), and the Brain Research Program through the National Research Foundation of Korea (NRF) funded by the Ministry of Science, ICT and Future Planning (NRF-2013R1A1A2011570).

References

Achard, S., Salvador, R., Whitcher, B., Suckling, J., and Bullmore, E. (2006). A resilient, low-frequency, small-world human brain functional network with highly connected association cortical hubs. *J. Neurosci.* 26, 63–72. doi: 10.1523/JNEUROSCI.3874-05.2006

Bai, F., Xie, C., Watson, D. R., Shi, Y., Yuan, Y., Wang, Y., et al. (2011). Aberrant hippocampal subregion networks associated with the classifications of aMCI subjects: a longitudinal resting-state study. *PLoS ONE* 6:e29288. doi: 10.1371/journal.pone.0029288

Bianchetti, A., and Trabucchi, M. (2001). Clinical aspects of Alzheimer's disease. *Aging Clin. Exp. Res.* 13, 221–230. doi: 10.1007/BF03351480

Boyle, P. A., Wilson, R. S., Aggarwal, N. T., Tang, Y., and Bennett, D. A. (2006). Mild cognitive impairment: risk of Alzheimer disease and rate of cognitive decline. *Neurology* 67, 441–445. doi: 10.1212/01.wnl.0000228244.10416.20

Braak, H., and Braak, E. (1991). Neuropathological stageing of Alzheimer-related changes. *Acta Neuropathol.* 82, 239–259. doi: 10.1007/BF00308809

Bullmore, E., and Sporns, O. (2009). Complex brain networks: graph theoretical analysis of structural and functional systems. *Nat. Rev. Neurosci.* 10, 186–198. doi: 10.1038/nrn2575

Celone, K. A., Calhoun, V. D., Dickerson, B. C., Atri, A., Chua, E. F., Miller, S. L., et al. (2006). Alterations in memory networks in mild cognitive impairment and Alzheimer's disease: an independent component analysis. *J. Neurosci.* 26, 10222–10231. doi: 10.1523/JNEUROSCI.2250-06.2006

Colizza, V., Flammini, A., Serrano, M. A., and Vespignani, A. (2006). Detecting rich-club ordering in complex networks. *Nat. Phys.* 2, 110–115. doi: 10.1038/nphys209

Delbeuck, X., van der Linden, M., and Collette, F. (2003). Alzheimer' Disease as a Disconnection Syndrome? *Neuropsychol. Rev.* 13, 79–92. doi: 10.1023/A:1023832305702

Della-Maggiore, V., Chau, W., Peres-Neto, P. R., and McIntosh, A. R. (2002). An empirical comparison of SPM preprocessing parameters to the analysis of fMRI data. *Neuroimage* 17, 19–28. doi: 10.1006/nimg.2002.1113

Dickerson, B., Salat, D., Greve, D., Chua, E., Rand-Giovannetti, E., Rentz, D., et al. (2005). Increased hippocampal activation in mild cognitive impairment compared to normal aging and AD. *Neurology* 65, 404–411. doi: 10.1212/01.wnl.0000171450.97464.49

Fischer, P., Jungwirth, S., Zehetmayer, S., Weissgram, S., Hoenigschnabl, S., Gelpi, E., et al. (2007). Conversion from subtypes of mild cognitive impairment to Alzheimer dementia. *Neurology* 68, 288–291. doi: 10.1212/01.wnl.0000252358.03285.9d

Folstein, M. F., Folstein, S. E., and McHugh, P. R. (1975). "Mini-mental state": a practical method for grading the cognitive state of patients for the clinician. *J. Psychiatr. Res.* 12, 189–198. doi: 10.1016/0022-3956(75)90026-6

Förstl, H., and Kurz, A. (1999). Clinical features of Alzheimer's disease. *Eur. Arch. Psychiatry Clin. Neurosci.* 249, 288–290. doi: 10.1007/s004060050101

Fox, N. C., Crum, W. R., Scahill, R. I., Stevens, J. M., Janssen, J. C., and Rossor, M. N. (2001). Imaging of onset and progression of Alzheimer's disease with voxel-compression mapping of serial magnetic resonance images. *Lancet* 358, 201–205. doi: 10.1016/S0140-6736(01)05408-3

Hagmann, P., Cammoun, L., Gigandet, X., Meuli, R., Honey, C. J., Wedeen, V. J., et al. (2008). Mapping the structural core of human cerebral cortex. *PLoS Biol.* 6:e159. doi: 10.1371/journal.pbio.0060159

Hämäläinen, A., Pihlajamäki, M., Tanila, H., Hänninen, T., Niskanen, E., Tervo, S., et al. (2007). Increased fMRI responses during encoding in mild cognitive impairment. *Neurobiol. Aging* 28, 1889–1903. doi: 10.1016/j.neurobiolaging.2006.08.008

Hughes, C. P., Berg, L., Danziger, W. L., Coben, L. A., and Martin, R. L. (1982). A new clinical scale for the staging of dementia. *Br. J. Psychiatry* 140, 566–572. doi: 10.1192/bjp.140.6.566

Jack, C. R. Jr., and Holtzman, D. M. (2013). Biomarker modeling of Alzheimer's disease. *Neuron* 80, 1347–1358. doi: 10.1016/j.neuron.2013.12.003

Kang, Y., and Na, D. (2003). *Seoul Neuropsychological Screening Battery*. Incheon: Human Brain Research & Consulting Co.

Kendi, A. K., Lehericy, S., Luciana, M., Ugurbil, K., and Tuite, P. (2008). Altered diffusion in the frontal lobe in Parkinson disease. *Am. J. Neuroradiol.* 29, 501–505. doi: 10.3174/ajnr.A0850

Kim, H., and Na, D. L. (1999). BRIEF REPORT normative data on the Korean version of the Boston naming test. *J. Clin. Exp. Neuropsychol.* 21, 127–133. doi: 10.1076/jcen.21.1.127.942

Lezak, M. (1983). *Neuropsychological Assessment*. New York, NY: Oxford University Press.

Lo, C.-Y., Wang, P.-N., Chou, K.-H., Wang, J., He, Y., and Lin, C.-P. (2010). Diffusion tensor tractography reveals abnormal topological organization in structural cortical networks in Alzheimer's disease. *J. Neurosci.* 30, 16876–16885. doi: 10.1523/JNEUROSCI.4136-10.2010

Maldjian, J. A., Laurienti, P. J., Kraft, R. A., and Burdette, J. H. (2003). An automated method for neuroanatomic and cytoarchitectonic atlas-based interrogatino of fMRi data sets. *Neuroimage* 19, 1233–1239. doi: 10.1016/S1053-8119(03)00169-1

McAuley, J. J., da Fontoura Costa, L., and Caetano, T. S. (2007). Rich-club phenomenon across complex network hierarchies. *Appl. Phys. Lett.* 91, 084103. doi: 10.1063/1.2773951

McKhann, G., Drachman, D., Folstein, M., Katzman, R., Price, D., and Stadlan, E. M. (1984). Clinical diagnosis of Alzheimer's disease Report of the NINCDS–ADRDA Work Group* under the auspices of department of health and human services task force on Alzheimer's disease. *Neurology* 34, 939–939. doi: 10.1212/WNL.34.7.939

Mennes, M., Zuo, X.-N., Kelly, C., Di Martino, A., Zang, Y.-F., Biswal, B., et al. (2011). Linking inter-individual differences in neural activation and behavior to intrinsic brain dynamics. *Neuroimage* 54, 2950–2959. doi: 10.1016/j.neuroimage.2010.10.046

Miller, S. L., Fenstermacher, E., Bates, J., Blacker, D., Sperling, R. A., and Dickerson, B. C. (2008). Hippocampal activation in adults with mild cognitive impairment predicts subsequent cognitive decline. *J. Neurol. Neurosurg. Psychiatry* 79, 630–635. doi: 10.1136/jnnp.2007.124149

Morris, J. C. (1993). The clinical dementia rating (CDR): current version and scoring rules. *Neurology* 43, 2412–2414. doi: 10.1212/WNL.43.11.2412-a

Petersen, R. C. (2004). Mild cognitive impairment as a diagnostic entity. *J. Intern. Med.* 256, 183–194. doi: 10.1111/j.1365-2796.2004.01388.x

Petersen, R. C., Smith, G. E., Waring, S. C., Ivnik, R. J., Tangalos, E. G., and Kokmen, E. (1999). Mild cognitive impairment: clinical characterization and outcome. *Arch. Neurol.* 56, 303–308. doi: 10.1001/archneur.56.3.303

Rubinov, M., and Sporns, O. (2010). Complex network measures of brain connectivity: uses and interpretations. *Neuroimage* 52, 1059–1069. doi: 10.1016/j.neuroimage.2009.10.003

Sanz-Arigita, E. J., Schoonheim, M. M., Damoiseaux, J. S., Rombouts, S. A., Maris, E., Barkhof, F., et al. (2010). Loss of 'small-world' networks in Alzheimer's disease: graph analysis of FMRI resting-state functional connectivity. *PLoS ONE* 5:e13788. doi: 10.1371/journal.pone.0013788

Scahill, R. I., Schott, J. M., Stevens, J. M., Rossor, M. N., and Fox, N. C. (2002). Mapping the evolution of regional atrophy in Alzheimer's disease: unbiased analysis of fluid-registered serial MRI. *Proc. Natl. Acad. Sci. U.S.A.* 99, 4703–4707. doi: 10.1073/pnas.052587399

Sohn, W. S., Yoo, K., Na, D. L., and Jeong, Y. (2014). Progressive changes in hippocampal resting-state connectivity across cognitive impairment: a cross-sectional study from normal to alzheimer disease. *Alzheimer Dis. Ass. Disord.* 28, 239–246. doi: 10.1097/WAD.0000000000000027

Stam, C., de Haan, W., Daffertshofer, A., Jones, B., Manshanden, I., van Walsum, A. V. C., et al. (2009). Graph theoretical analysis of magnetoencephalographic functional connectivity in Alzheimer's disease. *Brain* 132, 213–224. doi: 10.1093/brain/awn262

Stam, C., Jones, B., Nolte, G., Breakspear, M., and Scheltens, P. (2007). Small-world networks and functional connectivity in Alzheimer's disease. *Cereb. Cortex* 17, 92–99. doi: 10.1093/cercor/bhj127

Storey, E., Slavin, M. J., and Kinsella, G. J. (2002). Patterns of cognitive impairment in Alzheimer's disease: assessment and differential diagnosis. *Front. Biosci.* 7, e155–184. doi: 10.2741/storey

Strogatz, S. H. (2001). Exploring complex networks. *Nature* 410, 268–276. doi: 10.1038/35065725

Sun, Y., Yin, Q., Fang, R., Yan, X., Wang, Y., Bezerianos, A., et al. (2014). Disrupted functional brain connectivity and its association to structural connectivity in amnestic mild cognitive impairment and Alzheimer's disease. *PLoS ONE* 9:e96505. doi: 10.1371/journal.pone.0096505

Sunderland, T., Hampel, H., Takeda, M., Putnam, K. T., and Cohen, R. M. (2006). Biomarkers in the diagnosis of Alzheimer's disease: are we ready? *J. Geriatr. Psychiatry Neurol.* 19, 172–179. doi: 10.1177/0891988706291088

Supekar, K., Menon, V., Rubin, D., Musen, M., and Greicius, M. D. (2008). Network analysis of intrinsic functional brain connectivity in Alzheimer's disease. *PLoS Comput. Biol.* 4:e1000100. doi: 10.1371/journal.pcbi.1000100

Thompson, P. M., Hayashi, K. M., de Zubicaray, G., Janke, A. L., Rose, S. E., Semple, J., et al. (2003). Dynamics of gray matter loss in Alzheimer's disease. *J. Neurosci.* 23, 994–1005.

Tijms, B. M., Wink, A. M., de Haan, W., van der Flier, W. M., Stam, C. J., Scheltens, P., et al. (2013). Alzheimer's disease: connecting findings from graph theoretical studies of brain networks. *Neurobiol. Aging* 34, 2023–2036. doi: 10.1016/j.neurobiolaging.2013.02.020

Trojanowski, J. Q., Vandeerstichele, H., Korecka, M., Clark, C. M., Aisen, P. S., Petersen, R. C., et al. (2010). Update on the biomarker core of the Alzheimer's Disease Neuroimaging Initiative subjects. *Alzheimer Dement.* 6, 230–238. doi: 10.1016/j.jalz.2010.03.008

Tzourio-Mazoyer, N., Landeau, B., Papathanassiou, D., Crivello, F., Etard, O., Delcroix, N., et al. (2002). Automated anatomical labeling of activations in SPM using a macroscopic anatomical parcellation of the MNI MRI single-subject brain. *Neuroimage* 15, 273–289. doi: 10.1006/nimg.2001.0978

Wang, L., Zang, Y., He, Y., Liang, M., Zhang, X., Tian, L., et al. (2006). Changes in hippocampal connectivity in the early stages of Alzheimer's disease: evidence from resting state fMRI. *Neuroimage* 31, 496–504. doi: 10.1016/j.neuroimage.2005.12.033

Xie, T., and He, Y. (2011). Mapping the Alzheimer's brain with connectomics. *Front. Psychiatry* 2:77. doi: 10.3389/fpsyt.2011.00077

Yoo, K., Sohn, W. S., and Jeong, Y. (2013). Tool-use practice induces changes in intrinsic functional connectivity of parietal areas. *Front. Hum. Neurosci.* 7:49. doi: 10.3389/fnhum.2013.00049

Zhang, Y., Schuff, N., Jahng, G.-H., Bayne, W., Mori, S., Schad, L., et al. (2007). Diffusion tensor imaging of cingulum fibers in mild cognitive impairment and Alzheimer disease. *Neurology* 68, 13–19. doi: 10.1212/01.wnl.0000250326.77323.01

Zhou, Y., Dougherty J. H. Jr., Hubner, K. F., Bai, B., Cannon, R. L., and Hutson, R. K. (2008). Abnormal connectivity in the posterior cingulate and hippocampus in early Alzheimer's disease and mild cognitive impairment. *Alzheimer Dement.* 4, 265–270. doi: 10.1016/j.jalz.2008.04.006

11

Effects of Cognitive Training on Resting-State Functional Connectivity of Default Mode, Salience, and Central Executive Networks

Weifang Cao[1†], Xinyi Cao[2†], Changyue Hou[1], Ting Li[3], Yan Cheng[2], Lijuan Jiang[2], Cheng Luo[1], Chunbo Li[2,4,5*] and Dezhong Yao[1]*

[1] Key Laboratory for NeuroInformation of Ministry of Education, Center for Information in Medicine, High-Field Magnetic Resonance Brain Imaging Key Laboratory of Sichuan Province, School of Life Science and Technology, University of Electronic Science and Technology of China, Chengdu, China, [2] Shanghai Key Laboratory of Psychotic Disorders, Shanghai Mental Health Center, Shanghai Jiao Tong University School of Medicine, Shanghai, China, [3] Shanghai Changning Mental Health Center, Shanghai, China, [4] Bio-X Institutes, Key Laboratory for the Genetics of Developmental and Neuropsychiatric Disorders, Ministry of Education, Shanghai Jiao Tong University, Shanghai, China, [5] Brain Science and Technology Research Center, Shanghai Jiao Tong University, Shanghai, China

Edited by:
Alessio Avenanti,
Alma Mater Studiorum – University of Bologna, Italy

Reviewed by:
Antonio Gallo,
Second University of Naples, Italy
Jason S. Nomi,
University of Miami, USA

***Correspondence:**
Cheng Luo
chengluo@uestc.edu.cn;
Chunbo Li
chunbo_li@163.com

† These authors have contributed equally to this work.

Neuroimaging studies have documented that aging can disrupt certain higher cognitive systems such as the default mode network (DMN), the salience network and the central executive network (CEN). The effect of cognitive training on higher cognitive systems remains unclear. This study used a 1-year longitudinal design to explore the cognitive training effect on three higher cognitive networks in healthy older adults. The community-living healthy older adults were divided into two groups: the multi-domain cognitive training group (24 sessions of cognitive training over a 3-months period) and the wait-list control group. All subjects underwent cognitive measurements and resting-state functional magnetic resonance imaging scanning at baseline and at 1 year after the training ended. We examined training-related changes in functional connectivity (FC) within and between three networks. Compared with the baseline, we observed maintained or increased FC within all three networks after training. The scans after training also showed maintained anti-correlation of FC between the DMN and CEN compared to the baseline. These findings demonstrated that cognitive training maintained or improved the functional integration within networks and the coupling between the DMN and CEN in older adults. Our findings suggested that multi-domain cognitive training can mitigate the aging-related dysfunction of higher cognitive networks.

Keywords: aging, cognitive training, resting-state fMRI, functional connectivity, brain network

INTRODUCTION

As people age, they experience cognitive decline, which involves working memory, executive function and attention, among other functions, and this occurs with particular frequency in late life, resulting in an increasingly poor quality of life (Hedden and Gabrieli, 2004; Grady, 2012). To postpone the cognitive decline associated with aging, increasing numbers of studies have conducted interventions with older adults, focusing on cognitive training and physical exercise (Park and Bischof, 2013; Tanigawa et al., 2014). Results of neuropsychological studies have demonstrated benefits of cognitive functions after interventions in old adults, including improvements in working memory capacity, reasoning, and processing speed (Neely and Backman, 1995; Oswald et al., 2006; Bamidis et al., 2015; Leung et al., 2015). Our previous study has also demonstrated that the effects of interventions on cognition are maintained at 1 year after the training ended (Cheng et al., 2012). On the other hand, neuroimaging studies have proved that multi-domain training affects the spontaneous brain activity in healthy older adults, for example, altered regional homogeneity of spontaneous fluctuations in temporal gyrus and cerebellum, enhanced amplitude of low frequency fluctuations in frontal gyrus and cerebellum (Yin et al., 2014; Zheng et al., 2015). In another study, improved memory performance during memory task after training has been shown to associate with increased brain activation in the prefrontal, temporal, and parietal area in older adults (Kirchhoff et al., 2012). Also, the reduction in functional connection (FC) between the superior parietal cortex and inferior temporal lobe is observed after training in older adults, which is associated with training success (Strenziok et al., 2014). These findings suggest that the interventions bring about not only enhanced behavioral outcomes but improvement of the brain function in older adults (Kraft, 2012; Bamidis et al., 2014).

Recent studies suggest that functional brain networks, a higher level of organization of brain regions, are needed to better understand improved cognitive function after intervention (Langer et al., 2013; Bamidis et al., 2014). Using functional magnetic resonance imaging (fMRI), more than ten functional brain networks constituted of spatially distinct brain regions have been identified either at specific tasks (Calhoun et al., 2009) or at rest, including the default mode network (DMN), the salience network (SN) and the central executive network (CEN; Smith et al., 2009; Luo et al., 2012). Three (DMN, SN, and CEN) of these stable networks have been considered the 'core' neurocognitive networks for understanding higher cognitive functions and have received the most attention in cognitive studies (Sridharan et al., 2008; Bressler and Menon, 2010; Luo et al., 2011, 2014b). The DMN, which includes mainly the posterior cingulate cortex (PCC), medial prefrontal cortex (MPFC) and inferior parietal lobe (IPL), is involved in self-referential and autobiographical memory functions (Raichle et al., 2001; Buckner et al., 2008). The SN includes the bilateral anterior insula (AI) and dorsal anterior cingulate cortex, and it is associated with detecting internal and external events salient to homeostasis. In contrast, the CEN, composed of the dorsolateral frontal and parietal neocortices, is engaged in cognitively demanding tasks, such as decision making and working memory (Seeley et al., 2007). Many studies have indicated that these three networks, along with the disruption of FC within network and the anti-correlation between the DMN and CEN, are strongly affected by normal aging and Alzheimer's disease, which is associated with cognitive impairments (Meunier et al., 2009; Wu et al., 2011; Onoda et al., 2012; Tomasi and Volkow, 2012; Cao et al., 2014).

Previous studies have shown that brain networks are affected by interventions, such as the DMN and CEN, associated with improved behavioral outcomes and cognitive performances (Patel et al., 2013; Bamidis et al., 2014; Luo et al., 2014a; Tang and Posner, 2014). For instance, intervention studies, including either cognitive or physical training, reveal changes in the resting-state FC within the DMN and CEN in healthy adults (Voss et al., 2010, 2013; Taylor et al., 2013). Interventions have also been conducted on older adults to investigate the changes in brain networks that subserve cognitive function (Voss et al., 2010; Bamidis et al., 2014; Luo et al., 2016). A study of multimodal intervention in older adults has shown improved resting-state FC between the MPFC and medial temporal lobe in the DMN after training, suggesting an association with better cognitive performance (Li et al., 2014). Increases in cerebral blood flow and resting-state FC within the DMN and CEN are also observed after complex cognitive training in healthy seniors (Chapman et al., 2015). In addition, a study also demonstrated the decreased FC between the DMN and CEN after working memory training in health adults (Takeuchi et al., 2013). These findings suggest that training can affect FC of certain brain networks, such as DMN, CEN. However, no study has investigated the effects of multi-domain cognitive training on resting-state FC within and among the three networks (DMN, SN, and CEN) in older adults.

The purpose of this study is to explore the effects of cognitive training on resting-state FCs within and between the three networks in old adults. We hypothesized that multi-domain cognitive training would result in changes of resting-state FC within and among the three networks in healthy older adults, which might be beneficial for counteracting decreased integration within network and impaired coupling between networks with aging. In our work, we investigated the resting-state FC of three networks using seed-based FC analysis at baseline and at 1 year after training ended. The relationship between cognitive improvements and the changes of FC was also analyzed.

MATERIALS AND METHODS

Participants

The current work included 40 healthy older adults from two randomized groups [the multi-domain training group ($n = 23$) and the control group ($n = 17$)], who were recruited through a dispatched notice/broadcasting by the local institute of community service in three community centers around Tongji Hospital in Shanghai from March 2008 to April 2008. After a personal interview with professional interviewers, all participants then underwent cognitive measurements and fMRI scanning. The inclusion criteria included the following: age (65–75 years); educational year (more than 1 year); normal hearing, vision, or communication status; normal functional capacity; living independently in the community; score on the Chinese version of the Mini-Mental State Examination (MMSE) of 19 or above [the lower cut-off point of the MMSE score is due to the lower educational level in China (Li et al., 2006)]; and being free of neurological or psychiatric disorders and of brain injury. Exclusion criteria included the following: obvious cognitive decline, a diagnosis of AD; serious neurological or psychiatric disorders such as major depressive disorder, brain cancer, and schizophrenia. One left-handed subject in the multi-domain training group was included due to the absence of a relationship between the training-related changes and handedness (Mackey et al., 2013). This study was approved by the Ethical Committee of the East China Normal University. All participants gave written informed consent, and they were not provided monetary compensation for their participation in this study.

Neuropsychological Measurements

Interventions

Cognitive training employed a randomized, controlled design. The multi-domain training group was divided into a small group, and the training procedure took place in a classroom in Tongji Hospital. All participants received 24 sessions of cognitive training over a 3-months period at a frequency of twice a week. The multi-domain cognitive training targeted memory, reasoning, and problem-solving strategies using approaches such as visual-spatial map reading, handcraft making, healthy living, and physical exercise. Each session lasted 60 min. A lecture about a common disease in aging people was presented during the first 15 min of each session. Then, the trainer taught the participants about a special cognitive strategy or technique via slide lecture during the second 30 min. The newly practiced skills were consolidated by dealing with some real-life problems during the last 15 min. The wait-list control group served as a match for the social contact associated with cognitive training. The multi-domain training group and the control group attended a lecture about healthy living every 2 months. More details about the training are provided in our previous study (Cheng et al., 2012).

Cognitive Measurements

To evaluate the effects of intervention on cognitive function, composite outcome measurements were created, including the Repeatable Battery for the Assessment of Neuropsychological Status (RBANS, Form A), which shows good validity and reliability in a Chinese community-living elderly sample (Lim et al., 2010; Cheng et al., 2011), the trail-making test (TMT; Ashendorf et al., 2008), the visual reasoning test (Xiao et al., 2002) and the Color Word Stroop test (CWST; van Boxtel et al., 2001). All measurements were conducted at baseline and at 1 year after training.

To examine the effect of cognitive training on cognition, we compared the pre- and post-training changes between the multi-domain cognitive group and the control group using one-way analyses of covariance (ANCOVAs) with the differences between the 1-year post-test and baseline measurements as dependent variables and scores at baseline as covariates to exclude the possibility that any pre-existing difference in the measures between the groups affected the results of each measure ($p < 0.05$). In addition, two-sample t-tests were applied to investigate the differences in cognition measurements at baseline between the two groups. The confounding covariates, including age, gender and education years, were regressed in all statistical analyses.

Data Acquisition

All functional and structural imaging data were acquired using a Siemens 3T MRI scanner (Erlangen, Germany) at East China Normal University, Shanghai, China. All participants underwent scanning twice, at baseline and at 1 year after training. To minimize head motion, we fixed the subjects' heads using foam pads. Resting-state functional images were collected using a single-shot, gradient-recalled echo planar imaging sequence [repetition time (TR) = 2000 ms, echo time (TE) = 25 ms and flip angle (FA) = 90°, field of view (FOV) = 240 mm × 240 mm, in-plane matrix = 64 × 64, slice thickness = 5 mm, voxel size = 3.75 mm × 3.75 mm × 5 mm], generating 32 slices. The functional scanning lasted for 310 s, yielding a total of 155 volumes. To ensure magnetic field stabilization, the first five volumes were discarded. During the resting-state scanning, the subjects were asked to lie with their eyes closed, not to fall asleep, and not to think of anything in particular. Axial T1-weighted anatomical images were acquired using a magnetisation-prepared rapid gradient-echo sequence, generating 160 slices (TR = 1900 ms, TE = 3.43 ms, FA = 90°, matrix size = 256 × 256, FOV = 240 mm × 240 mm, slice thickness = 1 mm, voxel size = 0.9375 mm × 0.9375 mm × 1 mm).

Data Preprocessing

Resting-State fMRI Data

Imaging data preprocessing was performed using the SPM8 software package[1]. First, all imaging data were corrected for the slice-timing and realigned for head movement correction. Accounting for the effect of head motion on the FC analysis, we excluded all the participants whose head movement exceeded 1 mm or 1°. Furthermore, we also calculated the framewise displacement (FD) given by

$$FD_i = \left|\Delta d_{ix}\right| + \left|\Delta d_{iy}\right| + \left|\Delta d_{iz}\right| + |\Delta\alpha_i| + |\Delta\beta_i| + |\Delta\gamma_i|, \quad (1)$$

where i is the i-th time point and

$$\Delta d_{ix} = d_{(i-1)x} - d_{ix}(similarly for d_{iy}, d_{iz}, \alpha_i, \beta_i, \gamma_i). \quad (2)$$

The FD_0 was set to zero and rotational displacements were converted from degrees to millimeters (Power et al., 2012). Then, the resulting functional data were normalized to the Montreal Neurological Institute (MNI) template using a 12-parameter affine transformation (resampled to 3 mm × 3 mm × 3 mm). Finally, the imaging data were spatially smoothed with a 6-mm full-width at half maximum (FWHM) Gaussian kernel. We applied a temporal band-pass filter (the frequency range of 0.01 and 0.08 Hz) to reduce the low frequency drift and high frequency physiological noise (Fox et al., 2005; Jiang et al., 2015; Luo et al., 2015). Several nuisance covariates including white matter (WM) signal, cerebrospinal fluid (CSF) signal, global signal, and six head motion parameters were also removed from the time course of all brain voxels using a multiple linear regression analysis.

[1]http://www.fil.ion.ucl.ac.uk/spm/

Preprocessing of T1-Weighted Images

Previous studies provided the evidence of the loss of gray matter volume (GMV) with aging and of the potential effects on the functional results (Damoiseaux et al., 2008). In the present study, we increased the reliability of resting-state fMRI analysis by controlling for the GMV. The T1-weighted images were preprocessed using the voxel-based morphometry (VBM8[2]) toolbox in SPM8. The native T1-weighted image was normalized to MNI space using an exponentiated lie algebra (DARTEL) approach. The resulting images were then segmented into gray matter (GM), WM and CSF. For each subject, the GMV of the whole brain was calculated.

Functional Connectivity Analysis

To evaluate our hypothesis, a seed-based FC analysis was performed to examine the training effect on FC within and between the DMN, SN, and CEN. Three seeds were selected based on previous studies: the PCC (0, −52, 20), the right AI (38, 26, −10) and the right dorsolateral prefrontal cortex [right DLPFC (44, 36, 20)] to constitute the DMN, SN, and CEN, respectively (Fransson, 2006; Seeley et al., 2007; Luo et al., 2011). The average signal of spherical regions with nine-millimeter diameter centered at the three seeds was extracted. The FC map for each network was obtained by calculating Pearson correlation coefficient between the average time course of seed and each voxel in the whole brain for each subject. A Fisher z-transformation was used to convert the correlation coefficient of each voxel to a normal distribution (Shao et al., 2012; Chen et al., 2015). Thus, the individual z-score maps were obtained for each seed and subject. A one-sample t-test was used to identify the within-group FC map for each network. The significance level was set at $p < 0.05$ (FDR-corrected, cluster size > 621 mm^3).

Statistical Analysis

To evaluate the training effect on FC within and between the three networks, a whole-brain voxel-wise 2 (between-subject factor: training and control groups) × 2 (within-subject factor: baseline and 1-year after training ending) repeated analysis of variance (ANOVA) was performed using the explicit mask from the union set of the one-sample t-test results of three networks, by controlling for the whole brain GMV, as well as age, gender, education years and FD as confounding covariates. This analysis was performed using SPM8, and the significance level was set at $p < 0.05$ (cluster size > 621 mm^3). *Post hoc* comparisons (paired t-tests) were carried out for each significant interaction effect to clarify the effect of training on FC for each group.

Neural Correlate Analysis

To explore the relationship between FC and cognitive measurements, z-transformed connectivity values were extracted from regions that showed significant training-related effect, and the difference between the baseline and post-test was computed. Partial correlations were performed between the changes of resting-state FC and the pre- and post-training differences in the scores on the cognitive measures, while controlling for age, gender, and education years.

[2]http://dbm.neuro.uni-jena.de/

RESULTS

Demographic and Neuropsychological Tests

At baseline, 23 subjects (one left-handed) from the multi-domain training group and 17 subjects from the control group underwent cognitive measurements and the fMRI scanning. Eighteen subjects in the multi-domain training group and 14 in the control group finished both the cognitive measurements and the fMRI scanning at 1 year after the intervention, and they were involved in the final analysis. A total of eight participants withdrew (one death, two cancers, one operation, and four rejecting scanning). No significant differences in age, gender, education years, FD and MMSE score were found between the multi-domain training group and the control group ($p > 0.05$; **Table 1**).

No significant differences in all cognitive measurements were found at baseline between the two groups ($p > 0.05$; **Table 2**). However, the multi-domain training group showed significant improvements in performance on language ($p = 0.036$) and delayed memory ($p = 0.027$) and marginally significant improvement on the RBANS total score ($p = 0.058$) at 1-year after training compared to the baseline (**Table 2**).

The Effect of Cognitive Training on Networks

Three networks were constituted by seed-based FC analysis, seeding at the PCC for the DMN, at the right AI for the SN and at the right DLPFC for the CEN. The DMN mainly involved the PCC/precuneus, VMPFC, DMPFC, bilateral IPL, bilateral temporal lobe, cerebellar lobule IX and crus II (Supplementary Figure S1). The SN mainly included the bilateral AI, DMPFC, dACC, and bilateral TPJ (Supplementary Figure S2), and the CEN was composed of the DLPFC, DMPFC, and IPL, all bilaterally (Supplementary Figure S3).

TABLE 1 | Demographic information about the subjects at different timepoints.

		Multi-domain training group	Control group	p
Age (year)	Baseline	70.61 ± 3.29	68.59 ± 3.24	0.838
(mean ± SD)	One-year post-test	72.39 ± 3.43	70.85 ± 4.05	0.782
Gender (male)	Baseline	23 (16)	17 (9)	0.283
	One-year post-test	18 (13)	14 (9)	0.631
Education (year)	Baseline	10.91 ± 3.65	10.64 ± 3.06	0.452
(mean ± SD)	One-year post-test	11.11 ± 4.25	10.09 ± 3.34	0.383
MMSE	Baseline	27.57 ± 2.57	28.17 ± 1.94	0.505
(mean ± SD)	One-year post-test	27.72 ± 2.16	27.85 ± 2.31	0.900
FD	Baseline	0.12 ± 0.04	0.14 ± 0.05	0.448
(mean ± SD)	One-year post-test	0.12 ± 0.04	0.16 ± 0.07	0.068

FD, Framewise displacement; MMSE, the Mini-Mental State Examination; SD, standard deviation.

TABLE 2 | Baseline and 1-year post-test scores for psychological measures (mean ± SD).

	Multi-domain training		Contorl			
	Baseline	One-year Post-test	Baseline	One-year Post-test	P^a	P^b
RBANS total score	93.17 ± 16.10	106.94 ± 12.90	93.07 ± 15.00	99.57 ± 13.75	0.058	0.971
Immediate memory	86.22 ± 16.45	103.17 ± 23.35	84.00 ± 14.34	100.5 ± 14.33	0.695	0.694
Visuospatial	106.78 ± 12.86	103.9 ± 11.56	106.86 ± 19.05	103.00 ± 16.81	0.981	0.922
Language	92.44 ± 12.92	101.00 ± 8.39	93.29 ± 7.12	95.86 ± 5.86	**0.036***	0.861
Attention	90.67 ± 19.39	94.94 ± 15.17	91.5 ± 15.25	88.93 ± 15.24	0.22	0.776
Delayed memory	98.28 ± 18.86	118.50 ± 12.41	99.00 ± 13.13	110.21 ± 14.80	**0.027***	0.999
The CWST						
Color interfere	20.16 ± 13.95	27.33 ± 17.01	14.57 ± 7.62	23.85 ± 14.33	0.884	0.125
Word interfere	38.61 ± 15.56	39.89 ± 17.35	39.71 ± 14.10	42.00 ± 19.00	0.669	0.642
The Visual Reasoning Test	5.78 ± 1.35	6.56 ± 1.89	5.86 ± 2.74	5.93 ± 2.46	0.169	0.894
The TMT						
Trail A complete time	79.50 ± 23.60	73.72 ± 33.93	87.21 ± 37.37	77.07 ± 29.22	0.739	0.381
Trail B complete time	157.89 ± 55.41	138.5 ± 48.27	153.5 ± 68.11	142.57 ± 49.6	0.634	0.830

**p*<0.05. *CWST, Color Word Stroop test; RBANS, Repeatable Battery for the Assessment of Neuropsychological Status; TMT, Trail Making test.* [a]*One-way ANCOVAs with differences between 1-year post-test and baseline in psychological measures as dependent variables, by controlling for scores of the psychological measures at baseline, age, gender and education years as covariates.* [b]*Two sample t-test with scores of the psychological measures at baseline as dependent variables, by controlling for age, gender, and education years as covariates.*

The 2 × 2 repeated measure ANOVA revealed significant interactions ($p < 0.05$) for FC within and between networks. In this study, this analysis was performed for the FCs that showed no significant difference between the training and control groups at baseline, because a training-related effect was the only possibility.

The ANOVA revealed the significant interactions for the FC within the DMN [PCC - left superior frontal gyrus (SFG) and PCC - cerebellar lobule IX]; within the SN (right AI - right middle/posterior insula, and right AI - left frontoinsula) and within the CEN (right DLPFC - bilateral DLPFC and right DLPFC - right SFG). *Post hoc* comparison demonstrated that some connections showed increased or maintained FC in the training group but decreased FC in the control group, including those between the PCC and the left SFG and between the PCC and cerebellar lobule IX within the DMN, between the right AI and left frontoinsula within the SN, and between the right DLPFC and the bilateral DLPFC and between the right DLPFC and the right SFG within the CEN (**Figure 1**; **Table 3**). In addition, we observed increased FC between the right AI and right middle/posterior insula in the control group but maintained FC after training in the training group (**Figure 1**; **Table 3**).

Our results also revealed significant interactions in the FCs between networks, including between DMN and CEN and between DMN and SN. *Post hoc* comparisons showed that the anti-correlations between the DMN and CEN were maintained or increased after training, including an increase in the anti-correlation between the PCC and the left DLPFC in the training group, while this correlation was maintained in control group; meanwhile, the anti-correlation between the PCC and the right DLPFC was maintained in training group and decreased in the control group. For the seed at the right DLPFC, the anti-correlation between the right DLPFC and left IPL was maintained in the training group and increased in the control group. For the connection between the DMN and SN, the connectivity between the PCC and the right putamen was maintained in the training group and decreased in the control group (**Figure 2**; **Table 3**).

The Correlation between Cognitive Measures and Resting-State fMRI

We found a significant relationship between the changes in FC (between the two fMRI sessions) and the improvements in cognitive performances ($p < 0.05$, uncorrected). As shown in **Figure 3**, the increased FC between the right DLPFC and the right SFG had a slim positive correlation with the RBANS test scores in the multi-domain training group (**Figure 3A**). The increased FC between the right AI and the right middle/posterior insula predicted poorer delayed memory and RBANS scores in the control group (**Figures 3B,C**).

DISCUSSION

In the present study, we used resting-state fMRI analysis to examine the effects of multi-domain cognitive training on FC within and among three networks (DMN, SN, and CEN). Consistent with our *a priori hypothesis*, changes in resting-state FC within and among the three networks were found at the 1-year after multi-domain cognitive training ended in training group compared to the wait-list control group. After training, the maintained or increased anterior–posterior and interhemispheric FCs within network, including PCC - left SFG (DMN), PCC - cerebellar lobule IX (DMN), right AI - left AI (SN), and right DLPFC - left DLPFC (CEN), were observed in the training group, while these FCs decreased in the control group. Compared to the control group, the training group showed increased or maintained anti-correlated FC between DMN and CEN (PCC - DLPFC

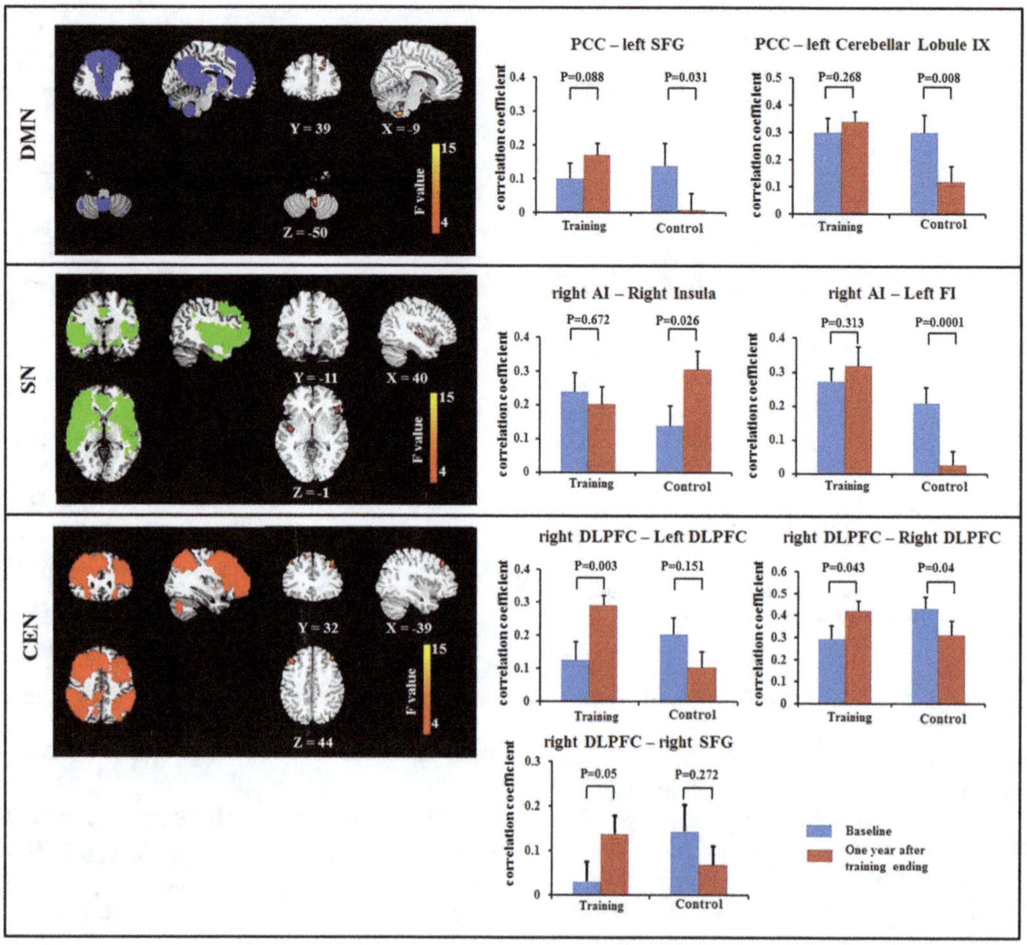

FIGURE 1 | Results of Resting-state functional connectivity (FC) within the DMN (top), within the SN (middle) and within the CEN (bottom) using a voxel-based 2 × 2 repeated ANOVA analysis (p < 0.05, cluster size > 621 mm^3). Bars at the right show the mean correlation coefficient of significantly altered FC within networks in training and control groups at the baseline (blue) and 1-year after training ended (red). CEN, Central executive network; DMN, default mode network; DLPFC, dorsolateral prefrontal cortex; FI, frontoinsula; PCC, posterior cingulate cortex; SFG, superior frontal gyrus; SN, salience network. The left side of the image corresponds to the right side of the subject.

TABLE 3 | Brain areas showing significant interactions for resting-state functional connectivity using a 2 (between-subject factor: training and control groups) × 2 (within-subject factor: baseline and 1-year after training ended) repeated ANOVA.

Seed	Brain region	BA	MNI coordinate			*F*-score	Cluster size (mm^3)
			X	*Y*	*Z*		
PCC	Left dorsolateral prefrontal lobe	20	−33	15	24	18.64	2187
	Left cerebellar lobule IX		−6	−51	−54	16.2	2241
	Right putamen	9	18	15	−9	13.17	1377
	Right dorsolateral prefrontal lobe		51	0	30	12.86	1782
	Left superior frontal gyrus	20	−24	36	39	11.66	1323
Right AI	Right insula	45	30	−9	−18	15.82	4644
	Left frontoinsula	45	−51	33	−12	11.67	2538
Right DLPFC	Right superior frontal cortex	11	15	27	54	13.30	3186
	Left dorsolateral prefrontal cortex	9	−39	30	42	12.78	1647
	Left inferior parietal lobe		−30	−63	30	13	1431
	Right superior frontal gyrus		42	27	42	12.12	2970

BA, Broadmann area; CEN, central executive network; DMN, default mode network; SN, salience network; DLPFC, dorsolateral prefrontal cortex; AI, anterior insula; PCC, posterior cingulate cortex.

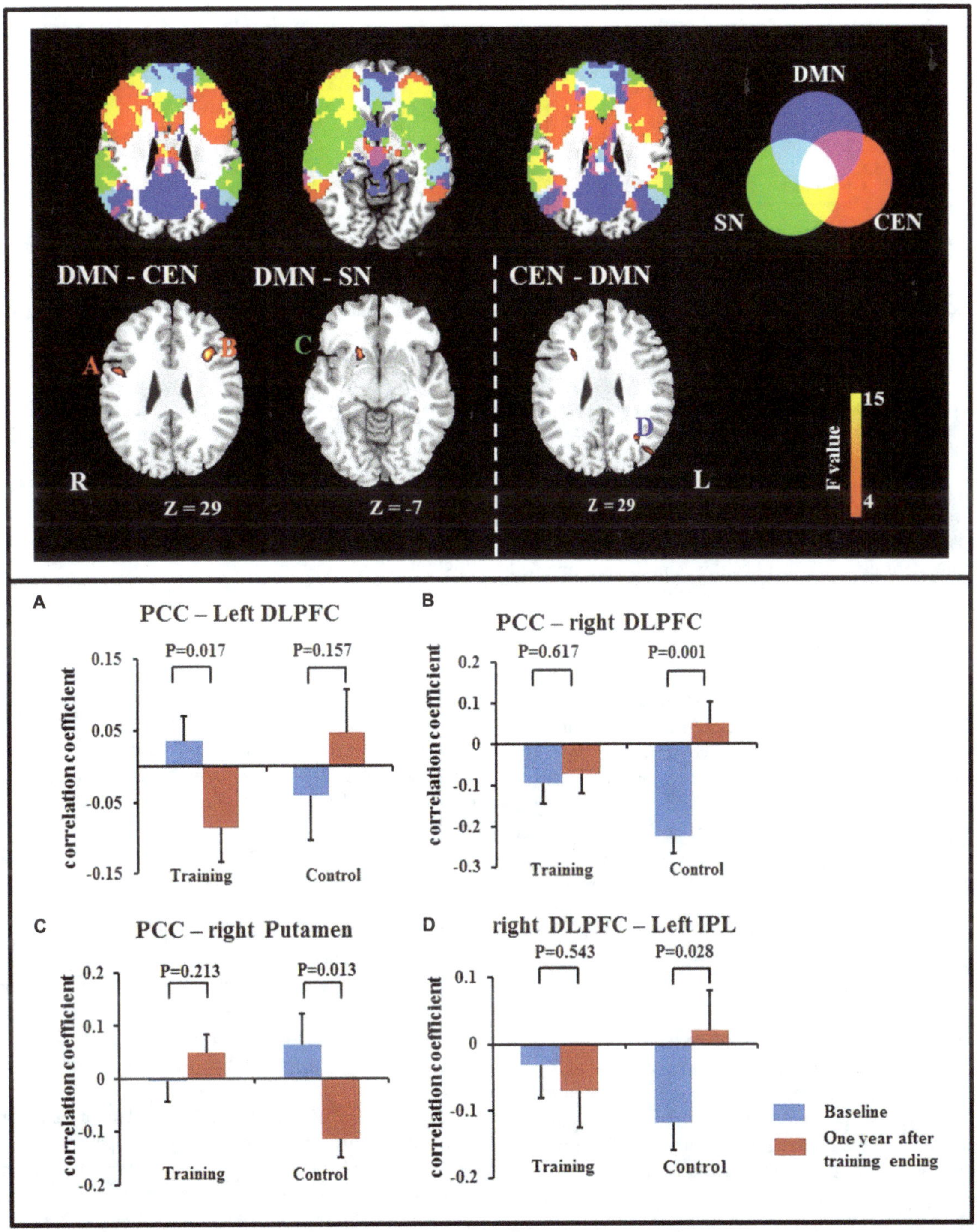

FIGURE 2 | Significant differences in FC were observed between DMN and CEN (A,B), between DMN and SN (C), and between CEN and DMN (D) using a voxel-based 2 × 2 repeated measure ANOVA (p < 0.05, cluster size > 621 mm^3). Bars at the bottom show the mean correlation coefficient of significant altered FC between networks in training and control groups at the baseline (blue) and 1-year after training ended (red). CEN, Central executive network; DMN, default mode network; DLPFC, dorsolateral prefrontal cortex; IPL, inferior parietal lobe; PCC, posterior cingulate cortex; SN, salience network.

and DLPFC - IPL). The coupling between DMN and SN (PCC - putamen) was also maintained in training group, but decreased in the control group. These findings suggested that multi-domain cognitive training might counteract decreased integration within network and impaired coupling between networks with aging.

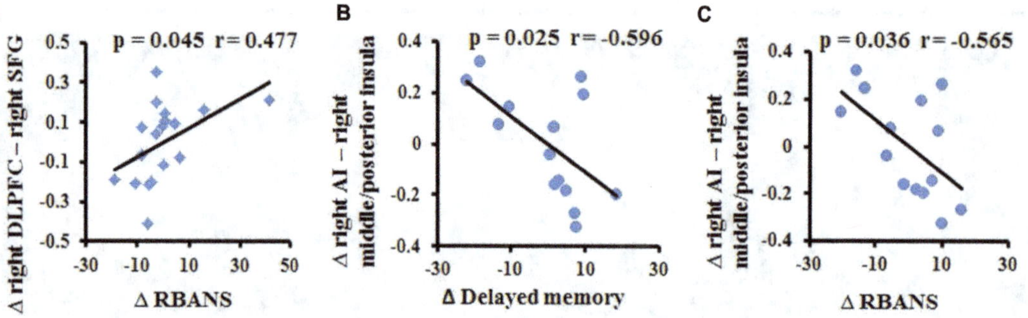

FIGURE 3 | Correlation between the change in resting-state FC and the change in cognitive performance in the multi-domain training group (A) and in the control group (B,C).

Training Effects on FC within Networks

This study found training-related enhanced integration of FC within the DMN, SN, and CEN. In particular, we observed that FCs between PCC and SFG and between PCC and cerebellar lobule IX were maintained in the multi-domain training group, but decreased in the control group. Previous studies have provided consistent evidence that healthy aging is accompanied by decreased FC within the DMN, particularly an anterior–posterior disruption of FC (Andrews-Hanna et al., 2007; Mevel et al., 2013). The decreased FC between the PCC and the SFG in the control group was consistent with previous findings, highlighting age-related disruption of connectivity at rest along the anterior–posterior axis of the DMN (Andrews-Hanna et al., 2007). The role of the cerebellum in cognitive function has been accepted. For example, lobule IX has been mentioned in association with DMN (Habas et al., 2009), and the FC between DMN nodes (PCC and MPFC) and cerebellar regions has been described as modified by aging and by diseases such as dementia (Bernard et al., 2013; Guo et al., 2015). Unlike the decreased FC with normal aging in the control group, multi-domain cognitive training maintained these FCs from the PCC to the SFG and to lobule IX of the cerebellum, suggesting that cognitive training might resist or postpone age-related disruption of FC within the DMN. In the CEN, we also observed increased FC between the right DLPFC and the frontal lobe (bilateral DLPFC and right SFG) at 1 year after training compared with baseline in the multi-domain training group, while these FCs decreased in the control group. These frontal regions have been found to be involved in executive and cognitive function (Ridderinkhof et al., 2004; Grady, 2012), such as working memory, and to be activated by tasks related to these function when the age-related effects were investigated (Grady, 2012). The frontal lobe is known to be affected by training (Park and Bischof, 2013). In addition, the change of FC between the right DLPFC and the right SFG was slight positively correlated with the improvement on the RBANS test in the training group. Thus, we presumed that the multi-domain training might have positive effects on improvement of behavior via enhancing the FC. However, a larger sample size should be considered to verify the relationship between the FC and cognitive function. A recent study of complex cognitive training in healthy seniors also found increased resting-state FC of the DMN and CEN, as well as increased cerebral blood flow (Chapman et al., 2015). Consistent with those reports, our results showed changes in intranetwork FC in the DMN and CEN after cognitive training. These findings might suggest that the cognitive training enhanced integration of FC within networks, resulting in the improvement of cognitive function.

Recent studies demonstrated that the decreased FC within the SN is an important feature of normal aging and is associated with the cognitive impairments (Onoda et al., 2012; He et al., 2013). Consistent with previous studies, we found decreased FC between the right AI and the left frontoinsula in the control group between the two timepoints scanned. However, the FC was maintained in the training group, as indicated by the absence of a difference between the FC values from before and after multi-domain cognitive training. In addition, we observed the FC between the right AI and right middle/posterior insula was maintained in the training group, but increase in the control group. The right AI, as a key node of the SN, is involved in cognitive function; by contrast, the middle/posterior insula serves in sensorimotor functions (Kurth et al., 2010). The increased FC between the right AI and right middle/posterior insula might indicate the disrupted function of the insula, likely reflecting an association with the cognitive decline in old adults. Here, we observed the negative correlation between the increase in the FC between the right anterior and right middle/posterior insula and the improvement of delayed memory and RBANS scores in the control group, probably implicating the relationship between the FC within the SN and the cognition. Thus, we speculated that cognitive training enhanced integration of the SN to retain at least some of the cognitive performance.

Training-Related Changes of FC between Networks

The triple network model of the DMN, SN, and CEN has been used to understand cognitive dysfunction in neurological and psychiatric disorders (Menon, 2011). A previous study provided evidence for a decrease in the anti-correlation between DMN and CEN in normal aging (Wu et al., 2011).

Here, we found that the aging-sensitive anti-correlation between DMN and CEN was maintained after training. A higher anti-correlation between DMN and CEN was also found after working memory training in healthy adults (Takeuchi et al., 2013). In addition, the disruption of SN and DMN connectivity has been observed in dementia (Zhou et al., 2010). Here, the connection between the DMN and SN was maintained in the training group, but decreased in the control group. Our results might also suggest that the anti-correlation of DMN and CEN is relatively sensitive to cognitive training.

Limitations

Interpreting the present findings requires the consideration of a few key limitations. First, our demographic characteristics, such as sample size and educational level, might affect the generalisability of the results. A larger sample size and a more consistent educational level among the subjects are necessary to verify the effect of cognitive training on the resting-state FC of three networks. Second, because the imaging data were not acquired at intermediate stages and or immediately after the completion of training completion, the effects of training on FCs within and between networks at additional intermediate timepoints and immediately after the completion of training are not studied. Third, we considered the effects of brain atrophy on FC in this work. However, the other focal damage (i.e., vascular lesions) is prevalent in the population and may have contributed to our findings. Fourth, the effects of cognitive training on resting-state FCs of three networks were observed in our study. This result suggested that the training was valid in the current population; however, further work should be performed to verify these conclusions in other populations. Finally, another control group of younger subjects should be considered in future work to determine whether the effects of cognitive training are specific to older adults.

CONCLUSION

We found changes in resting-state FC within networks and between the three networks at 1 year post-training, perhaps reflecting that cognitive training enhanced integration within network and maintenance of segregation between DMN and CEN. Our findings provide evidence that multi-domain cognitive training could mitigate the age-related functional alterations involving DMN, SN and CEN, thereby helping older adults maintain brain health.

AUTHOR CONTRIBUTIONS

Conceived and designed the work: WC, Cheng Luo, Chunbo Li, DY. Acquired the data: YC, XC, TL, LJ. Analyzed the data: WC, CH, XC, YC. Wrote the paper: WC, Cheng Luo. All authors revised the work for important intellectual content. All of the authors have read and approved the manuscript.

ACKNOWLEDGMENTS

This project was funded by the National Nature Science Foundation of China (81330032, 81371505, 91232725, 81271547, and 30770769), the Science and Technology Commission of Shanghai Municipality (134119a2501, 13dz2260500) and SHSMU-ION Research Center for Brain Disorders. This study was also sponsored by the '111' project of China (No. B12027).

REFERENCES

Andrews-Hanna, J. R., Snyder, A. Z., Vincent, J. L., Lustig, C., Head, D., Raichle, M. E., et al. (2007). Disruption of large-scale brain systems in advanced aging. *Neuron* 56, 924–935. doi: 10.1016/j.neuron.2007.10.038

Ashendorf, L., Jefferson, A. L., O'Connor, M. K., Chaisson, C., Green, R. C., and Stern, R. A. (2008). Trail Making Test errors in normal aging, mild cognitive impairment, and dementia. *Arch. Clin. Neuropsychol.* 23, 129–137. doi: 10.1016/j.acn.2007.11.005

Bamidis, P. D., Fissler, P., Papageorgiou, S. G., Zilidou, V., Konstantinidis, E. I., Billis, A. S., et al. (2015). Gains in cognition through combined cognitive and physical training: the role of training dosage and severity of neurocognitive disorder. *Front. Aging Neurosci.* 7:152. doi: 10.3389/fnagi.2015.00152

Bamidis, P. D., Vivas, A. B., Styliadis, C., Frantzidis, C., Klados, M., Schlee, W., et al. (2014). A review of physical and cognitive interventions in aging. *Neurosci. Biobehav. Rev.* 44, 206–220. doi: 10.1016/j.neubiorev.2014.03.019

Bernard, J. A., Peltier, S. J., Wiggins, J. L., Jaeggi, S. M., Buschkuehl, M., Fling, B. W., et al. (2013). Disrupted cortico-cerebellar connectivity in older adults. *Neuroimage* 83C, 103–119. doi: 10.1016/j.neuroimage.2013.06.042

Bressler, S. L., and Menon, V. (2010). Large-scale brain networks in cognition: emerging methods and principles. *Trends Cogn Sci.* 14, 277–290. doi: 10.1016/j.tics.2010.04.004

Buckner, R. L., Andrews-Hanna, J. R., and Schacter, D. L. (2008). The brain's default network: anatomy, function, and relevance to disease. *Ann. N. Y. Acad. Sci.* 1124, 1–38. doi: 10.1196/annals.1440.011

Calhoun, V. D., Eichele, T., and Pearlson, G. (2009). Functional brain networks in schizophrenia: a review. *Front. Hum. Neurosci.* 3:17. doi: 10.3389/neuro.09.017.2009

Cao, W., Luo, C., Zhu, B., Zhang, D., Dong, L., Gong, J., et al. (2014). Resting-state functional connectivity in anterior cingulate cortex in normal aging. *Front. Aging Neurosci.* 6:280. doi: 10.3389/fnagi.2014.00280

Chapman, S. B., Aslan, S., Spence, J. S., Hart, J. J. Jr., Bartz, E. K., Didehbani, N., et al. (2015). Neural mechanisms of brain plasticity with complex cognitive training in healthy seniors. *Cereb. Cortex* 25, 396–405. doi: 10.1093/cercor/bht234

Chen, X., Duan, M., Xie, Q., Lai, Y., Dong, L., Cao, W., et al. (2015). Functional disconnection between the visual cortex and the sensorimotor cortex suggests a potential mechanism for self-disorder in schizophrenia. *Schizophr. Res.* 166, 151–157. doi: 10.1016/j.schres.2015.06.014

Cheng, Y., Wu, W., Feng, W., Wang, J., Chen, Y., Shen, Y., et al. (2012). The effects of multi-domain versus single-domain cognitive training in non-demented older people: a randomized controlled trial. *BMC Med.* 10:30. doi: 10.1186/1741-7015-10-30

Cheng, Y., Wu, W., Wang, J., Feng, W., Wu, X., and Li, C. (2011). Reliability and validity of the repeatable battery for the assessment of neuropsychological status in community-dwelling elderly. *Arch. Med. Sci.* 7, 850–857. doi: 10.5114/aoms.2011.25561

Damoiseaux, J. S., Beckmann, C. F., Arigita, E. J., Barkhof, F., Scheltens, P., Stam, C. J., et al. (2008). Reduced resting-state brain activity in the "default network" in normal aging. *Cereb. Cortex* 18, 1856–1864. doi: 10.1093/cercor/bhm207

Fox, M. D., Snyder, A. Z., Vincent, J. L., Corbetta, M., Van Essen, D. C., and Raichle, M. E. (2005). The human brain is intrinsically organized into dynamic, anticorrelated functional networks. *Proc. Natl. Acad. Sci. U.S.A.* 102, 9673–9678. doi: 10.1073/pnas.0504136102

Fransson, P. (2006). How default is the default mode of brain function? Further evidence from intrinsic BOLD signal fluctuations. *Neuropsychologia* 44, 2836–2845. doi: 10.1016/j.neuropsychologia.2006.06.017

Grady, C. (2012). The cognitive neuroscience of ageing. *Nat. Rev. Neurosci.* 13, 491–505. doi: 10.1038/nrn3256

Guo, W., Liu, F., Zhang, Z., Liu, G., Liu, J., Yu, L., et al. (2015). Increased cerebellar functional connectivity with the default-mode network in unaffected siblings of schizophrenia patients at rest. *Schizophr. Bull.* 41, 1317–1325. doi: 10.1093/schbul/sbv062

Habas, C., Kamdar, N., Nguyen, D., Prater, K., Beckmann, C. F., Menon, V., et al. (2009). Distinct cerebellar contributions to intrinsic connectivity networks. *J. Neurosci.* 29, 8586–8594. doi: 10.1523/JNEUROSCI.1868-09.2009

He, X., Qin, W., Liu, Y., Zhang, X., Duan, Y., Song, J., et al. (2013). Abnormal salience network in normal aging and in amnestic mild cognitive impairment and Alzheimer's disease. *Hum. Brain Mapp.* 35, 3446–3464. doi: 10.1002/hbm.22414

Hedden, T., and Gabrieli, J. D. (2004). Insights into the ageing mind: a view from cognitive neuroscience. *Nat. Rev. Neurosci.* 5, 87–96. doi: 10.1038/nrn1323

Jiang, S., Luo, C., Liu, Z., Hou, C., Wang, P., Dong, L., et al. (2015). Altered local spontaneous brain activity in juvenile myoclonic epilepsy: a preliminary resting-state fMRI study. *Neural Plast.* 2015:635196. doi: 10.1155/2016/3547203

Kirchhoff, B. A., Anderson, B. A., Barch, D. M., and Jacoby, L. L. (2012). Cognitive and neural effects of semantic encoding strategy training in older adults. *Cereb. Cortex* 22, 788–799. doi: 10.1093/cercor/bhr129

Kraft, E. (2012). Cognitive function, physical activity, and aging: possible biological links and implications for multimodal interventions. *Neuropsychol. Dev. Cogn. B Aging Neuropsychol. Cogn.* 19, 248–263. doi: 10.1080/13825585.2011.645010

Kurth, F., Zilles, K., Fox, P. T., Laird, A. R., and Eickhoff, S. B. (2010). A link between the systems: functional differentiation and integration within the human insula revealed by meta-analysis. *Brain Struct. Funct.* 214, 519–534. doi: 10.1007/s00429-010-0255-z

Langer, N., von Bastian, C. C., Wirz, H., Oberauer, K., and Jancke, L. (2013). The effects of working memory training on functional brain network efficiency. *Cortex* 49, 2424–2438. doi: 10.1016/j.cortex.2013.01.008

Leung, N. T., Tam, H. M., Chu, L. W., Kwok, T. C., Chan, F., Lam, L. C., et al. (2015). Neural plastic effects of cognitive training on aging brain. *Neural Plast.* 2015:535618. doi: 10.1155/2015/535618

Li, C., Wu, W., Jin, H., Zhang, X., Xue, H., He, Y., et al. (2006). Successful aging in Shanghai, China: definition, distribution and related factors. *Int. Psychogeriatr.* 18, 551–563. doi: 10.1017/S1041610205002966

Li, R., Zhu, X., Yin, S., Niu, Y., Zheng, Z., Huang, X., et al. (2014). Multimodal intervention in older adults improves resting-state functional connectivity between the medial prefrontal cortex and medial temporal lobe. *Front. Aging Neurosci.* 6:39. doi: 10.3389/fnagi.2014.00039

Lim, M. L., Collinson, S. L., Feng, L., and Ng, T. P. (2010). Cross-cultural application of the repeatable battery for the assessment of neuropsychological status (rbans): performances of elderly Chinese Singaporeans. *Clin. Neuropsychol.* 24, 811–826. doi: 10.1080/13854046.2010.490789

Luo, C., Li, Q., Lai, Y., Xia, Y., Qin, Y., Liao, W., et al. (2011). Altered functional connectivity in default mode network in absence epilepsy: a resting-state fMRI study. *Hum. Brain Mapp.* 32, 438–449. doi: 10.1002/hbm.21034

Luo, C., Qiu, C., Guo, Z., Fang, J., Li, Q., Lei, X., et al. (2012). Disrupted functional brain connectivity in partial epilepsy: a resting-state fMRI study. *PLoS ONE* 7:e28196. doi: 10.1371/journal.pone.0028196

Luo, C., Tu, S., Peng, Y., Gao, S., Li, J., Dong, L., et al. (2014a). Long-term effects of musical training and functional plasticity in salience system. *Neural Plast.* 2014:180138. doi: 10.1155/2014/180138

Luo, C., Yang, T., Tu, S., Deng, J., Liu, D., Li, Q., et al. (2014b). Altered intrinsic functional connectivity of the salience network in childhood absence epilepsy. *J. Neurol. Sci.* 339, 189–195. doi: 10.1016/j.jns.2014.02.016

Luo, C., Zhang, X., Cao, X., Gan, Y., Li, T., Cheng, Y., et al. (2016). The lateralization of intrinsic networks in the aging brain implicates the effects of cognitive training. *Front. Aging Neurosci.* 8:32. doi: 10.3389/fnagi.2016.00032

Luo, C., Zhang, Y., Cao, W., Huang, Y., Yang, F., Wang, J., et al. (2015). Altered structural and functional feature of striato-cortical circuit in benign epilepsy with centrotemporal spikes. *Int. J. Neural. Syst.* 25:1550027. doi: 10.1142/S0129065715500276

Mackey, A. P., Miller Singley, A. T., and Bunge, S. A. (2013). Intensive reasoning training alters patterns of brain connectivity at rest. *J. Neurosci.* 33, 4796–4803. doi: 10.1523/JNEUROSCI.4141-12.2013

Menon, V. (2011). Large-scale brain networks and psychopathology: a unifying triple network model. *Trends Cogn. Sci.* 15, 483–506. doi: 10.1016/j.tics.2011.08.003

Meunier, D., Achard, S., Morcom, A., and Bullmore, E. (2009). Age-related changes in modular organization of human brain functional networks. *Neuroimage* 44, 715–723. doi: 10.1016/j.neuroimage.2008.09.062

Mevel, K., Landeau, B., Fouquet, M., La Joie, R., Villain, N., Mezenge, F., et al. (2013). Age effect on the default mode network, inner thoughts, and cognitive abilities. *Neurobiol. Aging* 34, 1292–1301. doi: 10.1016/j.neurobiolaging.2012.08.018

Neely, A. S., and Backman, L. (1995). Effects of multifactorial memory training in old age: generalizability across tasks and individuals. *J. Gerontol. B Psychol. Sci. Soc. Sci.* 50, 134–140. doi: 10.1093/geronb/50B.3.P134

Onoda, K., Ishihara, M., and Yamaguchi, S. (2012). Decreased functional connectivity by aging is associated with cognitive decline. *J. Cogn. Neurosci.* 24, 2186–2198. doi: 10.1162/jocn_a_00269

Oswald, W. D., Gunzelmann, T., Rupprecht, R., and Hagen, B. (2006). Differential effects of single versus combined cognitive and physical training with older adults: the SimA study in a 5-year perspective. *Eur. J. Ageing* 3, 179–192. doi: 10.1007/s10433-006-0035-z

Park, D. C., and Bischof, G. N. (2013). The aging mind: neuroplasticity in response to cognitive training. *Dialogues Clin. Neurosci.* 15, 109–119.

Patel, R., Spreng, R. N., and Turner, G. R. (2013). Functional brain changes following cognitive and motor skills training: a quantitative meta-analysis. *Neurorehabil. Neural Repair* 27, 187–199. doi: 10.1177/1545968312461718

Power, J. D., Barnes, K. A., Snyder, A. Z., Schlaggar, B. L., and Petersen, S. E. (2012). Spurious but systematic correlations in functional connectivity MRI networks arise from subject motion. *Neuroimage* 59, 2142–2154. doi: 10.1016/j.neuroimage.2011.10.018

Raichle, M. E., MacLeod, A. M., Snyder, A. Z., Powers, W. J., Gusnard, D. A., and Shulman, G. L. (2001). A default mode of brain function. *Proc. Natl. Acad. Sci. U.S.A.* 98, 676–682. doi: 10.1073/pnas.98.2.676

Ridderinkhof, K. R., van den Wildenberg, W. P., Segalowitz, S. J., and Carter, C. S. (2004). Neurocognitive mechanisms of cognitive control: the role of prefrontal cortex in action selection, response inhibition, performance monitoring, and reward-based learning. *Brain Cogn.* 56, 129–140. doi: 10.1016/j.bandc.2004.09.016

Seeley, W. W., Menon, V., Schatzberg, A. F., Keller, J., Glover, G. H., Kenna, H., et al. (2007). Dissociable intrinsic connectivity networks for salience processing and executive control. *J. Neurosci.* 27, 2349–2356. doi: 10.1523/JNEUROSCI.5587-06.2007

Shao, J., Myers, N., Yang, Q., Feng, J., Plant, C., Bohm, C., et al. (2012). Prediction of Alzheimer's disease using individual structural connectivity networks. *Neurobiol. Aging* 33, 2756–2765. doi: 10.1016/j.neurobiolaging.2012.01.017

Smith, S. M., Fox, P. T., Miller, K. L., Glahn, D. C., Fox, P. M., Mackay, C. E., et al. (2009). Correspondence of the brain's functional architecture during activation and rest. *Proc. Natl. Acad. Sci. U.S.A.* 106, 13040–13045. doi: 10.1073/pnas.0905267106

Sridharan, D., Levitin, D. J., and Menon, V. (2008). A critical role for the right fronto-insular cortex in switching between central-executive and default-mode networks. *Proc. Natl. Acad. Sci. U.S.A.* 105, 12569–12574. doi: 10.1073/pnas.0800005105

Strenziok, M., Parasuraman, R., Clarke, E., Cisler, D. S., Thompson, J. C., and Greenwood, P. M. (2014). Neurocognitive enhancement in older adults: comparison of three cognitive training tasks to test a hypothesis of training transfer in brain connectivity. *Neuroimage* 85(Pt 3), 1027–1039. doi: 10.1016/j.neuroimage.2013.07.069

Takeuchi, H., Taki, Y., Nouchi, R., Hashizume, H., Sekiguchi, A., Kotozaki, Y., et al. (2013). Effects of working memory training on functional connectivity and cerebral blood flow during rest. *Cortex* 49, 2106–2125. doi: 10.1016/j.cortex.2012.09.007

Tang, Y. Y., and Posner, M. I. (2014). Training brain networks and states. *Trends Cogn. Sci.* 18, 345–350. doi: 10.1016/j.tics.2014.04.002

Tanigawa, T., Takechi, H., Arai, H., Yamada, M., Nishiguchi, S., and Aoyama, T. (2014). Effect of physical activity on memory function in older adults with mild Alzheimer's disease and mild cognitive impairment. *Geriatr. Gerontol. Int.* 14, 758–762. doi: 10.1111/ggi.12159

Taylor, V. A., Daneault, V., Grant, J., Scavone, G., Breton, E., Roffe-Vidal, S., et al. (2013). Impact of meditation training on the default mode network during a restful state. *Soc. Cogn. Affect. Neurosci.* 8, 4–14. doi: 10.1093/scan/nsr087

Tomasi, D., and Volkow, N. D. (2012). Aging and functional brain networks. *Mol. Psychiatry* 17, 549–458. doi: 10.1038/mp.2011.81

van Boxtel, M. P., ten Tusscher, M. P., Metsemakers, J. F., Willems, B., and Jolles, J. (2001). Visual determinants of reduced performance on the Stroop color-word test in normal aging individuals. *J. Clin. Exp. Neuropsychol.* 23, 620–627. doi: 10.1076/jcen.23.5.620.1245

Voss, M. W., Erickson, K. I., Prakash, R. S., Chaddock, L., Kim, J. S., Alves, H., et al. (2013). Neurobiological markers of exercise-related brain plasticity in older adults. *Brain Behav. Immun.* 28, 90–99. doi: 10.1016/j.bbi.2012.10.021

Voss, M. W., Prakash, R. S., Erickson, K. I., Basak, C., Chaddock, L., Kim, J. S., et al. (2010). Plasticity of brain networks in a randomized intervention trial of exercise training in older adults. *Front. Aging Neurosci.* 2:32. doi: 10.3389/fnagi.2010.00032

Wu, J. T., Wu, H. Z., Yan, C. G., Chen, W. X., Zhang, H. Y., He, Y., et al. (2011). Aging-related changes in the default mode network and its anti-correlated networks: a resting-state fMRI study. *Neurosci. Lett.* 504, 62–67. doi: 10.1016/j.neulet.2011.08.059

Xiao, S., Yao, P., Li, X., and Zhang, M. (2002). Neuropsychological testing profiles of patients with Alzheimer's Disease and mild cognitive impairment: a case-control study. *Hong Kong J. Psychiatry* 12, 2–5.

Yin, S., Zhu, X., Li, R., Niu, Y., Wang, B., Zheng, Z., et al. (2014). Intervention-induced enhancement in intrinsic brain activity in healthy older adults. *Sci. Rep.* 4:7309. doi: 10.1038/srep07309

Zheng, Z., Zhu, X., Yin, S., Wang, B., Niu, Y., Huang, X., et al. (2015). Combined cognitive-psychological-physical intervention induces reorganization of intrinsic functional brain architecture in older adults. *Neural Plast* 2015:713104. doi: 10.1155/2015/713104

Zhou, J., Greicius, M. D., Gennatas, E. D., Growdon, M. E., Jang, J. Y., Rabinovici, G. D., et al. (2010). Divergent network connectivity changes in behavioural variant frontotemporal dementia and Alzheimer's disease. *Brain* 133, 1352–1367. doi: 10.1093/brain/awq075

12

Neurovascular and Neurometabolic Derailment in Aging and Alzheimer's Disease

Cátia F. Lourenço[1], *Ana Ledo*[1], *Cândida Dias*[1], *Rui M. Barbosa*[1,2] *and João Laranjinha*[1,2*]

[1] *Center for Neuroscience and Cell Biology, University of Coimbra, Coimbra, Portugal,* [2] *Faculty of Pharmacy, University of Coimbra, Coimbra, Portugal*

Edited by:
Enrique Cadenas, University of Southern California, USA

Reviewed by:
Paula I. Moreira, University of Coimbra, Portugal
Giuseppe Poli, University of Torino, Italy

***Correspondence:**
João Laranjinha, Faculty of Pharmacy, Center for Neuroscience and Cell Biology, University of Coimbra, Health Sciences Campus, Azinhaga de Santa Comba, 3000-548 Coimbra, Portugal
laranjin@ci.uc.pt

The functional and structural integrity of the brain requires local adjustment of blood flow and regulated delivery of metabolic substrates to meet the metabolic demands imposed by neuronal activation. This process—neurovascular coupling—and ensued alterations of glucose and oxygen metabolism—neurometabolic coupling—are accomplished by concerted communication between neural and vascular cells. Evidence suggests that neuronal-derived nitric oxide (•NO) is a key player in both phenomena. Alterations in the mechanisms underlying the intimate communication between neural cells and vessels ultimately lead to neuronal dysfunction. Both neurovascular and neurometabolic coupling are perturbed during brain aging and in age-related neuropathologies in close association with cognitive decline. However, despite decades of intense investigation, many aspects remain poorly understood, such as the impact of these alterations. In this review, we address neurovascular and neurometabolic derailment in aging and Alzheimer's disease (AD), discussing its significance in connection with •NO-related pathways.

Keywords: neurovascular coupling, neurometabolism, nitric oxide, Alzheimer's disease, aging

Introduction

The proper function of the brain depends critically upon constant and regulated blood supply. Despite representing only 2% of total body mass in the adult human, the brain is an energy expensive organ, consuming *circa* one fifth of the available oxygen and glucose (Zlokovic, 2011). Upon neural excitation, local metabolic rate may increase as much as 50% relative to basal values depending on the intensity of stimulation (Shulman and Rothman, 1998). Paradoxically, the intrinsic energy reserves are minimal (Kealy et al., 2013), which implies that, to assure an appropriate balance, changes in blood supply must be attuned to the physiological demands imposed by neural activation with high temporal and regional precision. The accomplishment of such interplay depends on the complex and concerted communication between neurons, astrocytes, pericytes, microglia, and vascular cells. Active neurons generate signals that are transduced at blood vessels to locally adjust blood flow and guarantee efficient delivery of bioenergetic substrates—a process termed neurovascular coupling. Furthermore, the profile of neuronal activity is closely associated with glucose and oxygen metabolism—neurometabolic coupling.

Neurovascular coupling has been a matter of intense investigation over the last decades and is yet not fully understood. Nonetheless, there are generally accepted propositions, such as (1) the process relies on glutamate-dependent pathways, in a feed-forward mechanism; (2) likely several molecules and/or pathways cooperate to translate the need for substrates imposed by the neuronal activity into changes in cerebral blood flow, and (3) the underlying mechanisms can be distinct throughout the brain areas, reflecting specificities of the neuronal networks. Amongst several molecules proposed to mediate neurovascular coupling, nitric oxide (•NO), a free radical intercellular messenger, has emerged as an attractive candidate (Iadecola, 1993). In the brain, •NO is produced upon glutamatergic activation by the neuronal isoform of nitric oxide synthase (nNOS), which is physically anchored and functionally coupled to the NMDA-type glutamate receptor (Christopherson et al., 1999). Nitric oxide is endowed with peculiar physicochemical properties (radical nature, small size, diffusibility, hydrophobicity), that determine a diversity of biological targets and pathways in which it is involved (for review Winkler and Luer, 1998; Guix et al., 2005).

Despite some inconsistent observations, ample evidence suggests that •NO plays a critical role in neurovascular coupling, particularly in the hippocampus and cerebellum (Rancillac et al., 2006; Lourenço et al., 2014a). Direct and *in vivo* data show that •NO is a direct mediator of the process, bridging neurons and blood vessels. The simultaneous monitoring of •NO fluctuations and CBF changes during glutamatergic activation, coupled to pharmacological approaches, strengthens the notion that •NO produced by neurons can diffuse toward neighboring blood vessels and promote vasodilation via activation of soluble guanylate cyclase (sGC). In turn, the involvement of endothelial-derived •NO appears to be negligible (Lourenço et al., 2014a). In addition to participating in neuron-to-blood vessel signaling pathways, •NO may be involved in the regulation of ensued processes, such as neurometabolic coupling. Nitric oxide can regulate energy metabolism/cellular respiration by interfering with several signaling pathways. For instance, at low nM concentrations •NO regulates mitochondrial respiration by inhibiting cytochrome c oxidase (CcO) in competition with O_2 (Rossignol et al., 2003; Moncada and Bolaños, 2006; Antunes and Cadenas, 2007). This competitive process allows not only for the fine tuning of mitochondrial respiration, but may also facilitate O_2 distribution from the microvasculature to sites of up-regulated energetic demand (Giulivi, 2003; Victor et al., 2009) or modulate production of mitochondrial-derived signaling molecules such as superoxide and hydrogen peroxide (Cadenas, 2004). Nonetheless, when •NO fluxes are increased in biological systems in concurrence with an unbalanced redox environment, production of •NO-derived reactive species such as peroxynitrite can significantly perturb mitochondrial function by inhibiting complex I of the mitochondrial respiratory chain, aconitase and Mn-superoxide dismutase (Brown, 2007). This Dr. Jekyll and Mr. Hyde type of bioactivity can also be observed for glycolysis, where •NO has been shown to boost glycolytic turnover in a cGMP dependent mechanism in astrocytes (but not neurons) (Bolanos et al., 2008) while gluteraldehyde-3-phosphate dehydrogenase can be inhibited by nitration (Palamalai and Miyagi, 2010).

Interestingly, the impact of •NO on brain metabolic status can reflect upon neurovascular coupling. Variations in O_2 concentration can alter vascular tone, both by affecting the synthesis of the vasoactive messengers (including •NO itself), and by altering the levels of lactate and adenosine, which modulate pathways underlying neurovascular coupling (Gordon et al., 2008; Attwell et al., 2010).

In sum, neuronal activity produces •NO, a messenger that diffuses to blood vessels inducing vasodilation. Consequently, increased delivery of energy substrates impacts local neuronal metabolism and function. Therefore, the two processes, neuronal activity-dependent CBF increase and oxygen and glucose utilization by active neural cells are inextricably linked, establishing a functional metabolic axis in brain, the neurovascular-neuroenergetic coupling axis. Nitric oxide is a master regulator of this axis. The perturbation of this •NO-driven regulatory cycle can trigger a sequence of events that may ultimately lead to neuronal dysfunction. Ample evidence supports the notion that alterations of the regulatory mechanisms involved in neurovascular and neurometabolic coupling lead to neuronal dysfunction and disease, as discussed in the following sections.

Dysfunction in Neurovascular Coupling During Brain Aging and Alzheimer's Disease

It is increasingly accepted that brain aging and age-associated diseases, such as Alzheimer's disease (AD), share some common histological and pathophysiological alterations that, ultimately, underlie compromised cognitive status. The possible contribution of abnormal cerebrovascular function to progressive functional decline has been vigorously emphasized and is nowadays well recognized. However, the putative triggers of this dysfunction remain a matter of extensive debate (Zlokovic, 2011; Kalaria, 2012; de la Torre, 2012). Age is the most relevant risk factor for the sporadic form of AD, the leading cause of dementia in the elderly. Although AD results predominantly from neurodegenerative changes, there is a growingly recognized contribution of well-defined decline in cerebrovascular parameters (Girouard and Iadecola, 2006). Between 60 and 90% of AD patients exhibit cerebrovascular pathologies including cerebral amyloid angiopathy, microinfarcts and ischemic lesions, blood–brain barrier disruption,and microvascular degeneration (Jellinger and Mitter-Ferstl, 2003; Bell and Zlokovic, 2009). Converging on this idea, the ethiopathogenetic role of a spectrum of chronic vascular disorders such as hypertension, hypercholesterolemia and type 2 diabetes has been proven to be present in the pathogenesis of AD (Kalaria, 2012).

The alterations in cerebrovascular function in aging and AD can be reflected by both chronic brain hypoperfusion and altered neurovascular coupling. Numerous clinical studies, based on evaluation of resting CBF in human subjects, unanimously recognize a negative correlation between global CBF and age (Krejza et al., 1999; Schultz et al., 1999; Fisher et al., 2013; Fabiani et al., 2014). Also, several lines of evidence support cerebral hypoperfusion as a preclinical condition in AD and one of the most accurate predictors for developing AD. Studies of brain function during behavioral tasks suggest age-related differences in activation, as well as differences between patients with AD and age-matched control subjects, revealing a close correlation with cognitive decline (Alsop et al., 2000; Ruitenberg et al., 2005; Xu et al., 2007). A significant observation is that the BOLD signal evaluated by fMRI during an associative encoding task is reduced in individuals carrying the APOE-ε4 allele, a recognized risk factor for sporadic AD (Fleisher et al., 2009).

However, whereas the correlation between cerebrovascular changes and cognitive decline has been firmly established, the neurobiological link between the two is still poorly defined, as is the causality (Iadecola, 2004). Evidence for cerebrovascular changes resulting in neuronal damage, hastening neurodegeneration, is clear but it is also known that neurogenic factors can underlie cerebrovascular dysfunction. Amyloid β peptide (Aβ), the main component of the amyloid plaques found in AD, may play a major role in cerebrovascular impairment, as it is known to disrupt the physiological mechanisms regulating CBF. Elevations of Aβ levels in rodent models of AD are associated with lower resting CBF and impaired vasodilatory responses in cerebral circulation (Iadecola et al., 1999; Niwa et al., 2002), including neurovascular coupling (Niwa et al., 2000a). Additionally, Aβ peptides can impair endothelium-dependent relaxation and enhance vasoconstriction (Thomas et al., 1996; Niwa et al., 2000b, 2001) by either promoting oxidative stress in the vascular cells (Hamel et al., 2008) and/or inhibiting the production of neuronal-derived vasodilating messengers (Iadecola, 2004) such as •NO (Venturini et al., 2002).

In an attempt to help clarify this controversy, we have observed age-dependent impairment of •NO-dependent neurovascular coupling both in rodent models of AD and aging. Furthermore, we found that this dysfunction appears to be primarily of cerebrovascular rather than neuronal origin. These studies were carried out in a triple transgenic mouse model of AD (3xTg-AD mice) and in Fisher 344 rats (widely used in brain aging studies). By simultaneously measuring •NO and CBF in the hippocampus, we observed that glutamate-evoked increase in CBF was diminished during aging and AD, despite the fact that •NO signaling remains almost unaltered. The effect of aging/AD on •NO-dependent CBF changes is summarized in **Figure 1**. Data obtained in 3xTg-AD mice revealed a shift in the CBF changes coupled to the •NO temporal dynamic elicited by glutamatergic activation. This is reflected by the increased delay on the onset of CBF increase (**Figure 1C**), as well as by the decrease in the amplitude of CBF change. The later leads to the abolishment of the correlation between •NO and CBF observed in control animals (**Figure 1B**). Similar observations were obtained during aging in F344 rats, with CBF changes declining 39% from 6 to 12 months, and a further 36% from 12 to 23 months, with no significant decrease in •NO signaling (unpublished data). Of note, the deterioration of the neurovascular coupling in both cases preceded an obvious impairment in cognitive function as accessed by behavior tests.

Overall, these results strengthen the notion of cerebrovascular dysfunction as a fundamental process underlying AD pathophysiology and brain aging. That is, while neuronal •NO signaling remains functional it is not conveniently transduced into vasodilation at blood vessels. Amongst the potential causes, changes of the redox environment in blood vessels may result in the quenching of •NO, impeding it's binding to sGC. In fact,

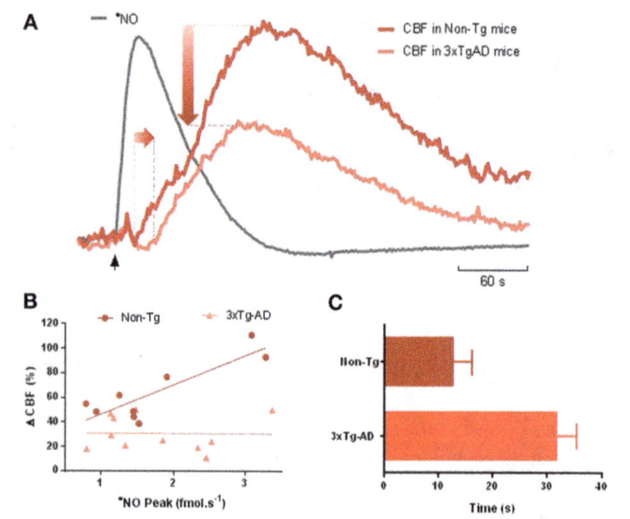

FIGURE 1 | Impairment of nitric oxide-dependent neurovascular coupling in AD. (A) Representative recordings of the simultaneous measurements of •NO concentration dynamics and CBF changes in the hippocampus of 12 months-old Non-Tg mice and 3xTg-AD mice in response to L-glutamate. L-glutamate (0.5 nmol, 1 s) was locally applied at time indicated by the black vertical arrow. The measurements were performed using •NO selective microelectrodes and Laser Doppler flowmetry as previously described (Lourenço et al., 2014a). The temporal dynamic of •NO is roughly identical in both strains and thus only a representative trace is presented (gray line). The CBF change coupled to the transient •NO increase showed a temporal delay and decrease in amplitude in 3xTg-AD mice (light red line) as compared to Non-Tg mice (dark red line). **(B)** The linear relationship between •NO peak amplitude and the amplitude CBF change observed in Non-Tg mice ($p = 0.003$) was lost in 3xTg-AD mice ($p = 0.981$). In the former, the linear regression showed an $R^2 = 0.735$ and a slope of 24% CBF/fmol s^{-1} •NO. **(C)** Delay between the onset of •NO transient and the onset of the CBF change in 12-months old 3xTg-AD mice and Non-Tg mice. Values represent the mean ± SEM ($p = 0.001$).

previous reports show that vascular oxidative stress may have serious implications in cerebrovascular function (reviewed in Hamel et al., 2008).

A deep understanding of the underlying mechanisms by which altered cerebrovascular function influences AD neuropathology has not yet been achieved. Nevertheless, in accordance with the hypothesis prompted by the vascular-driven theory of AD, cerebrovascular dysfunction and consequent hypoperfusion is suggested to be linked to (1) enhanced β-secretase protein expression, which potentiates Aβ overproduction and altered phosphorylated tau (Velliquette et al., 2005; Koike et al., 2010); (2) faulty clearance of Aβ peptides, favoring accumulation in the brain (Girouard and Iadecola, 2006) and (3) reduced supply of metabolic substrates and neurometabolic dysfunction.

Altered Neurometabolism in Brain Aging and Alzheimer's Disease

Brain aging is accompanied by widespread metabolic alterations associated with cognitive decline that connect with the so called "metabolic syndrome" (Barzilai et al., 2012).

Components of metabolic syndrome such as insulin resistance or hypercholesterolemia are predictors of accelerated cognitive decline and dementia, particularly AD (Haralampos et al., 2008). The pathways linking these metabolic alterations and the decay of cognitive function are still poorly understood, but mitochondrial dysfunction has been identified as a link between the two. Besides changes in neurotransmission processes (decrease in glutamate and GABA), brain aging and AD are associated with perturbations of primary energy metabolism (use of glucose and lactate) as well as in the turnover of lipid membranes (Castegna et al., 2004; Mohmmad Abdul and Butterfield, 2005; Bader Lange et al., 2008; Duarte et al., 2014). Mitochondria play an essential role in cellular respiration and are responsible not only for the production of ATP, but also for Ca^{2+} buffering, production and removal of reactive oxygen species, as well as of signaling molecules that regulate cell cycle, proliferation and apoptosis (for review Yin et al., 2014). The brain's consumption of glucose is primarily driven by the constant need to maintain ionic gradients in pre- and post-synaptic compartments in order to sustain excitability, as well as to maintain transmembrane lipid asymmetries (Harris et al., 2012). Considering the high energetic demand of this organ and it's excitability requirements, deregulation of optimal mitochondrial performance can significantly impact neurometabolism and function.

During the past decades, intensive research has shown that brain energy metabolism in impaired during the progression of AD (de Leon et al., 1983; Mosconi et al., 2005; Reiman et al., 2005; Scholl et al., 2011; Yin et al., 2014). Amyloidosis, or more specifically plaque pathology (Gearing et al., 1995), although present in roughly 90% of AD patients, is not in itself sufficient to account for the disease and many authors have reported that amyloid load may not necessarily correlate with dementia (Gearing et al., 1995; Hsia et al., 1999; Mucke et al., 2000; Swerdlow et al., 2014). As the amyloid cascade hypothesis of AD has evolved over the years, the concept of plaque as the causal factor of disease has given way to the notion that soluble forms of Aβ oligomers are in fact the toxic moiety (Lesne and Kotilinek, 2005; Walsh et al., 2005; Lesne et al., 2006). These oligomers have been shown to compromise the function of organelles such as the mitochondria.

Thus, the concept that mitochondrial dysfunction is a key contributor to the onset and progression of AD has become firmly consolidated and the "mitochondrial cascade hypothesis" has gained significant ground, especially with regards to late-onset AD (Chaturvedi and Flint Beal, 2013; Swerdlow et al., 2014). This hypothesis is sustained not only on the fact that both Aβ and hyperphosphorylated tau are capable of altering mitochondrial function, but also takes into account the major risk factor for sporadic AD—age. One important consequence of biological aging is the accumulation of somatic mtDNA mutations, which contribute to physiological decline and neurodegenerative disease (Lin et al., 2002). The impact of these point mutations on each individual as they age will be influenced by inherited and environmental factors (Wallace, 1992; Swerdlow et al., 2014).

Studies in both animal models and AD patients have shown that Aβ is capable of inhibiting the complexes of the mitochondrial respiratory chain, as well as the TCA cycle enzyme α-ketogluterate dehydrogenase (Casley et al., 2002; Manczak et al., 2006). Impairment of oxidative phosphorylation (OxPhos) is mainly due to the inhibition or decreased activity of CcO, which, along with ATP synthase, is known to be oxidized in the brains of AD patients (Kish et al., 1992; Mutisya et al., 1994; Maurer et al., 2000). Furthermore, mitochondrial dysfunction promotes tangle formation in AD by contributing to tau phosphorylation (Melov et al., 2007).

Using high resolution respirometry for evaluation of O_2 consumption rates (OCR) in intact hippocampal slices obtained from 3xTg-AD mice and age-matched controls (**Figure 2A**) we have observed an age-dependent impairment of OxPhos in old-aged animals which tends to be more evident in old-aged 3xTg-AD (**Figure 2B**). Both basal and maximal O_2 consumption rates decrease as a function of age in both genotypes. More relevantly, the sparing capacity has diminished in both old-age groups, implying a lower capacity to respond to energy-demanding situations (such as increased excitability) with adequate increase OxPhos to supply ATP. Decrease in basal tissue OCR was further revealed when we determined the drop in $[O_2]$ from the surrounding media to the tissue core (**Figure 2C**), which was significantly smaller in old-age 3TgAD animals. This drop in $[O_2]$ is expected to positively correlate with the metabolic activity state of the tissue. Of note is the fact that this 3xTg-AD model, although expressing a progressive AD phenotype as expected to occur in humans (Oddo et al., 2003), is a model of familiar AD and not sporadic AD. As such, it is not surprising to us to find that the major contributor to changes in OxPhos is actually age and not genotype. Sporadic AD is not associated with deterministic gene mutations, although some genetic influences have been identified, such as the APOE-ε4 variant (Corder et al., 1993; Swerdlow, 2007).

Hypometabolism in AD is most likely more than a mere consequence of the cellular and functional degeneration (decreased brain function would obviously require less energy substrate supply)—recent observations suggest that optimal glucose utilization is impaired in early asymptomatic stages of the disease and may contribute or precipitate AD neuropathology. Data collected from both clinical and animal model research strongly suggest that significant decrease in brain metabolism occurs well before any clinical manifestation of AD, namely measurable cognitive decline (for review Petrella et al., 2003).

Changes in the concentration dynamics of •NO in the brain may contribute to altered neurometabolism in aging and AD. In structures of the CNS intimately linked to memory and learning, such as the hippocampus, •NO is produced by neurons upon activation of glutamatergic synapses (Ledo et al., 2005, 2015; Lourenço et al., 2011, 2014b). Besides its obvious role as a neuromodulator, acting namely as a retrograde messenger in plasticity phenomena associated with memory and learning (Prast and Philippu, 2001), •NO has been looked upon as a master regulator of neurometabolism, as discussed above. Alongside or as a consequence of inhibition of the mitochondrial electron transporting chain (Antunes and Cadenas, 2007), •NO has also been shown to boost glycolytic rate and glucose uptake (reviewed in Almeida et al., 2005). One can hypothesize that

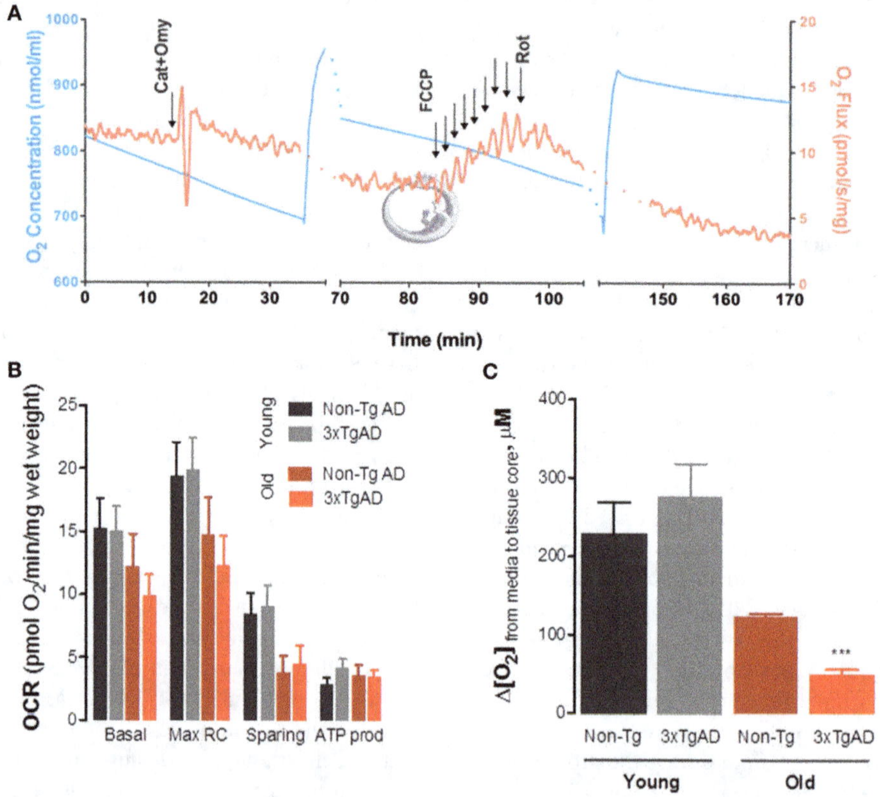

FIGURE 2 | Changes in mitochondrial oxidative phosphorylation in intact hippocampal slices from 3xTg-AD mice and Non-Tg mice show significant effect of aging on basal and maximal respiratory rates as well as sparing capacity. We developed a protocol that enabled us to evaluate OxPhos in intact hippocampal slices obtained from young and old-aged mice. Using a high-resolution respirometer (Oxygraph-2K, by Oroboros Instruments, Austria) we determined O_2 consumption rates (OCR) or O_2 flux (red line in **A**). Due to high O_2 requirement of hippocampal slices, experiments were performed at high $[O_2]$ and chambers were re-oxygenated throughout the experiment (blue line in **A**). Basal OCR was obtained in BSA-supplemented media containing 10 mM glucose+pyruvate. Carboxyatractyloside and oligomycin (CAT+Omy; 12.5 µM and 20 µg/mL) were then added to determine OCR not dependent on ATP production (leak). Maximal respiratory rate was achieved by titration with FCCP (20 µM), following which non-mitochondrial respiration was determined by adding rotenone (Rot, 2.2 µM). From each recording we determined the OCR values presented in **(B)**. Two-Way ANOVA analysis revealed a significant effect of age on both maximal ($F = 4.69$; $P = 0.0368$) and sparing capacity ($F = 7.39$; $^{***}p = 0.01$). In **(C)** one can observe that the drop in $[O_2]$ from the medium bathing the hippocampal slice (aCSF bubbled with $95\%O_2/5\%CO_2$ gas mixture, at 32°C) is significantly decreased in old-aged 3xTg-AD, further supporting respirometry data showing decrease in basal metabolic rate. This drop was determined electrochemically using carbon fiber microelectrodes held at −0, 8 V vs. Ag/AgCl and lowered from the perfusion media into the slice core gradually (see Ledo et al., 2005 for detailed description).

changes in either •NO concentration dynamics or cellular redox environment toward a more oxidative status (which promotes production of reactive oxygen and nitrogen species), not only detours •NO from its physiological role but also precipitates the production of highly oxidative and nitrosative sprecies such as peroxynitrite and dinitrogen trioxide (Heinrich et al., 2013). In line with this hypothesis, increase in tyrosine nitration is observed in the brains of AD patients when compared to healthy age-matched individuals, indicating changes in •NO bioactivity (Fernandez-Vizarra et al., 2004).

Using hippocampal slices to measure both NMDA-evoked •NO production and changes in O_2 profiles in the CA1 subregion, we have previously shown that •NO may act as a modulator of neurometabolic rate upon stimulation of glutamatergic transmission (Ledo et al., 2010). In hippocampal slices obtained from old-age 3xTg-AD mice, and looking specifically at the CA1 pyramidal layer, we observe decreased •NO upon activation of NMDA receptor (unpublished data), which most likely results from changes in •NO bioavailability due to its rapid reaction with species such as superoxide radical to produce peroxynitrite. As a consequence, we also observed that the tight coupling between neuronal-•NO and inhibition of O_2 consumption as shown in healthy subjects is lost, suggesting that •NO is no longer capable or available to act as the master regulator of neurometabolic coupling.

Conclusion

An increasing amount of evidence supports the notion that Alzheimer's disease is a multifaceted pathology that goes far beyond the amyloid pathology. As a major risk factor for AD, aging shares many common features associated with functional decline, namely neurovascular and neurometabolic alterations. Although the causal role of these changes in AD pathology remains controversial, it seems increasingly certain that they significantly impact the progression of neuronal dysfunction. Furthermore, the imbalance in the regulation of the neurovascular and neurometabolic coupling, resulting from cerebrovascular dysfunction, appear to be precocious events in neurodegeneration and brain aging. This shift in paradigm and the role of vascular redox status of brain microcirculation may be crucial for development of adequate therapeutically strategies that hamper cognition defects and neurodegeneration.

Acknowledgments

This work was supported by FEDER funds through the Programa Operacional Factores de Competitividade—COMPETE and National funds via FCT—Fundação para a Ciência e a Tecnologia under project(s) PTDC/BBB-BQB/3217/2012 and PTDC/BIA-BCM/116576/2010. Strategic project UID/NEU/04539/2013. CFL acknowledges FCT post-doctoral fellowship SFRH/BPD/82436/2011.

References

Almeida, A., Cidad, P., Delgado-Esteban, M., Fernandez, E., Garcia-Nogales, P., and Bolanos, J. P. (2005). Inhibition of mitochondrial respiration by nitric oxide: its role in glucose metabolism and neuroprotection. *J. Neurosci. Res.* 79, 166–171. doi: 10.1002/jnr.20281

Alsop, D. C., Detre, J. A., and Grossman, M. (2000). Assessment of cerebral blood flow in Alzheimer's disease by spin-labeled magnetic resonance imaging. *Ann. Neurol.* 47, 93–100. doi: 10.1002/1531-8249(200001)47:1<93::AID-ANA15>3.0.CO;2-8

Antunes, F., and Cadenas, E. (2007). The mechanism of cytochrome C oxidase inhibition by nitric oxide. *Front. Biosci.* 12:2118. doi: 10.2741/2118

Attwell, D., Buchan, A. M., Charpak, S., Lauritzen, M., Macvicar, B. A., and Newman, E. A. (2010). Glial and neuronal control of brain blood flow. *Nature* 468, 232–43. doi: 10.1038/nature09613

Bader Lange, M. L., Cenini, G., Piroddi, M., Abdul, H. M., Sultana, R., Galli, F., et al. (2008). Loss of phospholipid asymmetry and elevated brain apoptotic protein levels in subjects with amnestic mild cognitive impairment and Alzheimer disease. *Neurobiol. Dis.* 29, 456–464. doi: 10.1016/j.nbd.2007.11.004

Barzilai, N., Huffman, D. M., Muzumdar, R. H., and Bartke, A. (2012). The critical role of metabolic pathways in aging. *Diabetes* 61, 1315–1322. doi: 10.2337/db11-1300

Bell, R. D., and Zlokovic, B. V. (2009). Neurovascular mechanisms and blood-brain barrier disorder in Alzheimer's disease. *Acta Neuropathol.* 118, 103–113. doi: 10.1007/s00401-009-0522-3

Bolanos, J. P., Delgado-Esteban, M., Herrero-Mendez, A., Fernandez-Fernandez, S., and Almeida, A. (2008). Regulation of glycolysis and pentose-phosphate pathway by nitric oxide: impact on neuronal survival. *Biochim. Biophys. Acta* 1777, 789–793. doi: 10.1016/j.bbabio.2008.05.179

Brown, G. C. (2007). Nitric oxide and mitochondria. *Front. Biosci.* 12:2122. doi: 10.2741/2122

Cadenas, E. (2004). Mitochondrial free radical production and cell signaling. *Mol. Aspects Med.* 25, 17–26. doi: 10.1016/j.mam.2004.02.005

Casley, C. S., Land, J. M., Sharpe, M. A., Clark, J. B., Duchen, M. R., and Canevari, L. (2002). Beta-amyloid fragment 25-35 causes mitochondrial dysfunction in primary cortical neurons. *Neurobiol. Dis.* 10, 258–267. doi: 10.1006/nbdi.2002.0516

Castegna, A., Lauderback, C. M., Mohmmad-Abdul, H., and Butterfield, D. A. (2004). Modulation of phospholipid asymmetry in synaptosomal membranes by the lipid peroxidation products, 4-hydroxynonenal and acrolein: implications for Alzheimer's disease. *Brain Res.* 1004, 193–197. doi: 10.1016/j.brainres.2004.01.036

Chaturvedi, R. K., and Flint Beal, M. (2013). Mitochondrial diseases of the brain. *Free Radic. Biol. Med.* 63, 1–29. doi: 10.1016/j.freeradbiomed.2013.03.018

Christopherson, K. S., Hillier, B. J., Lim, W. A., and Bredt, D. S. (1999). PSD-95 assembles a ternary complex with the N-methyl-D-aspartic acid receptor and a bivalent neuronal NO synthase PDZ domain. *J. Biol. Chem.* 274, 27467–27473. doi: 10.1074/jbc.274.39.27467

Corder, E. H., Saunders, A. M., Strittmatter, W. J., Schmechel, D. E., Gaskell, P. C., Small, G. W., et al. (1993). Gene dose of apolipoprotein E type 4 allele and the risk of Alzheimer's disease in late onset families. *Science* 261, 921–923. doi: 10.1126/science.8346443

de la Torre, J. C. (2012). Cerebral hemodynamics and vascular risk factors: setting the stage for Alzheimer's disease. *J. Alzheimers Dis.* 32, 553–567. doi: 10.3233/JAD-2012-120793

de Leon, M. J., Ferris, S. H., George, A. E., Christman, D. R., Fowler, J. S., Gentes, C., et al. (1983). Positron emission tomographic studies of aging and Alzheimer disease. *AJNR Am. J. Neuroradiol.* 4, 568–571.

Duarte, J. M., Schuck, P. F., Wenk, G. L., and Ferreira, G. C. (2014). Metabolic disturbances in diseases with neurological involvement. *Aging Dis.* 5, 238–255. doi: 10.14336/AD.2014.0500238

Fabiani, M., Gordon, B. A., Maclin, E. L., Pearson, M. A., Brumback-Peltz, C. R., Low, K. A., et al. (2014). Neurovascular coupling in normal aging: a combined optical, ERP and fMRI study. *Neuroimage* 85(Pt 1), 592–607. doi: 10.1016/j.neuroimage.2013.04.113

Fernandez-Vizarra, P., Fernandez, A. P., Castro-Blanco, S., Encinas, J. M., Serrano, J., Bentura, M. L., et al. (2004). Expression of nitric oxide system in clinically evaluated cases of Alzheimer's disease. *Neurobiol. Dis.* 15, 287–305. doi: 10.1016/j.nbd.2003.10.010

Fisher, J. P., Hartwich, D., Seifert, T., Olesen, N. D., McNulty, C. L., Nielsen, H. B., et al. (2013). Cerebral perfusion, oxygenation and metabolism during exercise in young and elderly individuals. *J. Physiol.* 591(Pt 7), 1859–1870. doi: 10.1113/jphysiol.2012.244905

Fleisher, A. S., Podraza, K. M., Bangen, K. J., Taylor, C., Sherzai, A., Sidhar, K., et al. (2009). Cerebral perfusion and oxygenation differences in Alzheimer's disease risk. *Neurobiol. Aging* 30, 1737–1748. doi: 10.1016/j.neurobiolaging.2008.01.012

Gearing, M., Mirra, S. S., Hedreen, J. C., Sumi, S. M., Hansen, L. A., and Heyman, A. (1995). The Consortium to Establish a Registry for Alzheimer's Disease (CERAD). Part X. Neuropathology confirmation of the clinical diagnosis of Alzheimer's disease. *Neurology* 45(3 Pt 1), 461–466. doi: 10.1212/WNL.45.3.461

Girouard, H., and Iadecola, C. (2006). Neurovascular coupling in the normal brain and in hypertension, stroke, and Alzheimer disease. *J. Appl. Physiol.* 100, 328–335. doi: 10.1152/japplphysiol.00966.2005

Giulivi, C. (2003). Characterization and function of mitochondrial nitric-oxide synthase. *Free Radic. Biol. Med.* 34, 397–408. doi: 10.1016/S0891-5849(02)01298-4

Gordon, G. R., Choi, H. B., Rungta, R. L., Ellis-Davies, G. C., and MacVicar, B. A. (2008). Brain metabolism dictates the polarity of astrocyte control over arterioles. *Nature* 456, 745–79. doi: 10.1038/nature07525

Guix, F. X., Uribesalgo, I., Coma, M., and Munoz, F. J. (2005). The physiology and pathophysiology of nitric oxide in the brain. *Prog. Neurobiol.* 76, 126–152. doi: 10.1016/j.pneurobio.2005.06.001

Hamel, E., Nicolakakis, N., Aboulkassim, T., Ongali, B., and Tong, X. K. (2008). Oxidative stress and cerebrovascular dysfunction in mouse models of Alzheimer's disease. *Exp. Physiol.* 93, 116–120. doi: 10.1113/expphysiol.2007.038729

Haralampos, J. M., Matilda, F., and Sotirios, G. (2008). Metabolic syndrome and Alzheimer's disease: a link to a vascular hypothesis? *CNS Spectr.* 13, 606–613. doi: 10.1017/S1092852900016886

Harris, J. J., Jolivet, R., and Attwell, D. (2012). Synaptic energy use and supply. *Neuron* 75, 762–777. doi: 10.1016/j.neuron.2012.08.019

Heinrich, T. A., da Silva, R. S., Miranda, K. M., Switzer, C. H., Wink, D. A., and Fukuto, J. M. (2013). Biological nitric oxide signaling: chemistry and terminology (NO chemical biology and terminology). *Br. J. Pharmacol.* 169, 1417–1429. doi: 10.1111/bph.12217

Hsia, A. Y., Masliah, E., McConlogue, L., Yu, G. Q., Tatsuno, G., Hu, K., et al. (1999). Plaque-independent disruption of neural circuits in Alzheimer's disease mouse models. *Proc. Natl. Acad. Sci. U.S.A.* 96, 3228–3233. doi: 10.1073/pnas.96.6.3228

Iadecola, C. (1993). Regulation of the cerebral microcirculation during neural activity: is nitric oxide the missing link? *Trends Neurosci.* 16, 206–214. doi: 10.1016/0166-2236(93)90156-G

Iadecola, C. (2004). Neurovascular regulation in the normal brain and in Alzheimer's disease. *Nat. Rev. Neurosci.* 5, 347–360. doi: 10.1038/nrn1387

Iadecola, C., Zhang, F., Niwa, K., Eckman, C., Turner, S. K., Fischer, E., et al. (1999). SOD1 rescues cerebral endothelial dysfunction in mice overexpressing amyloid precursor protein. *Nat. Neurosci.* 2, 157–161. doi: 10.1038/5715

Jellinger, K. A., and Mitter-Ferstl, E. (2003). The impact of cerebrovascular lesions in Alzheimer disease–a comparative autopsy study. *J. Neurol.* 250, 1050–1055. doi: 10.1007/s00415-003-0142-0

Kalaria, R. N. (2012). Cerebrovascular disease and mechanisms of cognitive impairment: evidence from clinicopathological studies in humans. *Stroke* 43, 2526–2534. doi: 10.1161/strokeaha.112.655803

Kealy, J., Bennett, R., and Lowry, J. P. (2013). Simultaneous recording of hippocampal oxygen and glucose in real time using constant potential amperometry in the freely-moving rat. *J. Neurosci. Methods* 215, 110–120. doi: 10.1016/j.jneumeth.2013.02.016

Kish, S. J., Bergeron, C., Rajput, A., Dozic, S., Mastrogiacomo, F., Chang, L. J., et al. (1992). Brain cytochrome oxidase in Alzheimer's disease. *J. Neurochem.* 59, 776–779. doi: 10.1111/j.1471-4159.1992.tb09439.x

Koike, M. A., Green, K. N., Blurton-Jones, M., and Laferla, F. M. (2010). Oligemic hypoperfusion differentially affects tau and amyloid-{beta}. *Am. J. Pathol.* 177, 300–310. doi: 10.2353/ajpath.2010.090750

Krejza, J., Mariak, Z., Walecki, J., Szydlik, P., Lewko, J., and Ustymowicz, A. (1999). Transcranial color Doppler sonography of basal cerebral arteries in 182 healthy subjects: age and sex variability and normal reference values for blood flow parameters. *AJR Am. J. Roentgenol.* 172, 213–218. doi: 10.2214/ajr.172.1.9888770

Ledo, A., Barbosa, R., Cadenas, E., and Laranjinha, J. (2010). Dynamic and interacting profiles of *NO and O2 in rat hippocampal slices. *Free Radic. Biol. Med.* 48, 1044–1050. doi: 10.1016/j.freeradbiomed.2010.01.024

Ledo, A., Barbosa, R., Gerhardtt, G., Cadenas, E., and Laranjinha, J. (2005). Concentration dynamics of nitric oxide in rat hippocampal subregions evoked by stimulation of the NMDA glutamate receptor. *Proc. Natl. Acad. Sci. U.S.A.* 102, 17483–17488. doi: 10.1073/pnas.0503624102

Ledo, A., Lourenço, C. F., Caetano, M., Barbosa, R. M., and Laranjinha, J. (2015). Age-associated changes of nitric oxide concentration dynamics in the central nervous system of fisher 344 rats. *Cell. Mol. Neurobiol.* 35, 33–44. doi: 10.1007/s10571-014-0115-0

Lesne, S., Koh, M. T., Kotilinek, L., Kayed, R., Glabe, C. G., Yang, A., et al. (2006). A specific amyloid-beta protein assembly in the brain impairs memory. *Nature* 440, 352–357. doi: 10.1038/nature04533

Lesne, S., and Kotilinek, L. (2005). Amyloid plaques and amyloid-beta oligomers: an ongoing debate. *J. Neurosci.* 25, 9319–9320. doi: 10.1523/JNEUROSCI.3246-05.2005

Lin, M. T., Simon, D. K., Ahn, C. H., Kim, L. M., and Beal, M. F. (2002). High aggregate burden of somatic mtDNA point mutations in aging and Alzheimer's disease brain. *Hum. Mol. Genet.* 11, 133–145. doi: 10.1093/hmg/11.2.133

Lourenço, C. F., Ferreira, N. R., Santos, R. M., Lukacova, N., Barbosa, R. M., and Laranjinha, J. (2014b). The pattern of glutamate-induced nitric oxide dynamics *in vivo* and its correlation with nNOS expression in rat hippocampus, cerebral cortex and striatum. *Brain Res.* 1554, 1–11. doi: 10.1016/j.brainres.2014.01.030

Lourenço, C. F., Santos, R., Barbosa, R. M., Gerhardt, G., Cadenas, E., and Laranjinha, J. (2011). *In vivo* modulation of nitric oxide concentration dynamics upon glutamatergic neuronal activation in the hippocampus. *Hippocampus* 21, 622–630. doi: 10.1002/hipo.20774

Lourenço, C. F., Santos, R. M., Barbosa, R. M., Cadenas, E., Radi, R., and Laranjinha, J. (2014a). Neurovascular coupling in hippocampus is mediated via diffusion by neuronal-derived nitric oxide. *Free Radic. Biol. Med.* 73, 421–49. doi: 10.1016/j.freeradbiomed.2014.05.021

Manczak, M., Anekonda, T. S., Henson, E., Park, B. S., Quinn, J., and Reddy, P. H. (2006). Mitochondria are a direct site of A beta accumulation in Alzheimer's disease neurons: implications for free radical generation and oxidative damage in disease progression. *Hum. Mol. Genet.* 15, 1437–1449. doi: 10.1093/hmg/ddl066

Maurer, I., Zierz, S., and Möller, H. J. (2000). A selective defect of cytochrome c oxidase is present in brain of Alzheimer disease patients. *Neurobiol. Aging* 21, 455–462. doi: 10.1016/S0197-4580(00)00112-3

Melov, S., Adlard, P. A., Morten, K., Johnson, F., Golden, T. R., Hinerfeld, D., et al. (2007). Mitochondrial oxidative stress causes hyperphosphorylation of tau. *PLoS ONE* 2:e536 doi: 10.1371/journal.pone.0000536

Mohmmad Abdul, H., and Butterfield, D. A. (2005). Protection against amyloid beta-peptide (1-42)-induced loss of phospholipid asymmetry in synaptosomal membranes by tricyclodecan-9-xanthogenate (D609) and ferulic acid ethyl ester: implications for Alzheimer's disease. *Biochim. Biophys. Acta* 1741, 140–148. doi: 10.1016/j.bbadis.2004.12.002

Moncada, S., and Bolaños, J. P. (2006). Nitric oxide, cell bioenergetics and neurodegeneration. *J. Neurochem.* 97, 1676–189. doi: 10.1111/j.1471-4159.2006.03988.x

Mosconi, L., Tsui, W. H., De Santi, S., Li, J., Rusinek, H., Convit, A., et al. (2005). Reduced hippocampal metabolism in MCI and AD: automated FDG-PET image analysis. *Neurology* 64, 1860–1867. doi: 10.1212/01.WNL.0000163856.13524.08

Mucke, L., Yu, G. Q., McConlogue, L., Rockenstein, E. M., Abraham, C. R., and Masliah, E. (2000). Astroglial expression of human alpha(1)-antichymotrypsin enhances alzheimer-like pathology in amyloid protein precursor transgenic mice. *Am. J. Pathol.* 157, 2003–2010. doi: 10.1016/S0002-9440(10)64839-0

Mutisya, E. M., Bowling, A. C., and Beal, M. F. (1994). Cortical cytochrome oxidase activity is reduced in Alzheimer's disease. *J. Neurochem.* 63, 2179–2184. doi: 10.1046/j.1471-4159.1994.63062179.x

Niwa, K., Carlson, G. A., and Iadecola, C. (2000b). Exogenous A beta1-40 reproduces cerebrovascular alterations resulting from amyloid precursor protein overexpression in mice. *J. Cereb. Blood Flow Metab.* 20, 1659–1668. doi: 10.1097/00004647-200012000-00005

Niwa, K., Kazama, K., Younkin, S. G., Carlson, G. A., and Iadecola, C. (2002). Alterations in cerebral blood flow and glucose utilization in mice overexpressing the amyloid precursor protein. *Neurobiol. Dis.* 9, 61–68. doi: 10.1006/nbdi.2001.0460

Niwa, K., Porter, V. A., Kazama, K., Cornfield, D., Carlson, G. A., and Iadecola, C. (2001). A beta-peptides enhance vasoconstriction in cerebral circulation. *Am. J. Physiol. Heart Circ. Physiol.* 281, H2417–H2424.

Niwa, K., Younkin, L., Ebeling, C., Turner, S. K., Westaway, D., Younkin, S., et al. (2000a). Abeta 1-40-related reduction in functional hyperemia in mouse neocortex during somatosensory activation. *Proc. Natl. Acad. Sci. U.S.A.* 97, 9735–9740. doi: 10.1073/pnas.97.17.9735

Oddo, S., Caccamo, A., Shepherd, J. D., Murphy, M. P., Golde, T. E., Kayed, R., et al. (2003). Triple-transgenic model of Alzheimer's disease with plaques and tangles: intracellular Abeta and synaptic dysfunction. *Neuron* 39, 409–421. doi: 10.1016/S0896-6273(03)00434-3

Palamalai, V., and Miyagi, M. (2010). Mechanism of glyceraldehyde-3-phosphate dehydrogenase inactivation by tyrosine nitration. *Protein Sci.* 19, 255–62. doi: 10.1002/pro.311

Petrella, J. R., Coleman, R. E., and Doraiswamy, P. M. (2003). Neuroimaging and early diagnosis of Alzheimer disease: a look to the future. *Radiology* 226, 315–336. doi: 10.1148/radiol.2262011600

Prast, H., and Philippu, A. (2001). Nitric oxide as modulator of neuronal function. *Prog. Neurobiol.* 64, 51–68. doi: 10.1016/S0301-0082(00)00044-7

Rancillac, A., Rossier, J., Guille, M., Tong, X. K., Geoffroy, H., Amatore, C., et al. (2006). Glutamatergic control of microvascular tone by distinct GABA neurons in the cerebellum. *J. Neurosci.* 26, 6997–7006. doi: 10.1523/jneurosci.5515-05.2006

Reiman, E. M., Chen, K., Alexander, G. E., Caselli, R. J., Bandy, D., Osborne, D., et al. (2005). Correlations between apolipoprotein E epsilon4 gene dose and brain-imaging measurements of regional hypometabolism. *Proc. Natl. Acad. Sci. U.S.A.* 102, 8299–8302. doi: 10.1073/pnas.0500579102

Rossignol, R., Faustin, B., Rocher, C., Malgat, M., Mazat, J. P., and Letellier, T. (2003). Mitochondrial threshold effects. *Biochem. J.* 370(Pt 3), 751–62. doi: 10.1042/bj20021594

Ruitenberg, A., den Heijer, T., Bakker, S. L., van Swieten, J. C., Koudstaal, P. J., Hofman, A., et al. (2005). Cerebral hypoperfusion and clinical onset of dementia: the Rotterdam Study. *Ann. Neurol.* 57, 789–794. doi: 10.1002/ana.20493

Scholl, M., Almkvist, O., Axelman, K., Stefanova, E., Wall, A., Westman, E., et al. (2011). Glucose metabolism and PIB binding in carriers of a His163Tyr presenilin 1 mutation. *Neurobiol. Aging* 32, 1388–1399. doi: 10.1016/j.neurobiolaging.2009.08.016

Schultz, S. K., O'Leary, D. S., Boles Ponto, L. L., Watkins, G. L., Hichwa, R. D., and Andreasen, N. C. (1999). Age-related changes in regional cerebral blood flow among young to mid-life adults. *Neuroreport* 10, 2493–2496. doi: 10.1097/00001756-199908200-00011

Shulman, R. G., and Rothman, D. L. (1998). Interpreting functional imaging studies in terms of neurotransmitter cycling. *Proc. Natl. Acad. Sci. U.S.A.* 95, 11993–11998. doi: 10.1073/pnas.95.20.11993

Swerdlow, R. H. (2007). Is aging part of Alzheimer's disease, or is Alzheimer's disease part of aging? *Neurobiol. Aging* 28, 1465–1480. doi: 10.1016/j.neurobiolaging.2006.06.021

Swerdlow, R. H., Burns, J. M., and Khan, S. M. (2014). The Alzheimer's disease mitochondrial cascade hypothesis: progress and perspectives. *Biochim. Biophys. Acta* 1842, 1219–1231. doi: 10.1016/j.bbadis.2013.09.010

Thomas, T., Thomas, G., McLendon, C., Sutton, T., and Mullan, M. (1996). beta-Amyloid-mediated vasoactivity and vascular endothelial damage. *Nature* 380, 168–171. doi: 10.1038/380168a0

Velliquette, R. A., O'Connor, T., and Vassar, R. (2005). Energy inhibition elevates beta-secretase levels and activity and is potentially amyloidogenic in APP transgenic mice: possible early events in Alzheimer's disease pathogenesis. *J. Neurosci.* 25, 10874–10883. doi: 10.1523/JNEUROSCI.2350-05.2005

Venturini, G., Colasanti, M., Persichini, T., Fioravanti, E., Ascenzi, P., Palomba, L., et al. (2002). Beta-amyloid inhibits NOS activity by subtracting NADPH availability. *FASEB J.* 16, 1970–1972. doi: 10.1096/fj.02-0186fje

Victor, V. M., Nunez, C., D'Ocon, P., Taylor, C. T., Esplugues, J. V., and Moncada, S. (2009). Regulation of oxygen distribution in tissues by endothelial nitric oxide. *Circ. Res.* 104, 1178–1183. doi: 10.1161/circresaha.109.197228

Wallace, D. C. (1992). Mitochondrial genetics: a paradigm for aging and degenerative diseases? *Science* 256, 628–632. doi: 10.1126/science.1533953

Walsh, D. M., Klyubin, I., Shankar, G. M., Townsend, M., Fadeeva, J. V., Betts, V., et al. (2005). The role of cell-derived oligomers of Abeta in Alzheimer's disease and avenues for therapeutic intervention. *Biochem. Soc. Trans.* 33(Pt 5), 1087–1090. doi: 10.1042/BST20051087

Winkler, S. R., and Luer, M. S. (1998). Antiepileptic drug review: part 1. *Surg. Neurol.* 49, 449–452. doi: 10.1016/S0090-3019(97)00223-1

Xu, G., Antuono, P. G., Jones, J., Xu, Y., Wu, G., Ward, D., et al. (2007). Perfusion fMRI detects deficits in regional CBF during memory-encoding tasks in MCI subjects. *Neurology* 69, 1650–1656. doi: 10.1212/01.wnl.0000296941.06685.22

Yin, F., Boveris, A., and Cadenas, E. (2014). Mitochondrial energy metabolism and redox signaling in brain aging and neurodegeneration. *Antioxid. Redox Signal.* 20, 353–371. doi: 10.1089/ars.2012.4774

Zlokovic, B. V. (2011). Neurovascular pathways to neurodegeneration in Alzheimer's disease and other disorders. *Nat. Rev. Neurosci.* 12, 723–738. doi: 10.1038/nrn3114

13

Triad of Risk for Late Onset Alzheimer's: Mitochondrial Haplotype, APOE Genotype and Chromosomal Sex

Yiwei Wang[1] *and Roberta D. Brinton*[2]*

[1] *Department of Clinical Pharmacy, School of Pharmacy, University of Southern California, Los Angeles, CA, USA,*
[2] *Department of Pharmacology and Pharmaceutical Sciences, School of Pharmacy, University of Southern California, Los Angeles, CA, USA*

Edited by:
George E. Barreto,
Pontifical Xavierian University,
Colombia

Reviewed by:
Panteleimon Giannakopoulos,
University of Geneva, Switzerland
Russell H. Swerdlow,
University of Kansas, USA

Correspondence:
Roberta D. Brinton
rbrinton@usc.edu

Brain is the most energetically demanding organ of the body, and is thus vulnerable to even modest decline in ATP generation. Multiple neurodegenerative diseases are associated with decline in mitochondrial function, e.g., Alzheimer's, Parkinson's, multiple sclerosis and multiple neuropathies. Genetic variances in the mitochondrial genome can modify bioenergetic and respiratory phenotypes, at both the cellular and system biology levels. Mitochondrial haplotype can be a key driver of mitochondrial efficiency. Herein, we focus on the association between mitochondrial haplotype and risk of late onset Alzheimer's disease (LOAD). Evidence for the association of mitochondrial genetic variances/haplotypes and the risk of developing LOAD are explored and discussed. Further, we provide a conceptual framework that suggests an interaction between mitochondrial haplotypes and two demonstrated risk factors for Alzheimer's disease (AD), apolipoprotein E (APOE) genotype and chromosomal sex. We posit herein that mitochondrial haplotype, and hence respiratory capacity, plays a key role in determining risk of LOAD and other age-associated neurodegenerative diseases. Further, therapeutic design and targeting that involve mitochondrial haplotype would advance precision medicine for AD and other age related neurodegenerative diseases.

Keywords: mitochondria, haplogroup, Alzheimer's disease, APOE, sex

INTRODUCTION

A central role of mitochondria in age-related metabolic and neurodegenerative diseases has long been proposed, and an association between mitochondrial dysfunction and Alzheimer's disease has been long proposed across multiple investigative strategies from analysis of human tissue to cell model systems (Beal, 1996; Gibson et al., 2000; Trimmer et al., 2000; Swerdlow and Khan, 2004; Bubber et al., 2005; Wallace, 2005; Lin and Beal, 2006; Brinton, 2008, 2009; Khusnutdinova et al., 2008; Simpkins et al., 2008; Coskun et al., 2012; Brinton et al., 2015). The "mitochondrial cascade hypothesis", originally proposed by Swerdlow and Khan (2004) as an explanation for late onset Alzheimer's disease (LOAD), proposed that inherited mitochondrial genetic variations and mutations accumulated from aging should occupy the apex of the disease cascade. Briefly, this hypothesis maintained that mitochondrial genetic variations and mutations lead to deficient electron transport chain function, resulting in less ATP production, increased free radical production, disrupted

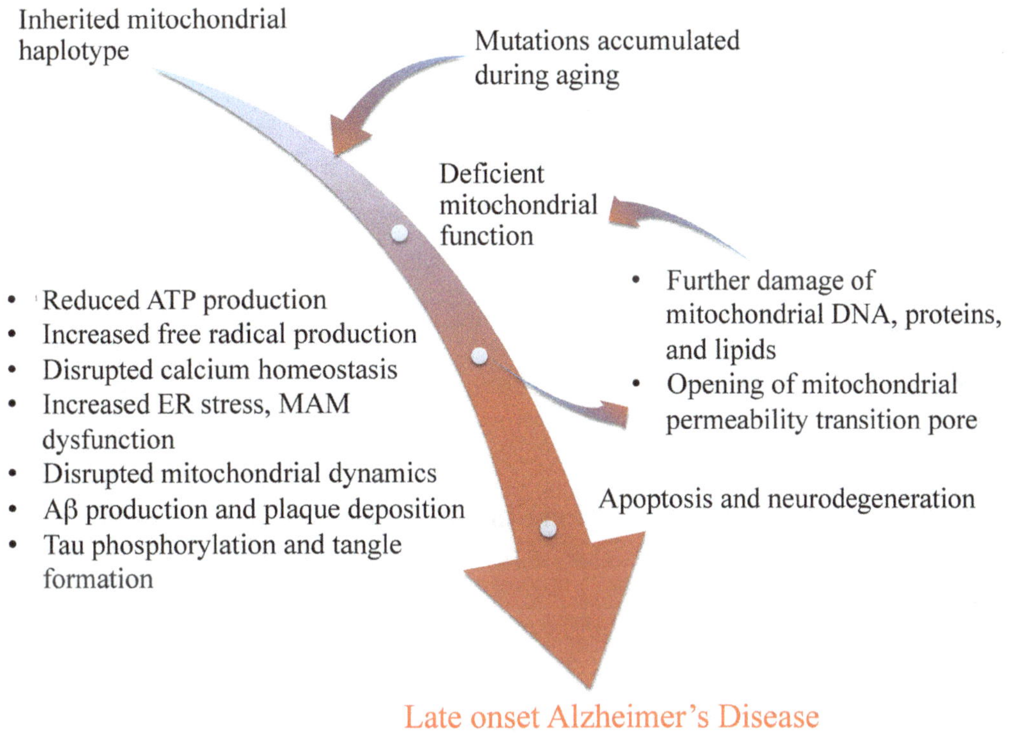

FIGURE 1 | Modified mitochondrial cascade of late-onset Alzheimer's disease (LOAD). Inherited mitochondrial genetic variations and accumulated mutations during aging lead to deficiency in mitochondrial functions, initiating a cascade of events including reduced ATP production, increased free radical formation and ER stress, disrupted mitochondrial associated membrane (MAM) function and mitochondrial dynamics, as well as amyloid beta plaque and tau tangle formation, which result in further damages of mitochondria and ultimately leads to apoptosis and neurodegeneration, such as LOAD.

calcium homeostasis, beta amyloid production and plaque deposition, and tau phosphorylation and tangle formation. These results in turn lead to further damage of mitochondrial DNA, proteins, and lipids, and the opening of mitochondrial permeability transition pore, which ultimately leads to cell death and neurodegeneration (see **Figure 1**). Recent studies also indicated disrupted crosstalk between mitochondria and endoplasmic reticulum (ER) via mitochondrial associated membrane (MAM), as well as abnormal mitochondrial dynamics in the etiology of Alzheimer's disease (AD; Trimmer et al., 2000; Baloyannis et al., 2004; Paillusson et al., 2013; Burté et al., 2015; Zhang et al., 2016; see **Figure 1**).

Here we review the link between mitochondrial dysfunction and the risk of AD, the contribution of mitochondrial genetic variances to the risk, and how the risk is modulated by other factors, such as apolipoprotein E (APOE) genotype and sex differences.

MITOCHONDRIAL GENOME AND HAPLOTYPES

Unlike many other organelles, mitochondria have their own genome. The human mitochondrial genome is a circular set of 16,569 base pairs encoding 37 genes. Thirteen of these genes encode protein subunits required for four of the five electron transport chain complexes: complex I (NADH ubiquinone oxidoreductase), complex III (cytochrome bc1 complex), complex IV (cytochrome c oxidase), and complex V (ATP synthase); two encode rRNAs for mitochondrial ribosomes (12S and 16S), and 22 encode tRNAs (see **Figure 2**).

Mitochondrial retention of their own genome throughout evolution solves two cell biology problems. First, the 13 electron transport subunits coded by mitochondrial DNA solves the problem that if they were generated by nuclear DNA, they would not cross the inner mitochondria membrane due to their high hydrophobicity (Popot and de Vitry, 1990). Second, the eukaryotic mitochondrial genome is transcribed and translated quite differently than the nuclear genome (Mercer et al., 2011). The genetic system of the mitochondria is transcribed as precursor polycistronic transcripts that are subsequently cleaved to generate mRNAs, tRNAs and rRNAs (Mercer et al., 2011). The mRNAs devoted to generating the 13 catalytic subunits required for oxidative phosphorylation are further translated using several non-universal codons unique to the mitochondrial translation machinery (Watanabe, 2010; Watanabe and Yokobori, 2011).

Like nuclear DNA, mitochondrial DNA undergoes mutation, though at a much higher rate (Miyata et al., 1982; Wallace et al., 1987), likely due to higher replication rate, a more

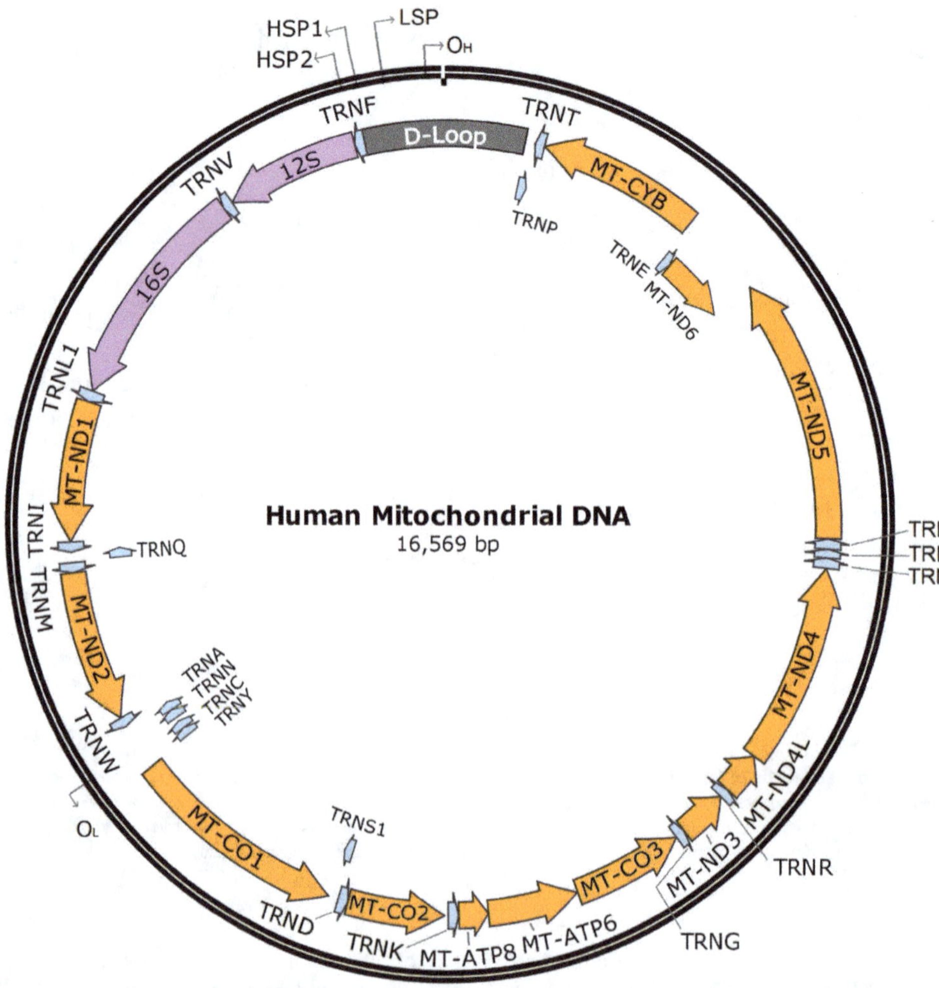

FIGURE 2 | Human mitochondrial DNA. Orange indicates protein-encoding genes (13), purple indicates mitochondrial rRNAs (2), blue indicates tRNAs (22), and gray indicates the D-loop. O_H: heavy strand origin, O_L: light strand origin, HSP1: major heavy strand promoter, HSP2: minor heavy strand promoter, LSP, light strand promoter.

mutagenic environment, and less efficient DNA repair (Xu et al., 2012). Unlike the nucleus, the mitochondrial DNA repair mechanism is largely limited to base excision repair. Mismatch as a result of either recombination or repair can lead to single nucleotide polymorphisms (SNPs).

Clusters of specific SNPs in the mitochondrial genome define mitochondrial haplogroups that reflect maternal lineage (Giles et al., 1980; Torroni et al., 1992). For example, the four lineages specific for sub-Saharan Africa are L0, L1, L2 and L3, and haplogroups A, B, C, D, G and F are common in Asia (Stewart and Chinnery, 2015). The major haplogroups within descendants of European ancestry are haplogroups H, I, J, K, M, T, U, V, W and X (Torroni et al., 1996). These haplogroups can be further classified into subhaplogroups or clustered together into superhaplogroups, such as superhaplogroup HV, JT, UK.

MITOCHONDRIAL DYSFUNCTION AND INCREASED RISK OF ALZHEIMER'S DISEASE

AD is a systemic disease with multiple etiologies (Morris et al., 2014). Early evidence linking mitochondrial dysfunction to AD dates back to a 1987 study by Sims et al. (1987), who found a reduced rate of oxygen uptake in the presence and absence of ADP in frontal neocortex of postmortem confirmed AD cases, indicating potential mitochondrial uncoupling in AD patients (Sims et al., 1987).

More direct evidence for the association between mitochondrial dysfunction and AD came later from studies on the activity of electron transport chain enzymes in AD patients and post mortem AD brain tissues. In the early 1990's, reduced cytochrome c oxidase (complex IV) activity was observed in both platelets and postmortem AD brain

(Parker et al., 1990, 1994). The reduction of cytochrome c activity in AD brain was later refined to the temporal cortex and hippocampus (Maurer et al., 2000). Supporting these findings, reduced mRNA levels of cytochrome c oxidase subunit 1 and 3 were observed in AD mid temporal gyrus and cytochrome c oxidase subunit 2 in AD hippocampus (Chandrasekaran et al., 1994; Aksenov et al., 1999). Furthermore, in both AD temporal and parietal cortices, protein levels of cytochrome c oxidase subunits were reduced, especially those encoded by mitochondria DNA (Kish et al., 1999). Although no reduction of cytochrome c oxidase content was observed in platelets of AD patients, cytoplasmic hybrids (cybrids) containing exogenous mitochondria extracted from platelets of AD patients showed less cytochrome c oxidase activity compared to cybrids harboring mitochondria from age-matched controls (Davis et al., 1997; Sheehan et al., 1997; Cardoso et al., 2004). Alternations in gene expression, protein level, and activity of other electron transport chain complexes have also been reported in AD tissues, though the evidence was less compelling and sometimes contradicted (Schagger and Ohm, 1995; Chandrasekaran et al., 1997; Aksenov et al., 1999; Kim et al., 2000; Bosetti et al., 2002; Bubber et al., 2005; Valla et al., 2006).

Upstream to electron transport chain, impairment of the tricarboxylic acid (TCA) cycle enzymes was observed in AD brain. Autopsy-confirmed AD brain had significantly reduced activity in pyruvate dehydrogenase complex, isocitrate dehydrogenase, and α-ketoglutarate dehydrogenase complex, whereas the activity of succinate dehydrogenase and malate dehydrogenase were increased (Bubber et al., 2005). The severity of enzyme activity impairment was also correlated with the clinical severity of Alzheimer's pathology (Bubber et al., 2005). Decreased mitochondrial respiratory capacity was consistent with the higher level of lactate and lower key substrates for TCA cycle in cerebrospinal fluid and blood in AD patients (Redjems-Bennani et al., 1998; Mancuso et al., 2003).

Consistent with deficits in mitochondrial respiratory capacity, AD brain had elevated levels of peroxidation products in the frontal cortex, as well as decreased levels of superoxide dismutase, a radical defensive enzyme, in the frontal cortex, hippocampus, and cerebellum (Richardson, 1993). Increased oxidative stress is consistent with free radical damage of mitochondrial components and loss of mitochondrial membrane potential as observed in cybrids harboring mitochondria with AD origin (Cassarino et al., 1998; Trimmer et al., 2000).

Besides altered bioenergetic capacity, the crosstalk between mitochondria and the ER via MAM, which regulates many key functions of mitochondria, such as calcium uptake, phospholipid exchange, intracellular trafficking, ER stress and mitochondrial biogenesis, was also disrupted in AD (Paillusson et al., 2013; Burté et al., 2015).

Beyond changes in mitochondrial function, distribution and morphology of mitochondria were also different in AD patients. Neurons from AD brain harbored mitochondria of smaller sizes and disrupted mitochondrial cristae morphology, and cybrids created using mitochondria from sporadic AD patients also showed swollen mitochondria and less cristae (Trimmer et al., 2000; Baloyannis et al., 2004). The fission and fusion cycle of mitochondria also seemed disrupted in the hippocampus of AD brain (Zhang et al., 2016). The number of mitochondria was also significantly reduced, likely as a result of increased mitochondria degradation, turnover and autophagy (Hirai et al., 2001).

AD has a pattern of maternal inheritance, where inheritance of AD from mothers are more frequent than from fathers (Duara et al., 1993). The observation of maternal pattern of Alzheimer's inheritance has been replicated over many decades by multiple groups, and has been linked to deficits in mitochondrial respiration and glucose metabolism apparently early in the aging process (Edland et al., 1996; Mosconi et al., 2011; Liu et al., 2013). In cognitively normal individuals, those with a maternal history of LOAD showed decline in platelet cytochrome c oxidase activity, compared to those with a paternal or no family history of the disease (Edland et al., 1996; Mosconi et al., 2011). In this same cohort, Mosconi et al. (2011) observed significantly lower brain glucose metabolism in persons with a maternal history of Alzheimer's relative to those with a paternal or no family history of the disease. These data coupled with maternal inheritance of the mitochondrial genome strongly support a role for mitochondrial genetic variances in the etiology of the disease.

MITOCHONDRIAL HAPLOTYPE IS ASSOCIATED WITH DIFFERENT RESPIRATORY, METABOLIC AND BIOENERGETIC PHENOTYPES

Mitochondrial genetic background can also affect metabolism and bioenergetic function. Resting metabolic rate (RMR) and total energy expenditure (TEE) were measured in 294 participants in the health, aging and body composition study (Health ABC; Tranah et al., 2011), including participants of cluster L, which contains common African haplogroups, and cluster N, which contains common European haplogroups (Tranah et al., 2011). Compared to N, cluster L had significantly lower RMR and TEE. Specifically, haplogroups L0, L2 and L3 had significantly lower RMR than haplogroup H and superhaplogroups UK and JT; haplogroup L3 had significantly lower TEE than haplogroup H and superhaplogroups UK and JT; haplogroup L2 had significantly lower TEE than haplogroup H and superhaplogroup JT (Tranah et al., 2011; see **Table 1**). In a cohort of healthy Spanish males, haplogroup J participants had significantly lower maximum oxygen consumption (VO_{2max}) than non-J participants (Marcuello et al., 2009). This difference was later confirmed in an independent cohort of healthy Spanish males, where haplogroup H was determined to be the driving force for the difference (Martínez-Redondo et al., 2010; see **Table 1**).

The underlying cellular mechanism of the observed differences across different mitochondrial haplogroups was

TABLE 1 | Mitochondrial haplogroups/superhaplogroups differentially associated with respiratory phenotypes.

	Relatively high	Relatively low	Reference
RMR	H, UK, JT	L2, L3, L3	Tranah et al. (2011)
TEE	H, UK, JT	L0, L2	Tranah et al. (2011)
VO_{2max}	H	J	Marcuello et al. (2009) and Martínez-Redondo et al. (2010)

Individuals of haplogroup/superhaplogroups H, UK and JT had higher rest metabolism rate (RMR), total energy differences (TEE) and/or VO_{2max} compared to individuals of cluster L and haplogroup J.

primarily elucidated using trans-mitochondrial cytoplasmic hybrids, or cybrids, which controlled for the nuclear genetic background to reveal mitochondrial variances. An early cybrids study using cultured A539 human lung carcinoma cells harboring either mitochondria of haplogroup H or T failed to identify any differences in bioenergetics function (Amo et al., 2008). However, differences in bioenergetics and mitochondrial function were identified in multiple later studies using different cell lines and mitochondrial haplogroups. Cybrids constructed from osteosarcoma 143B rho0 cells and platelets from healthy Spanish donors of either haplogroup H or superhaplogroup UK were investigated for mtDNA content (Gómez-Durán et al., 2010). Cybrids harboring UK superhaplogroup were found to have lower mtDNA content, lower mt-rRNA level, reduced protein synthesis, and decreased cytochrome c oxidase amount (Gómez-Durán et al., 2010). UK cybrids also had lower mitochondrial inner membrane potential and higher mitochondrial uncoupling, indicating potentially lower respiratory capacity and reduced ATP production (Gómez-Durán et al., 2010). Similar results were obtained in a later study in middle-age Caucasian males, where OXPHOS capacity normalized to citrate synthase content was found to be reduced by 24% in subjects with haplogroup U background comparing to those with haplogroup H background (Larsen et al., 2014). In 2013, cybrids constructed from human retinal epithelial cell line ARPE-19 and either haplogroup H or J mitochondria showed reduced ATP production and glycolysis in J cybrids (Kenney et al., 2013). In accordance with the observed reduction in mitochondrial respiration, J cybrids also showed lower ROS production (Kenney et al., 2013). Haplogroup J cybrids with chondrocyte nuclear genetic background also demonstrated lower NO levels than non-J cybrids (Fernández-Moreno et al., 2011). Similarly, major Asian mitochondrial haplogroups are also differentially associated with bioenergetic function (Lin et al., 2012). These associations identified in the human are also evident in animal models ranging from *Drosophila* to mice such that different mitochondrial genetic background is associated with differences in respiratory and metabolic phenotypes, electron transport chain enzyme activities and mitochondrial functions (Pichaud et al., 2012; Scheffler et al., 2012; Latorre-Pellicer et al., 2016).

Although different nuclear genetic background employed in the above studies make it difficult to compare the results across studies, this growing body of evidence supports mitochondrial genetic variance/haplotype as a key factor in the observed differences in bioenergetics and metabolism.

MITOCHONDRIAL GENETIC VARIANCES/HAPLOTYPES AND HAPLOGROUPS AND THE RISK OF ALZHEIMER'S DISEASE

In an early effort to assess the contribution of mitochondrial DNA variances to pathologies of neurodegenerative diseases, researchers identified a non-synonymous SNP in $tRNA^{Gln}$, mt4336C, that had an increased frequency in a Caucasian cohort of late onset Alzheimer's and Parkinson disease patients (Shoffner et al., 1993). The contribution of mt4336C was later confirmed in a different North American Caucasian cohort of AD patients (Hutchin and Cortopassi, 1995). Individuals harboring the mt4336C SNP also tended to harbor the mt16304C SNP, and had a more closely related D-loop sequence, which could be traced back to a single phylogenetic node (Shoffner et al., 1993; Hutchin and Cortopassi, 1995). However, two other studies did not confirm either mt4336C or mt16304C as a risk factor for developing AD in similar populations, when blood samples and leukocytes from clinically diagnosed patients were used instead of histopathologically confirmed postmortem AD brain tissues (Wragg et al., 1995; Zsurka et al., 1998). Today, mt16304C is known as a defining SNP for subhaplogroup H5, and mt4336C a defining SNP for subhaplogroup H5a. The above studies constituted the earliest debate over whether mitochondrial genetic variances can modify the risk of developing AD.

In fact, haplogroup H and superhaplogroup HV, which contains haplogroup H and its subhaplogroups, have been the most reported haplogroup in association with increased risk of developing AD (Chinnery et al., 2000; Edland et al., 2002; van der Walt et al., 2004, 2005; Elson et al., 2006; Fesahat et al., 2007; Mancuso et al., 2007; Maruszak et al., 2009, 2011; Santoro et al., 2010; Coto et al., 2011; Ridge et al., 2012; Fachal et al., 2015; see **Table 2**). A study based on 30 Iranian late onset Alzheimer's patients and 100 controls found that haplogroup H was significantly more abundant in the disease group (Fesahat et al., 2007; see **Table 2**). In a Spanish-Caucasian group, haplogroup H and its defining SNP mt7028C were enriched in LOAD patients compared to controls (Coto et al., 2011; see **Table 2**). In a large Caucasian cohort containing 422 late-onset AD patients and 318 neurologically healthy controls, researchers found that superhaplogroup HV, which contains haplogroup H, had significantly higher presence in LOAD than in control (Maruszak et al., 2011; see **Table 2**). Finally, a meta-analysis pooling data from five previous studies (some studies including early-onset AD patients) also confirmed the association between haplogroup H and superhaplogroup HV and the risk of developing AD (Maruszak et al., 2011; see **Table 2**).

When mitochondrial DNA was sequenced in greater depth, subhaplogroup H5 was significantly associated with AD compared to haplogroup H of central-northern Italians, (Santoro

TABLE 2 | Observed effects of mitochondrial superhaplogroup HV and haplogroup H on risk of Alzheimer's disease (AD).

Haplogroups	Observations	Reference
HV	Increased risk, especially in females	Maruszak et al. (2011)
	No effect	Elson et al. (2006), Maruszak et al. (2009) and Fachal et al. (2015)
H	Increased risk	Fesahat et al. (2007), Maruszak et al. (2009, 2011) and Coto et al. (2011)
	Defining SNP mt7028C increased risk	Coto et al. (2011)
	Defining SNP mt7028C increased risk in females only	van der Walt et al. (2004)
	H5 increased risk, especially in females	Santoro et al. (2010)
	H5 and APOE4 synergistically increased risk	Maruszak et al. (2011)
	H5a defining SNP mt4336C increased risk in APOE4 carriers	Edland et al. (2002)
	H6a1a and H6a1b decreased risk	Ridge et al. (2012)
	No effect	Chinnery et al. (2000), van der Walt et al. (2005), Mancuso et al. (2007) and Fachal et al. (2015)

Effects of haplogroup H defining single nucleotide polymorphisms (SNPs) and its subhaplogroups are listed under haplogroup H.

et al., 2010; see **Table 2**). However, from the Cache county study on aging and memory in Utah residents, subhaplogroups H6a1a and H6a1b were found to be protective against AD (Ridge et al., 2012; see **Table 2**). While the protective role of subhaplogroups H6a1a and H6a1b seems contradictory to the overall risk of haplogroup H, the data predict that the observed risks within haplogroup H may be driven by its subhaplogroups with H5 increases risk of LOAD whereas H6 reduces risk.

The second most studied superhaplogroup is UK, and its member haplogroups U and K, including their subhaplogroups (While haplogroup K is currently recognized as a branch of haplogroup U, early studies classified haplogroups U and K as two parallel haplogroups under superhaplogroup UK. For consistency of referring to previous studies, we will use the earlier classification system throughout this review article; see **Table 3**). In a Utah based ADNI cohort, superhaplogroup UK was identified as a risk factor for AD (Lakatos et al., 2010; see **Table 3**). These findings are in contrast to an earlier study conducted in a Poland-based Caucasian population, where no effect of superhaplogroup UK was observed (Maruszak et al., 2009; see **Table 3**). The disparity may be explained by differences in the distribution of specific subhaplogroups or SNPs in the studied populations. Specifically, while each of the three defining SNPs for haplogroup U (mt11467G, mt12308G and mt12372A) has been identified as a risk factor for AD (Lakatos et al., 2010), subhaplogroup U5a1 and SNP mt16224C, a haplogroup K defining SNP, were shown to be protective (Maruszak et al., 2011; see **Table 3**).

Another common European haplogroup studied for its association with AD is haplogroup T, where one study in French-Canadians found that the frequency of SNPs mt709A and mt15928A, both defining SNPs for haplogroup T, were three times higher in controls than in AD patients, suggesting a protective role of haplogroup T (Chagnon et al., 1999; see **Table 4**). However, the Health, Aging, and Body Composition (Health ABC) study found that haplogroup T had increased risk for dementia when compared to haplogroup H (Tranah et al., 2012). The Health ABC study also found that haplogroup J, also under superhaplogroup JT, was associated with significant decline in cognitive function compared to haplogroup H (Tranah et al., 2012).

In addition to major European haplogroups, several African and Asian haplogroups have also been reported to be associated with the AD or risk of dementia (see **Table 5**). For example,

TABLE 3 | Observed effects of mitochondrial superhaplogroup KU and haplogroups K and U on risk of AD.

Haplogroups	Observations	Reference
UK	Increased risk	Lakatos et al. (2010)
	Decreased risk in males	Maruszak et al. (2011)
	No effect	Maruszak et al. (2009) and Fachal et al. (2015)
K	Defining SNP mt16224C decreased risk	Maruszak et al. (2011)
	Decreased risk in APOE4 carriers	Carrieri et al. (2001) and Maruszak et al. (2011)
	No effect	Chinnery et al. (2000), van der Walt et al. (2005), Elson et al. (2006), Fesahat et al. (2007), Mancuso et al. (2007) and Maruszak et al. (2009)
U	Increased risk	Fesahat et al. (2007)
	Increased risk in males	van der Walt et al. (2004)
	Defining SNPs mt11467G, mt12308G, and mt12372A individually increased risk	Lakatos et al. (2010)
	Decreased risk in females	van der Walt et al. (2004)
	Decreased risk in APOE4 carriers	Carrieri et al. (2001)
	U5a1 decreases risk	Maruszak et al. (2011)
	No effect	Chinnery et al. (2000), van der Walt et al. (2005), Elson et al. (2006), Mancuso et al. (2007), Maruszak et al. (2009) and Fachal et al. (2015)

TABLE 4 | Observed effects of mitochondrial superhaplogroup JT and haplogroups J and T on risk of AD.

Haplogroups	Observations	Reference
JT	Decreased risk in females	Maruszak et al. (2011)
	No effect	Maruszak et al. (2009) and Fachal et al. (2015)
J	Decline in cognitive function comparing to H	Tranah et al. (2012)
	J2b defining SNP mt7476T, mt5633T, and mt15812A increased risk	Chagnon et al. (1999)
	No effect	Chinnery et al. (2000), van der Walt et al. (2005), Elson et al. (2006), Fesahat et al. (2007), Mancuso et al. (2007), Maruszak et al. (2009) and Fachal et al. (2015)
T	Increased risk for dementia comparing to H	Tranah et al. (2012)
	T defining SNP mt709A and mt15928A decreased risk	Chagnon et al. (1999)
	Decreased risk in females	Maruszak et al. (2011)
	No effect	Chinnery et al. (2000), van der Walt et al. (2005), Elson et al. (2006), Fesahat et al. (2007), Mancuso et al. (2007), Maruszak et al. (2009) and Fachal et al. (2015)

in an African American population, haplogroup L1 was found to have increased risk for developing dementia (Tranah et al., 2014). In Asians, subhaplogroups G2a, B4c1 and N9b1 were reported to be associated with AD in Japanese populations, and haplogroup B5 was reported to be associated with AD in Han Chinese (Takasaki, 2008, 2009; Bi et al., 2015; see **Table 5**).

As reviewed here, the field has not reached consensus on the effect of mitochondrial haplogroups on late onset AD (LOAD). Different sets of haplogroups are identified in different studies and different studies could identify opposite effects of the same mitochondrial haplotype on risk of LOAD. Moreover, multiple studies involving Caucasians of European descendant (European descents in UK and US, Tuscans, Spanish and Old order Amish from Indiana and Ohio) did not detect associations between any haplogroup and AD (Chinnery et al., 2000; van der Walt et al., 2005; Elson et al., 2006; Mancuso et al., 2007; Fachal et al., 2015; see **Tables 2–5**). While the controversy may be driven by differences in the distribution of subhaplogroups within the studied population or different DNA sources (e.g., postmortem brain tissue vs. peripheral blood), the discrepancies between studies also suggested that as intriguing as the results are, mitochondrial genetic variances are unlikely to be the sole driving force of LOAD. Further, the most consistent risk factor for LOAD is APOE genotype, but it alone is not an absolute determinant. Below, we determine the relationship between mitochondrial haplogroup and APOE genotype on risk of AD.

TABLE 5 | Association between some Asian mitochondrial haplogroups and the risk of Alzheimer's disease.

Haplogroups	Observations	References
L1	Increased risk	Tranah et al. (2014)
G2a	Increased risk	Takasaki (2008, 2009)
B4c1	Increased risk	Takasaki (2009)
N9b1	Increased risk	Takasaki (2009)
B5	Increases risk	Bi et al. (2015)

Studies listed in chronological order.

THE INTERACTION BETWEEN MITOCHONDRIAL HAPLOGROUP AND APOE GENOTYPE ON RISK OF AD

APOEε4 genotype is a widely recognized risk factor for AD, and has been repeatedly confirmed in the studies reviewed herein (Corder et al., 1993; Poirier et al., 1993; Rebeck et al., 1993; Saunders et al., 1993; Carrieri et al., 2001; Edland et al., 2002; Coto et al., 2011; Maruszak et al., 2011). Further, APOEε4 has been associated with mitochondrial dysfunction and glucose hypometabolism in brain (Reiman et al., 2001, 2004, 2005; Mosconi et al., 2004a,b,c, 2005, 2008; Valla et al., 2010; Wolf et al., 2013). Compared to non-carriers, APOEε4 carriers showed reduced cerebral parietal glucose metabolism among cognitive normal elderlies with family history of AD (Small et al., 1995, 2000). In APOEε4 positive MCI patients, reduced regional cerebral metabolic rate of glucose consumption (rCMRglc) was detected in temporoparietal and posterior cingulate cortex (Mosconi et al., 2004b). In AD patients, more severe hypometabolism was detected in the parietal, temporal, and cingulate areas in APOEε4 carriers than non-carriers (Mosconi et al., 2004c; Drzezga et al., 2005). Brain glucose hypometabolism was also more widespread in APOEε4 positive AD patients (Mosconi et al., 2004a). On the therapeutic side, mild-to-moderate AD patients who are APOEε4 carriers were shown to be less responsive to rosiglitazone, which can improve mitochondrial efficiency and glucose metabolism (Risner et al., 2006; Roses et al., 2007).

In longitudinal studies, APOEε4 carriers had significantly greater rCMRglc decline in the vicinity of temporal, posterior cingulate, and prefrontal cortex, basal forebrain, parahippocampal gyrus, and thalamus (Reiman et al., 2001; Mosconi et al., 2008). Decrease of glucose metabolism was also evident in young and middle-aged APOEε4 carriers in posterior cingulate, parietal, temporal, and prefrontal cortex, as well as thalamus (Reiman et al., 2004; Mosconi et al., 2008). The effect of APOEε4 allele has also been shown to be gene dose dependent with APOEε4

TABLE 6 | Three modes of interactions between APOEε4 status and mitochondrial haplogroups in modulating the risk of AD.

Interactions	Haplogroups/SNPs	Reference
Neutralizing	K	Carrieri et al. (2001) and Maruszak et al. (2011)
	U	Carrieri et al. (2001)
Enabling	mt4336C (H)	Edland et al. (2002)
Synergistic	H5	Maruszak et al. (2011)
	mt7028C (H)	Coto et al. (2011)

Haplogroups K and U could neutralize the risk of APOEε4 on AD. Haplogroup H defining SNP mt4336C was associated with LOAD in APOEε4 carriers only. Subhaplogroup H5 and haplogroup H defining SNP mt7028C could act synergistically with APOEε4 to increase the risk of LOAD.

homozygote carriers showing greater hypometabolic deficit relative to APOEε3/4 heterozygote carriers (Reiman et al., 2005).

At the cellular level, APOEε4 gene expression in human was associated with down-regulation of genes involved in mitochondrial oxidative phosphorylation and energy metabolism (Xu et al., 2006, 2007). APOEε4 gene expression was also found to be associated with lower mitochondrial cytochrome oxidase activity in posterior cingulate cortex among young adults with family history of AD (Valla et al., 2010). Neurons from humanized APOEε4 knock-in mice had significantly lower amount of all five electron transport chain complexes comparing to those from APOEε3 knock-in mice (Chen et al., 2011). Proteomic analysis revealed decreased expression of proteins involved in the TCA cycle, glucose, lipid and amino acid metabolism in APOEε4 knock-in mice (Shi et al., 2014). Further, cytochrome c levels were significantly lower in ApoEε4 mice compared with ApoEε3 mice (Shi et al., 2014). *In vitro* studies also suggested that truncated APOEε4 fragment can interact directly with mitochondria and cause mitochondrial dysfunction and neurotoxicity (Chang et al., 2005; Mahley et al., 2007). Given the association between decreased bioenergetic capacity in brain and the risk of AD, an interaction between APOE genotype and mitochondrial haplotypes is possible.

After stratifying by APOEε4 status, three interesting modes of interactions between APOEε4 status and mitochondrial haplogroups in modulating the risk of AD were apparent (see **Table 6**).

The first mode is a neutralizing effect of mitochondrial haplogroup on the effect of APOEε4 on risk of AD (see **Table 6**). Early studies identified a non-random association between mitochondrial haplogroup and APOEε4 status in AD patients (Carrieri et al., 2001). Specifically, while APOEε4 carriers had significantly higher odds ratio for AD, those belonging to haplogroups K and U did not, indicating a neutralizing effect of haplogroups K and U on the risk of APOEε4 gene status (Carrieri et al., 2001). The non-random distribution of mitochondrial haplogroups associated with APOEε4 status and the neutralizing effect of mitochondrial haplogroup K on APOEε4 were later confirmed by Maruszak et al. (2011).

The second mode is an enabling effect of APOEε4 on mitochondrial genetic variances as risk factors for AD (see **Table 6**). In non-APOEε4 carriers, SNP mt4336C (a defining SNP for subhaplogroup H5a) was not an AD risk factor, however, in APOEε4 carriers, the same SNP was a risk factor for AD (Edland et al., 2002). This study indicated that APOE genotype could explain the earlier disparity regarding the association between SNP mt4336C and AD (Shoffner et al., 1993; Hutchin and Cortopassi, 1995; Wragg et al., 1995; Zsurka et al., 1998).

A synergistic effect was also observed between APOEε4 and mitochondrial haplotypes (see **Table 6**). For example, SNP mt7028C, a defining SNP for haplogroup H, and subhaplogroup H5 were suggested to act synergistically with APOEε4 to increase risk for AD (Coto et al., 2011; Maruszak et al., 2011).

As with the association between mitochondrial haplotype and the risk of late onset AD, the interaction between APOEε4 and mitochondrial genetic variances in modulating the risk of late onset AD remains debatable. Multiple studies failed to identify any correlation between mitochondrial haplogroup and APOEε4 status or failed to identify an interaction between the two on the risk of developing AD (Zsurka et al., 1998; Chinnery et al., 2000; van der Walt et al., 2005; Mancuso et al., 2007; Lakatos et al., 2010; Santoro et al., 2010; Ridge et al., 2013). Collectively, these disparate findings on the association between mitochondrial

TABLE 7 | Sex differentiates effects of mitochondrial haplogroups on risk of AD.

Haplogroups/SNPs	Female	Male	Authors
H	Increased risk	No effect	Maruszak et al. (2009, 2011)
H5	Increased risk	No effect	Santoro et al. (2010)
HV	Increased risk	No effect	Maruszak et al. (2009, 2011)
T	Decreased risk	No effect	Maruszak et al. (2011)
JT	Decreased risk	No effect	Maruszak et al. (2011)
U	Decreased risk	Increased risk	van der Walt et al. (2004)
KU	No effect	Decreased risk	Maruszak et al. (2011)
mt7028C (H)	Increased risk	No effect	Maruszak et al. (2009)
mt13368A (T)	Decreased risk	No effect	Maruszak et al. (2011)
mt13708G (non-J)	No effect	Increased risk	Maruszak et al. (2009)
mt9055A (K)	No effect	Decreased risk	Maruszak et al. (2011)

Haplogroups and SNPs identified to have sex differences from literatures are listed. A possible haplogroup defined by the SNPs listed is indicated in the parenthesis following the SNP.

haplotype, APOE genotype, and risk of AD emphasize the importance of a precision medicine approach that considers mitochondrial genetic variance in combination with nuclear genetics.

MITOCHONDRIAL HAPLOGROUP AND SEX DIFFERENCES AND RISK OF ALZHEIMER'S DISEASE

Females are at greater lifetime risk for LOAD, and also have higher prevalence and incidence rate than all age-matched males (Brookmeyer et al., 1998; Mielke et al., 2014; Grimm et al., 2016). The higher risk for female is also evident in faster disease progression and greater burden of AD pathology (Aguero-Torres et al., 1998; Corder et al., 2004; Barnes et al., 2005; Skup et al., 2011; Kelly et al., 2013; Mielke et al., 2014; Grimm et al., 2016). While the underlying mechanism remains to be elucidated, increased mitochondrial oxidative stress may play a role (Schuessel et al., 2004; Mandal et al., 2012). Given the effect of mitochondrial genetic variances on mitochondrial function and risk of AD, it is of interest to identify any interaction between mitochondrial haplotypes and sex difference on risk of LOAD.

While almost all the reviewed studies recognized sex differences on risk of LOAD, only a few studied the effects of mitochondrial genetic variances in each sex (van der Walt et al., 2004; Maruszak et al., 2009, 2011; Santoro et al., 2010; see **Table 7**). Within these studies, some mitochondrial genetic variances were found to be associated with AD in females only (van der Walt et al., 2004; Maruszak et al., 2009, 2011; Santoro et al., 2010). Superhaplogroup JT, haplogroup T, a haplogroup T defining SNP mt13368A, a haplogroup U defining SNP 12308G and a non-H defining SNP mt7028T were found to exert protective effects only in females (van der Walt et al., 2004; Maruszak et al., 2011; see **Table 7**). Superhaplogroup HV, haplogroup H, subhaplogroup H5 and a haplogroup H defining SNP mt7028C were identified as risk factors for only in females (Maruszak et al., 2009, 2011; Santoro et al., 2010; see **Table 7**).

In contrast, some variances affected only males (see **Table 7**). Superhaplogroup UK, and SNP mt9055A, a defining SNP for haplogroup K, were found to be associated with reduced risk of AD in males, while SNP mt13708G (for many non-J haplogroups), and SNP mt10398A, a defining SNP for some subhaplogroups of U, were associated with increased risk only in males (van der Walt et al., 2004; Maruszak et al., 2009, 2011; see **Table 7**). Certain mitochondrial genetic variances also showed opposite effects in each sex. For example, haplogroup U was associated with increased risk in males but decreased risk in females (van der Walt et al., 2004; see **Table 7**).

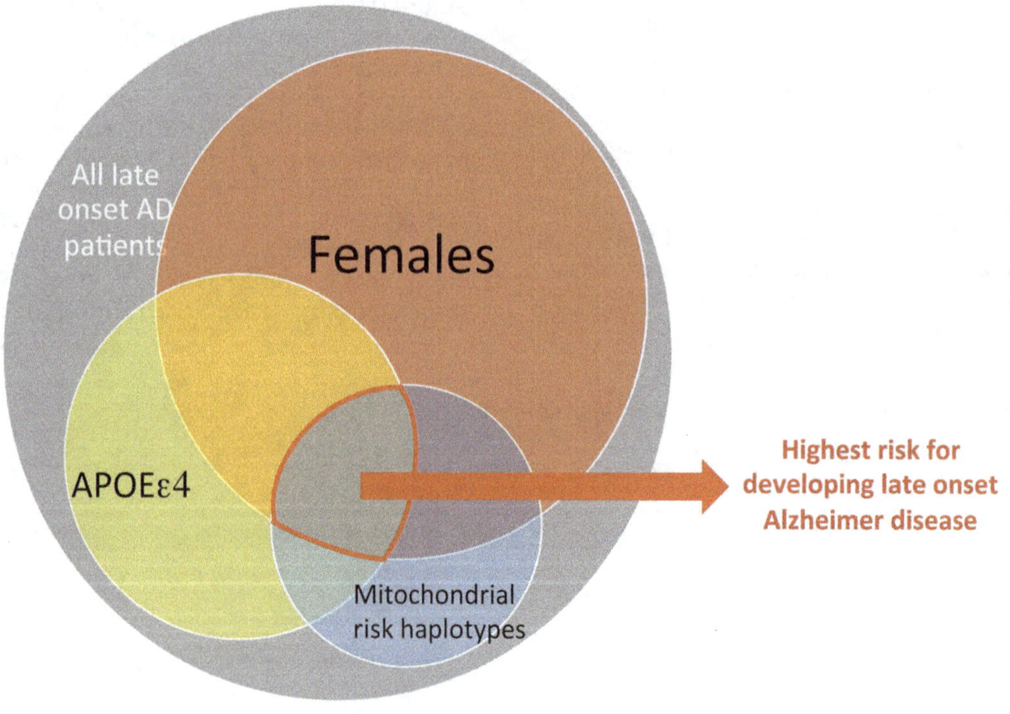

FIGURE 3 | A conceptual framework where the combination of mitochondrial and nuclear genetic risk factors plus sex as a higher risk factor for LOAD. Each of the three factors: sex, APOEε4 genotype and mitochondrial genetic variance has moderate risk for developing late onset AD, but constitutes a much higher risk when combined.

These results indicate that previously observed associations between mitochondrial haplogroups and AD could be driven by sex. Conversely, the effects observed in one sex could be diluted in the whole population, or be neutralized by the other sex, resulting in non-significant associations.

CONCLUSION AND PERSPECTIVES

Mounting evidence suggested a central role of mitochondrial dysfunction in the etiology of late onset AD. As reviewed above, disruption of mitochondrial bioenergetics, structure and dynamics have all been indicated in AD patients. Given the maternal pattern of inheritance of late onset AD and mitochondrial genome, herein we reviewed the association of mitochondrial genetic variances on bioenergetics, respiratory phenotypes and risk of developing LOAD. While the outcomes remain debatable, a large body of science supports an association between mitochondrial genetic variances and differences in bioenergetics and AD susceptibility. Several factors can help explain the disagreement. First, although most studies were conducted in descendants of European origin, the geographic distribution of participants were drastically different, which could result in diverse nuclear genetic background. Since mitochondria communicate extensively with the nucleus, uncontrolled nuclear background can potentially mask effects of mitochondrial genetic variances. Second, as we have reviewed, observations could be driven by certain subhaplogroups, thus results obtained from different populations may be biased by their dominant subhaplogroup. Third, given the heteroplasmic nature of the mitochondrial DNA, accumulated mutations throughout aging may be haplotype and tissue specific (Wallace, 2005), which could contribute to the discrepancies between studies that had different sources of mtDNA (e.g., brain tissues vs. peripheral blood samples; Wallace, 1994). And last, the criteria for mitochondrial haplogroup assignment evolved during the past two decades. Initial studies used haplotype assignment based on only 10 SNPs in the control region, whereas more recent studies used 138 SNPs across the whole human mitochondrial genome. As a result, some ambiguous assignments were resolved and more subhaplogroups were identified.

The data also indicate that mitochondrial haplotype is one factor among several that impacts risk of AD. This is consistent with the multifactorial nature of aging trajectories and risk for LOAD. A systems biology approach that integrates mitochondrial genetic variances and risk factors such as APOEε4 genotype and sex is a step towards resolving disparities across studies of mitochondrial haplotype and risk of neurodegenerative diseases associated with mitochondrial dysfunction (see **Figure 3**). More importantly, we propose a precision medicine approach, where nuclear genetic risk factors (especially APOEε4 genotype), mitochondrial haplotypes, and sex differences can be incorporated into future therapeutic designs for LOAD.

AUTHOR CONTRIBUTIONS

YW and RDB wrote and reviewed the manuscript together.

ACKNOWLEDGMENTS

This work was supported by: National Institute on Aging (NIA) grants R01AG032236 and P01AG026572 to RDB, Project 1 to RDB and YW.

REFERENCES

Aguero-Torres, H., Fratiglioni, L., Guo, Z., Viitanen, M., and Winblad, B. (1998). Prognostic factors in very old demented adults: a seven-year follow-up from a population-based survey in Stockholm. *J. Am. Geriatr. Soc.* 46, 444–452. doi: 10.1111/j.1532-5415.1998.tb02464.x

Aksenov, M. Y., Tucker, H. M., Nair, P., Aksenova, M. V., Butterfield, D. A., Estus, S., et al. (1999). The expression of several mitochondrial and nuclear genes encoding the subunits of electron transport chain enzyme complexes, cytochrome c oxidase and NADH dehydrogenase, in different brain regions in Alzheimer's disease. *Neurochem. Res.* 24, 767–774. doi: 10.1023/A:1020783614031

Amo, T., Yadava, N., Oh, R., Nicholls, D. G., and Brand, M. D. (2008). Experimental assessment of bioenergetic differences caused by the common European mitochondrial DNA haplogroups H and T. *Gene* 411, 69–76. doi: 10.1016/j.gene.2008.01.007

Baloyannis, S. J., Costa, V., and Michmizos, D. (2004). Mitochondrial alterations in Alzheimer's disease. *Am. J. Alzheimers Dis. Other Demen.* 19, 89–93. doi: 10.1177/153331750401900205

Barnes, L. L., Wilson, R. S., Bienias, J. L., Schneider, J. A., Evans, D. A., and Bennett, D. A. (2005). SEx differences in the clinical manifestations of Alzheimer disease pathology. *Arch. Gen. Psychiatry* 62, 685–691. doi: 10.1001/archpsyc.62.6.685

Beal, M. F. (1996). Mitochondria, free radicals and neurodegeneration. *Curr. Opin. Neurobiol.* 6, 661–666. doi: 10.1016/s0959-4388(96)80100-0

Bi, R., Zhang, W., Yu, D., Li, X., Wang, H. Z., Hu, Q. X., et al. (2015). Mitochondrial DNA haplogroup B5 confers genetic susceptibility to Alzheimer's disease in Han Chinese. *Neurobiol. Aging* 36, 1604.e7–1604.e16. doi: 10.1016/j.neurobiolaging.2014.10.009

Bosetti, F., Brizzi, F., Barogi, S., Mancuso, M., Siciliano, G., Tendi, E. A., et al. (2002). Cytochrome c oxidase and mitochondrial F1F0-ATPase (ATP synthase) activities in platelets and brain from patients with Alzheimer's disease. *Neurobiol. Aging* 23, 371–376. doi: 10.1016/s0197-4580(01)00314-1

Brinton, R. D. (2008). The healthy cell bias of estrogen action: mitochondrial bioenergetics and neurological implications. *Trends Neurosci.* 31, 529–537. doi: 10.1016/j.tins.2008.07.003

Brinton, R. D. (2009). Estrogen-induced plasticity from cells to circuits: predictions for cognitive function. *Trends Pharmacol. Sci.* 30, 212–222. doi: 10.1016/j.tips.2008.12.006

Brinton, R. D., Yao, J., Yin, F., Mack, W. J., and Cadenas, E. (2015). Perimenopause as a neurological transition state. *Nat. Rev. Endocrinol.* 11, 393–405. doi: 10.1038/nrendo.2015.82

Brookmeyer, R., Gray, S., and Kawas, C. (1998). Projections of Alzheimer's disease in the United States and the public health impact of delaying disease onset. *Am. J. Public Health* 88, 1337–1342. doi: 10.2105/ajph.88.9.1337

Bubber, P., Haroutunian, V., Fisch, G., Blass, J. P., and Gibson, G. E. (2005). Mitochondrial abnormalities in Alzheimer brain: mechanistic implications. *Ann. Neurol.* 57, 695–703. doi: 10.1002/ana.20474

Burté, F., Carelli, V., Chinnery, P. F., and Yu-Wai-Man, P. (2015). Disturbed mitochondrial dynamics and neurodegenerative disorders. *Nat. Rev. Neurol.* 11, 11–24. doi: 10.1038/nrneurol.2014.228

Cardoso, S. M., Proença, M. T., Santos, S., Santana, I., and Oliveira, C. R. (2004). Cytochrome c oxidase is decreased in Alzheimer's disease platelets. *Neurobiol. Aging* 25, 105–110. doi: 10.1016/s0197-4580(03)00033-2

Carrieri, G., Bonafè, M., De Luca, M., Rose, G., Varcasia, O., Bruni, A., et al. (2001). Mitochondrial DNA haplogroups and APOE4 allele are non-independent variables in sporadic Alzheimer's disease. *Hum. Genet.* 108, 194–198. doi: 10.1007/s004390100463

Cassarino, D. S., Swerdlow, R. H., Parks, J. K., Parker, W. D. Jr., and Bennett, J. P. Jr. (1998). Cyclosporin A increases resting mitochondrial membrane potential in SY5Y cells and reverses the depressed mitochondrial membrane potential of Alzheimer's disease cybrids. *Biochem. Biophys. Res. Commun.* 248, 168–173. doi: 10.1006/bbrc.1998.8866

Chagnon, P., Gee, M., Filion, M., Robitaille, Y., Belouchi, M., and Gauvreau, D. (1999). Phylogenetic analysis of the mitochondrial genome indicates significant differences between patients with Alzheimer disease and controls in a French-Canadian founder population. *Am. J. Med. Genet.* 85, 20–30. doi: 10.1002/(SICI)1096-8628(19990702)85:1<20::AID-AJMG6>3.0.CO;2-K

Chandrasekaran, K., Giordano, T., Brady, D. R., Stoll, J., Martin, L. J., and Rapoport, S. I. (1994). Impairment in mitochondrial cytochrome oxidase gene expression in Alzheimer disease. *Brain Res. Mol. Brain Res.* 24, 336–340. doi: 10.1016/0169-328x(94)90147-3

Chandrasekaran, K., Hatanpää, K., Rapoport, S. I., and Brady, D. R. (1997). Decreased expression of nuclear and mitochondrial DNA-encoded genes of oxidative phosphorylation in association neocortex in Alzheimer disease. *Brain Res. Mol. Brain Res.* 44, 99–104. doi: 10.1016/s0169-328x(96)00191-x

Chang, S., Ran Ma, T., Miranda, R. D., Balestra, M. E., Mahley, R. W., and Huang, Y. (2005). Lipid- and receptor-binding regions of apolipoprotein E4 fragments act in concert to cause mitochondrial dysfunction and neurotoxicity. *Proc. Natl. Acad. Sci. U S A* 102, 18694–18699. doi: 10.1073/pnas.0508254102

Chen, H. K., Ji, Z. S., Dodson, S. E., Miranda, R. D., Rosenblum, C. I., Reynolds, I. J., et al. (2011). Apolipoprotein E4 domain interaction mediates detrimental effects on mitochondria and is a potential therapeutic target for Alzheimer disease. *J. Biol. Chem.* 286, 5215–5221. doi: 10.1074/jbc.M110.151084

Chinnery, P. F., Taylor, G. A., Howell, N., Andrews, R. M., Morris, C. M., Taylor, R. W., et al. (2000). Mitochondrial DNA haplogroups and susceptibility to AD and dementia with Lewy bodies. *Neurology* 55, 302–304. doi: 10.1212/wnl.55.2.302

Corder, E., Saunders, A., Strittmatter, W., Schmechel, D., Gaskell, P., Small, G., et al. (1993). Gene dose of apolipoprotein E type 4 allele and the risk of Alzheimer's disease in late onset families. *Science* 261, 921–923. doi: 10.1126/science.8346443

Corder, E. H., Ghebremedhin, E., Taylor, M. G., Thal, D. R., Ohm, T. G., and Braak, H. (2004). The biphasic relationship between regional brain senile plaque and neurofibrillary tangle distributions: modification by age, sex and APOE polymorphism. *Ann. N Y Acad. Sci.* 1019, 24–28. doi: 10.1196/annals.1297.005

Coskun, P., Wyrembak, J., Schriner, S. E., Chen, H. W., Marciniack, C., Laferla, F., et al. (2012). A mitochondrial etiology of Alzheimer and Parkinson disease. *Biochim. Biophys. Acta* 1820, 553–564. doi: 10.1016/j.bbagen.2011.08.008

Coto, E., Gómez, J., Alonso, B., Corao, A. I., Díaz, M., Menéndez, M., et al. (2011). Late-onset Alzheimer's disease is associated with mitochondrial DNA 7028C/haplogroup H and D310 poly-C tract heteroplasmy. *Neurogenetics* 12, 345–346. doi: 10.1007/s10048-011-0295-4

Davis, R. E., Miller, S., Herrnstadt, C., Ghosh, S. S., Fahy, E., Shinobu, L. A., et al. (1997). Mutations in mitochondrial cytochrome c oxidase genes segregate with late-onset Alzheimer disease. *Proc. Natl. Acad. Sci. U S A* 94, 4526–4531. doi: 10.1073/pnas.94.9.4526

Drzezga, A., Riemenschneider, M., Strassner, B., Grimmer, T., Peller, M., Knoll, A., et al. (2005). Cerebral glucose metabolism in patients with AD and different APOE genotypes. *Neurology* 64, 102–107. doi: 10.1212/01.wnl.0000148478.39691.d3

Duara, R., Lopez-Alberola, R. F., Barker, W. W., Loewenstein, D. A., Zatinsky, M., Eisdorfer, C. E., et al. (1993). A comparison of familial and sporadic Alzheimer's disease. *Neurology* 43, 1377–1384. doi: 10.1212/wnl.43.7.1377

Edland, S. D., Silverman, J. M., Peskind, E. R., Tsuang, D., Wijsman, E., and Morris, J. C. (1996). Increased risk of dementia in mothers of Alzheimer's disease cases: evidence for maternal inheritance. *Neurology* 47, 254–256. doi: 10.1212/wnl.47.1.254

Edland, S. D., Tobe, V. O., Rieder, M. J., Bowen, J. D., McCormick, W., Teri, L., et al. (2002). Mitochondrial genetic variants and Alzheimer disease: a case-control study of the T4336C and G5460A variants. *Alzheimer Dis. Assoc. Disord.* 16, 1–7. doi: 10.1097/00002093-200201000-00001

Elson, J., Herrnstadt, C., Preston, G., Thal, L., Morris, C., Edwardson, J. A., et al. (2006). Does the mitochondrial genome play a role in the etiology of Alzheimer's disease? *Hum. Genet.* 119, 241–254. doi: 10.1007/s00439-005-0123-8

Fachal, L., Mosquera-Miguel, A., Pastor, P., Ortega-Cubero, S., Lorenzo, E., Oterino-Durán, A., et al. (2015). No evidence of association between common European mitochondrial DNA variants in Alzheimer, Parkinson and migraine in the Spanish population. *Am. J. Med. Genet. B Neuropsychiatr. Genet.* 168B, 54–65. doi: 10.1002/ajmg.b.32276

Fernández-Moreno, M., Tamayo, M., Soto-Hermida, A., Mosquera, A., Oreiro, N., Fernández-López, C., et al. (2011). mtDNA haplogroup J modulates telomere length and nitric oxide production. *BMC Musculoskelet. Disord.* 12:283. doi: 10.1186/1471-2474-12-283

Fesahat, F., Houshmand, M., Panahi, M. S., Gharagozli, K., and Mirzajani, F. (2007). Do haplogroups H and U act to increase the penetrance of Alzheimer's disease? *Cell. Mol. Neurobiol.* 27, 329–334. doi: 10.1007/s10571-006-9126-9

Gibson, G. E., Haroutunian, V., Zhang, H., Park, L. C., Shi, Q., Lesser, M., et al. (2000). Mitochondrial damage in Alzheimer's disease varies with apolipoprotein E genotype. *Ann. Neurol.* 48, 297–303. doi: 10.1002/1531-8249(200009)48:3<297::AID-ANA3>3.3.CO;2-Q

Giles, R. E., Blanc, H., Cann, H. M., and Wallace, D. C. (1980). Maternal inheritance of human mitochondrial DNA. *Proc. Natl. Acad. Sci. U S A* 77, 6715–6719. doi: 10.1073/pnas.77.11.6715

Gómez-Durán, A., Pacheu-Grau, D., López-Gallardo, E., Díez-Sánchez, C., Montoya, J., López-Pérez, M. J., et al. (2010). Unmasking the causes of multifactorial disorders: OXPHOS differences between mitochondrial haplogroups. *Hum. Mol. Genet.* 19, 3343–3353. doi: 10.1093/hmg/ddq246

Grimm, A., Mensah-Nyagan, A. G., and Eckert, A. (2016). Alzheimer, mitochondria and gender. *Neurosci. Biobehav. Rev.* 67, 89–101. doi: 10.1016/j.neubiorev.2016.04.012

Hirai, K., Aliev, G., Nunomura, A., Fujioka, H., Russell, R. L., Atwood, C. S., et al. (2001). Mitochondrial abnormalities in Alzheimer's disease. *J. Neurosci.* 21, 3017–3023.

Hutchin, T., and Cortopassi, G. (1995). A mitochondrial DNA clone is associated with increased risk for Alzheimer disease. *Proc. Natl. Acad. Sci. U S A* 92, 6892–6895. doi: 10.1073/pnas.92.15.6892

Kelly, R. D., Rodda, A. E., Dickinson, A., Mahmud, A., Nefzger, C. M., Lee, W., et al. (2013). Mitochondrial DNA haplotypes define gene expression patterns in pluripotent and differentiating embryonic stem cells. *Stem Cells* 31, 703–716. doi: 10.1002/stem.1313

Kenney, M. C., Chwa, M., Atilano, S. R., Pavlis, J. M., Falatoonzadeh, P., Ramirez, C., et al. (2013). Mitochondrial DNA variants mediate energy production and expression levels for CFH, C3 and EFEMP1 genes: implications for age-related macular degeneration. *PLoS One* 8:e54339. doi: 10.1371/journal.pone.0054339

Khusnutdinova, E., Gilyazova, I., Ruiz-Pesini, E., Derbeneva, O., Khusainova, R., Khidiyatova, I., et al. (2008). A mitochondrial etiology of neurodegenerative diseases: evidence from Parkinson's disease. *Ann. N Y Acad. Sci.* 1147, 1–20. doi: 10.1196/annals.1427.001

Kim, S. H., Vlkolinsky, R., Cairns, N., and Lubec, G. (2000). Decreased levels of complex III core protein 1 and complex V β chain in brains from patients with Alzheimer's disease and Down syndrome. *Cell. Mol. Life Sci.* 57, 1810–1816. doi: 10.1007/pl00000661

Kish, S. J., Mastrogiacomo, F., Guttman, M., Furukawa, Y., Taanman, J. W., Dozic, S., et al. (1999). Decreased brain protein levels of cytochrome oxidase subunits in Alzheimer's disease and in hereditary spinocerebellar ataxia disorders: a nonspecific change? *J. Neurochem.* 72, 700–707. doi: 10.1046/j.1471-4159.1999.0720700.x

Lakatos, A., Derbeneva, O., Younes, D., Keator, D., Bakken, T., Lvova, M., et al. (2010). Association between mitochondrial DNA variations and Alzheimer's disease in the ADNI cohort. *Neurobiol. Aging* 31, 1355–1363. doi: 10.1016/j.neurobiolaging.2010.04.031

Larsen, S., Díez-Sánchez, C., Rabøl, R., Ara, I., Dela, F., and Helge, J. W. (2014). Increased intrinsic mitochondrial function in humans with mitochondrial haplogroup H. *Biochim. Biophys. Acta* 1837, 226–231. doi: 10.1016/j.bbabio.2013.10.009

Latorre-Pellicer, A., Moreno-Loshuertos, R., Lechuga-Vieco, A. V., Sánchez-Cabo, F., Torroja, C., Acín-Pérez, R., et al. (2016). Mitochondrial and nuclear DNA matching shapes metabolism and healthy ageing. *Nature* 535, 561–565. doi: 10.1038/nature18618

Lin, M. T., and Beal, M. F. (2006). Mitochondrial dysfunction and oxidative stress in neurodegenerative diseases. *Nature* 443, 787–795. doi: 10.1038/nature 05292

Lin, T. K., Lin, H. Y., Chen, S. D., Chuang, Y. C., Chuang, J. H., Wang, P. W., et al. (2012). The creation of cybrids harboring mitochondrial haplogroups in the Taiwanese population of ethnic Chinese background: an extensive *in vitro* tool for the study of mitochondrial genomic variations. *Oxid. Med. Cell. Longev.* 2012:824275. doi: 10.1155/2012/824275

Liu, Z., Chen, H. H., Li, T. L., Xu, L., and Du, H. Q. (2013). A cross-sectional study on cerebrospinal fluid biomarker levels in cognitively normal elderly subjects with or without a family history of Alzheimer's disease. *CNS Neurosci. Ther.* 19, 38–42. doi: 10.1111/cns.12028

Mahley, R. W., Huang, Y., Fau-Weisgraber, K. H., and Weisgraber, K. H. (2007). Detrimental effects of apolipoprotein E4: potential therapeutic targets in Alzheimer's disease. *Curr. Alzheimer Res.* 4, 537–540. doi: 10. 2174/156720507783018334

Mancuso, M., Filosto, M., Bosetti, F., Ceravolo, R., Rocchi, A., Tognoni, G., et al. (2003). Decreased platelet cytochrome c oxidase activity is accompanied by increased blood lactate concentration during exercise in patients with Alzheimer disease. *Exp. Neurol.* 182, 421–426. doi: 10.1016/s0014-4886(03)00092-x

Mancuso, M., Nardini, M., Micheli, D., Rocchi, A., Nesti, C., Giglioli, N. J., et al. (2007). Lack of association between mtDNA haplogroups and Alzheimer's disease in Tuscany. *Neurol. Sci.* 28, 142–147. doi: 10.1007/s10072-007-0807-z

Mandal, P. K., Tripathi, M., and Sugunan, S. (2012). Brain oxidative stress: detection and mapping of anti-oxidant marker 'Glutathione' in different brain regions of healthy male/female, MCI and Alzheimer patients using non-invasive magnetic resonance spectroscopy. *Biochem. Biophys. Res. Commun.* 417, 43–48. doi: 10.1016/j.bbrc.2011.11.047

Marcuello, A., Martínez-Redondo, D., Dahmani, Y., Casajús, J. A., Ruiz-Pesini, E., Montoya, J., et al. (2009). Human mitochondrial variants influence on oxygen consumption. *Mitochondrion* 9, 27–30. doi: 10.1016/j.mito.2008. 10.002

Martínez-Redondo, D., Marcuello, A., Casajús, J. A., Ara, I., Dahmani, Y., Montoya, J., et al. (2010). Human mitochondrial haplogroup H: the highest VO2max consumer–is it a paradox? *Mitochondrion* 10, 102–107. doi: 10.1016/j. mito.2009.11.005

Maruszak, A., Canter, J. A., Styczynska, M., Zekanowski, C., and Barcikowska, M. (2009). Mitochondrial haplogroup H and Alzheimer's disease–is there a connection? *Neurobiol. Aging* 30, 1749–1755. doi: 10.1016/j.neurobiolaging. 2008.01.004

Maruszak, A., Safranow, K., Branicki, W., Gaw-da-Walerych, K., Pospiech, E., Gabryelewicz, T., et al. (2011). The impact of mitochondrial and nuclear DNA variants on late-onset Alzheimer's disease risk. *J. Alzheimers Dis.* 27, 197–210. doi: 10.3233/JAD-2011-110710

Maurer, I., Zierz, S., and Möller, H. J. (2000). A selective defect of cytochrome c oxidase is present in brain of Alzheimer disease patients. *Neurobiol. Aging* 21, 455–462. doi: 10.1016/s0197-4580(00)00112-3

Mercer, T. R., Neph, S., Dinger, M. E., Crawford, J., Smith, M. A., Shearwood, A. M., et al. (2011). The human mitochondrial transcriptome. *Cell* 146, 645–658. doi: 10.1016/j.cell.2011.06.051

Mielke, M. M., Vemuri, P., and Rocca, W. A. (2014). Clinical epidemiology of Alzheimer's disease: assessing sex and gender differences. *Clin. Epidemiol.* 6, 37–48. doi: 10.2147/CLEP.s37929

Miyata, T., Hayashida, H., Kikuno, R., Hasegawa, M., Kobayashi, M., and Koike, K. (1982). Molecular clock of silent substitution: at least six-fold preponderance of silent changes in mitochondrial genes over those in nuclear genes. *J. Mol. Evol.* 19, 28 35. doi: 10.1007/bf02100221

Morris, J. K., Honea, R. A., Vidoni, E. D., Swerdlow, R. H., and Burns, J. M. (2014). Is Alzheimer's disease a systemic disease? *Biochim. Biophys. Acta* 1842, 1340–1349. doi: 10.1016/j.bbadis.2014.04.012

Mosconi, L., de Leon, M., Murray, J., Lezi, E, Lu, J., Javier, E., et al. (2011). Reduced mitochondria cytochrome oxidase activity in adult children of mothers with Alzheimer's disease. *J. Alzheimers Dis.* 27, 483–490. doi: 10.3233/JAD-2011-110866

Mosconi, L., De Santi, S., Brys, M., Tsui, W. H., Pirraglia, E., Glodzik-Sobanska, L., et al. (2008). Hypometabolism and altered cerebrospinal fluid markers in normal apolipoprotein E E4 carriers with subjective memory complaints. *Biol. Psychiatry* 63, 609–618. doi: 10.1016/j.biopsych.2007.05.030

Mosconi, L., Herholz, K., Prohovnik, I., Nacmias, B., De Cristofaro, M. T., Fayyaz, M., et al. (2005). Metabolic interaction between ApoE genotype and onset age in Alzheimer's disease: implications for brain reserve. *J. Neurol. Neurosurg. Psychiatry* 76, 15–23. doi: 10.1136/jnnp.2003. 030882

Mosconi, L., Nacmias, B., Sorbi, S., De Cristofaro, M. T., Fayazz, M., Tedde, A., et al. (2004a). Brain metabolic decreases related to the dose of the ApoE e4 allele in Alzheimer's disease. *J. Neurol. Neurosurg. Psychiatry* 75, 370–376. doi: 10. 1136/jnnp.2003.014993

Mosconi, L., Perani, D., Sorbi, S., Herholz, K., Nacmias, B., Holthoff, V., et al. (2004b). MCI conversion to dementia and the APOE genotype: a prediction study with FDG-PET. *Neurology* 63, 2332–2340. doi: 10.1212/01. WNL.0000147469.18313.3B

Mosconi, L., Sorbi, S., Nacmias, B., De Cristofaro, M. T., Fayyaz, M., Bracco, L., et al. (2004c). Age and ApoE genotype interaction in Alzheimer's disease: an FDG-PET study. *Psychiatry Res.* 130, 141–151. doi: 10.1016/j.pscychresns.2003. 12.005

Paillusson, S., Stoica, R., Gomez-Suaga, P., Lau, D. H. W., Mueller, S., Miller, T., et al. (2013). There's something wrong with my MAM; the ER-mitochondria axis and neurodegenerative diseases. *Trends Neurosci.* 39, 146–157. doi: 10. 1016/j.tins.2016.01.008

Parker, W. D. Jr., Filley, C. M., and Parks, J. K. (1990). Cytochrome oxidase deficiency in Alzheimer's disease. *Neurology* 40, 1302–1303. doi: 10.1212/WNL. 40.8.1302

Parker, W. D. Jr., Parks, J., Filley, C. M., and Kleinschmidt-Demasters, B. K. (1994). Electron transport chain defects in Alzheimer's disease brain. *Neurology* 44, 1090–1096. doi: 10.1212/WNL.44.6.1090

Pichaud, N., Ballard, J. W., Tanguay, R. M., and Blier, P. U. (2012). Naturally occurring mitochondrial DNA haplotypes exhibit metabolic differences: insight into functional properties of mitochondria. *Evolution* 66, 3189–3197. doi: 10.1111/j.1558-5646.2012.01683.x

Poirier, J., Bertrand, P., Kogan, S., Gauthier, S., Davignon, J., and Bouthillier, D. (1993). Apolipoprotein E polymorphism and Alzheimer's disease. *Lancet* 342, 697–699. doi: 10.1016/0140-6736(93)91705-Q

Popot, J. L., and de Vitry, C. (1990). On the microassembly of integral membrane proteins. *Annu. Rev. Biophys. Biophys. Chem.* 19, 369–403. doi: 10. 1146/annurev.biophys.19.1.369

Rebeck, G. W., Reiter, J. S., Strickland, D. K., and Hyman, B. T. (1993). Apolipoprotein E in sporadic Alzheimer's disease: allelic variation and receptor interactions. *Neuron* 11, 575–580. doi: 10.1016/0896-6273(93)90070-8

Redjems-Bennani, N., Jeandel, C., Lefebvre, E., Blain, H., Vidailhet, M., and Guéant, J. L. (1998). Abnormal substrate levels that depend upon mitochondrial function in cerebrospinal fluid from Alzheimer patients. *Gerontology* 44, 300–304. doi: 10.1159/000022031

Reiman, E. M., Caselli, R. J., Chen, K., Alexander, G. E., Bandy, D., and Frost, J. (2001). Declining brain activity in cognitively normal apolipoprotein E epsilon 4 heterozygotes: a foundation for using positron emission tomography to efficiently test treatments to prevent Alzheimer's disease. *Proc. Natl. Acad. Sci. U S A* 98, 3334–3339. doi: 10.1073/pnas.061509598

Reiman, E. M., Chen, K., Alexander, G. E., Caselli, R. J., Bandy, D., Osborne, D., et al. (2004). Functional brain abnormalities in young adults at genetic risk for late-onset Alzheimer's dementia. *Proc. Natl. Acad. Sci. U S A* 101, 284–289. doi: 10.1073/pnas.2635903100

Reiman, E. M., Chen, K., Alexander, G. E., Caselli, R. J., Bandy, D., Osborne, D., et al. (2005). Correlations between apolipoprotein E epsilon4 gene dose and brain-imaging measurements of regional hypometabolism. *Proc. Natl. Acad. Sci. U S A* 102, 8299–8302. doi: 10.1073/pnas.0500579102

Richardson, J. S. (1993). Free radicals in the genesis of Alzheimer's disease. *Ann. N Y Acad. Sci.* 695, 73–76. doi: 10.1111/j.1749-6632.1993.tb23031.x

Ridge, P. G., Koop, A., Maxwell, T. J., Bailey, M. H., Swerdlow, R. H., Kauwe, J. S., et al. (2013). Mitochondrial haplotypes associated with biomarkers for Alzheimer's disease. *PLoS One* 8:e74158. doi: 10.1371/journal.pone. 0074158

Ridge, P. G., Maxwell, T. J., Corcoran, C. D., Norton, M. C., Tschanz, J. T., O'Brien, E., et al. (2012). Mitochondrial genomic analysis of late onset Alzheimer's disease reveals protective haplogroups H6A1A/H6A1B: the cache county study on memory in aging. *PLoS One* 7:e45134. doi: 10.1371/journal.pone.0045134

Risner, M. E., Saunders, A. M., Altman, J. F., Ormandy, G. C., Craft, S., Foley, I. M., et al. (2006). Efficacy of rosiglitazone in a genetically defined population with mild-to-moderate Alzheimer's disease. *Pharmacogenomics J.* 6, 246–254. doi: 10.1038/sj.tpj.6500369

Roses, A. D., Saunders, A. M., Huang, Y., Strum, J., Weisgraber, K. H., and Mahley, R. W. (2007). Complex disease-associated pharmacogenetics: drug efficacy, drug safety and confirmation of a pathogenetic hypothesis (Alzheimer's disease). *Pharmacogenomics J.* 7, 10–28. doi: 10.1038/sj.tpj.6500397

Santoro, A., Balbi, V., Balducci, E., Pirazzini, C., Rosini, F., Tavano, F., et al. (2010). Evidence for sub-haplogroup h5 of mitochondrial DNA as a risk factor for late onset Alzheimer's disease. *PLoS One* 5:e12037. doi: 10.1371/journal.pone.0012037

Saunders, A. M., Strittmatter, W. J., Schmechel, D., George-Hyslop, P. S., Pericak-Vance, M. A., Joo, S., et al. (1993). Association of apolipoprotein E allele ε4 with late-onset familial and sporadic Alzheimer's disease. *Neurology* 43, 1467–1467. doi: 10.1212/wnl.43.8.1467

Schagger, H., and Ohm, T. G. (1995). Human diseases with defects in oxidative phosphorylation. 2. F1F0 ATP-synthase defects in Alzheimer disease revealed by blue native polyacrylamide gel electrophoresis. *Eur. J. Biochem.* 227, 916–921. doi: 10.1111/j.1432-1033.1995.0916p.x

Scheffler, K., Krohn, M., Dunkelmann, T., Stenzel, J., Miroux, B., Ibrahim, S., et al. (2012). Mitochondrial DNA polymorphisms specifically modify cerebral beta-amyloid proteostasis. *Acta Neuropathol.* 124, 199–208. doi: 10.1007/s00401-012-0980-x

Schuessel, K., Leutner, S., Cairns, N. J., Müller, W. E., and Eckert, A. (2004). Impact of gender on upregulation of antioxidant defence mechanisms in Alzheimer's disease brain. *J. Neural Transm. (Vienna)* 111, 1167–1182. doi: 10.1007/s00702-004-0156-5

Sheehan, J. P., Swerdlow, R. H., Miller, S. W., Davis, R. E., Parks, J. K., Parker, W. D., et al. (1997). Calcium homeostasis and reactive oxygen species production in cells transformed by mitochondria from individuals with sporadic Alzheimer's disease. *J. Neurosci.* 17, 4612–4622.

Shi, L., Du, X., Zhou, H., Tao, C., Liu, Y., Meng, F., et al. (2014). Cumulative effects of the ApoE genotype and gender on the synaptic proteome and oxidative stress in the mouse brain. *Int. J. Neuropsychopharmacol.* 17, 1863–1879. doi: 10.1017/s1461145714000601

Shoffner, J. M., Brown, M. D., Torroni, A., Lott, M. T., Cabell, M. F., Mirra, S. S., et al. (1993). Mitochondrial DNA variants observed in alzheimer disease and parkinson disease patients. *Genomics* 17, 171–184. doi: 10.1006/geno.1993.1299

Simpkins, J. W., Yang, S.-H., Sarkar, S. N., and Pearce, V. (2008). Estrogen actions on mitochondria–Physiological and pathological implications. *Mol. Cell. Endocrinol.* 290, 51–59. doi: 10.1016/j.mce.2008.04.013

Sims, N. R., Finegan, J. M., Blass, J. P., Bowen, D. M., and Neary, D. (1987). Mitochondrial function in brain tissue in primary degenerative dementia. *Brain Res.* 436, 30–38. doi: 10.1016/0006-8993(87)91553-8

Skup, M., Zhu, H., Wang, Y., Giovanello, K. S., Lin, J. A., Shen, D., et al. (2011). Sex differences in grey matter atrophy patterns among AD and aMCI patients: results from ADNI. *Neuroimage* 56, 890–906. doi: 10.1016/j.neuroimage.2011.02.060

Small, G. W., Ercoli, L. M., Silverman, D. H., Huang, S. C., Komo, S., Bookheimer, S. Y., et al. (2000). Cerebral metabolic and cognitive decline in persons at genetic risk for Alzheimer's disease. *Proc. Natl. Acad. Sci. U S A* 97, 6037–6042. doi: 10.1073/pnas.090106797

Small, G. W., Mazziotta, J. C., Collins, M. T., Baxter, L. R., Phelps, M. E., Mandelkern, M. A., et al. (1995). APolipoprotein e type 4 allele and cerebral glucose metabolism in relatives at risk for familial alzheimer disease. *JAMA* 273, 942–947. doi: 10.1001/jama.273.12.942

Stewart, J. B., and Chinnery, P. F. (2015). The dynamics of mitochondrial DNA heteroplasmy: implications for human health and disease. *Nat. Rev. Genet.* 16, 530–542. doi: 10.1038/nrg3966

Swerdlow, R. H., and Khan, S. M. (2004). A "mitochondrial cascade hypothesis" for sporadic Alzheimer's disease. *Med. Hypotheses* 63, 8–20. doi: 10.1016/j.mehy.2003.12.045

Takasaki, S. (2008). Mitochondrial SNPs associated with Japanese centenarians, Alzheimer's patients and Parkinson's patients. *Comput. Biol. Chem.* 32, 332–337. doi: 10.1016/j.compbiolchem.2008.03.014

Takasaki, S. (2009). Mitochondrial haplogroups associated with Japanese centenarians, Alzheimer's patients, Parkinson's patients, type 2 diabetic patients and healthy non-obese young males. *J Genet Genomics* 36, 425–434. doi: 10.1016/s1673-8527(08)60132-0

Torroni, A., Huoponen, K., Francalacci, P., Petrozzi, M., Morelli, L., Scozzari, R., et al. (1996). Classification of european mtDNAs from an analysis of three european populations. *Genetics* 144, 1835–1850.

Torroni, A., Schurr, T. G., Yang, C. C., Szathmary, E. J., Williams, R. C., Schanfield, M. S., et al. (1992). Native American mitochondrial DNA analysis indicates that the Amerind and the Nadene populations were founded by two independent migrations. *Genetics* 130, 153–162.

Tranah, G. J., Manini, T. M., Lohman, K. K., Nalls, M. A., Kritchevsky, S., Newman, A. B., et al. (2011). Mitochondrial DNA variation in human metabolic rate and energy expenditure. *Mitochondrion* 11, 855–861. doi: 10.1016/j.mito.2011.04.005

Tranah, G. J., Nalls, M. A., Katzman, S. M., Yokoyama, J. S., Lam, E. T., Zhao, Y., et al. (2012). Mitochondrial DNA sequence variation associated with dementia and cognitive function in the elderly. *J. Alzheimers Dis.* 32, 357–372.

Tranah, G. J., Yokoyama, J. S., Katzman, S. M., Nalls, M. A., Newman, A. B., Harris, T. B., et al. (2014). Mitochondrial DNA sequence associations with dementia and amyloid-beta in elderly African Americans. *Neurobiol. Aging* 35, 442.e1–442.e8. doi: 10.1016/j.neurobiolaging.2013.05.023

Trimmer, P. A., Swerdlow, R. H., Parks, J. K., Keeney, P., Bennett, J. P. Jr., Miller, S. W., et al. (2000). Abnormal mitochondrial morphology in sporadic Parkinson's and Alzheimer's disease cybrid cell lines. *Exp. Neurol.* 162, 37–50. doi: 10.1006/exnr.2000.7333

Valla, J., Schneider, L., Niedzielko, T., Coon, K. D., Caselli, R., Sabbagh, M. N., et al. (2006). Impaired platelet mitochondrial activity in Alzheimer's disease and mild cognitive impairment. *Mitochondrion* 6, 323–330. doi: 10.1016/j.mito.2006.10.004

Valla, J., Yaari, R., Wolf, A. B., Kusne, Y., Beach, T. G., Roher, A. E., et al. (2010). Reduced posterior cingulate mitochondrial activity in expired young adult carriers of the APOE epsilon4 allele, the major late-onset Alzheimer's susceptibility gene. *J. Alzheimers Dis.* 22, 307–313. doi: 10.3233/JAD-2010-100129

van der Walt, J. M., Dementieva, Y. A., Martin, E. R., Scott, W. K., Nicodemus, K. K., Kroner, C. C., et al. (2004). Analysis of European mitochondrial haplogroups with Alzheimer disease risk. *Neurosci. Lett.* 365, 28–32. doi: 10.1016/j.neulet.2004.04.051

van der Walt, J. M., Scott, W. K., Slifer, S., Gaskell, P. C., Martin, E. R., Welsh-Bohmer, K., et al. (2005). Maternal lineages and alzheimer disease risk in the old order amish. *Hum. Genet.* 118, 115–122. doi: 10.1007/s00439-005-0032-x

Wallace, D. C. (1994). Mitochondrial DNA sequence variation in human evolution and disease. *Proc. Natl. Acad. Sci. U S A* 91, 8739–8746. doi: 10.1073/pnas.91.19.8739

Wallace, D. C. (2005). A mitochondrial paradigm of metabolic and degenerative diseases, aging, and cancer: a dawn for evolutionary medicine. *Annu. Rev. Genet.* 39, 359–407. doi: 10.1146/annurev.genet.39.110304.095751

Wallace, D. C., Ye, J. H., Neckelmann, S. N., Singh, G., Webster, K. A., and Greenberg, B. D. (1987). Sequence analysis of cDNAs for the human and bovine ATP synthase beta subunit: mitochondrial DNA genes sustain seventeen times more mutations. *Curr. Genet.* 12, 81–90. doi: 10.1007/bf00434661

Watanabe, K. (2010). Unique features of animal mitochondrial translation systems. *Proc. Jan. Acad. Ser. B Phys. Biol. Sci.* 86, 11–39. doi: 10.2183/pjab.86.11

Watanabe, K., and Yokobori, S. (2011). tRNA modification and genetic code variations in animal mitochondria. *J. Nucleic Acids* 2011:623095. doi: 10.4061/2011/623095

Wolf, A. B., Caselli, R. J., Reiman, E. M., and Valla, J. (2013). APOE and neuroenergetics: an emerging paradigm in Alzheimer's disease. *Neurobiol. Aging* 34, 1007–1017. doi: 10.1016/j.neurobiolaging.2012.10.011

Wragg, M. A., Talbot, C. J., Morris, J. C., Lendon, C. L., and Goate, A. M. (1995). No association found between Alzheimer's disease and a mitochondrial tRNA glutamine gene variant. *Neurosci. Lett.* 201, 107–110. doi: 10.1016/0304-3940(95)12146-3

Xu, P. T., Li, Y. J., Qin, X. J., Kroner, C., Green-Odlum, A., Xu, H., et al. (2007). A SAGE study of apolipoprotein E3/3, E3/4 and E4/4 allele-specific gene expression in hippocampus in Alzheimer disease. *Mol. Cell. Neurosci.* 36, 313–331. doi: 10.1016/j.mcn.2007.06.009

Xu, P. T., Li, Y. J., Qin, X. J., Scherzer, C. R., Xu, H., Schmechel, D. E., et al. (2006). Differences in apolipoprotein E3/3 and E4/4 allele-specific gene expression in hippocampus in Alzheimer disease. *Neurobiol. Dis.* 21, 256–275. doi: 10.1016/j.nbd.2005.07.004

Xu, S., Schaack, S., Seyfert, A., Choi, E., Lynch, M., and Cristescu, M. E. (2012). High mutation rates in the mitochondrial genomes of daphnia pulex. *Mol. Biol. Evol.* 29, 763–769. doi: 10.1093/molbev/msr243

Zhang, L., Trushin, S., Christensen, T. A., Bachmeier, B. V., Gateno, B., Schroeder, A., et al. (2016). Altered brain energetics induces mitochondrial fission arrest in Alzheimer's Disease. *Sci. Rep.* 6:18725. doi: 10.1038/srep18725

Zsurka, G., Kálmán, J., Császár, A., Raskó, I., Janka, Z., and Venetianer, P. (1998). No mitochondrial haplotype was found to increase risk for Alzheimer's disease. *Biol. Psychiatry* 44, 371–373. doi: 10.1016/s0006-3223(97)00461-7

14

Orbitofrontal Cortex and the Early Processing of Visual Novelty in Healthy Aging

David A. S. Kaufman[1], Cierra M. Keith[1] and William M. Perlstein[2,3,4]*

[1] Department of Psychology, Saint Louis University, St. Louis, MO, USA, [2] Department of Clinical and Health Psychology, University of Florida, Gainesville, FL, USA, [3] Department of Psychiatry, University of Florida, Gainesville, FL, USA, [4] VA RR&D Brain Rehabilitation Research Center of Excellence, Malcom Randall Veterans Administration Medical Center, Gainesville, FL, USA

Edited by:
Junfeng Sun,
Shanghai Jiao Tong University, China

Reviewed by:
Shulan Hsieh,
National Cheng Kung University, Taiwan
Ling Li,
University of Electronic Science and Technology of China, China

***Correspondence:**
David A. S. Kaufman
dkaufma3@slu.edu

Event-related potential (ERP) studies have previously found that scalp topographies of attention-related ERP components show frontal shifts with age, suggesting an increased need for compensatory frontal activity to assist with top-down facilitation of attention. However, the precise neural time course of top-down attentional control in aging is not clear. In this study, 20 young (mean: 22 years) and 14 older (mean: 64 years) adults completed a three-stimulus visual oddball task while high-density ERPs were acquired. Colorful, novel distracters were presented to engage early visual processing. Relative to young controls, older participants exhibited elevations in occipital early posterior positivity (EPP), approximately 100 ms after viewing colorful distracters. Neural source models for older adults implicated unique patterns of orbitofrontal cortex (OFC; BA 11) activity during early visual novelty processing (100 ms), which was positively correlated with subsequent activations in primary visual cortex (BA 17). Older adult EPP amplitudes and OFC activity were associated with performance on tests of complex attention and executive function. These findings are suggestive of age-related, compensatory neural changes that may driven by a combination of weaker cortical efficiency and increased need for top-down control over attention. Accordingly, enhanced early OFC activity during visual attention may serve as an important indicator of frontal lobe integrity in healthy aging.

Keywords: ERPs, aging, oddball, orbitofrontal cortex, attention, sLORETA

INTRODUCTION

The ability to orient to new stimuli and respond with flexibility to a changing environment is a crucial skill (Barceló et al., 2002). One way to simulate environmental change and examine cognitive control involves the introduction of an unexpected novel stimulus, which intends to capture and divert attention (de Fockert et al., 2004; Barcelo et al., 2006). In cognitive neuroscience, the oddball paradigm has been frequently used to assess neural responses to irregularly occurring, novel stimuli (Friedman, 2003). Although it is a relatively simple task involving response to an infrequent target stimulus presented amongst more common standard stimuli, it has been interpreted as a probe for frontal cortex activity (Fabiani and Friedman, 1995). Huettel and McCarthy (2004) theorized that activation of the prefrontal cortex during the oddball paradigm can be associated with inhibition and modification of behavioral response strategies. Given the infrequency of targets, oddball tasks foster a predominantly passive response style that must be overcome when targets are detected. Accordingly, optimization of attentional processing during these tasks requires synchronization between bottom-up and top-down processing systems.

Top-down processing assists in the voluntary discrimination of relevant stimuli from distractors (Gazzaley et al., 2005). Normal aging is associated with increases in distractibility, which may be due to increased difficulty filtering irrelevant sensory information during attentional processing (McDowd and Filion, 1992; Chao and Knight, 1997; Alain and Woods, 1999; Fabiani et al., 2006). This inhibitory deficit hypothesis is commonly cited as an influential factor driving age-related cognitive decline (Hasher and Zacks, 1988; Gazzaley and D'Esposito, 2007). Age-related changes in attentional control are often linked to frontal lobe structures, which undergo structural and functional compromise in healthy aging (Raz et al., 2005). However, older adults also exhibit declines with bottom-up sensory processing (Carp et al., 2011), which can also contribute to age-related declines in visual attention. While many studies have suggested that enhanced activity in frontal lobe structures helps to compensate for age-related declines in sensory processing (Reuter-Lorenz and Cappell, 2008; Li et al., 2013), it remains unclear exactly how top-down mechanisms of control are coordinated.

The neural time course of attentional processing can be examined with high temporal resolution using electrophysiological methods. Visual oddball studies have frequently reported event-related potentials (ERPs) that highlight age-related differences in attention. In particular, target-related P3 components (also referred to as P300 or P3b) demonstrate increased latency in older adults, while overall amplitudes decrease with age (Polich, 2007; Friedman, 2008). In young adults, target-related P3 amplitudes are typically maximal over parietal electrode sites, yet in older adults these amplitudes decrease at both parietal and central locations, while often preserving higher amplitudes over frontal sites. This has often been interpreted as an age-related "frontal shift" with regard to neural resources necessary for processing attentional targets (Fabiani and Friedman, 1995; Friedman et al., 1993). When infrequent distracters are incorporated into oddball paradigms, they evoke a different type of P3 response (often referred to as P3a or novelty P3), which reflects a more rapid detection of novel, task-irrelevant events (Simons and Perlstein, 1997). Distracter-related P3 amplitudes are maximal over frontocentral sites, and increase when the target recognition is more difficult (Katayama and Polich, 1999; Polich and Comerchero, 2003). Although the shift in target-related P3 amplitudes has often presumed a link with frontal lobe structures, imaging studies suggest that a broader network of neural sources give rise to this component, including prefrontal cortex, temporal-parietal junction, lateral parietal cortex, and anterior cingulate (Bedowski et al., 2004).

While many studies have investigated age-related frontal shifts in P3 potentials, effects of aging on early visual sensory (or "exogenous") ERPs have received less attention. This omission is important, as recent studies have revealed that frontal lobe structures may influence visual processing in very early time windows (80–150 ms). Using a combination of Magnetoencephalography (MEG) and Functional magnetic resonance imaging (fMRI) methods, Bar et al. (2006) found that the orbitofrontal cortex (OFC) exhibited differential activity that predicted successful recognition of visual objects, beginning approximately 80 ms after the object appeared. These authors took their findings to suggest that the OFC may receive coarse visual inputs following initial sensory processing which can then be used to make predictions that guide subsequent visual processing that is more specialized (Bar, 2009). Indeed, some cells in the OFC appear to be particularly sensitive to visual novelty, showing selective activation between 80–120 ms post-stimulus (Rolls et al., 2005). While few studies have reported age-related changes that occur in these early sensory processing stages, De Sanctis et al. (2008) observed increased N1 amplitude in older adults, along with enhanced early frontal cortical activation. These results suggest that older adults may enhance frontal activity during early visual processing in order increase their top-down control over visual attention.

In the current study, a three-stimulus oddball paradigm was used to examine early processing of visual novelty in young and older adults. Scalp ERP results were analyzed for early sensory processing and subjected to source localization. Distracter novelty was manipulated during the task, which presented either monochrome or colorful distractors in different trial blocks. Color distracters were presented in order to evoke early visual cortex activity associated with color feature selection, which can be observed as a large posterior negativity, beginning approximately 140 ms post-stimulus and localized to occipital cortex (Hillyard and Anllo-Vento, 1998). Given the proposed role of the OFC in novelty processing and top-down regulation of attention, it was hypothesized that this structure would become differentially involved during the early processing of distracters (80–120 ms). In particular, this early OFC activation was expected to precede visual cortex activations associated with color feature processing. In line with prior studies reporting age-related decline in visual attention, older adults were expected to rely on greater levels of OFC involvement during early processing of colorful distracters. In addition to the oddball paradigm, participants completed several neuropsychological tasks, so that age-related changes could be interpreted in the broader context of executive functioning.

MATERIALS AND METHODS

Participants

A total of 34 participants (20 younger, 14 older) were recruited from advertisements in the local community and undergraduate psychology courses. Demographic characteristics are presented in **Table 1**. Participants were matched across all characteristics except for age, in which younger participants had a mean age (± SD) of 22.1 years (± 3.1) and older participants had a mean age of 64.4 years (± 9.5). Neuropsychological

TABLE 1 | Demographic and cognitive data for younger and older participants.

	Younger (*n* = 20)		Older (*n* = 14)		
	Mean	(SD)	Mean	(SD)	*p*
Demographics					
Age (years)	22.1	(3.1)	64.4	(9.5)	*<0.001*
Education (years)	15.4	(1.7)	17.1	(3.3)	ns
Female (%)	50	–	43	–	ns
Right-handed (%)	85	–	86	–	ns
Cognitive functioning					
MMSE	28.9	(1.1)	28.7	(1.3)	ns
Digit symbol coding (Total)	87.7	(12.2)	77.4	(11.7)	*0.02*
Stroop word reading (sec)	101.4	(15.0)	99.5	(13.5)	ns
Stroop color naming (sec)	80.0	(14.0)	72.6	(15.9)	ns
Stroop color word naming (sec)	46.9	(12.6)	38.8	(11.9)	ns
Trails A (sec)	20.8	(4.7)	27.7	(10.6)	*0.01*
Trails B (sec)	47.0	(15.4)	63.8	(28.7)	*0.03*
WCST Categories completed	6.0	0.0	5.6	(1.3)	ns
WCST Total errors	15.1	(9.6)	17.6	(16.7)	ns
WCST Perseverative responses	8.6	(4.3)	10.3	(10.4)	ns
WCST Perseverative errors	7.9	(3.8)	9.8	(8.9)	ns
WCST Set failure	0.1	(0.3)	0.3	(0.7)	ns

MMSE, Mini-Mental State Examination; WCST, Wisconsin Card Sorting Test.

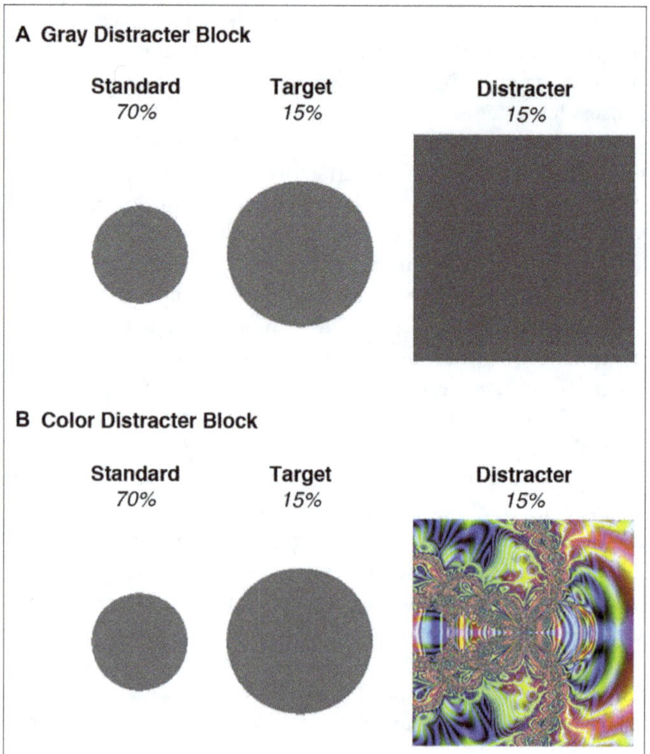

FIGURE 1 | Stimuli used in the two blocks of the oddball task. (A) All stimuli in the gray distracter block were comprised of an identical gray color. **(B)** Standards and targets in the color distracter block were identical to those presented in the gray distracter block, but the distracters consisted of unique colorful fractal designs.

testing revealed that older adults had comparable levels of cognition (MMSE), inhibition (Stroop), and feedback-dependent problem solving (Wisconsin Card Sorting Test). However, older adults were significantly slower on tasks of complex attention and set-shifting (Digit Symbol Coding, Trails A and B). Potential participants (3 young, 1 older) were excluded from the study because they endorsed a history of substance abuse or dependence, acquired brain disorders (e.g., traumatic brain injury), neurological disorders, or color-blindness. Participants provided written informed consent according to procedures established by the University of Florida Health Science Center Institutional Review Board and were provided either $20 or course extra credit for study participation.

Event-Related Potential Stimuli and Task

Stimuli and procedures for the three-stimulus oddball task were adapted from Polich and Comerchero (2003). Standard stimuli, to which the participants were told not to respond, consisted of small gray circles measuring 2" in diameter. Target stimuli were medium-sized gray circles, measuring 3", and participants were instructed to press a button when they saw these stimuli. Distracter stimuli, to which the participants were told not to respond, consisted of large squares measuring 4.5" in diameter. Because distracters were deviant from standards and targets in these two characteristics (size, shape), the amount of visual attention devoted to these distracters was optimized (Polich and Comerchero, 2003; Sawaki and Katayama, 2007). Distracter novelty was further manipulated by stimulus features contained within the large squares. Half of the distracters were gray, like the targets and standards, and were identical in appearance throughout the experiment. The other distracters contained colorful fractal designs that were unique and only occurred once over the course of the experiment (see **Figure 1** for an example). Mean (± SD) luminance intensity for the color distracter slides were 24.1 cd/m^2 (± 9.3), which did not deviate substantially from that of gray distracters (23.1 cd/m^2). Thus color and gray distracters had similar physical properties (size, luminance), despite their differences in chromatic features.

A total of 600 stimuli were randomly presented in four blocks of 150. Seventy percentage were standard stimuli (small circles), 15% were targets (medium circles), and 15% were distracters (large squares). Each stimulus was presented for 75 ms, with a 2 s inter-stimulus interval. Color and gray distracters were presented in different trial blocks to examine the block-related effects of distracter type on behavioral and electrophysiological data. Presentation order of color and gray distracter blocks was counterbalanced across participants such that half of the participants completed the color distracter blocks first and third, while the other participants completed color distracter blocks second and fourth. A practice task consisting of 10 stimuli (6 standards, 2 targets, and 2 gray distracters) was presented in advance to ascertain that all participants were able to discriminate targets from standards. The practice task was repeated as needed until all participants achieved 8 out of 10 correct responses.

Electrophysiological Data Recording, Reduction, and Measurement

Electroencephalographram data were recorded from the scalp using a 64-channel system (Electrical Geodesics, Inc., Eugene, Oregon) running Net Station Software. Impedance of electrodes was maintained below 50 kΩ. EEG was initially referenced to the vertex and recorded continuously at 250 Hz, with on-line band-pass filtering from 0.1 to 100 Hz. Electroencephalogram data were then re-referenced to an average reference off-line and digitally low-pass filtered at 30 Hz. Eye movement and blink artifacts were corrected using spatial filtering methods (Scherg, 1990). The mean (± SD) amplitude used for rejection was a lenient 110 μV (± 16), in order to maximize the number of trials that could be included in averaging without introducing artifacts. The maximum allowable amplitude settings for each trial were individualized for each participant (as recommended by Luck, 2005), but did not differ by group, $t_{(32)} = 0.25$, $p > 0.80$. Point-to-point transitions were not allowed to exceed 75 μV. Of the 64 electrodes used to collect data, less than 2% were interpolated during analysis in order to correct for artifacts.

Individual-subject stimulus-locked averages were derived separately for standard, target, and distracter stimuli in each of the two distracter blocks. Error trials were excluded from ERP analysis. Epochs were extracted from a window of 200 ms prior- to 800 ms post-stimulus presentation and baseline-corrected (200 ms prior to stimulus onset) before subject averaging and analysis. Four occipital electrodes corresponding with O1, O2, PO7, and PO8 were used to examine early posterior positivity (EPP; EGI sensors: 32, 37, 40, 45).

Early Posterior Negativity (EPN) was maximal over medial occipital sites, particularly for younger adults, so three medial occipital electrodes corresponding with O1, O2, and Oz were used to quantify this component (EGI sensors: 37, 40, 38). Four midline electrodes corresponding with FCz, Cz, CPz, Pz were chosen for measurement and analysis of P3 responses (EGI sensors: 4, 65, 30, 34). ERP components were analyzed using adaptive mean amplitude and peak latency scoring protocols in Net Station Software. The adaptive mean algorithm identified a peak within each selected time window and then defined a new time window around this peak for scoring the mean voltage. Time windows used for scoring the different ERP components were as follows: Lateral EPP: 80–130 ms (adaptive mean: 8 ms pre- to 8 ms post-peak), Midline EPN: 100–220 ms (adaptive mean: 8 ms pre- to 8 ms post-peak), and P3: 300–650 ms (adaptive mean: 120 ms pre- to 120 ms post-peak).

Data Analysis

Visual inspection of the oddball task data for normality revealed a considerable positive skew. We, therefore, applied the arcsine correction for all error rate data (Neter et al., 1985) and subjected them to a 2-Distracter (gray, color) × 3-Stimulus (standard, target, distracter) repeated measures analysis of variance (ANOVA). For analyses of oddball task response time (RT), median RTs were employed for correct responses (Ratcliff, 1993) and compared between distracter conditions via dependent sample *t*-tests.

Because of their broad scalp distribution, P3 mean amplitudes and peak latencies were examined with 2-Distracter (gray, color) × 3-Stimulus (standard, target, distracter) × 4-Electrode Site (Fcz, Cz, Cpz, Pz) repeated measures ANOVAs. EPP and EPN components were subjected to 2-Distracter (gray, color) × 3-Stimulus (standard, target, distracter) repeated measures ANOVAs, using data from the average electrodes in which each ERP component showed maximal amplitude (Picton et al., 2000). Orthogonal ("Helmert") planned contrasts were used in these ANOVAs such that stimulus comparisons were made in the following order: (1) standards vs. targets and distracters; and (2) targets vs. distracters. When applicable, difference waves were calculated by subtracting one condition of interest from another (e.g., color distracters—gray distracters). In order to isolate scalp ERP signals associated with color distracter processing, difference waves were calculated for each stimulus type, such that trials from the gray distracter block were subtracted from trials in the color distracter block.

When necessary to decompose ANOVA results, follow-up *post hoc* comparisons were made using Bonferroni corrections for multiple comparisons. The Huynh-Feldt epsilon adjustment was used for all repeated measures ANOVAs with greater than 1 degree of freedom; uncorrected degrees of freedom and corrected *p*-values are reported.

Neural Source Analysis

Source localization was examined using a realistic finite difference forward model of head conductivity (based on a typical adult head MRI from the Montreal Neurological Institute). A dense dipole set was used in GeoSource 2.0 Software (Electrical Geodesics Inc.), which includes 2447 source dipoles (*x*, *y*, *z* triples) in 7 mm^3 voxels of gray matter, following the method of Pascual-Marqui et al. (1994). The linear inverse solution was computed using the constraints of sLORETA.

Brodmann areas (BAs) were examined using "source montages" defined by the Talairach coordinates (Waters and Tucker, 2013). All dipoles in the brain were represented by a triple regional source, consisting of three dipoles in the *x*, *y*, and *z* orthogonal orientations. The net equivalent dipole for each BA source region was computed as the vector sum of the *x*, *y*, *z* triples for the voxels contained within that region. Particular BAs were selected for statistical analysis based on our predictions that OFC and visual cortex would both be active during the early time windows corresponding to scalp ERP components. Thus BA 11 and BA 17 were selected as *a priori* regions of interest, with neural time course activations for these two regions extracted as the root mean square (RMS) of the *x*, *y*, *z* orthogonal orientations. Consistent with other methods used to examine neural source effects (Lamm et al., 2013; Waters and Tucker, 2013), these two source regions were noted to exhibit changes in source intensity (above an arbitrary threshold) that was observably coincident with the temporal features of the scalp ERP. Mean amplitudes from these source waveforms were then calculated for particular time windows of interest (100 ms, 140 ms), and subjected to difference wave calculation in a manner similar to scalp ERP components of interest.

RESULTS

Oddball Task Performance

Accuracy and RT data from the oddball task were subjected to separate 2-Distracter × 3-Stimulus ANOVAs. With regard to task accuracy, planned contrasts revealed a main effect of distracter type, such that participants made more errors to infrequent stimuli than standards, [$F_{(1,32)} = 47.8$, $p < 0.001$, $\eta^2 = 0.60$], while distracters evoked more errors than targets [$F_{(1,32)} = 18.3$, $p < 0.001$, $\eta^2 = 0.36$]. There was no main effect of group for accuracy. Errors were much more common for trials in the color distracter blocks than gray distracter blocks [$F_{(1,32)} = 69.4$, $p < 0.001$, $\eta^2 = 0.69$], with high error rates for distracters (21.0%), followed by targets (6.1%), and standards (2.0%) in the color distracter block. With regard to target RT, there were no main effects of group or distracter type or Group × Distracter interaction.

Event-Related Potential Data

Within the gray distracter block, standard stimuli waveforms contained an average (± SD) of 165.5 ± 22.9 trials, while target waveforms contained 35.5 ± 5.1 trials and distracter waveforms contained 34.0 ± 4.9. Within the color distracter block, standard stimuli waveforms contained an average (± SD) of 165.7 ± 23.9 trials, while target waveforms contained 34.8 ± 5.2 trials and distracter waveforms contained 34.6 ± 5.2. A Group (2) × Distracter (2) × Stimulus (3) ANOVA confirmed that younger and older participants did not differ in their number of trials that were acceptable for analysis. Furthermore, distracter type did not influence the number of trials comprising the waveforms (main effect and interaction with stimulus type were nonsignificant). Stimulus-locked ERP waveforms taken from lateral and medial occipital sites can be seen in **Figure 2**.

Early Posterior Positivity (EPP)

EPP activity was maximal over lateral occipital sites. While there was no main effect of group, planned contrasts revealed that EPP amplitude exhibited a significant Group × Distracter × Stimulus interaction. Older adults exhibited larger EPP for color distracters than younger adults, even though other stimuli showed no group differences, $F_{(1,32)} = 8.9, p < 0.01, \eta^2 = 0.22$.

In order to better isolate scalp ERP signals associated with color distracter processing, difference waves were calculated for each stimulus type, such that trials from gray distracter blocks were subtracted from those with color distracters. This resulted in the following EPP difference wave categories: (1) standard color-gray; (2) target color-gray; and (3) distracter color-gray. A Group (2) × Stimulus (3) ANOVA confirmed that the color-related enhancement of distracter EPP was only seen in older adults, $F_{(1,32)} = 15.7, p < 0.001, \eta^2 = 0.33$. **Figure 3A** shows these effects by graphing the standardized EPP amplitudes (i.e., color-gray difference waves) for each stimulus across groups.

EPP latencies peaked between 100–112 ms across conditions. There was a significant main effect of group, such that EPP amplitudes peaked earlier for older adults, $F_{(1,32)} = 4.3, p < 0.05, \eta^2 = 0.12$. A Distracter × Stimulus interaction revealed that EPP peak latency was shorter for color distracters than gray, while other stimuli did not differ as a function of distracter block, $F_{(1,32)} = 6.1, p < 0.05, \eta^2 = 0.16$.

Early Posterior Negativity (EPN)

EPN activity was maximal over medial occipital sites. There was a main effect of group, with older adults exhibiting larger EPN than younger adults, $F_{(1,32)} = 12.8, p = 0.001, \eta^2 = 0.29$. Planned contrasts revealed that EPN amplitude exhibited significant a distracter × stimulus type interaction, such that color distracters evoked larger EPN than gray distracters, $F_{(1,32)} = 25.1, p = 0.001, \eta^2 = 0.44$. However, this interaction did not differ as a function of group, and no other effects on EPN were significant.

EPN difference waves were calculated for each stimulus type, following the same procedures employed for EPP difference waves. A Group (2) × Stimulus (3) ANOVA confirmed a strong main effect of stimulus, such that color distracters evoked larger EPN amplitudes than targets or standards, $F_{(1,32)} = 43.3$, $p < 0.001$. This color-related enhancement of distracter EPN did not differ as a function of group, $F_{(1,32)} = 0.1$, $p > 0.72$. **Figure 3B** shows these effects by plotting the standardized EPN amplitudes (i.e., color-gray difference waves) for each stimulus across groups.

EPN latencies peaked between 140–160 ms across conditions. Planned contrasts revealed a Distracter × Stimulus interaction, such that EPN peak latency was shorter for distracters than targets and standards, but only in color distracter block, $F_{(1,32)} = 6.7$, $p < 0.05$, $\eta^2 = 0.17$. Thus EPN latency did not vary as a function of group.

P3

P3 activity had a broad distribution and could be seen across multiple midline sites. Planned contrasts revealed a significant Group (2) × Distracter (2) × Stimulus (3) × Site (4) interaction, such that older patients exhibited larger centrofrontal P3 amplitude for targets and distracters relative standards in the color distracter block [$F_{(1,32)} = 10.0$, $p < 0.01$, $\eta^2 = 0.24$]. This effect can be visualized when comparing the P3 voltage distribution maps in **Figure 2**, which demonstrate enhanced centrofrontal P3 amplitude for older adults relative to younger controls.

Midline P3 latencies peaked between 380–450 ms across conditions. Planned contrasts of peak latencies revealed a main effect of stimulus, such that target P3 latencies were longer than those evoked by distracters [$F_{(1,32)} = 14.4, p = 0.001, \eta^2 = 0.29$], or standards [$F_{(1,32)} = 6.7, p < 0.05, \eta^2 = 0.17$]. While there was no main effect of group, group interacted with stimulus [$F_{(1,32)} = 13.1, p = 0.001, \eta^2 = 0.29$], such that older adults had P3 latencies that were longer for infrequent stimuli (targets and distracters) relative to young adults.

Neural Source Modeling

In order to estimate neural sources associated with the early sensory effects of color distracters, difference waves for each stimulus were subjected to sLORETA analysis. Visual

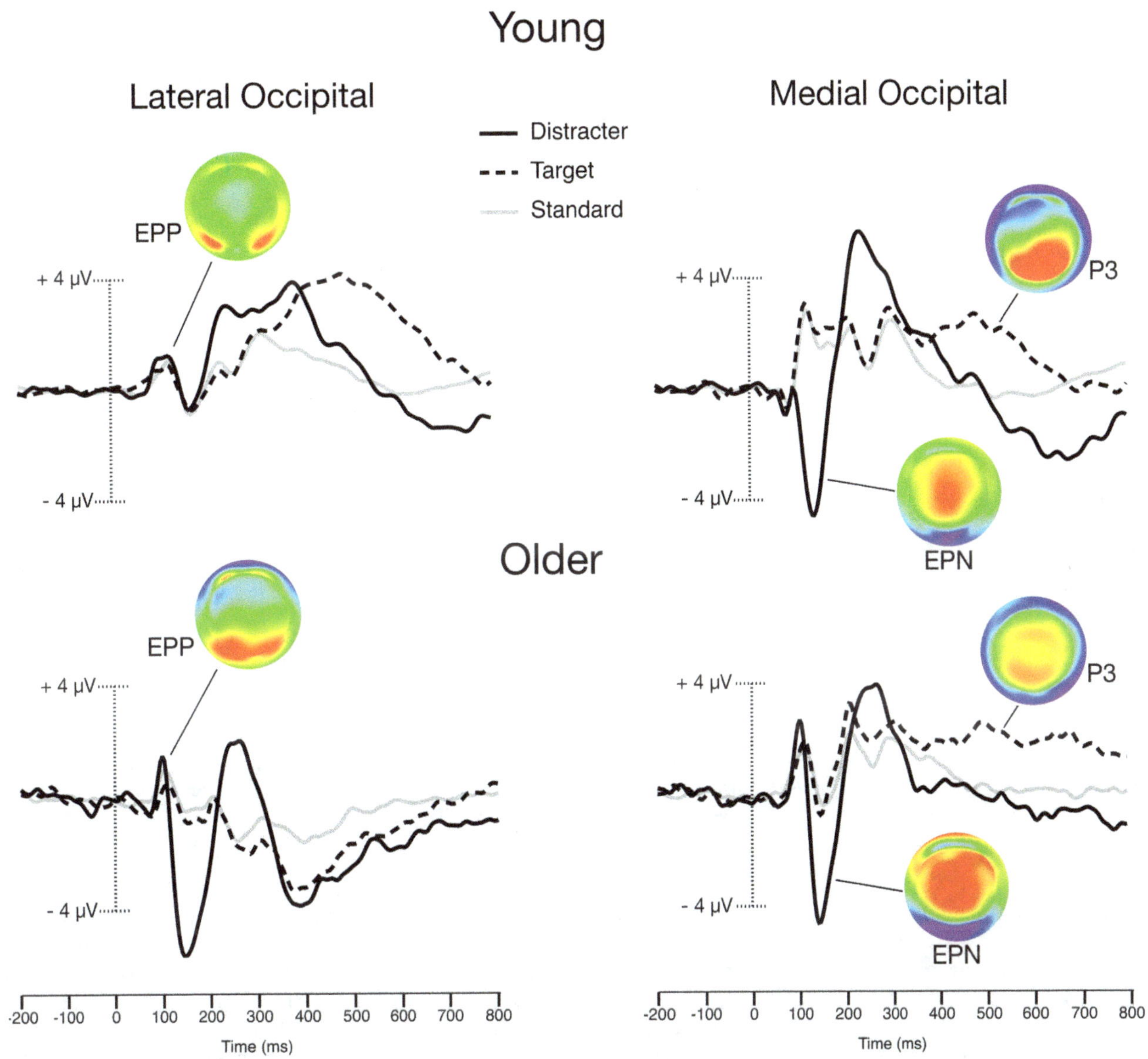

FIGURE 2 | Grand-averaged Event-related potentials (ERPs) from the color distracter block trials. Scalp maps illustrate the peak amplitudes of color distracter processing for early posterior positivity (EPP; 100 ms), Early Posterior Negativity (EPN; 140 ms), and P3 (400 ms). Lateral occipital waveforms were averaged from O1, O2, PO7, and PO8 electrodes. Medial occipital waveforms were averaged from O1, O2, and Oz electrodes.

examination of sLORETA source models revealed distracter-related activations in visual cortex (BA 17) and OFC (BA 11) regions within the first 200 ms post-stimulus. For each BA region of interest, the RMS of each dipole's three orientations was calculated, as shown in the source waveforms in **Figure 4**. For both age groups, activity began to increase in visual cortex regions approximately 80 ms post-stimulus, peaked around 140 ms, and then decreased back down to baseline around 200 ms post-stimulus. In order to quantify these activations, mean source amplitudes were scored for visual cortex ROIs during the beginning (100 ms) and peak activation (140 ms) portions of this time window. It should be noted that this early time window corresponds to the peak latency of the scalp EPP, while the later time window corresponds to the peak latency of the scalp EPN. Shortly after the initial increase in visual cortex activity, small activations can be seen in OFC between 90–110 ms post-stimulus. Accordingly, mean source amplitudes were scored for the OFC during the peak of this frontal activation (100 ms), which also overlaps in time with the scalp EPP. No distinct neural activations were evoked by color distracters during the P3 time window (350–600 ms); thus, no source models were generated for P3 components.

Cortical source activations for each stimulus were then subjected to difference wave contrasts (color-gray distracter), in a manner similar to EPP and EPN scalp waveforms.

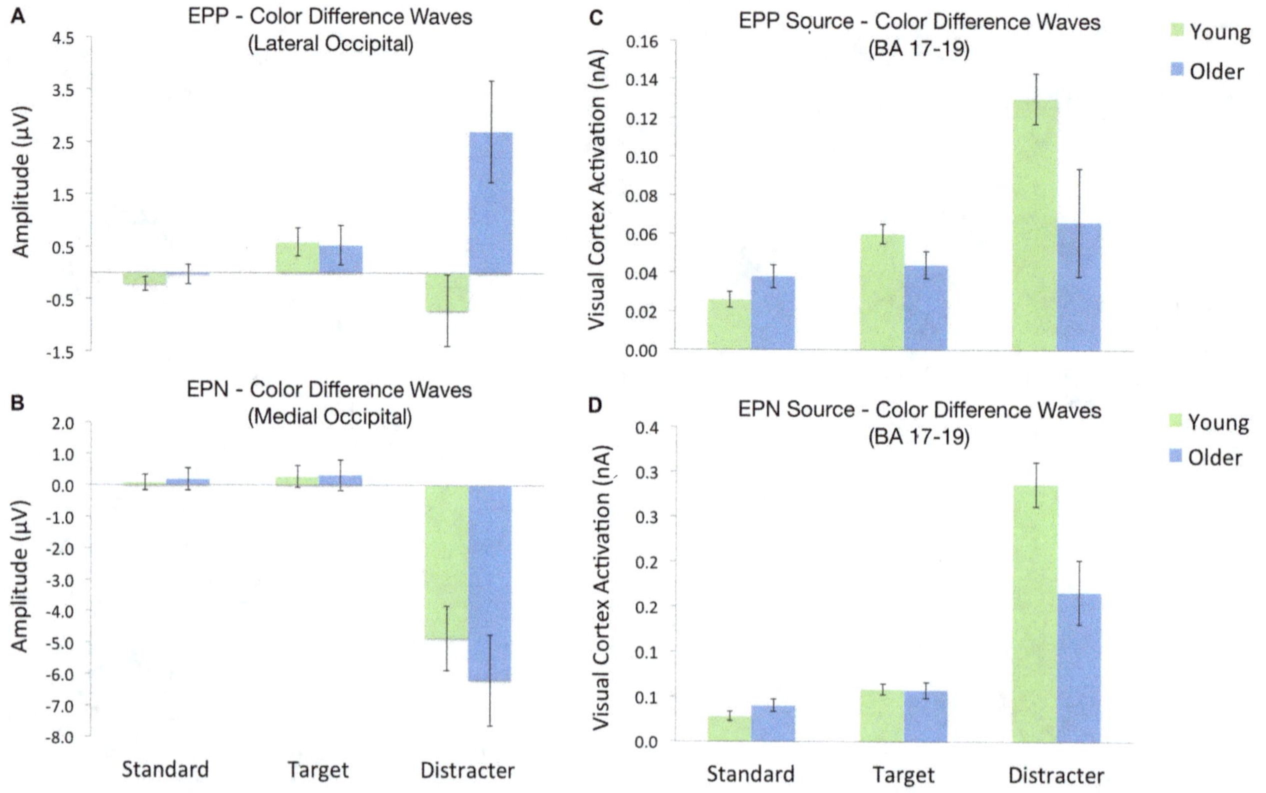

FIGURE 3 | ERP amplitudes and source activations across each oddball stimulus. Each value depicts the contrast between stimuli in the color and gray distracter blocks (i.e., color-gray difference waves). **(A)** EPP amplitudes across lateral occipital electrodes. **(B)** EPN amplitudes across medial occipital electrodes. **(C)** Visual cortex source activity during the EPP time window. **(D)** Visual cortex source activity during the EPN time window.

Activations from BA 17 were subjected to separate Group (2) × Stimulus (3) ANOVAs for the early (100 ms) and later (140 ms) time windows of visual processing. Visual source activations in the EPP time window (100 ms) revealed a Group × Stimulus interaction, such that older adults exhibited decreased visual cortex activity for color distracters relative to younger adults, despite the fact that standards and targets evoked equal activity between groups, $F_{(1,32)} = 8.1$, $p < 0.01$, $\eta^2 = 0.20$. Likewise, the EPN time window (140 ms) also showed this interaction, with younger adults exhibiting greater visual cortex activity for color distracters, $F_{(1,32)} = 5.5$, $p < 0.05$, $\eta^2 = 0.15$. Thus despite the fact that color distracters evoked larger scalp EPP amplitudes in older adults, visual cortex activations were stronger in younger adults during both EPP and EPN time windows, as shown in **Figures 3C,D**.

Neural source activations were found to be associated with scalp ERP components, but the relationships between EPP and source activity differed as a function of age. Older adults showed a positive correlation between early primary visual cortex activity (100 ms) and color distracter EPP ($r = 0.60$, $p < 0.05$), such that stronger visual cortex activity correlated with larger scalp signals for color distracters. Additionally, early OFC activation (100 ms) correlated with EPP amplitude in older adults ($r = 0.69$, $p < 0.01$). In this same time window, younger adults showed no relationships between EPP and neural sources in the visual cortex or OFC. EPN amplitude was correlated with visual cortex activations (140 ms) similarly for older ($r = -0.64$, $p < 0.05$) and younger adults ($r = -0.68$, $p = 0.001$).

Neural source activations from OFC were also subjected to Group (2) × Stimulus (3) ANOVA to examine the effects of color distracters. Unlike visual cortex regions, the strength of source signal in the OFC did not vary significantly as a function of group, $F_{(1,32)} = 0.54$, $p > 0.46$, and there were no Group × Stimulus interactions, $F_{(1,32)} = 0.16$, $p > 0.68$. However, older adults showed a significant relationship between early OFC and visual cortex activity, such that early (100 ms) OFC activations correlated with subsequent (140 ms) visual cortex activations ($r = 0.61$, $p < 0.05$). Young adults did not show this association. RMS source waveforms extracted from dipoles in these regions reveal the neural time course of OFC and visual cortex activity, as seen in **Figure 4**. Older adults exhibited an early peak of OFC activation approximately 100 ms post-stimulus, followed by a subsequent peak of visual cortex activation approximately 140 ms post-stimulus. Younger adults did not show this early OFC activation or any association between OFC and visual cortex during early visual processing.

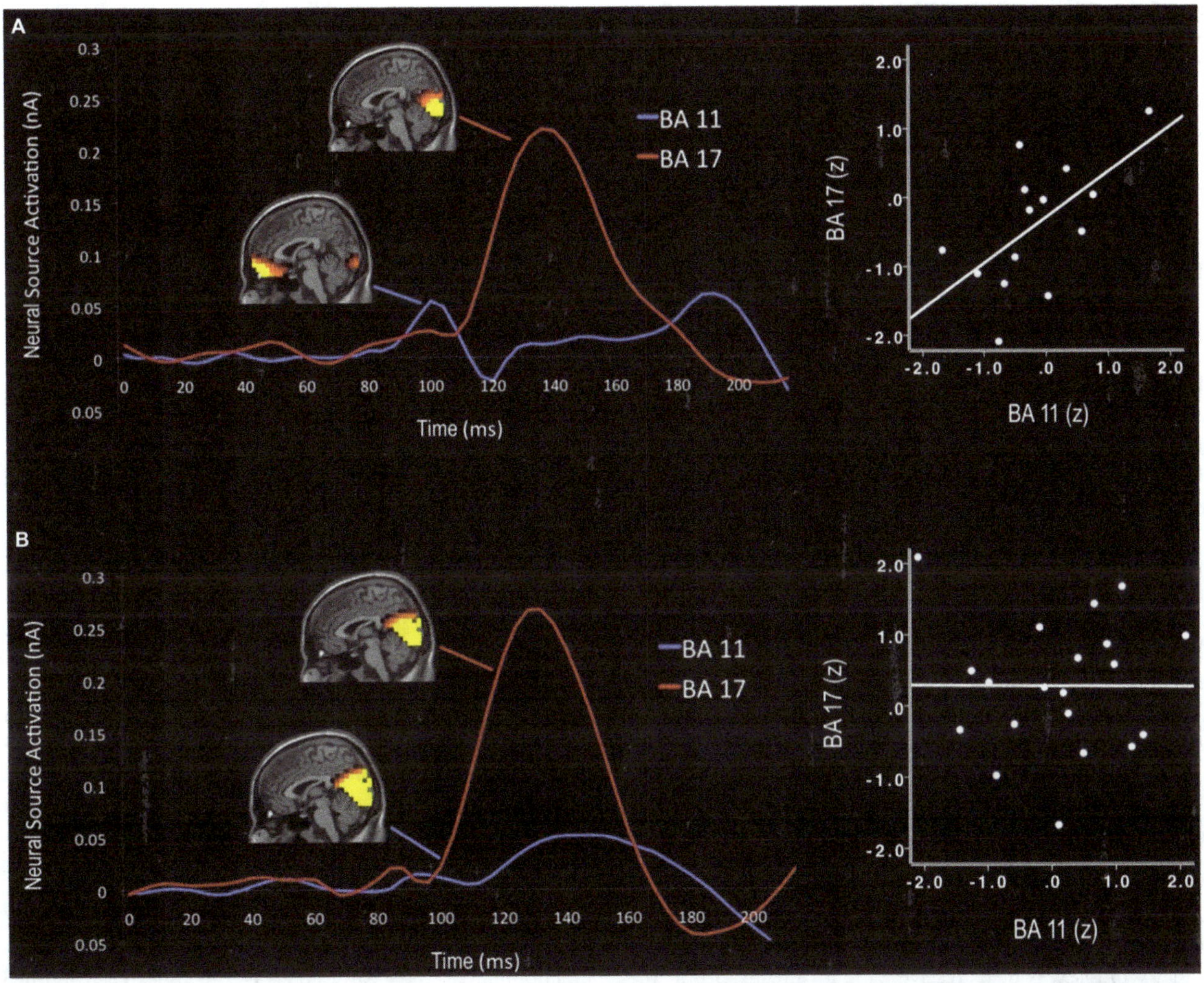

FIGURE 4 | Neural time course of distracter color-gray difference waves for older (A) and younger adults (B). Activation maps display cortical activity at 100 ms and 140 ms that was preferential for color-related distracter processing. Early orbitofrontal cortex (OFC; BA 11) activations predicted subsequent visual cortex activity (BA 17) in older adults, but not for younger adults. Note: Scales visible source activations differ for each time window (100 ms: visible range = 0.06–0.10 nA; 140 ms: visible range = 0.15–0.25 nA).

Correlations with Executive Function

In older adults, several scores from several neuropsychological tests were associated with scalp ERPs and source activations. For older adults, the total number of errors on the WCST was positively correlated with color distracter EPP amplitude ($r = 0.60$, $p < 0.05$). Early OFC activations (100 ms) correlated with scores from Digit Symbol Coding ($r = 0.67$, $p < 0.01$) and Stroop Color Word Naming ($r = 0.54$, $p < 0.05$). Additionally, subsequent visual cortex activations (140 ms) correlated with Digit Symbol Coding ($r = 0.76$, $p < 0.01$). Thus better executive function in older adults was associated with enhanced early processing of color distracters—larger scalp EPP, enhanced OFC activations (100 ms), and enhanced visual cortex activations (140 ms).

Younger adults showed a different pattern of relationships between neuropsychological measures and color distracter processing. No tests were correlated with scalp ERPs in young adults. Early visual cortex activations (100 ms) correlated with scores from Stroop Color Word Naming ($r = 0.54$, $p < 0.05$), while subsequent visual cortex activations (140 ms) correlated with completion time from Trails B ($r = -0.45$, $p < 0.05$). OFC activations were not associated with any of the neuropsychological measures. Therefore, better executive function in younger adults was correlated with enhanced processing of color distracters in the visual cortex, but not the OFC.

DISCUSSION

This study examined age-related differences in visual novelty processing. Occipital electrodes revealed two early sensory ERPs that were selectively enhanced by colorful distracters in the oddball task. An EPP peaked at 100 ms in lateral occipital electrodes, while an early posterior negativity (EPN) peaked at

140 ms in medial occipital electrodes. Enhancement of the EPN was expected, since this component is associated with color feature processing (Hillyard and Anllo-Vento, 1998). However, older adults also exhibited amplified sensory processing of colorful distracters prior to the EPN. This occurred during an earlier stage of visual attention (100 ms after stimulus onset), and was associated with increased activity in primary visual cortex and OFC. Older adults' OFC activity during this early time window was correlated with subsequent visual cortex activity (140 ms), suggesting that the OFC may have been engaged to help facilitate visual recognition of the colorful distracters. In contrast, young adults did not exhibit any early (100 ms) enhanced processing in scalp EPP or neural source activity. Cells in the OFC have been shown to respond selectively to novel visual stimuli, as early as 80 ms following stimulus onset (Rolls et al., 2005). The function of this early activity may be to direct attention toward unexpected or salient stimuli that require further processing (Petrides et al., 2002). When incoming sensory information is ambiguous, perceptual decisions may benefit from "predictive coding", in which the brain maintains an internal template in order to better anticipate forthcoming perceptions (Summerfield et al., 2006). Consistent with this view, the OFC appears to be synchronized with early (80 ms) and later (130 ms) visual cortex processing (Bar et al., 2006), in order to enhance processing in sensory cortex and improve recognition success. Until recently, the neuroanatomical connections necessary to explain this effect have not been clear. However, it appears that magnocellular pathways provide rapid feed-forward (occipital to OFC) and feed-backward (OFC to fusiform) pathways on a timescale that would facilitate object recognition (Kveraga et al., 2007). It has also been proposed that a subcortical route may project visual information to the OFC from the pulvinar complex, which receives input directly from the retina (Pessoa and Adolphs, 2010). With either pathway, it would appear that early projections reaching the OFC within 100 ms would provide only coarse visual information (e.g., limited spatial frequency and contrast). However, even this basic level of representation appears to be sufficient to activate a minimal set of perceptual expectations in the OFC, which can then influence subsequent bottom-up visual processing to facilitate recognition (Bar et al., 2006; Kveraga et al., 2007).

In the later stage of color feature processing (140 ms), EPN amplitude was amplified for both groups in response to colorful distracters, which appears to have been driven by broad increases throughout primary and secondary visual cortices (BA 17–19). Young adults had greater activation in visual cortex during this stage of processing than older adults. Weaker ERP correlates of visual processing have been observed in other visual detection studies (Czigler et al., 2006), and support a general notion that visual processing isless efficient in healthy aging. Thus the current findings support prior claims that healthy aging is associated with neural dedifferentiation of visual processing networks (Grady et al., 1994; Madden et al., 2004; Carp et al., 2011; Burianova et al., 2013).

In line with prior oddball studies focusing on P3 potentials, older adults demonstrated a "frontal shift" in their P3 responses to targets and distracters. In older adults, colorful distracters evoked larger P3 amplitudes in centrofrontal sites, even though their anterior P3 responses had longer latencies than young adults. This finding has been documented using ERP methods (e.g., Fabiani and Friedman, 1995), as well as functional neuroimaging (Davis et al., 2008). One implication of these findings is that the anterior shift in neural recruitment reflects compensation to offset age-related declines in posterior brain function. Frontal regions like the OFC may become active earlier in older adults in order to enhance top-down organization of sensory information, which becomes less efficient with age (Burianova et al., 2013).

The involvement of OFC in early processing of visual novelty has interesting implications for our understanding of cognitive aging. While generally appreciated for its role in emotional processing and decision-making (Bechara et al., 2000), the OFC plays a broader role in generating expectations about incoming information (Petrides et al., 2002). Additionally, such findings may be relevant to the inhibitory deficit hypothesis of cognitive aging. While often associated with emotional control over behavior, the OFC plays a prominent role in regulating inhibitory control (Bari and Robbins, 2013). Recent studies have supported a role for OFC in executive functions needed to dissociate between two perceptually similar actions during response conflict (Bryden and Roesch, 2015). In particular, dopamine regulation of OFC may play a critical role in facilitating proper inhibitory control when behavioral flexibility is required (Cheng and Li, 2013).

It is noteworthy that the older adults in the current study were not cognitively impaired. They did not differ from young adults in overall cognitive status or general levels of executive functioning, yet their early OFC activity appeared to influence subsequent bottom-up visual processing. Given the correlations between neural source activity and cognitive tests, it appears that greater OFC involvement in top-down regulation of attention was associated with broader neuropsychological benefits in healthy aging. Unlike the older group, young adults did not show relationships between early OFC activity and executive function, even though early visual cortex activations were associated with better executive function. Due to the greater activity of visual cortex in this group, it is likely that their visual recognition processing was more efficient and needed less compensatory assistance from the OFC. Older adults relied more on the OFC to provide predictive coding at the earliest stage of visual processing, such that they could perform the task successfully despite weaker visual cortex activations. Importantly, this tendency in our older adult sample appeared to be adaptive, as greater levels of this OFC activation was correlated with greater levels of executive function.

In summary, the current study revealed age-related differences in the early sensory processing of novel stimuli. Older adults had enhanced scalp signals corresponding to an early stage of visual processing (100 ms), which correlated with neural activity in both primary visual cortex and OFC. Consistent with prior findings on posterior cortex dedifferentiation, older adults required enhanced OFC activation in order to compensate for reduced visual processing efficiency. This early compensatory OFC activity in older adults predicted subsequent feature processing in visual cortex (140 ms) and was associated with greater levels of complex attention and executive function. Thus older adults benefited from greater top-down control during visual processing. These findings lend support for models of cognitive aging that account for both neural dedifferentiation and compensatory neural reorganization. Future studies are needed to explore the underlying neural dynamics and connectivity between the OFC and visual cortex, and determine the degree to which these findings generalize to older individuals with more significant levels of neural dedifferentiation or cognitive decline.

ETHICS STATEMENT

The study was approved by the University of Florida, Health Sciences Institutional Review Board.

AUTHOR CONTRIBUTIONS

DASK, Data collection, analysis, manuscript writing; CMK, Manuscript writing; WMP, Manuscript writing and oversight.

REFERENCES

Alain, C., and Woods, D. L. (1999). Age-related changes in processing auditory stimuli during visual attention: evidence for deficits in inhibitory control and sensory memory. *Psychol. Aging* 14, 507–519. doi: 10.1037/0882-7974.14.3.507

Bar, M. (2009). The proactive brain: memory for predictions. *Philos. Trans. R. Soc. Lond. B Biol. Sci.* 364, 1235–1243. doi: 10.1098/rstb.2008.0310

Bar, M., Kassam, K. S., Ghuman, A. S., Boshyan, J., Schmid, A. M., Dale, A. M., et al. (2006). Top-down facilitation of visual recognition. *Proc. Natl. Acad. Sci. U S A* 103, 449–454. doi: 10.1073/pnas.0507062103

Barcelo, F., Escera, C., Corral, M. J., and Periánez, J. A. (2006). Task switching and novelty processing activate a common neural network for cognitive control. *J. Cogn. Neurosci.* 18, 1734–1748. doi: 10.1162/jocn.2006.18.10.1734

Barceló, F., Periáñez, J. A., and Knight, R. T. (2002). Think differently: a brain orienting response to task novelty. *Neuroreport* 13, 1887–1892. doi: 10.1097/00001756-200210280-00011

Bari, A., and Robbins, T. W. (2013). Inhibition and impulsivity: behavioral and neural basis of response control. *Prog. Neurobiol.* 108, 44–79. doi: 10.1016/j.pneurobio.2013.06.005

Bechara, A., Damasio, H., and Damasio, A. R. (2000). Emotion, decision making and the orbitofrontal cortex. *Cereb. Cortex* 10, 295–307. doi: 10.1093/cercor/10.3.295

Bedowski, C., Prvulovic, D., Goebel, R., Zanella, F. E., and Linden, D. E. (2004). Attentional systems in target and distracter processing: a combined ERP and fMRI study. *Neuroimage* 22, 530–540. doi: 10.1016/j.neuroimage.2003.12.034

Bryden, D. W., and Roesch, M. R. (2015). Executive control signals in orbitofrontal cortex during response inhibition. *J. Neurosci.* 35, 3903–3914. doi: 10.1523/JNEUROSCI.3587-14.2015

Burianova, H., Lee, Y., Grady, C. L., and Moscovitch, M. (2013). Age-related dedifferentiation and compensatory changes in the functional network underlying face processing. *Neurobiol. Aging* 34, 2759–2767. doi: 10.1016/j.neurobiolaging.2013.06.016

Carp, J., Park, J., Polk, T. A., and Park, D. C. (2011). Age differences in neural distinctiveness revealed by multi-voxel pattern analysis. *Neuroimage* 56, 736–743. doi: 10.1016/j.neuroimage.2010.04.267

Chao, L. L., and Knight, R. T. (1997). Prefrontal deficits in attention and inhibitory control with aging. *Cereb. Cortex* 7, 63–69. doi: 10.1093/cercor/7.1.63

Cheng, J. T., and Li, J. S. (2013). Intra-orbitofrontal cortex injection of haloperidol removes the beneficial effect of methylphenidate on reversal learning of spontaneously hypertensive rats in an attentional set-shifting task. *Behav. Brain Res.* 15, 148–154. doi: 10.1016/j.bbr.2012.11.006

Czigler, I., Pató, L., Poszet, E., and Balázs, L. (2006). Age and novelty: event-related potentials to visual stimuli within an auditory oddball–visual detection task. *Int. J. Psychophysiol.* 62, 290–299. doi: 10.1016/j.ijpsycho.2006.05.008

Davis, S. W., Dennis, N. A., Daselaar, S. M., Fleck, M. S., and Cabeza, R. (2008). Que PASA? The posterior-anterior shift in aging. *Cereb. Cortex* 18, 1201–1209. doi: 10.1093/cercor/bhm155

de Fockert, J., Rees, G., Frith, C., and Lavie, N. (2004). Neural correlates of attentional capture in visual search. *J. Cogn. Neurosci.* 16, 751–759. doi: 10.1162/089892904970762

De Sanctis, P., Katz, R., Wylie, G. R., Sehatpour, P., Alexopoulos, G. S., and Foxe, J. J. (2008). Enhanced and bilateralized visual sensory processing in the ventral stream may be a feature of normal aging. *Neurobiol. Aging* 29, 1576–1586. doi: 10.1016/j.neurobiolaging.2007.03.021

Fabiani, M., and Friedman, D. (1995). Changes in brain activity patterns in aging: the novelty oddball. *Psychophysiology* 32, 579–594. doi: 10.1111/j.1469-8986.1995.tb01234.x

Fabiani, M., Low, K. A., Wee, E., Sable, J. J., and Gratton, G. (2006). Reduced suppression or labile memory? Mechanisms of inefficient filtering of irrelevant information in older adults. *J. Cogn. Neurosci.* 18, 637–650. doi: 10.1162/jocn.2006.18.4.637

Friedman, D. (2003). Cognition and aging: a highly selective overview of event-related potential (ERP) data. *J. Clin. Exp. Neuropsychol.* 25, 702–720. doi: 10.1076/jcen.25.5.702.14578

Friedman, D. (2008). "The components of aging," in *Oxford Handbook of Event-Related Potential Components*, eds S. L. Luck and E. S. Kappenman (New York, NY: Oxford University Press), 513–536.

Friedman, D., Simpson, G., and Hamberger, M. (1993). Age-related changes in scalp topography to novel and target stimuli. *Psychophysiology* 30, 383–396. doi: 10.1111/j.1469-8986.1993.tb02060.x

Gazzaley, A., Cooney, J. W., McEvoy, K., Knight, R. T., and D'Esposito, M. (2005). Top-down enhancement and suppression of the magnitude and speed of neural activity. *J. Cogn. Neurosci.* 17, 507–517. doi: 10.1162/0898929053279522

Gazzaley, A., and D'Esposito, M. (2007). Top-down modulation and normal aging. *Ann. N Y Acad. Sci.* 1097, 67–83. doi: 10.1196/annals.1379.010

Grady, C. L., Maisog, J. M., Horwitz, B., Ungerleider, L. G., Mentis, M. J., Salerno, J. A., et al. (1994). Age-related changes in cortical blood flow activation during visual processing of faces and location. *J. Neurosci.* 14, 1450–1462.

Hasher, L., and Zacks, R. T. (1988). "Working memory, comprehension and aging: a review and a new view," in *The Psychology of Learning and Motivation*, ed. G. H. Bower (New York, NY: Academic Press), 193–225.

Hillyard, S. A., and Anllo-Vento, L. (1998). Event-related brain potentials in the study of visual selective attention. *Proc. Natl. Acad. Sci. U S A* 95, 781–787. doi: 10.1073/pnas.95.3.781

Huettel, S. A., and McCarthy, G. (2004). What is odd in the oddball task? Prefrontal cortex is activated by dynamic changes in response strategy. *Neuropsychologia* 42, 379–386. doi: 10.1016/j.neuropsychologia.2003.07.009

Katayama, J., and Polich, J. (1999). Auditory and visual P300 topography from a 3 stimulus paradigm. *Clin. Neurophysiol.* 110, 463–468. doi: 10.1016/s1388-2457(98)00035-2

Kveraga, K., Boshyan, J., and Bar, M. (2007). Magnocellular projections as the trigger of top-down facilitation in recognition. *J. Neurosci.* 27, 13232–13240. doi: 10.1523/jneurosci.3481-07.2007

Lamm, C., Pine, D. S., and Fox, N. A. (2013). Impact of negative affectively charged stimuli and response style on cognitive-control-related neural activation: an ERP study. *Brain Cogn.* 83, 234–243. doi: 10.1016/j.bandc.2013.07.012

Li, L., Gratton, C., Fabiani, M., and Knight, R. T. (2013). Age-related frontoparietal changes during the control of bottom-up and top-down attention: an ERP study. *Neurobiol. Aging* 34, 477–488. doi: 10.1016/j.neurobiolaging.2012.02.025

Luck, S. J. (2005). *An Introduction to the Event-Related Potential Technique.* Cambridge, MA: The MIT Press.

Madden, D. J., Whiting, W. L., Provenzale, J. M., and Huettel, S. A. (2004). Age-related changes in neural activity during visual target detection measured by fMRI. *Cereb. Cortex* 14, 143–155. doi: 10.1093/cercor/bhg113

McDowd, J. M., and Filion, D. L. (1992). Aging, selective attention and inhibitory processes: a psychophysiological approach. *Psychol. Aging* 7, 65–71. doi: 10.1037/0882-7974.7.1.65

Neter, J., Wasserman, W., and Kutner, M. H. (1985). *Applied Linear Statistical Models: Regression, Analysis of Variance, and Experimental Designs*, 2nd Edn. Homewood, IL: R.D. Irwin.

Pascual-Marqui, R. D., Michel, C. M., and Lehmann, D. (1994). Low-resolution electromagnetic tomography: a new method for localizing activity in the brain. *Int. J. Psychophysiol.* 18, 49–65. doi: 10.1016/0167-8760(84)90014-x

Pessoa, L., and Adolphs, R. (2010). Emotion processing and the amygdala: from a 'low road' to 'many roads' of evaluating biological significance. *Nat. Rev. Neurosci.* 11, 773–783. doi: 10.1038/nrn2920

Petrides, M., Alivisatos, B., and Frey, S. (2002). Differential activation of the human orbital, mid-ventrolateral and mid-dorsolateral prefrontal cortex during the processing of visual stimuli. *Proc. Natl. Acad. Sci. U S A* 99, 5649–5654. doi: 10.1073/pnas.072092299

Picton, T. W., Bentin, S., Berg, P., Donchin, E., Hillyard, S. A., Johnson, R. Jr., et al. (2000). Guidelines for using human event-related potentials to study cognition: recording standards and publication criteria. *Psychophysiology* 37, 127–152. doi: 10.1017/s0048577200000305

Polich, J. (2007). Updating P300: an integrative theory of P3a and P3b. *Clin. Neurophysiol.* 118, 2128–2148. doi: 10.1016/j.clinph.2007.04.019

Polich, J., and Comerchero, M. D. (2003). P3a from visual stimuli: typicality, task and topography. *Brain Topogr.* 15, 141–152. doi: 10.1023/A:1022637732495

Ratcliff, R. (1993). Methods for dealing with reaction time outliers. *Psychol. Bull.* 114, 510–532. doi: 10.1037/0033-2909.114.3.510

Raz, N., Kindenberger, U., Rodrigue, K. M., Kennedy, K. M., Head, D., Williamson, A., et al. (2005). Regional brain changes in aging healthy adults: general trends, individual differences and modifiers. *Cereb. Cortex* 15, 1676–1689. doi: 10.1093/cercor/bhi044

Reuter-Lorenz, P. A., and Cappell, K. A. (2008). Neurocognitive aging and the compensation hypothesis. *Curr. Dir. Psychol. Sci.* 17, 177–182. doi: 10.1111/j.1467-8721.2008.00570.x

Rolls, E. T., Browning, A. S., Inoue, K., and Hernadi, I. (2005). Novel visual stimuli activat a population of neurons in the primate orbitofrontal cortex. *Neurobiol. Learn. Mem.* 84, 111–123. doi: 10.1016/j.nlm.2005.05.003

Sawaki, R., and Katayama, J. (2007). Difficulty of discrimination modulates attentional capture for deviant information. *Psychophysiology* 44, 374–382. doi: 10.1111/j.1469-8986.2007.00506.x

Scherg, M. (1990). "Fundamentals of dipole source potential analysis," in *Auditory Evoked Magnetic Fields and Electric Potentials. Advances in Audiology*, (Vol. 6) eds F. Grandori and M. Hoke (Basel: Karger), 65–78.

Simons, R. F., and Perlstein, W. M. (1997). "A tale of two reflexes: an ERP analysis of prepulse inhibition and orienting," in *Attention and Orienting: Sensory and Motivational Processes*, eds R. F. Simons and P. J. Lang (Mahwah, NJ: Lawrence Erlbaum Associates, Inc.), 229–255.

Summerfield, C., Enger, T., Greene, M., Koechlin, E., Mangels, J., and Hirsch, J. (2006). Predictive codes for forthcoming perception in the frontal cortex. *Science* 314, 1311–1314. doi: 10.1126/science.1132028

Waters, A. C., and Tucker, D. M. (2013). Positive and negative affect in adolescent self-evaluation: psychometric information in single trials used to generate dimension-specific ERPs and neural source models. *Psychophysiology* 50, 538–549. doi: 10.1111/psyp.12035

15

Oxidized Cholesterol as the Driving Force Behind the Development of Alzheimer's Disease

Paola Gamba†, Gabriella Testa†, Simona Gargiulo, Erica Staurenghi, Giuseppe Poli and Gabriella Leonarduzzi*

Department of Clinical and Biological Sciences, School of Medicine, University of Turin, Orbassano, Torino, Italy

Edited by:
Enrique Cadenas,
University of Southern California, USA

Reviewed by:
Giuseppe Valacchi,
University of Ferrara, Italy
João Laranjinha,
University of Coimbra, Portugal

***Correspondence:**
Giuseppe Poli,
Department of Clinical and Biological Sciences, School of Medicine, University of Turin, San Luigi Hospital, 10043 Orbassano, Torino, Italy
giuseppe.poli@unito.it

†These authors have contributed equally to this work.

Alzheimer's disease (AD), the most common neurodegenerative disorder associated with dementia, is typified by the pathological accumulation of amyloid Aβ peptides and neurofibrillary tangles (NFT) within the brain. Considerable evidence indicates that many events contribute to AD progression, including oxidative stress, inflammation, and altered cholesterol metabolism. The brain's high lipid content makes it particularly vulnerable to oxidative species, with the consequent enhancement of lipid peroxidation and cholesterol oxidation, and the subsequent formation of end products, mainly 4-hydroxynonenal and oxysterols, respectively from the two processes. The chronic inflammatory events observed in the AD brain include activation of microglia and astrocytes, together with enhancement of inflammatory molecule and free radical release. Along with glial cells, neurons themselves have been found to contribute to neuroinflammation in the AD brain, by serving as sources of inflammatory mediators. Oxidative stress is intimately associated with neuroinflammation, and a vicious circle has been found to connect oxidative stress and inflammation in AD. Alongside oxidative stress and inflammation, altered cholesterol metabolism and hypercholesterolemia also significantly contribute to neuronal damage and to progression of AD. Increasing evidence is now consolidating the hypothesis that oxidized cholesterol is the driving force behind the development of AD, and that oxysterols are the link connecting the disease to altered cholesterol metabolism in the brain and hypercholesterolemia; this is because of the ability of oxysterols, unlike cholesterol, to cross the blood brain barrier (BBB). The key role of oxysterols in AD pathogenesis has been strongly supported by research pointing to their involvement in modulating neuroinflammation, Aβ accumulation, and cell death. This review highlights the key role played by cholesterol and oxysterols in the brain in AD pathogenesis.

Keywords: Alzheimer's disease, oxidative stress, inflammation, oxidized cholesterol, oxysterols

Abbreviations: α-EPOX, 5α, 6α-epoxicholesterol; β-EPOX, 5β, 6β-epoxicholesterol; 24-OH, 24-hydroxycholesterol; 25-OH, 25-hydroxycholesterol; 4β-OH, 4β-hydroxycholestrerol; 7β-OH, 7β-hydroxycholesterol; 7α-OH, 7α-hydroxycholesterol; 7-OH-4-C, 7α-hydroxy-3-oxo-4-cholestenoic acid; 7-K, 7-ketocholesterol; ABCA1, ATP-binding cassette transporter A1; ABCG1, ATP-binding cassette transporter G1; AD, Alzheimer's disease; ApoE, apolipoprotein E; APP, amyloid precursor protein; Aβ, amyloid β; BACE1, beta-site amyloid precursor protein cleaving enzyme 1; BBB, blood-brain barrier; CNS, central nervous system; CSF, cerebrospinal fluid; CYP27A1, 27-hydroxylase; CYP46A1, 24-hydroxylase; LPS, lipopolisaccaride; LXR, liver X receptor; NF-κB, nuclear factor-κB; NFT, neurofibrillary tangles; NO, nitric oxide; PSEN1, presenilin 1; PSEN2, presenilin 2; RNS, reactive nitrose species; ROS, reactive oxygen species; TLR, Toll-like receptor.

Introduction

Alzheimer's disease (AD) is the most common age-related neurodegenerative disorder associated with dementia, and the progressive deterioration of mental capacities. It is a complex disease characterized by progressive memory impairment, cognitive deficit, and personality changes; these symptoms are due to substantial synaptic and neuronal loss occuring in specific brain areas, especially in the neocortex, hippocampus, and other subcortical regions. Brains from AD patients show distinct neuropathological features, which we now know are the hallmarks of the disease: extracellular deposits of amyloid β (Aβ) peptides in the form of senile plaques, Aβ deposits in the cerebral blood vessels, and intracellular inclusion of neurofibrillary tangles (NFT) composed of hyperphosphorylated tau protein (Querfurth and LaFerla, 2010; Chopra et al., 2011).

One of the events that promotes AD pathogenesis is the abnormal processing of amyloid precursor protein (APP), which leads to excess production of Aβ peptides through the sequential enzymatic actions of beta-site APP cleaving enzyme 1 (BACE1), a β-secretase, and γ-secretase, both enzymes of the amiloidogenic pathway. An imbalance between the production and clearance of Aβ peptides in the brain, and their aggregation, cause Aβ to accumulate, with subsequent formation of senile plaques. Depending on the site of γ-secretase cleavage, two major forms of Aβ are generated: a peptide of 40 amino acids ($A\beta_{1-40}$), and one of 42 amino acids ($A\beta_{1-42}$). $A\beta_{1-42}$ is the predominant species of Aβ in senile plaques, and the insoluble oligomers and intermediate amyloids are its most neurotoxic forms (Walsh and Selkoe, 2007). Aβ oligomers are hypothesized to cause neuronal damage and cognitive failure by generating free radicals, as well as mitochondrial oxidative damage, synaptic failure, and inflammatory changes in AD brains (Oddo et al., 2003; Mattson, 2004; Reddy and Beal, 2005; Castellani et al., 2010). Different assembly states of Aβ, and its accumulation in different cellular compartments, can then affect critical pathways, thereby facilitating the development of tau pathology. Experimental evidence confirms that Aβ accumulation precedes and drives NFT formation (Götz et al., 2001; Lewis et al., 2001).

Besides aging, which is the most obvious risk factor for the disease, a number of theories point to other risk factors, such as culture, lifestyle, head injury, and genetics. Other risk factors are associated with vascular disease, including hypercholesterolemia, hypertension, atherosclerosis, coronary heart disease, smoking, obesity, and diabetes (Mayeux, 2003). Some evidence suggests that the dietary intake of homocysteine-related vitamins (vitamin B12 and folate), antioxidants (vitamins C and E), unsaturated fatty acids, and also a moderate alcohol intake, especially in the form of wine, may reduce the risk of AD (Luchsinger and Mayeux, 2004).

Although environmental factors increase the risk of AD, this disease can also be caused by various gene mutations (Gatz et al., 2006). In this contest, mutation in the genes *APP*, presenilin 1 (*PSEN1*), and presenilin 2 (*PSEN2*) accounts for most cases of the familial (or early-onset) form of AD, by increasing the production and aggregation of Aβ and amyloid plaque formation (Tanzi and Bertram, 2005). Conversely, the apolipoprotein E (*ApoE*) gene is an important genetic risk factor for the sporadic (or late-onset) form of AD (Raber et al., 2004). The contribution of other candidate genes is probably less important, and none has been verified. A possible explanation for this difficulty in clarifying the genetic background might be that the sporadic form of AD is not a uniform disease entity, and that several susceptibility-enhancing genes may act in concert, each conferring only a small increase in risk, in a complex interaction with environmental factors.

However, although the pathophysiology of AD is still not clearly understood, considerable evidence indicates that many events participate in the development and progression of the disease, including oxidative stress, inflammation, glial cell activation, dysregulation of metal ions and calcium, presence of ApoEε4, altered cholesterol metabolism, and dysregulation of intercellular communication among brain cells (Quintanilla et al., 2012).

Oxidative Stress in AD Pathogenesis

It has been extensively reported that free radicals are pathologically important in neurodegenerative diseases, and that the brain tissue is exposed to oxidative damage during the development of AD, already from its early onset (Smith et al., 2000, 2010; Mariani et al., 2005; Zhu et al., 2005; Reynolds et al., 2007). Because age is a significant risk factor for AD, it is also widely accepted that oxidative stress increases with age leading to the accumulation of oxidative damage in biomolecules (Butterfield and Kanski, 2001; Martin and Grotewiel, 2006; Jacob et al., 2013).

The brain is particularly vulnerable to oxidative damage for numerous reasons, but chiefly because it utilizes about 25% of the respired oxygen, with a consequent increase of free radicals; it also contains high concentrations of catalytic iron and lipids, which are easily oxidized by free radicals. Further, the brain contains relatively low levels of antioxidants and antioxidant defense enzymes, and is thus not very efficient at removing free radicals (Ansari and Scheff, 2010; Mazzetti et al., 2015). Because the brain has a high lipid content, it is extremely vulnerable to oxidative species, with the consequent enhancement of lipid peroxidation and cholesterol oxidation, and the subsequent formation of end products, mainly 4-hydroxynonenal and oxysterols, respectively from the two processes (Sottero et al., 2009; Reed, 2011).

Within the brain, neurons are the cells most vulnerable to excess reactive oxygen species (ROS) and reactive nitrose species (RNS), and their survival depends on the antioxidant action of astrocytes. Astrocytes are very important for normal brain function, because of their ability to actively promote neuroprotection, in particular by releasing glutathione, which protects neurons from oxidative stress (Shih et al., 2003). However, neurons can also defend themselves through an intrinsic mechanism of antioxidant defense involving the glucose metabolism (Fernandez-Fernandez et al., 2012).

AD brains display high levels of oxidative stress, and a direct association between free radical generation and the presence of

Aβ plaques has been shown both in living AD mouse models and in human AD tissue (McLellan et al., 2003). However, it is still not clear whether oxidative stress is a cause or a consequence of the neuropathology associated with AD (Zhu et al., 2007; Bonda et al., 2010; Smith et al., 2010; Luque-Contreras et al., 2014). In support of its being a cause, it has been proposed that oxidative stress precedes the onset of clinical and pathological AD symptoms, including Aβ deposition, NFT formation, vascular malfunction, and cognitive decline (Nunomura et al., 2001; Praticò et al., 2001). In this connection, in a triple-transgenic mouse model of AD, mimicking AD progression in humans, the levels of antioxidants (glutathione and vitamin E) were found to be decreased, and the extent of lipid peroxidation increased, before the appearance of senile plaques and NFT (Resende et al., 2008). Moreover, as a prominent early event, oxidative stress is believed to contribute to tau hyperphosphorylation in neurons (Su et al., 2010) and, of note, it has been observed that neuritic and cored amyloid plaques show evidence of oxidatively modified Aβ (Head et al., 2002). Conversely, Aβ is a potent promoter of oxidative stress, since it is a potent generator of both ROS (Ding et al., 2007) and RNS (Combs et al., 2001). Within the Aβ sequence, it has been suggested that methionine 35 plays an important role in promoting oxidative activity. When this amino acid is replaced by cysteine, the oxidative stress induced by Aβ is greatly attenuated (Butterfield and Boyd-Kimball, 2005; Butterfield et al., 2013). In this connection, it has also been proposed that the amyloid oligomers may insert themselves into the lipid bilayer, causing lipid peroxidation and, consequently, oxidative damage to proteins and other biomolecules (Butterfield et al., 2001). Aβ oligomers are, indeed, the strongest inducers of oxidative stress among all Aβ species (Tamagno et al., 2006; Naylor et al., 2008). Generation of free radicals, altered membrane properties, as well as disturbed calcium homeostasis, may also underlie the apoptotic effect of Aβ oligomers (Malaplate-Armand et al., 2006). It has also been observed, not only in cultured neurons but also *in vivo* using the double transgenic model of AD (APP/PS1), that Aβ causes an increase in oxidative stress that leads to phosphorylation of p38, which in turn phosphorylates tau at its T231 residue (Giraldo et al., 2014).

Mitochondrial dysfunction is another feature of AD pathogenesis (Castellani et al., 2002). Defects in the mitochondria are typically defects of the electron transport chain; these contribute both to the hyperproduction of a variety of ROS, and to the deficiency of several key enzymes responsible for oxidative metabolism that, in turn, cause cell damage and eventual death (Cottrell et al., 2001). Moreover, it has been shown that oxidative species, through mitochondrial impairment, cause tau hyperphosphorylation leading to neuron and synapse loss (Melov et al., 2007). Mitochondrial dysfunction and oxidative damage have been investigated in triple-transgenic mice that develop both Aβ and tau disorders. These mice exhibited increased oxidative stress, manifested by increased hydrogen peroxide production and lipid peroxidation (Yao et al., 2009; Reddy, 2011).

APP and Aβ have also been associated with dysfunctional consequences for mitochondrial homeostasis and cell death (Manczak et al., 2006). APP impairs mitochondrial energy metabolism, thus causing mitochondrial abnormalities leading to ROS production (Anandatheerthavarada et al., 2003); accumulation of APP in the mitochondrial import channel then potentially inhibits mitochondrial import (Reddy et al., 2004). Aβ is also considered a potent mitochondrial poison, especially affecting the synaptic pool. It appears that Aβ enters the mitochondria, induces free radical generation, disrupts the electron transport chain, and ultimately causes mitochondrial dysfunction (Mungarro-Menchaca et al., 2002). Aβ, then, inhibits key mitochondrial enzymes in the brain and in isolated mitochondria (Caspersen et al., 2005; Reddy and Beal, 2008), and cytochrome c oxidase is also specifically attacked (Crouch et al., 2005). A recent study on the transgenic mouse brain confirmed that Aβ accumulates in neuronal mitochondria, thus affecting mitochondrial function, as shown by increased mitochondrial permeability, the decline of both respiratory function and cytochrome c oxidase activity, and increased mitochondrial oxidative stress (Du et al., 2010).

An association between ApoEε4 and oxidative stress-mediated damage in AD has been also suggested. Despite playing a beneficial role, by maintaining lipid homeostasis and redox balance, ApoE can also contribute to oxidative damage in an isoform-dependent manner, the ApoEε4 isoform being the most harmful in AD (Luque-Contreras et al., 2014). The *ApoEε4* genotype is also involved in mitochondrial dysfunction (Chang et al., 2005), and might be a risk for potential antioxidant system loss in AD (Shea et al., 2002).

Alterations in cerebrovascular regulation have recently been ascribed to the early stages of AD, and the vascular endothelium is also a target for oxidative stress leading to endothelium dysfunction (Iadecola, 2004; Park et al., 2008). Chronic hypoperfusion may thus play an important role in the pathophysiology of AD, because it induces oxidative stress, and over time this damage could initiate mitochondrial failure (Sochocka et al., 2013). A recent study has shown that inhibition of NADPH oxidase activity can mitigate cognitive impairment in rodent models of hypoperfusion (Kim et al., 2012). Oxidative stress is intimately associated with neuroinflammation, and there has been found to be a vicious circle connecting oxidative stress and inflammation in AD (Rosales-Corral et al., 2010; Quintanilla et al., 2012; Joshi and Praticò, 2015). It has been observed that the redox status modulates inflammatory factors involvement in signaling processes, which are critical mediators of oxidative stress and inflammation, causing neurodegeneration (Mrak and Griffin, 2005; Kierdorf et al., 2010). Activation of glial cells and increased cytokine production is also induced by oxidative stress and, in turn, glial activation leads to the release of other neurotoxic factors such as ROS and nitric oxide (NO), which further exacerbate neuronal damage (Town et al., 2005; Block et al., 2007; Michelucci et al., 2009; von Bernhardi et al., 2010). Consequently, the resultant cellular damage amplifies the inflammatory response, with glial activation and leukocyte recruitment, leading to further inflammation in the AD brain (**Figure 1**).

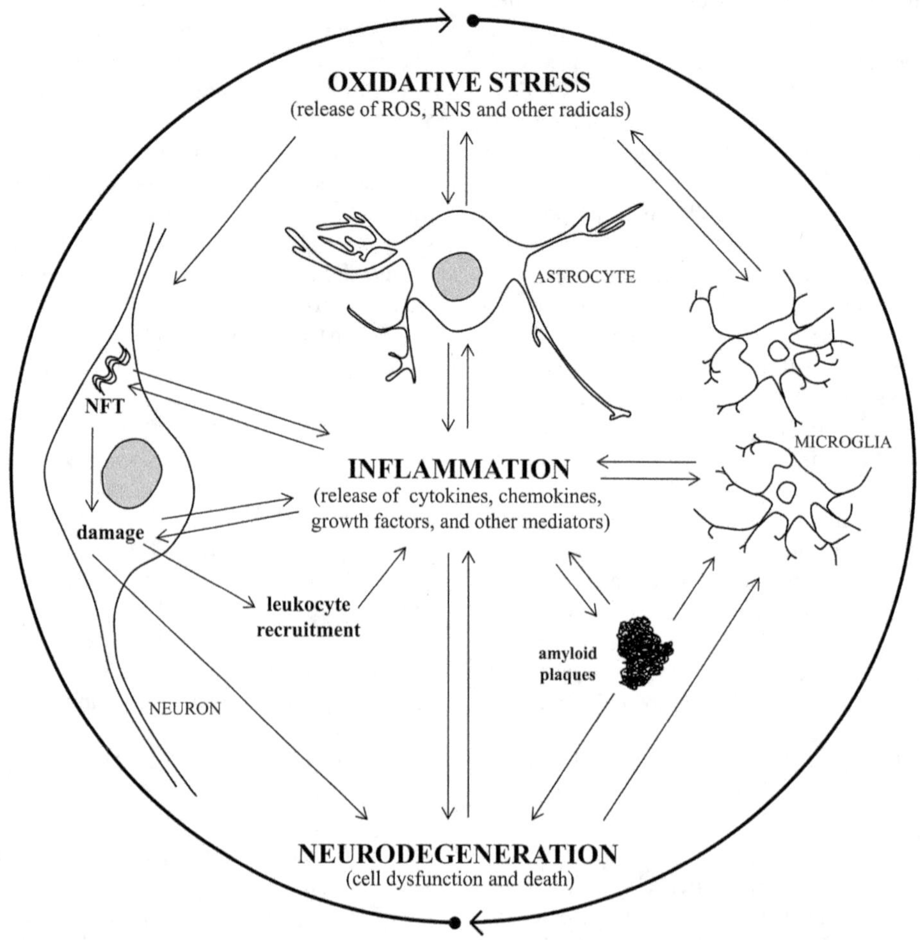

FIGURE 1 | A vicious circle connects oxidative stress, inflammation, and neurodegeneration in Alzheimer's disease (AD). Oxidative stress damage and inflammatory response are closely associated with AD, causing neurodegeneration. Oxidative stress induces activation of microglia and astrocytes with a consequent increase of pro-inflammatory mediator production and, in turn, glial activation leads to toxic radical release, exacerbating neuronal damage. Consequently, the resultant cellular damage amplifies the inflammatory response, with glial activation and leukocyte recruitment, leading to further inflammation in the AD brain. The release of inflammatory cytokines leads to amyloid plaque and neurofibrillary tangle (NFT) formation, that triggers inflammatory molecule release and causes neuronal damage, with consequent neurodegeneration.

Inflammation in AD Pathogenesis

Besides oxidative stress damage, inflammatory responses are also closely associated with AD pathology. Inflammation occurs in pathologically vulnerable regions of the AD brain, with increased expression of acute-phase proteins and pro-inflammatory molecules, which create a chronic and self-sustaining inflammatory process, involving activated glia cells, and stressed neurons (Mrak and Griffin, 2005; Perry et al., 2010; Morales et al., 2014). Thus chronic inflammation plays a basic role in the progression of neuropathological changes in AD, resulting in neuronal dysfunction and death. The importance of neuroinflammation has emerged from several studies of AD brains, which have evidenced the activation and proliferation of glial cells, together with enhanced release of inflammatory mediators (cytokines, chemokines, growth factors, and other mediators) and free-radical-mediated oxidative stress (ROS, NO, and other radicals) (Glass et al., 2010; Heneka et al., 2010; McGeer and McGeer, 2010; Holmes and Butchart, 2011; Azizi and Mirshafiey, 2012; Rubio-Perez and Morillas-Ruiz, 2012; Lyman et al., 2014; Figueiredo-Pereira et al., 2015). Microglia are key players in the disease process, and once activated they present cell-surface antigens commonly present on monocytes and macrophages (Latta et al., 2014). Microglial activation thus leads to the initiation of an innate immune response, dominated by the release of pro-inflammatory cytokines (Town et al., 2005; Mrak, 2012; Weitz and Town, 2012). Incidental to this is also the phagocytosis of fibrils and large aggregates of Aβ, suggesting an initial neuroprotective defense mechanism (D'Andrea et al., 2004; Colton and Wilcock, 2010). Further, microglia can also secrete a number of soluble factors, such as glia-derived neurotrophic factor, which are potentially beneficial to the survival of neurons (Liu and Hong, 2003). Although the initial purpose of microglial activation is to counteract the detrimental effects induced by the pathological features, it subsequently leads to the release of high concentrations of neurotoxic factors, such as inflammatory molecules, NO, ROS, proteolitic enzymes, complementary factors, and excitatory amino acids, which further exacerbate cell damage (Michelucci et al., 2009). Moreover, in later stages of the disease, the overproduction of inflammatory cytokines makes the microglia phagocytically inactive, especially against insoluble oligomers and high concentrations of Aβ (Hickman et al., 2008; Krabbe et al., 2013).

A growing body of evidence also suggests that the central nervous system (CNS) and systemic inflammation cannot be viewed in isolation. Systemic inflammation might exarcerbate behavioral symptoms and accelerate AD progression by increasing the production of local pro-inflammatory cytokines and chemokines, as well as of ROS and NO (Holmes, 2013). The detrimental effects of peripheral inflammatory molecules in the brain of AD patients chiefly occur because these mediators can easily enter the brain, together with infiltrating leukocytes, thanks to increased permeability of the blood-brain barrier (BBB) as the disease progresses (Leoni et al., 2003; Popescu et al., 2009; Takeda et al., 2014). Attention is also now being paid to the participation of Toll-like receptors (TLRs) in inflammation and neurodegeneration. The recruitment of TLRs contributes to inflammation by amplifying the release of inflammatory molecules, thus playing an important role in the impact of inflammation on neuronal function and death (Drouin-Ouellet and Cicchetti, 2012).

However, it also remains unclear in the case of inflammation whether this process is a cause or a consequence of AD. Clinical and experimental studies support the appearance of neuroinflammatory changes already at the early stages of AD, even before the formation of extracellular Aβ deposits and intracellular NFT accumulation (Sheng et al., 2000). The release of pro-inflammatory cytokines and enzymes could affect the normal behavior of neuronal cells, leading to cell dysfunction and abnormalities such as Aβ peptides and NFT accumulation, events in the pathway leading to neuronal degeneration. Inflammatory molecules, and a number of stress conditions, enhance APP levels and the amyloidogenic processing of APP to induce $A\beta_{1-42}$ peptide production. This, in turn, inhibits the formation of the soluble APP fraction that seems to have a neuronal protective effect (Fassbender et al., 2000; Misonou et al., 2000). Conversely, it has been demonstrated that intraneuronal Aβ and soluble Aβ oligomers activate microglia in the earliest stages of AD, even before senile plaque and NFT formation, in particular when cells are stressed (Ferretti and Cuello, 2011; Khandelwal et al., 2011). Moreover, Aβ and NFT have also been shown to trigger the release by activated glia cells of pro-inflammatory mediators, free radicals, and other neurotoxic substances, implying that the development of AD leads to the initiation of several self-propagating cycles (Vukic et al., 2009; Morales et al., 2013). Fibrillar Aβ can also activate microglia by binding to cell membranes via specific receptors, including a multi-receptor complex involving CD36, $\alpha_6\beta_1$-integrin, and CD47 (Verdier et al., 2004; Yu and Ye, 2015), while the disruption of the *APP* gene and of its proteolytic products delays and decreases microglial activation (DeGiorgio et al., 2002). Once activated, microglia may also recruit and activate astrocytes, which actively enhance the inflammatory response to extracellular Aβ deposits (Jo et al., 2014). Aggregated amyloid fibrils and neurotoxic inflammatory molecules, secreted by glial cells, intensify neuronal dysfunction and death, either alone or in concert (Brown and Bal-Price, 2003; Findeis, 2007). In this context, activated glia cells and the released inflammatory molecules, together with other components of the immune response, are often present in proximity to neurons and areas of amyloid plaque (Abbas et al., 2002; Serrano-Pozo et al., 2013). Of note, microglia have also been suggested to be preferentially associated with certain types of amyloid deposits (D'Andrea et al., 2004). Furthermore, astrocytes are known to play a critical role in Aβ clearance, in providing trophic support to neurons, and in forming a protective barrier between Aβ deposits and neurons. The presence of large numbers of astrocytes associated with Aβ plaques suggests that these lesions induce the release of chemotactic molecules that mediate astrocyte recruitment. However, it has been suggested that astrocytes could also be a source for Aβ peptides, because they overexpress BACE1 in response to chronic stress (Roßner et al., 2005; Wang et al., 2011). While Aβ has been widely demonstrated to be pro-inflammatory, the association between microglial activation and tau pathology development is still not supported by direct evidence, since neurofibrillary disorder occurs both in the presence and absence of neuroinflammation (Streit et al., 2014), and intraneuronal NFT lesions usually precede the formation of Aβ aggregates (Braak and Del Tredici, 2004).

Although it has been reported that microglia and astrocytes actively promote disease development, and play pivotal roles in amyloid deposition (Wegiel et al., 2004), conversely it has also been reported that microglia are protective and may remove amyloid deposits, thus having no effect on AD development (Simard et al., 2006; Grathwohl et al., 2009). Moreover, and interestingly, it has been suggested that infiltrating macrophages from the circulation, rather than microglia, play a central role in clearing Aβ deposits in cerebral amyloid angiopathy (Hawkes and McLaurin, 2009), but that these cells can also play a determinant role in AD development (Gate et al., 2010; Rezai-Zadeh et al., 2011).

Of note, while neurons were traditionally believed to be passive bystanders in neuroinflammation, some recent evidence suggests that not only astrocytes and microglia, but also neurons themselves, contribute to the chronic inflammation in AD, by serving as a source of inflammatory molecules (Tchelingerian et al., 1994; Yan et al., 1995; Murphy et al., 1999; Suzuki et al., 1999; Acarin et al., 2000; Heneka and O'Banion, 2007; Rubio-Perez and Morillas-Ruiz, 2012; Ramesh et al., 2013). An increase in pro-inflammatory molecule expression has also been observed in human neuroblastoma SH-SY5Y cells after incubation with some cholesterol oxidation products (known as oxysterols) potentially implicated in AD pathogenesis (Testa et al., 2014).

Brain Cholesterol Metabolism and AD

The human brain contains approximately 25% of the body's cholesterol; this is essential for its normal functioning, being a major component of neuronal cell membranes and an essential factor in membrane fluidity. In the adult brain, cholesterol is mostly present in its non-esterified form; however, small amounts of desmosterol and cholesteryl ester are also present. The brain is separated from the peripheral circulation by the BBB, which prevents the dietary intake of cholesterol being transported from the circulation to the brain, since lipoproteins do not cross the BBB. This means that nearly all the brain cholesterol is synthesized *de novo* within the CNS, from 3-hydroxy-3-methyl-glutaryl-coenzyme A reductase, through a complex series of reactions involving more than 20 enzymes; cholesterol metabolism is, thus, regulated independently of that in the peripheral tissues (Vance et al., 2005; Dietschy, 2009). Because neurons do not efficiently synthesize cholesterol, they rely on astrocytes as an external source. Astrocytes meet neuronal cholesterol demands by secreting ApoE-cholesterol complexes, which are transported to the neurons for their development and function. On note, ApoE transcription is regulated by 24-hydroxycholesterol (24-OH) released by the neurons via the liver X receptor (LXR), this cholesterol oxidation product being one of its natural ligands (Pfrieger, 2003; Nieweg et al., 2009). LXR is a nuclear receptor that regulates the expression of specific genes involved in cholesterol efflux and metabolism, such as ATP-binding cassette transporters A1 and G1 (*ABCA1* and *ABCG1*), and *ApoE* (Sodhi and Singh, 2013).

ApoE is the brain's principal cholesterol-carrier protein; through its receptors it regulates the redistribution and homeostasis of cholesterol within the brain. Humans express three naturally-occurring alleles of the *ApoE* gene: ε2, ε3, and ε4. Murine studies have shown that astrocytes and microglia are the primary ApoE secreting cells in the brain, but neurons can express ApoE under conditions of excitotoxic injury (Xu et al., 2006).

The association between ApoE polymorphism and AD is presumably related to disorders in cholesterol transport. In this connection, it has been found that receptors recognizing ApoE are widely expressed in the brain of AD patients. Of note, AD is accelerated in ApoEε4 individuals: those who are homozygous for the ε4 allelic variant of ApoE have a 50–90% higher chance of developing AD by age 85 years than those carrying ε2 and ε3, showing that this ApoE isoform is one of the major risk factors for AD (Puglielli et al., 2003; Evans et al., 2004; Bu, 2009; Kim et al., 2009a; Martins et al., 2009; Schipper, 2011). However, the mechanisms whereby ApoE isoforms affect the risk of AD are still obscure. One hypothesis is that ApoEε4 protein accelerates the uptake of cholesterol-rich particles by the vasculature, leading to more rapid disease progression: compared to ApoEε4, ApoEε2 and ApoEε3 proteins show reduced receptor binding.

Although ApoE facilitates intracellular Aβ degradation by microglia, reducing intracellular cholesterol levels (Lee et al., 2011) by accelerating its clearance by binding Aβ and forming a stable complex (Sagare et al., 2007; Jiang et al., 2008), ApoE is, conversely, essential for Aβ aggregation and deposition, promoting Aβ fibrillization and plaque formation, as well as tau hyperphosphorylation and NFT formation (Cam and Bu, 2006; Bu, 2009; Marzolo and Bu, 2009). Of note, in the AD-affected brain, ApoE colocalizes with cholesterol and fibrillar Aβ in senile plaques (Burns et al., 2003b). It has also been shown that the *ApoEε4* genotype enhances Aβ production and Aβ fibril formation *in vitro*, as well as in transgenic mice with mutated APP, more than in mice expressing ApoEε3 (Holtzman et al., 2000; Carter et al., 2001; Ye et al., 2005). In addition, ApoEε4 synergizes with Aβ toxicity (Ji et al., 2002). Conversely, a striking reduction in amyloid deposits has been observed in all brain regions of ApoE-null mice (Bales et al., 1999). It has also been suggested that, in AD patients with ApoEε4, a decreased ability to clear Aβ contributes to increasing Aβ accumulation and amyloid plaque formation (Deane et al., 2008). In addition, ApoE may mediate Aβ cell internalization, by binding to the low density lipoprotein receptor-related protein (LRP; Herz and Beffert, 2000). Further, like APP, ApoE also undergoes cleavage, and ApoEε4 is more susceptible to cleavage than is ApoEε3. Fragments of ApoE, such as Aβ, can be toxic, causing AD-like neurotoxicity in mouse models (Harris et al., 2003; Brecht et al., 2004); the lipid-binding region of ApoE is required for this toxicity (Chang et al., 2005).

Accumulating evidence also supports a key role for human ApoE in modulating neuroinflammation (Maezawa et al., 2006c; Keene et al., 2011; Tai et al., 2015). Many studies have reported that ApoEε4 induces a detrimental neuroinflammatory phenotype, both in peripheral and CNS inflammation. *In vitro* data, using microglia isolated from ApoE transgenic mice, has demonstrated *ApoE* genotype-specific modulation of TLR4/lipopolisaccaride (LPS) induced inflammation. In particular, LPS-induced pro-inflammatory cytokines are more strongly expressed in ApoEε4 and ApoEε3 (Maezawa et al., 2006b). Moreover, in microglia treated with LPS/interferon γ, pro-inflammatory cytokine levels were higher, and anti-inflammatory cytokine levels were lower, in ApoEε4 compared to ApoEε3. Unlike what occurs in microglia, in astrocytes TLR4/LPS-induced secretion of pro-inflammatory cytokines follows the pattern: ApoEε2 > ApoEε3 > ApoEε4 via differential nuclear factor-κB (NF-κB) activation (Maezawa et al., 2006a). With regard to ApoE modulation of Aβ-induced neuroinflammation, the available results are scarse. It has been demonstrated that impaired ApoEε4 function modulates the effects induced by Aβ on inflammatory receptor signaling, by amplifying the detrimental pathway TLR4-p38α and suppressing the beneficial pathway interleukin-4R-nuclear receptor (Tai et al., 2015). Importantly, ApoE also modulates BBB function, by a process that may be considered neuroinflammatory. It has been observed that a lack of murine ApoE combined with the expression of ApoEε4, but not of ApoEε2 nor ApoEε3, leads to BBB breakdown by activating the pro-inflammatory pathway cyclophilin A-NF-κB-matrix metalloproteinase 9 in pericytes. Consequently, blood-derived neurotoxic proteins are taken up by neurons, and microvascular and cerebral blood flows are reduced. It has been shown that the vascular defects in ApoE-deficient and ApoEε4-expressing mice precede neuronal dysfunction and can initiate neurodegenerative changes (Bell et al., 2012).

In addition to ApoE, other LXR-responsive genes involved in cholesterol efflux are the *ABCA1* and *ABCG1* (Voloshyna and Reiss, 2011). ABCA1 is reported to be involved in ApoE metabolism and Aβ production, as well as in the modulation of amyloid plaque formation in the CNS (Koldamova et al., 2010; Kim et al., 2011). A close correlation between Aβ and ABCA1 levels has been demonstrated, since, in cultured astrocytes, Aβ inhibits ABCA1 expression (Canepa et al., 2011). In addition, it has also been shown that AD transgenic mice lacking ABCA1 develop increased Aβ levels and senile plaques, in the absence of changes in APP processing (Wahrle et al., 2004). By contrast, in transgenic mice overexpressing ABCA1, the increased ABCA1 function significantly decreases Aβ deposition (Wahrle et al., 2008). Another ABC transporter, ABCA7, has been found to stimulate cellular cholesterol efflux to ApoE-containing particles in the same way as ABCA1 (Chan et al., 2008).

Cholesterol transport and homeostasis are thus closely linked to multiple aspects of Aβ biology, since cholesterol levels influence the production and deposition of the pathogenic Aβ peptides (Burns et al., 2003a; Hughes et al., 2014; Lane-Donovan et al., 2014). Cholesterol has indeed been shown to directly modulate the processing of APP in neuronal cell cultures (Ehehalt et al., 2003), probably by promoting β-secretase activity (Xiong et al., 2008). However, the mechanisms whereby cholesterol affects Aβ production and deposition are still not fully understood. A change in membrane properties and distribution of cholesterol has been suggested as a possible mechanism (Shobab et al., 2005). Cholesterol is mainly concentrated in membrane microdomains termed lipid rafts, which are considered to be the site of the amyloidogenic pathway (Cordy et al., 2006; Vetrivel and Thinakaran, 2010). Further, it has been shown that cellular cholesterol, especially when levels in the membrane are elevated, binds directly to APP at its C terminal transmembrane domain (Harris, 2008; Beel et al., 2010); as a consequence of the binding APP is inserted into the phospholipid monolayers of the lipid rafts and other organelles, where β- and γ-secretases reside (Wahrle et al., 2002; Beel et al., 2010). The amyloidogenic pathway of APP processing is thus linked to cholesterol levels in these microdomains: β- and γ-secretase activities are stimulated by high, and inhibited by low levels of cholesterol (Grimm et al., 2008; Xiong et al., 2008). Conversely, in the non-amyloidogenic pathway, APP is processed by α-secretase in non-raft domains, and this event is promoted by a decreased cellular cholesterol level (Reid et al., 2007). Moreover, α-secretase can be forced to associate with lipid rafts thus inactivating the amyloidogenic pathway (Harris et al., 2009). Of note, it has also been suggested that high levels of non-esterified cholesterol alone might not affect APP processing, while the conversion of free cholesterol to esterified cholesterol might up-regulate APP processing and Aβ generation (Puglielli et al., 2001). Conversely, inhibition of the enzyme acyl-coenzyme A:cholesterol acyl-transferase 1, which esterifies cholesterol, leads to the formation of smaller amounts of cholesteryl esters and Aβ (Bhattacharyya and Kovacs, 2010). These observations suggest that the balance between non-esterified and esterified cholesterol is a fundamental point controlling the amyloidogenic pathway.

It has also been shown that increased cholesterol levels in the lipid bilayers favor Aβ binding to cell membranes (Kakio et al., 2001). Additionally, cholesterol interacts with the peptide as soon as it inserts into the lipid bilayer, and accelerates its recruitment and oligomerization (Fantini and Yahi, 2010). Indeed, cholesterol enhances Aβ to form neurotoxic aggregates (Yanagisawa, 2005), and binds avidly to Aβ protofibrils at level of lipid rafts where fibrillogenesis of these peptides has been proposed to take place (Kakio et al., 2002; Harris, 2008). Conversely, other research has demonstrated that cholesterol decreases the Aβ-induced changes in structure and morphology of lipid rafts, hindering β-sheet formation in membranes, and thereby reducing peptide insertion, aggregation, and cytotoxicity (Arispe and Doh, 2002; Curtain et al., 2003; Qiu et al., 2011).

The effect of Aβ on cholesterol metabolism has also been investigated: Aβ, especially the oligomeric rather than the monomeric form, may alter the intracellular trafficking and homeostasis of cholesterol, by promoting the release from the cells of cholesterol and other lipids, in the form of Aβ-lipid complexes (Michikawa et al., 2001). It has also been reported that Aβ fibrils down-regulate cholesterol metabolism in cultured neurons (Gong et al., 2002). Additionally, the intracellular domain of APP, which is released upon γ-secretase cleavage of APP, may act as a transcriptional suppressor of LRP1, leading to the down-regulation of cellular cholesterol uptake (Liu et al., 2007) and synaptic failure (Koudinov and Koudinova, 2005), as well as enhancement of tau phosphorylation (Fan et al., 2001). It has also been shown that extracellular cholesterol accumulates in the senile plaques of AD patients, and in transgenic mice expressing the Swedish Alzheimer mutation APP751, by binding to aggregated Aβ (Mori et al., 2001).

Given the above considerations, it appears that cholesterol distribution and trafficking within brain cells, rather than the total amount of cholesterol in the neurons, play key roles in APP processing and in the amyloid cascade during AD progression. Conversely, Aβ may affect cellular cholesterol dynamics, such as transport, distribution, and binding, which in turn have a variety of effects on AD-related pathologic changes leading to neurodegeneration.

A number of epidemiological studies also suggest a positive correlation between hypercholesterolemia and susceptibility to AD, in particular in individuals with the *ApoEε4* genotype, which influences cholesterol metabolism, although this relationship is still the subject of considerable controversy (Shobab et al., 2005; Panza et al., 2006; Jenner et al., 2010; Wood et al., 2014; Luckhoff et al., 2015).

Elevated dietary cholesterol has been reported to increase senile plaque formation in numerous animal models. In double transgenic (APP/PS) mice, consumption of a high-cholesterol diet (7 weeks) elevated Aβ deposition in the CNS (Refolo et al., 2000). In addition, in transgenic mice, a typical Western diet (1% cholesterol), increased Aβ accumulation and plaque burden, particularly in the dentate gyrus of the hippocampus (Hooijmans et al., 2007). APP23 mice fed a high-fat/high-cholesterol diet for 4 months showed the AD phenotype. This resulted in significantly worse memory deficits than in the same mice fed with a normal diet (Fitz et al., 2010). Furthermore, studies using New Zealand white rabbits have demonstrated that a diet inducing hypercholesterolemia doubles the Aβ concentration in the hippocampal cortex (Sparks et al., 2000). In addition to increasing Aβ, cholesterol-enriched diets increased tau phosphorylation and oxidative stress in rabbit brains (Ghribi et al., 2006; Jaya Prasanthi et al., 2008). It has also been shown that cholesterol colocalizes with fibrillar Aβ in the amyloid plaques of transgenic mice (Burns et al., 2003b). Conversely, a study on guinea pigs showed that lowering total cholesterol profile by administering statins decreased cerebral Aβ production and accumulation (Fassbender et al., 2001).

Although systemic lipoprotein carrying cholesterol cannot cross the BBB, oxysterols, formed during oxidative stress, can cross the BBB, partly because they may have damaging effects on the BBB's integrity and function (Dias et al., 2014). This consideration supports the idea that oxysterols are the link between hypercholesterolemia and AD.

The Involvement of Oxysterols in AD Pathogenesis

To maintain cholesterol homeostasis in the brain, and because the brain cannot degrade cholesterol, there must be a mechanism to eliminate excess cholesterol, transporting it through the BBB into the systemic circulation, thus preventing its accumulation. The most important such mechanism operates via the conversion of cholesterol to oxysterols. Cholesterol is converted into the relatively polar oxysterol 24-OH, which is produced in the brain almost exclusively by cholesterol 24-hydroxylase (CYP46A1) expressed in neurons, and which, unlike cholesterol itself, diffuses across the BBB into the systemic circulation. To a lesser extent, cholesterol is also converted into 27-OH in the brain by cholesterol 27-hydroxylase (CYP27A1), and then into 7α-hydroxy-3-oxo-4-cholestenoic acid (7-OH-4-C) by the enzyme CYP7B; crossing the BBB, 7-OH-4-C reaches the liver where it is eliminated (Björkhem, 2006; Meaney et al., 2007; Björkhem et al., 2009). However, most 27-OH has been found to flow from the systemic circulation into the brain, since it can cross the BBB; here it acts as an important link between extracerebral and intracerebral pools of cholesterol, and may contribute to the negative effects of hypercholesterolemia in the brain (Heverin et al., 2005; Björkhem, 2006; Sharma et al., 2008). A further oxysterol, 7β-hydroxycholesterol (7β-OH), derives from cholesterol oxidation in the brain, following its interaction with APP and Aβ (Nelson and Alkon, 2005). In addition to those oxysterols, others including 7α-hydroxycholesterol (7α-OH), 4β-hydroxycholestrerol (4β-OH), 5α, 6α- and 5β, 6β-epoxicholesterol (α- and β-EPOX) and 7-ketocholesterol (7-K), have recently been identified post-mortem in human AD brains, and their concentrations compared across the disease states (Hascalovici et al., 2009). Of note, the study authors observed that the levels of potentially amyloidogenic sterol species derived from the auto-oxidation of cholesterol, like β-EPOX, were higher at the mild cognitive impairment disease stage. Oxysterols have also been identified in mouse brains and, in addition to the above cited cholesterol derivatives, consistent levels of 25-hydroxycholesterol (25-OH) were found (Ahonen et al., 2014). Increased levels of 24-OH, 7-K, and β-EPOX have also been detected in areas of the rat hippocampus undergoing gliosis and neuroinflammation, after excitotoxic injury (He et al., 2006; Kim et al., 2010). Further, because oxysterols can cross the BBB, the flux of more than 20 cholesterol metabolites between brain and circulation has very recently been verified in 20 patients. Differences in concentrations, between jugular and forearm veins, of 18 oxysterols, 5 cholestenoic acids and 3 cholenoic acids were measured. The study reported that 24-OH and 7-OH-4-C, of enzymatic origin, but also 6-oxo-5α-hydroxycholesterol, 7β-OH, 7-K, which are formed from cholesterol by ROS, are exported from the brain, while 27-OH is imported into brain (Iuliano et al., 2015). Of these cholesterol metabolites, that exported in the largest quantities is 24-OH. Two other cholesterol metabolites, 7α, 25-dihydroxycholest-4-en-3-one and 7α, (25R)26-hydroxycholest-4-en-3-one, were reported to be exported from the brain (Crick et al., 2015b). Oxysterols and cholestenoic acids have also been identified and quantified in mouse cerebrospinal fluid (CSF), and the findings compared with concentrations of the same metabolites found in the plasma, in order to clarify cholesterol metabolism. Concentrations of oxysterols were lower in the CSF than in the plasma, but 7α, 24-dihydroxycholesterol and 7α, 24-dihydroxycholest-4-en-3-one, both of enzymatic origin, were only identified in the CSF (Crick et al., 2015a). These data clearly demonstrate that there are several routes by which cholesterol metabolites may be exported or imported from the brain (**Figure 2**).

The idea has therefore gained ground that, owing to their ability, unlike cholesterol, to cross the BBB, oxysterols might be the missing link between altered brain cholesterol metabolism and AD pathogenesis, as well as between hypercholesterolemia and AD (Gamba et al., 2012). Although this means that the brain can eliminate excess amounts of oxysterols, it could conversely allow toxic amounts of these compounds, present in the bloodstream, to accumulate in the brain, as in the case of 27-OH. The key role of oxysterols in AD pathogenesis has been strongly supported by the last decade's research, pointing to the involvement of these oxysterols in the amyloid cascade.

To date, although contradictory results could obviously arise from future findings on the other cholesterol metabolites found in the brain, the oxysterols most widely considered to be potentially implicated in the pathogenesis of AD are 24-OH and 27-OH, both of enzymatic origin (Iuliano, 2011; Jeitner et al., 2011; Leoni and Caccia, 2011; Gamba et al., 2012; Hughes et al., 2013; Marwarha and Ghribi, 2014; Noguchi et al., 2014; **Table 1**).

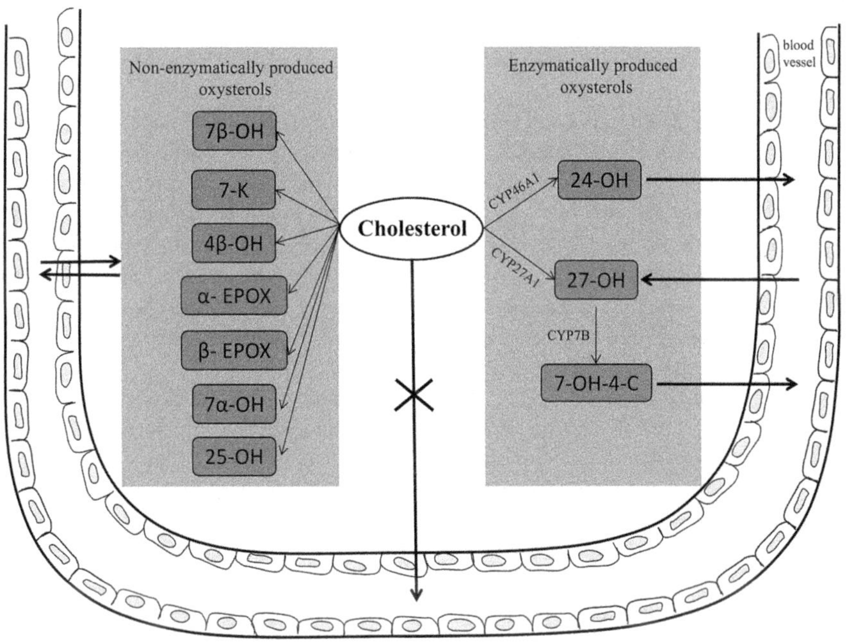

FIGURE 2 | Enzymatically and non-enzymatically produced oxysterols in AD brain and their fluxes across the blood brain barrier (BBB). In neuronal cells, cholesterol is converted into 24-hydroxycholesterol (24-OH) by the enzyme CYP46A1; 24-OH, unlike cholesterol, diffuses across the BBB into the systemic circulation. To a lesser extent, cholesterol is also converted into 27-hydroxycholesterol (27-OH) by the enzyme CYP27A1, and then into 7α-hydroxy-3-oxo-4-cholestenoic acid (7-OH-4-C) by the enzyme CYP7B; crossing the BBB, 7-OH-4-C reaches the liver where it is eliminated. However, most 27-OH flows from the circulation into the brain, since it can cross the BBB. In addition, other oxysterols, such as 7β-hydroxycholesterol (7β-OH), 7-ketocholesterol (7-K), 7α-hydroxycholesterol (7α-OH), 4β-hydroxycholestrerol (4β-OH), 5α, 6α- and 5β, 6β-epoxicholesterol (α- and β-EPOX), and 25-hydroxycholesterol (25-OH), have been found in AD brain deriving from brain cholesterol autoxidation. Potentially these oxysterols, as well as other cholesterol metabolites, can cross the BBB.

TABLE 1 | 24-hydroxycholesterol and 27-hydroxycholesterol levels in Alzheimer's disease patients compared with healthy controls.

Oxysterol	Levels of oxysterol in AD subjects compared with control subjects	Reference
24-hydroxycholesterol	↓ Brain levels	Heverin et al. (2004)
	↑ CSF levels	Papassotiropoulos et al. (2002), Schönknecht et al. (2002) and Leoni et al. (2004)
	↓ Plasma levels	Bretillon et al. (2000) and Kölsch et al. (2004)
	↑ Plasma levels	Lütjohann et al. (2000)
	= Plasma levels	Iuliano et al. (2010)
27-hydroxycholesterol	↑ Brain levels	Heverin et al. (2004) and Shafaati et al. (2011)
	↑ CSF levels	Leoni et al. (2004)
	↓ Plasma levels	Kölsch et al. (2004)
	= Plasma levels	Iuliano et al. (2010)

CSF, cerebrospinal fluid.

Higher levels of 24-OH than in unaffected individuals have been found in the peripheral circulation and CSF of early-stage AD patients, suggesting that cholesterol turnover in the brain increases during the neurodegenerative changes of AD (Lütjohann et al., 2000; Papassotiropoulos et al., 2002; Kölsch et al., 2004). Conversely, plasma levels of 24-OH were lower in patients with later stages of AD than in unaffected individuals, suggesting that the rate of cholesterol transport slows as the disease progresses (Bretillon et al., 2000; Kölsch et al., 2004). These apparently contradictory results may be rationalized by considering that increased plasma levels of 24-OH reflect ongoing neurodegeneration and/or demyelinization, whereas decreased plasma levels in later stages reflect a selective loss of neuronal cells expressing the enzyme CYP46A1 (Björkhem and Meaney, 2004). The decrease of 24-OH in the AD brain may also be the result of an increase in total free cholesterol (likely derived from cell membrane collapse and widespread myelin release) that exceeds the brain's capacity to convert it to 24-OH (Vaya and Schipper, 2007). However, it has been observed that, in glial cells, and especially around senile plaques, there is an ectopic induction of CYP46A1, leading to some 24-OH production, but without compensating for the decrease of that oxysterol (Bogdanovic et al., 2001; Brown et al., 2004). Another study, however, has found that plasma levels of 24-OH and 27-OH in AD patients are not significantly different from control values (Iuliano et al., 2010). A small fraction of total 24-OH excretion occurs via the CSF, and the 24-OH concentration is increased in the CSF of AD patients, probably reflecting neuronal damage and loss rather then metabolically active neuronal cells (Schönknecht et al., 2002; Leoni et al., 2004).

It has also been reported that, in critical areas of post-mortem AD brains, as well as in aged mice expressing the Swedish Alzheimer mutation APP751, 24-OH levels are decreased and those of 27-OH increased (Heverin et al., 2004). Increased levels of 27-OH were also found in the brains of patients carrying the Swedish APP670/671 mutation (Shafaati et al., 2011). As a consequence of neuron loss, expression of CYP27A1 may also be reduced; however, 27-OH levels remain elevated because CYP27A1 is also expressed in astrocytes and oligodendrocytes, leading to *in situ* generation of 27-OH (Brown et al., 2004). Accumulation of 27-OH in the brain is also due to the increased flux of this oxysterol across the BBB, because of either hypercholesterolemia associated to oxidative stress (Björkhem, 2006), or damaged BBB integrity (Leoni et al., 2003). There is a positive correlation between levels of cholesterol and those of 27-OH in the circulation, and the high flux of 27-OH from the peripheral circulation into the brain suggests that this oxysterol may be the link between hypercholesterolemia and AD. An alternative explanation for the accumulation of 27-OH is reduced activity of CYP7B, the neuronal enzyme responsible for 27-OH metabolism; this reduction arises from the reduced CYP7B expression in the brain of AD patients, because of neuron loss (Yau et al., 2003). Moreover, high CSF levels of 27-OH were found in mild cognitive impairment and AD patients (Leoni et al., 2004).

From these considerations, it is clear that the balance between 24-OH and 27-OH levels is important. Oxysterol homeostasis in the brain is tightly regulated, specific levels being maintained in various brain regions. For example, the 27-OH:24-OH ratio is ~1:8 in the frontal cortex, 1:5 in the occipital cortex, and 1:10 in the basal ganglia, and the increased ratio of 27-OH to 24-OH in AD brains is consistent with AD pathogenesis. Thus it is likely that reduced levels of 24-OH may accelerate disease progression, and that the increased levels of 27-OH may be insufficient to compensate for this: the shift in balance between the two oxysterols might lead to increased generation and accumulation of Aβ with consequent neurodegeneration (Heverin et al., 2004; Björkhem, 2006; Björkhem et al., 2009). In a retrospective study on cardiovascular patients with evidence of cerebrovascular disease, higher plasma levels of 24-OH and a higher 24-OH/27-OH ratio were found to be associated with the development of incidental cognitive impairment over 8 years of follow-up (Hughes et al., 2012). However, opinions still differ about the involvement of 24-OH and 27-OH in APP processing and Aβ production.

To date, the conversion of cholesterol into 24-OH, by inducing CYP46A1 activity, has been considered to exert a protective action on the brain, mainly by regulating cholesterol homeostasis and favoring the efflux of its excess from the brain to the blood, but also by preventing Aβ generation (Björkhem et al., 2009). Astrocytes are sensitive to levels of 24-OH, which regulates the expression of LXR-responsive genes involved in cholesterol homeostasis (i.e., *ABCA1*, *ABCG1* and *ApoE*) (Abildayeva et al., 2006). Indeed, 24-OH acts as an endogenous ligand of LXR. Conversely, it has been reported that brain accumulation of 27-OH antagonizes the preventive effect of 24-OH on generation of Aβ and that it is potentially toxic (Shafaati et al., 2011). Since the flux of 27-OH across the BBB increases under conditions of hypercholesterolemia (Björkhem, 2006), or in the case of increased BBB permeability (Leoni et al., 2003), the inhibitory effect of 24-OH on Aβ generation would consequently be reduced.

Studies on human neuroblastoma cells and on brain tissues have somewhat clarified the different effects of 24-OH and 27-OH on APP levels and processing: 24-OH may favor the non-amyloidogenic pathway, with consequent inhibition of Aβ formation, whereas 27-OH is thought to stimulate the amyloidogenic pathway, with production of Aβ as well as tau hyperphosphorylation (Bu, 2009; Prasanthi et al., 2009; Marwarha et al., 2010). However, the mechanisms underlying their different effects are still unclear.

In human SH-SY5Y neuroblastoma cells, 24-OH appears to exert a unique modulatory effect on APP processing: it directly increases α-secretase activity, as well as elevating the α/β-secretase activity ratio; conversely, 27-OH enhances the generation of Aβ (Famer et al., 2007). *In vitro* experiments suggest that 24-OH reduces Aβ production, by down-regulating APP trafficking via enhancement of the complex formation of APP, also up-regulating glucose-regulated protein 78 in the endoplasmic reticulum. The inhibitory effect of 24-OH was reduced in glucose-regulated protein 78 knockdowned cells (Urano et al., 2013). In rat primary cortical neurons, both 24-OH and 27-OH were found to be inhibitors of Aβ secretion, 24-OH being approximately 1000 times more potent than 27-OH (Brown et al., 2004). SH-SY5Y cells incubated with 27-OH release higher levels of $A\beta_{1-42}$ and APP as well as of BACE1. Conversely, cells incubated with 24-OH do not release increased $A\beta_{1-42}$ levels, and are associated with increased levels of sAPPα, suggesting that 24-OH favors APP processing via the non-amyloidogenic pathway (Prasanthi et al., 2009). Another study, on hippocampal slices from adult rabbits, found that 27-OH increases Aβ accumulation by reducing levels of insulin-like growth factor 1, a neurotrophic factor that promotes neurogenesis and has a neuroprotective effect (Sharma et al., 2008). This oxysterol has also been found to increase both BACE1 and Aβ levels in retinal pigment epithelial cells (Dasari et al., 2010). In neuronal SK-N-BE cells, 24-OH and 27-OH have both been shown to enhance expression and activity of the β-secretase of the amyloidogenic pathway of APP processing, leading to increased Aβ generation and accumulation in those cells (Gamba et al., 2014; **Table 2**).

24-OH has also been reported to be neurotoxic, but this effect may depend on its concentration. It has been demonstrated that high concentrations of 24-OH (25–50 μM) caused cell death when added to undifferentiated or differentiated SH-SY5Y cells: the effect was mediated by increased generation of

TABLE 2 | Effects of 24-hydroxycholesterol and 27-hydroxycholesterol on the amyloidogenic pathway.

Oxysterol	Dosage	Effects	Experimental model	Reference
24-hydroxycholesterol	C = 10 μM	↓ Aβ production	Primary culture of rat cortical neurons	Brown et al. (2004)
	C = 5 μM	↑ α-secretase activity ↓ β-secretase activity	Undifferentiated human neuroblastoma cell line SH-SY5Y	Famer et al. (2007)
	C = 10 μM	↑ α-secretase activity no effect on APP, BACE1 and Aβ level	Undifferentiated human neuroblastoma cell line SH-SY5Y	Prasanthi et al. (2009)
	C = 1–10 μM	↑ APP level ↓ Aβ production no effect on β-secretase activity	Undifferentiated SH-SY5Y cells and Chinese hamster ovary (CHO) cells	Urano et al. (2013)
	C = 1 μM	↑ APP level and Aβ production ↑ α-secretase level ↑ β-secretase level and activity	Differentiated human neuroblastoma cell line SK-N-BE	Gamba et al. (2014)
27-hydroxycholesterol	C = 1–15 μM	↓ Aβ production	Primary culture of rat cortical neurons	Brown et al. (2004)
	C = 5 μM	No effect on α- and β-secretase activity	Undifferentiated human neuroblastoma cell line SH-SY5Y	Famer et al. (2007)
	C = 10 μM	↑ Aβ production ↑ APP and BACE1 level	Undifferentiated human neuroblastoma cell line SH-SY5Y	Prasanthi et al. (2009)
	C = 10–25 μM	↑ Aβ production ↑ BACE1 level	Retinal pigmented epithelial cells ARPE-19	Dasari et al. (2010)
	C = 5 μM	↑ Aβ production ↑ BACE1 level and activity	Undifferentiated human neuroblastoma cell line SH-SY5Y	Marwarha et al. (2013)
	C = 1 μM	↑ APP level and Aβ production ↑ α-secretase level ↑ β- and γ-secretase level and activity	Differentiated human neuroblastoma cell line SK-N-BE	Gamba et al. (2014)

Aβ, amyloid β; APP, amyloid precursor protein; BACE1, beta-site amyloid precursor protein cleaving enzyme 1.

free radicals (Kölsch et al., 2001). High concentrations of 24-OH (50 μM) also induce necroptosis, a form of programmed necrosis in neuronal SH-SY5Y cells (Yamanaka et al., 2011). In contrast, pretreatment of human neuroblastoma SH-SY5Y cells with sub-lethal concentrations of 24-OH induces adaptive responses, and protects the cells against subsequent cytotoxic stress induced by 7-K treatment, via transcriptional activation of the LXR signaling pathway. The cytoprotective effects of 24-OH disappeared in LXRβ-knockdowned cells, suggesting that this nuclear receptor may play a key role in the 24-OH-induced adaptive response. Adaptive responses are also induced by other oxysterols, such as 25-OH and 27-OH, both ligands of LXR, similarly to 24-OH (Okabe et al., 2013). However, in our recent studies, a very low concentration (1 μM) of 24-OH was found to markedly potentiate both the apoptotic and the necrogenic effects exerted by the $A\beta_{1-42}$ peptide, on two human differentiated neuronal cell lines (SK-N-BE and NT-2) (Gamba et al., 2011), but also on human dental pulp progenitor cells differentiated into neuron-like cells (Testa et al., 2012). 24-OH appeared to interact with $A\beta_{1-42}$ by strongly increasing intracellular ROS steady-state levels, an action not exerted by either 27-OH or 7β-OH (Gamba et al., 2011). This evidence supports the opinion that Aβ must form oligomers in order to induce neurotoxicity, and that the latter process is probably enhanced by redox imbalance. Additionally, 50 μM 24-OH has been shown to enhance the neurotoxic effect of the $A\beta_{1-42}$ peptide in the human differentiated neuroblastoma cell line MSN, as well as augmenting ROS generation (Ferrera et al., 2008). Although in many of the various *in vitro* tests performed in our laboratory, 27-OH (1 μM) did not display neurotoxicity, in terms of necrosis and apoptosis (Gamba et al., 2011), conversely, the toxicity of 27-OH (5–20 μM) has been demonstrated in astrocyte cells (C6 cells). This oxysterol increased ROS levels and decreased antioxidant defense system levels, with consequent decrease of cell viability. In addition, 27-OH down-regulated the expression of the nuclear factor E2-related factor 2 signaling pathway (Ma et al., 2015).

It is known that hypertension is a risk factor for AD, and that angiotensin converting enzyme activity is increased in AD brains. In this connection, it has been suggested that 27-OH might up-regulate the renin-angiotensin system in AD brains. A positive correlation between angiotensin converting enzyme activity in the CSF, and both plasma and CSF levels of 27-OH, has been shown, as well as an increased production of angiotensinogen in rat primary neurons, astrocytes, and human neuroblastoma cells treated with 27-OH (Mateos et al., 2011).

Moreover, 7β-OH has been found to be neurotoxic at very low concentrations on cultured rat hippocampal neuronal cells, and may therefore contribute to neurodegeneration in AD brains. In the same study, it has also been shown that Aβ can oxidize cholesterol to form 7β-OH in a highly efficient mechanism and more actively than APP. Oxidation of cholesterol was accompanied by hydrogen peroxide production, suggesting that Aβ could contribute to the oxidative damage observed in AD (Nelson and Alkon, 2005). 7β-OH causes re-arrangement of the liquid-ordered phase which results in the formation of lipid rafts (Wang et al., 2008; Mitomo et al., 2009); it is also a potent inhibitor of α protein kinase C, an enzyme critical for memory consolidation and synaptic plasticity that is implicated in AD (Nelson and Alkon, 2005). Another oxysterol that might derive from the autoxidation of cellular cholesterol released during neurodegeneration is 7α-OH, which appeared to be responsible for SH-SY5Y cell death (Kölsch et al., 2000); a further possibility is 7-K. 7-K has been shown to enhance mitochondrial dysfunction in the neuronal PC12 cell line, leading to cell death (Kim et al., 2006; Kim and Lee, 2010; Jang and Lee, 2011). It has also been reported that incorporation of 7-K to lipid raft domains of plasma membranes triggers apoptotic signaling; α-tochopherol (vitamin E) reduces the cytotoxicity of 7-K by inhibiting its distribution to the lipid raft domains (Berthier et al., 2004; Royer et al., 2009). It has recently been suggested that 25-OH is an important regulator of cholesterol metabolism, as well as of humoral immunity (Diczfalusy, 2013; Waltl et al., 2013). Of note, it has also been hypothesized that Aβ deposition is not a central event in AD, but rather is subservient to 25-OH. Confirming this hypothesis, it has been observed that, in a large cohort of AD patients, specific *25-hydroxylase* haplotypes were associated with a complete absence of Aβ deposits in the brain, despite all other aspects of AD pathology being present (Papassotiropoulos et al., 2005). This suggests that neuroinflammation and 25-hydroxylase activation precede Aβ generation in the sequence of events leading to the disease. An interesting study on different immortalized, tumoral and normal cells of the CNS has found that oxysterols oxidized at C4, such as 4α-OH and 4β-OH, have no effect on cell viability and almost no effect on cell growth; conversely, oxysterols oxidized at C7, such as 7-K, 7α-OH, and 7β-OH, inhibit cell growth and decrease viability through their cytotoxic activity. These data suggest that 4α-OH and 4β-OH, the only oxysterols identified as having cytostatic properties, may be of some interest for attempts to counteract cell proliferation (Nury et al., 2013).

Oxysterols have also been shown to modify specific sites of the Aβ peptide thus enhancing Aβ aggregation and its neurotoxicity. Following Aβ modification at Lys-16, peptide aggregates were formed faster than in the case of modification at Lys-28 or at Asp-1 (Usui et al., 2009).

Further, evidence has emerged that Aβ has predominant cholesterol oxidase activity, particularly in the presence of divalent cations such as Cu^{2+}. Significantly elevated levels of 4-cholesten-3-one were reported in brains of Aβ transgenic mice and in brain tissue of AD patients (Puglielli et al., 2005; Yoshimoto et al., 2005).

The interaction of Aβ with cell membranes is the crucial event in AD pathogenesis. Of note, there is less evidence to date on the negative effects of oxysterols on Aβ binding to the cell membranes. Because the orientation of oxysterols in the cell membrane differs from that of cholesterol, they are less able to condense lipids, thus modifying some physical properties of membrane, including raft domains; it has thus been suggested that oxysterols may facilitate Aβ interaction with cell membranes. The effects of 7-K and 7β-OH on enhancing Aβ insertion into the lipid bilayer, by decreasing intermolecular cohesive interaction, have been demonstrated (Kim and Frangos, 2008). Using a model membrane, it was shown that 25-OH and 7-K render the membrane more sensitive to Aβ, in contrast to the role played by cholesterol, which inhibits Aβ's interaction with membranes. 7-K facilitated Aβ's localization in the membrane, while 25-OH stimulated the peptide's insertion but lead to membrane modification. In addition, the higher potential of $A\beta_{1-42}$, compared to $A\beta_{1-40}$, to interact with the membrane has also been demonstrated (Phan et al., 2013). Further, it is hypothesized that increased oxysterol concentrations, mainly of 7-K, but also of 24-OH and β-EPOX, may enhance exocytosis and neurotransmitter release in damaged areas of the brain, thereby aggravating neuronal excitotoxicity (Ma et al., 2010). Further, in our study we observed that 24-OH, 27-OH, and 7β-OH markedly enhanced the binding of $A\beta_{1-42}$ on membranes of human differentiated neuronal cell lines (SK-N-BE and NT-2), by up-regulating CD36 and β1-integrin receptors (Gamba et al., 2011), two components of the multireceptor complex CD36/β1-integrin/CD47, through which Aβ peptide binds to cell membranes (Verdier et al., 2004; Yu and Ye, 2015). This event might favor the accumulation of the toxic $A\beta_{1-42}$ peptide into neurons.

Although oxysterols have been analyzed for their involvement in neurotoxicity and Aβ production during AD progression, their role as natural ligands for LXR is now emerging (e.g., 24-OH, 27-OH, 22-OH, 25-OH, 4β-OH, and 7α-OH) (Vaya and Schipper, 2007). Indeed, astrocytes are sensitive to 24-OH-mediated up-regulation of ApoE, a LXR-target gene involved in cholesterol efflux (Abildayeva et al., 2006). Moreover, it has been reported that 27-OH prevents Aβ generation from primary human neurons, not by modulating α-, β-, or γ-secretase, but rather by overexpressing LXR-responsive genes (*ABCA1*, *ABCG1* and *ApoE*) (Kim et al., 2009b). Moreover, incubation of primary brain cells with 22-OH significantly reduced Aβ secretion in a dose-dependent manner, while ABCA1 expression and cholesterol efflux were induced (Koldamova et al., 2003).

Recent *in vitro* evidence also suggests that 24-OH and 27-OH might contribute to decreasing the influx of Aβ peptide into the brain across the BBB, increasing expression of the ABCB1 transporter in brain capillary endothelial cells, resulting in protection from peripheral Aβ entry (Saint-Pol et al., 2013). Of note, ABCB1 has never been described as an LXR target gene, and other nuclear receptors might control its transcription. Conversely, treatment of brain pericytes with 24-OH up-regulated ABCA1 expression that was correlated with an increase of cholesterol efflux, whereas 24-OH treatment did not reduce the pericytes' ability to accumulate Aβ in the cells (Saint-Pol et al., 2012). The clearance of Aβ might also be mediated through microglia-induced phagocytosis of Aβ, which depends on LXR activation (Terwel et al., 2011).

Of note, LXR activation not only regulates cholesterol homeostasis, and Aβ peptide transport and clearance, but also neuroinflammation. Studies have shown that LXR activation inhibits inflammatory gene expression, pointing to the ability of LXRs to inactivate promoters of pro-inflammatory genes

(Wang et al., 2002; Cao et al., 2007; Zelcer et al., 2007; Sodhi and Singh, 2013; Steffensen et al., 2013). Moreover, LXR activation may prevent neuroinflammation, by indirectly down-regulating TLR target genes. However, although LXR-activating oxysterols might reduce membrane cholesterol content and inflammation, they may also activate opposing pathways, and induce inflammation independently of LXRs. In our very recent study, we observed that 27-OH, 24-OH, and 7β-OH enhanced inflammatory molecule expression in human neuroblastoma SH-SY5Y cells via TLR4/cyclooxygenase-2/membrane bound prostaglandin E synthase; this clearly indicates that oxysterols may promote neuroinflammation in AD (Testa et al., 2014).

Although it can be assumed that oxysterols may increase the activation of microglia promoting their phagocytosis, there is less evidence to date on their effects on microglial phagocytosis during neuroninflammation. The phagocytosis of fibrils and large aggregates of Aβ by microglia is an important neuroprotective mechanism for Aβ peptide clearance (D'Andrea et al., 2004; Colton and Wilcock, 2010) but, in later stages of AD, the increased inflammatory molecule release makes the microglia phagocytically inactive leading to neuronal death (Hickman et al., 2008; Krabbe et al., 2013). Among the receptors promoting Aβ phagocytosis and clearance by microglia, the CD36 scavenger receptor appears to be involved and its increased expression may be crucial in preventing AD (Verdier et al., 2004; Yu and Ye, 2015): CD36 initiates a signaling cascade that promotes microglial activation and recruitment to β-amyloid deposits in the brain (Stuart et al., 2007). Concernig sterols, it has been shown that cholesterol (20 μM) and α-EPOX (20 μM) do not interfere with CD36 membrane distribution but both compounds were found to up-regulate the total CD36 levels in the mouse microglial cell line BV-2 potentiating phagocytosis in LPS-stimulated cells (Račková, 2013). Moreover, treatment with methyl-β-cyclodextrin, a reagent able to remove cholesterol from cell membranes, inhibited phagocytosis in LPS-activated microglia, indirectly supporting the potential role of sterols in phagocytosis (Churchward and Todd, 2014).

Conclusion

This review has pointed up the vicious circle connecting oxidative stress and inflammation in AD. Alongside oxidative stress and neuroinflammation, altered cholesterol metabolism in the brain and hypercholesterolemia also significantly contribute to AD pathogenesis. Thanks to consistent research evidence, it is now believed that oxidized cholesterol is the driving force behind the development of AD and that oxysterols are the link connecting altered cholesterol metabolism and hypercholesterolemia to this neurodegenerative disease. Oxysterols play a fundamental role, by enhancing inflammation, Aβ generation and accumulation, and neuron death.

The involvement of oxysterols in AD pathogenesis, and the analysis of such products in the plasma and CSF, may contribute to clarifying the role of cholesterol metabolism in AD; ultimately, it may be helpful in developing therapeutic strategies to prevent or slow AD pathogenesis.

Acknowledgments

This work was supported by the CRT Foundation (Turin) and the University of Turin (Italy).

References

Abbas, N., Bednar, I., Mix, E., Marie, S., Paterson, D., Ljungberg, A., et al. (2002). Up-regulation of the inflammatory cytokines IFN-gamma and IL-12 and down-regulation of IL-4 in cerebral cortex regions of APP(SWE) transgenic mice. *J. Neuroimmunol.* 126, 50–57. doi: 10.1016/s0165-5728(02)00050-4

Abildayeva, K., Jansen, P. J., Hirsch-Reinshagen, V., Bloks, V. W., Bakker, A. H., Ramaekers, F. C., et al. (2006). 24(S)-hydroxycholesterol participates in a liver X receptor-controlled pathway in astrocytes that regulates apolipoprotein E-mediated cholesterol efflux. *J. Biol. Chem.* 281, 12799–12808. doi: 10.1074/jbc.m601019200

Acarin, L., González, B., and Castellano, B. (2000). Neuronal, astroglial and microglial cytokine expression after an excitotoxic lesion in the immature rat brain. *Eur. J. Neurosci.* 12, 3505–3520. doi: 10.1046/j.1460-9568.2000.00226.x

Ahonen, L., Maire, F. B., Savolainen, M., Kopra, J., Vreeken, R. J., Hankemeier, T., et al. (2014). Analysis of oxysterols and vitamin D metabolites in mouse brain and cell line samples by ultra-high-performance liquid chromatography-atmospheric pressure photoionization-mass spectrometry. *J. Chromatogr. A.* 1364, 214–222. doi: 10.1016/j.chroma.2014.08.088

Anandatheerthavarada, H. K., Biswas, G., Robin, M. A., and Avadhani, N. G. (2003). Mitochondrial targeting and a novel transmembrane arrest of Alzheimer's amyloid precursor protein impairs mitochondrial function in neuronal cells. *J. Cell. Biol.* 161, 41–54. doi: 10.1083/jcb.200207030

Ansari, M. A., and Scheff, S. W. (2010). Oxidative stress in the progression of Alzheimer disease in the frontal cortex. *J. Neuropathol. Exp. Neurol.* 69, 155–167. doi: 10.1097/NEN.0b013e3181cb5af4

Arispe, N., and Doh, M. (2002). Plasma membrane cholesterol controls the cytotoxicity of Alzheimer's disease AbetaP (1-40) and (1-42) peptides. *FASEB J.* 16, 1526–1536. doi: 10.1096/fj.02-0829com

Azizi, G., and Mirshafiey, A. (2012). The potential role of proinflammatory and antiinflammatory cytokines in Alzheimer disease pathogenesis. *Immunopharmacol. Immunotoxicol.* 34, 881–895. doi: 10.3109/08923973.2012.705292

Bales, K. R., Verina, T., Cummins, D. J., Du, Y., Dodel, R. C., Saura, J., et al. (1999). Apolipoprotein E is essential for amyloid deposition in the APP (V717F) transgenic mouse model of Alzheimer's disease. *Proc. Natl. Acad. Sci. U S A* 96, 15233–15238. doi: 10.1073/pnas.96.26.15233

Beel, A. J., Sakakura, M., Barrett, P. J., and Sanders, C. R. (2010). Direct binding of cholesterol to the amyloid precursor protein: An important interaction in lipid-Alzheimer's disease relationships? *Biochim Biophys. Acta* 1801, 975–982. doi: 10.1016/j.bbalip.2010.03.008

Bell, R. D., Winkler, E. A., Singh, I., Sagare, A. P., Deane, R., Wu, Z., et al. (2012). Apolipoprotein E controls cerebrovascular integrity via cyclophilin A. *Nature* 485, 512–516. doi: 10.1038/nature11087

Berthier, A., Lemaire-Ewing, S., Prunet, C., Monier, S., Athias, A., Bessède, G., et al. (2004). Involvement of a calcium-dependent dephosphorylation of BAD associated with the localization of Trpc-1 within lipid rafts in 7-ketocholesterol-induced THP-1 cell apoptosis. *Cell Death Differ.* 11, 897–905. doi: 10.1038/sj.cdd.4401434

Bhattacharyya, R., and Kovacs, D. M. (2010). ACAT inhibition and amyloid beta reduction. *Biochim. Biophys. Acta* 1801, 960–965. doi: 10.1016/j.bbalip.2010.04.003

Björkhem, I. (2006). Crossing the barrier: oxysterols as cholesterol transporters and metabolic modulators in the brain. *J. Intern. Med.* 260, 493–508. doi: 10.1111/j.1365-2796.2006.01725.x

Björkhem, I., and Meaney, S. (2004). Brain cholesterol: long secret life behind a barrier. *Arterioscler. Thromb. Vasc. Biol.* 24, 806–815. doi: 10.1161/01.atv.0000120374.59826.1b

Björkhem, I., Cedazo-Minguez, A., Leoni, V., and Meaney, S. (2009). Oxysterols and neurodegenerative diseases. *Mol. Aspects Med.* 30, 171–179. doi: 10.1016/j.mam.2009.02.001

Block, M. L., Zecca, L., and Hong, J. S. (2007). Microglia-mediated neurotoxicity: uncovering the molecular mechanisms. *Nat. Rev. Neurosci.* 8, 57–69. doi: 10.1038/nrn2038

Bogdanovic, N., Bretillon, L., Lund, E. G., Diczfalusy, U., Lannfelt, L., Winblad, B., et al. (2001). On the turnover of brain cholesterol in patients with Alzheimer's disease. Abnormal induction of the cholesterol-catabolic enzyme CYP46 in glial cells. *Neurosci. Lett.* 314, 45–48. doi: 10.1016/s0304-3940(01)02277-7

Bonda, D. J., Wang, X., Perry, G., Nunomura, A., Tabaton, M., Zhu, X., et al. (2010). Oxidative stress in Alzheimer disease: a possibility for prevention. *Neuropharmacology* 59, 290–294. doi: 10.1016/j.neuropharm.2010.04.005

Brecht, W. J., Harris, F. M., Chang, S., Tesseur, I., Yu, G. Q., Xu, Q., et al. (2004). Neuron-specific apolipoprotein e4 proteolysis is associated with increased tau phosphorylation in brains of transgenic mice. *J. Neurosci.* 24, 2527–2534. doi: 10.1523/jneurosci.4315-03.2004

Bretillon, L., Sidén, A., Wahlund, L. O., Lütjohann, D., Minthon, L., Crisby, M., et al. (2000). Plasma levels of 24S-hydroxycholesterol in patients with neurological diseases. *Neurosci. Lett.* 293, 87–90. doi: 10.1016/s0304-3940(00)01466-x

Brown, G. C., and Bal-Price, A. (2003). Inflammatory neurodegeneration mediated by nitric oxide, glutamate and mitochondria. *Mol. Neurobiol.* 27, 325–355. doi: 10.1385/mn:27:3:325

Brown, J. 3rd, Theisler, C., Silberman, S., Magnuson, D., Gottardi-Littell, N., Lee, J. M., et al. (2004). Differential expression of cholesterol hydroxylases in Alzheimer's disease. *J. Biol. Chem.* 279, 34674–34681. doi: 10.1074/jbc.m402324200

Braak, H., and Del Tredici, K. (2004). Alzheimer's disease: intraneuronal alterations precede insoluble amyloid-beta formation. *Neurobiol. Aging* 25, 713–718. doi: 10.1016/j.neurobiolaging.2003.12.015

Bu, G. (2009). Apolipoprotein E and its receptors in Alzheimer's disease: pathways, pathogenesis and therapy. *Nat. Rev. Neurosci.* 10, 333–344. doi: 10.1038/nrn2620

Burns, M. P., Noble, W. J., Olm, V., Gaynor, K., Casey, E., LaFrancois, J., et al. (2003b). Co-localization of cholesterol, apolipoprotein E and fibrillar Abeta in amyloid plaques. *Brain Res. Mol. Brain Res.* 110, 119–125. doi: 10.1016/s0169-328x(02)00647-2

Burns, M., Gaynor, K., Olm, V., Mercken, M., LaFrancois, J., Wang, L., et al. (2003a). Presenilin redistribution associated with aberrant cholesterol transport enhances beta-amyloid production in vivo. *J. Neurosci.* 23, 5645–5649.

Butterfield, D. A., and Boyd-Kimball, D. (2005). The critical role of methionine 35 in Alzheimer's amyloid beta-peptide (1-42)-induced oxidative stress and neurotoxicity. *Biochim. Biophys. Acta* 1703, 149–156. doi: 10.1016/j.bbapap.2004.10.014

Butterfield, D. A., and Kanski, J. (2001). Brain protein oxidation in age-related neurodegenerative disorders that are associated with aggregated proteins. *Mech. Ageing Dev.* 122, 945–962. doi: 10.1016/s0047-6374(01)00249-4

Butterfield, D. A., Drake, J., Pocernich, C., and Castegna, A. (2001). Evidence of oxidative damage in Alzheimer's disease brain: central role for amyloid beta-peptide. *Trends Mol. Med.* 7, 548–554. doi: 10.1016/s1471-4914(01)02173-6

Butterfield, D. A., Swomley, A. M., and Sultana, R. (2013). Amyloid β-peptide (1-42)-induced oxidative stress in Alzheimer disease: importance in disease pathogenesis and progression. *Antioxid. Redox Signal.* 19, 823–835. doi: 10.1089/ars.2012.5027

Cam, J. A., and Bu, G. (2006). Modulation of beta-amyloid precursor protein trafficking and processing by the low density lipoprotein receptor family. *Mol. Neurodegener.* 18, 1–8. doi: 10.1186/1750-1326-1-8

Canepa, E., Borghi, R., Viña, J., Traverso, N., Gambini, J., Domenicotti, C., et al. (2011). Cholesterol and amyloid-A: evidence for a cross-talk between astrocytes and neuronal cells. *J. Alzheimers Dis.* 25, 645–653. doi: 10.3233/JAD-2011-110053

Cao, G., Bales, K. R., DeMattos, R. B., and Paul, S. M. (2007). Liver X receptor-mediated gene regulation and cholesterol homeostasis in brain: relevance to Alzheimer's disease therapeutics. *Curr. Alzheimer Res.* 4, 179–184. doi: 10.2174/156720507780362173

Carter, D. B., Dunn, E., McKinley, D. D., Stratman, N. C., Boyle, T. P., Kuiper, S. L., et al. (2001). Human apolipoprotein E4 accelerates beta-amyloid deposition in APPsw transgenic mouse brain. *Ann. Neurol.* 50, 468–475. doi: 10.1002/ana.1134

Caspersen, C., Wang, N., Yao, J., Sosunov, A., Chen, X., Lustbader, J. W., et al. (2005). Mitochondrial Abeta: a potential focal point for neuronal metabolic dysfunction in Alzheimer's disease. *FASEB J.* 19, 2040–2041. doi: 10.1096/fj.05-3735fje

Castellani, R. J., Rolston, R. K., and Smith, M. A. (2010). Alzheimer disease. *Dis. Mon.* 56, 484–546. doi: 10.1016/j.disamonth.2010.06.001

Castellani, R., Hirai, K., Aliev, G., Drew, K. L., Nunomura, A., Takeda, A., et al. (2002). Role of mitochondrial dysfunction in Alzheimer's disease. *J. Neurosci. Res.* 70, 357–360. doi: 10.1002/jnr.10389

Chan, S. L., Kim, W. S., Kwok, J. B., Hill, A. F., Cappai, R., Rye, K. A., et al. (2008). ATP-binding cassette transporter A7 regulates processing of amyloid precursor protein in vitro. *J. Neurochem.* 106, 793–804. doi: 10.1111/j.1471-4159.2008.05433.x

Chang, S., ran Ma, T., Miranda, R. D., Balestra, M. E., Mahley, R. W., and Huang, Y. (2005). Lipid- and receptor-binding regions of apolipoprotein E4 fragments act in concert to cause mitochondrial dysfunction and neurotoxicity. *Proc. Natl. Acad. Sci. U S A* 102, 18694–18699. doi: 10.1073/pnas.0508254102

Chopra, K., Misra, S., and Kuhad, A. (2011). Current perspectives on pharmacotherapy of Alzheimer's disease. *Expert Opin. Pharmacother.* 12, 335–350. doi: 10.1517/14656566.2011.520702

Churchward, M. A., and Todd, K. G. (2014). Statin treatment affects cytokine release and phagocytic activity in primary cultured microglia through two separable mechanisms. *Mol. Brain* 7:85. doi: 10.1186/s13041-014-0085-7

Colton, C., and Wilcock, D. M. (2010). Assessing activation states in microglia. *CNS Neurol. Disord. Drug Targets* 9, 174–191. doi: 10.2174/187152710791012053

Combs, C. K., Karlo, J. C., Kao, S. C., and Landreth, G. E. (2001). β-amyloid stimulation of microglia anti monocytes results in TNFα-dependent expression of inducible nitric oxide synthase and neuronal apoptosis. *J. Neurosci.* 21, 1179–1188.

Cordy, J. M., Hooper, N. M., and Turner, A. J. (2006). The involvement of lipid rafts in Alzheimer's disease. *Mol. Membr. Biol.* 23, 111–122. doi: 10.1080/09687860500496417

Cottrell, D. A., Blakely, E. L., Johnson, M. A., Ince, P. G., and Turnbull, D. M. (2001). Mitochondrial enzyme-deficient hippocampal neurons and choroidal cells in AD. *Neurology* 57, 260–264. doi: 10.1212/wnl.57.2.260

Crick, P. J., Beckers, L., Baes, M., Van Veldhoven, P. P., Wang, Y., and Griffiths, W. J. (2015a). The oxysterol and cholestenoic acid profile of mouse cerebrospinal fluid. *Steroids* doi: 10.1016/j.steroids.2015.02.021 [Epub ahead of print]

Crick, P. J., William Bentley, T., Abdel-Khalik, J., Matthews, I., Clayton, P. T., Morris, A. A., et al. (2015b). Quantitative charge-tags for sterol and oxysterol analysis. *Clin. Chem.* 61, 400–411. doi: 10.1373/clinchem.2014.231332

Crouch, P. J., Blake, R., Duce, J. A., Ciccotosto, G. D., Li, Q. X., Barnham, K. J., et al. (2005). Copper-dependent inhibition of human cytochrome c oxidase by a dimeric conformer of amyloid-beta1-42. *J. Neurosci.* 25, 672–679. doi: 10.1523/jneurosci.4276-04.2005

Curtain, C. C., Ali, F. E., Smith, D. G., Bush, A. I., Masters, C. L., and Barnham, K. J. (2003). Metal ions, pH and cholesterol regulate the interactions of Alzheimer's disease amyloid-beta peptide with membrane lipid. *J. Biol. Chem.* 278, 2977–2982. doi: 10.1074/jbc.m205455200

D'Andrea, M. R., Cole, G. M., and Ard, M. D. (2004). The microglial phagocytic role with specific plaque types in the Alzheimer disease brain. *Neurobiol. Aging* 25, 675–683. doi: 10.1016/j.neurobiolaging.2003.12.026

Dasari, B., Prasanthi, J. R., Marwarha, G., Singh, B. B., and Ghribi, O. (2010). The oxysterol 27-hydroxycholesterol increases β-amyloid and oxidative stress in retinal pigment epithelial cells. *BMC Ophthalmol.* 10:22. doi: 10.1186/1471-2415-10-22

Deane, R., Sagare, A., Hamm, K., Parisi, M., Lane, S., Finn, M. B., et al. (2008). ApoE isoform-specific disruption of amyloid beta peptide clearance from mouse brain. *J. Clin. Invest.* 118, 4002–4013. doi: 10.1172/JCI36663

DeGiorgio, L. A., Shimizu, Y., Chun, H. S., Kim, Y. S., Sugama, S., Son, J. H., et al. (2002). Amyloid precursor protein gene disruption attenuates degeneration of substantia nigra compacta neurons following axotomy. *Brain Res.* 938, 38–44. doi: 10.1016/s0006-8993(02)02483-6

Dias, I. H., Polidori, M. C., and Griffiths, H. R. (2014). Hypercholesterolaemia-induced oxidative stress at the blood-brain barrier. *Biochem. Soc. Trans.* 42, 1001–1005. doi: 10.1042/BST20140164

Diczfalusy, U. (2013). On the formation and possible biological role of 25-hydroxycholesterol. *Biochimie* 95, 455–460. doi: 10.1016/j.biochi.2012.06.016

Dietschy, J. M. (2009). Central nervous system: cholesterol turnover, brain development and neurodegeneration. *Biol. Chem.* 390, 287–293. doi: 10.1515/BC.2009.035

Ding, Q., Dimayuga, E., and Keller, J. N. (2007). Oxidative damage, protein synthesis and protein degradation in Alzheimer's disease. *Curr. Alzheimer Res.* 4, 73–79. doi: 10.2174/156720507779939788

Drouin-Ouellet, J., and Cicchetti, F. (2012). Inflammation and neurodegeneration: the story 'retolled'. *Trends Pharmacol. Sci.* 33, 542–551. doi: 10.1016/j.tips.2012.07.002

Du, H., Guo, L., Yan, S., Sosunov, A. A., McKhann, G. M., and Yan, S. S. (2010). Early deficits in synaptic mitochondria in an Alzheimer's disease mouse model. *Proc. Natl. Acad. Sci. U S A* 107, 18670–18675. doi: 10.1073/pnas.1006586107

Ehehalt, R., Keller, P., Haass, C., Thiele, C., and Simons, K. (2003). Amyloidogenic processing of the Alzheimer beta-amyloid precursor protein depends on lipid rafts. *J. Cell. Biol.* 160, 113–123. doi: 10.1083/jcb.200207113

Evans, R. M., Hui, S., Perkins, A., Lahiri, D. K., Poirier, J., and Farlow, M. R. (2004). Cholesterol and APOE genotype interact to influence Alzheimer disease progression. *Neurology* 62, 1869–1871. doi: 10.1212/01.wnl.0000125323.15458.3f

Famer, D., Meaney, S., Mousavi, M., Nordberg, A., Björkhem, I., and Crisby, M. (2007). Regulation of alpha- and beta-secretase activity by oxysterols: cerebrosterol stimulates processing of APP via the alpha-secretase pathway. *Biochem. Biophys. Res. Commun.* 359, 46–50. doi: 10.1016/j.bbrc.2007.05.033

Fan, Q. W., Yu, W., Senda, T., Yanagisawa, K., and Michikawa, M. (2001). Cholesterol-dependent modulation of tau phosphorylation in cultured neurons. *J. Neurochem.* 76, 391–400. doi: 10.1046/j.1471-4159.2001.00063.x

Fantini, J., and Yahi, N. (2010). Molecular insights into amyloid regulation by membrane cholesterol and sphingolipids: common mechanisms in neurodegenerative diseases. *Expert Rev. Mol. Med.* 12:e27. doi: 10.1017/s1462399410001602

Fassbender, K., Masters, C., and Beyreuther, K. (2000). Alzheimer's disease: an inflammatory disease? *Neurobiol. Aging* 21, 433–436. doi: 10.1016/S0197-4580(00)00147-0

Fassbender, K., Simons, M., Bergmann, C., Stroick, M., Lütjohann, D., Keller, P., et al. (2001). Simvastatin strongly reduces levels of Alzheimer's disease beta-amyloid peptides Abeta 42 and Abeta 40 in vitro and in vivo. *Proc. Natl. Acad. Sci. U S A* 98, 5856–5861. doi: 10.1073/pnas.081620098

Fernandez-Fernandez, S., Almeida, A., and Bolaños, J. P. (2012). Antioxidant and bioenergetic coupling between neurons and astrocytes. *Biochem. J.* 443, 3–11. doi: 10.1042/bj20111943

Ferrera, P., Mercado-Gómez, O., Silva-Aguilar, M., Valverde, M., and Arias, C. (2008). Cholesterol potentiates beta-amyloid-induced toxicity in human neuroblastoma cells: involvement of oxidative stress. *Neurochem. Res.* 33, 1509–1517. doi: 10.1007/s11064-008-9623-y

Ferretti, M. T., and Cuello, A. C. (2011). Does a pro-inflammatory process precede Alzheimer's disease and mild cognitive impairment? *Curr. Alzheimer Res.* 8, 164–174. doi: 10.2174/1567211213451702050

Figueiredo-Pereira, M. E., Rockwell, P., Schmidt-Glenewinkel, T., and Serrano, P. (2015). Neuroinflammation and J2 prostaglandins: linking impairment of the ubiquitin-proteasome pathway and mitochondria to neurodegeneration. *Front. Mol. Neurosci.* 7:104. doi: 10.3389/fnmol.2014.00104

Findeis, M. A. (2007). The role of amyloid β peptide 42 in Alzheimer's disease. *Pharmacol. Ther.* 116, 266–286. doi: 10.1016/j.pharmthera.2007.06.006

Fitz, N. F., Cronican, A., Pham, T., Fogg, A., Fauq, A. H., Chapman, R., et al. (2010). LXR agonist treatment ameliorates amyloid pathology and memory deficits caused by high fat diet in APP23 mice. *J. Neurosci.* 30, 6862–6872. doi: 10.1523/JNEUROSCI.1051-10.2010

Gamba, P., Guglielmotto, M., Testa, G., Monteleone, D., Zerbinati, C., Gargiulo, S., et al. (2014). Up-regulation of β-amyloidogenesis in neuron-like human cells by both 24- and 27-hydroxycholesterol: protective effect of N-acetyl-cysteine. *Aging Cell.* 13, 561–572. doi: 10.1111/acel.12206

Gamba, P., Leonarduzzi, G., Tamagno, E., Guglielmotto, M., Testa, G., Sottero, B., et al. (2011). Interaction between 24-hydroxycholesterol, oxidative stress and amyloid-β in amplifying neuronal damage in Alzheimer's disease: three partners in crime. *Aging Cell* 10, 403–417. doi: 10.1111/j.1474-9726.2011.00681.x

Gamba, P., Testa, G., Sottero, B., Gargiulo, S., Poli, G., and Leonarduzzi, G. (2012). The link between altered cholesterol metabolism and Alzheimer's disease. *Ann. N Y Acad. Sci.* 1259, 54–64. doi: 10.1111/j.1749-6632.2012.06513.x

Gate, D., Rezai-Zadeh, K., Jodry, D., Rentsendorj, A., and Town, T. (2010). Macrophages in Alzheimer's disease: the blood-borne identity. *J. Neural Transm.* 117, 961–970. doi: 10.1007/s00702-010-0422-7

Gatz, M., Reynolds, C. A., Fratiglioni, L., Johansson, B., Mortimer, J. A., Berg, S., et al. (2006). Role of genes and environments for explaining Alzheimer disease. *Arch. Gen. Psychiatry* 63, 168–174. doi: 10.1001/archpsyc.63.2.168

Ghribi, O., Larsen, B., Schrag, M., and Herman, M. M. (2006). High cholesterol content in neurons increases BACE, A-amyloid and phosphorylated tau levels in rabbit hippocampus. *Exp. Neurol.* 200, 460–467. doi: 10.1016/j.expneurol.2006.03.019

Giraldo, E., Lloret, A., Fuchsberger, T., and Viña, J. (2014). Aβ and tau toxicities in Alzheimer's are linked via oxidative stress-induced p38 activation: protective role of vitamin E. *Redox Biol.* 2, 873–877. doi: 10.1016/j.redox.2014.03.002

Glass, C. K., Saijo, K., Winner, B., Marchetto, M. C., and Gage, F. H. (2010). Mechanisms underlying inflammation in neurodegeneration. *Cell* 140, 918–934. doi: 10.1016/j.cell.2010.02.016

Gong, J. S., Sawamura, N., Zou, K., Sakai, J., Yanagisawa, K., and Michikawa, M. (2002). Amyloid beta-protein affects cholesterol metabolism in cultured neurons: implications for pivotal role of cholesterol in the amyloid cascade. *J. Neurosci. Res.* 70, 438–446. doi: 10.1002/jnr.10347

Götz, J., Chen, F., van Dorpe, J., and Nitsch, R. M. (2001). Formation of neurofibrillary tangles in P301l tau transgenic mice induced by Abeta 42 fibrils. *Science* 293, 1491–1495. doi: 10.1126/science.1062097

Grathwohl, S. A., Kälin, R. E., Bolmont, T., Prokop, S., Winkelmann, G., Kaeser, S. A., et al. (2009). Formation and maintenance of Alzheimer's disease beta-amyloid plaques in the absence of microglia. *Nat. Neurosci.* 12, 1361–1363. doi: 10.1038/nn.2432

Grimm, M. O., Grimm, H. S., Tomic, I., Beyreuther, K., Hartmann, T., and Bergmann, C. (2008). Independent inhibition of Alzheimer disease beta- and gamma-secretase cleavage by lowered cholesterol levels. *J. Biol. Chem.* 283, 11302–11311. doi: 10.1074/JBC.M801520200

Harris, B., Pereira, I., and Parkin, E. (2009). Targeting ADAM10 to lipid rafts in neuroblastoma SH-SY5Y cells impairs amyloidogenic processing of the amyloid precursor protein. *Brain Res.* 1296, 203–215. doi: 10.1016/j.brainres.2009.07.105

Harris, F. M., Brecht, W. J., Xu, Q., Tesseur, I., Kekonius, L., Wyss-Coray, T., et al. (2003). Carboxyl-terminal-truncated apolipoprotein E4 causes Alzheimer's disease-like neurodegeneration and behavioral deficits in transgenic mice. *Proc. Natl. Acad. Sci. U S A* 100, 10966–10971. doi: 10.1073/pnas.1434398100

Harris, J. R. (2008). Cholesterol binding to amyloid-beta fibrils: a TEM study. *Micron* 39, 1192–1196. doi: 10.1016/j.micron.2008.05.001

Hascalovici, J. R., Vaya, J., Khatib, S., Holcroft, C. A., Zukor, H., Song, W., et al. (2009). Brain sterol dysregulation in sporadic AD and MCI: relationship to heme oxygenase-1. *J. Neurochem.* 110, 1241–1253. doi: 10.1111/j.1471-4159.2009.06213.x

Hawkes, C. A., and McLaurin, J. (2009). Selective targeting of perivascular macrophages for clearance of beta-amyloid in cerebral amyloid angiopathy. *Proc. Natl. Acad. Sci. U S A* 106, 1261–1266. doi: 10.1073/pnas.0805453106

He, X., Jenner, A. M., Ong, W. Y., Farooqui, A. A., and Patel, S. C. (2006). Lovastatin modulates increased cholesterol and oxysterol levels and has a neuroprotective effect on rat hippocampal neurons after kainate injury. *J. Neuropathol. Exp. Neurol.* 65, 652–663. doi: 10.1097/01.jnen.0000225906.82428.69

Head, E., Lott, I. T., Cribbs, D. H., Cotman, C. W., and Rohn, T. T. (2002). Beta-amyloid deposition and neurofibrillary tangle association with caspase activation in Down syndrome. *Neurosci. Lett.* 330, 99–103. doi: 10.1016/s0304-3940(02)00705-x

Heneka, M. T., and O'Banion, M. K. (2007). Inflammatory processes in Alzheimer's disease. *J. Neuroimmunol.* 184, 69–91. doi: 10.1016/j.jneuroim.2006.11.017

Heneka, M. T., O'Banion, M. K., Terwel, D., and Kummer, M. P. (2010). Neuroinflammatory processes in Alzheimer's disease. *J Neural Transm.* 117, 919–947. doi: 10.1007/s00702-010-0438-z

Herz, J., and Beffert, U. (2000). Apolipoprotein E receptors: linking brain development and Alzheimer's disease. *Nat. Rev. Neurosci.* 1, 51–58. doi: 10.1038/35036221

Heverin, M., Bogdanovic, N., Lütjohann, D., Bayer, T., Pikuleva, I., Bretillon, L., et al. (2004). Changes in the levels of cerebral and extracerebral sterols in the brain of patients with Alzheimer's disease. *J. Lipid Res.* 45, 186–193. doi: 10.1194/jlr.m300320-jlr200

Heverin, M., Meaney, S., Lütjohann, D., Diczfalusy, U., Wahren, J., and Björkhem, I. (2005). Crossing the barrier: net flux of 27-hydroxycholesterol into the human brain. *J. Lipid Res.* 46, 1047–1052. doi: 10.1194/jlr.m500024-jlr200

Hickman, S. E., Allison, E. K., and El Khoury, J. (2008). Microglial dysfunction and defective beta-amyloid clearance pathways in aging Alzheimer's disease mice. *J. Neurosci.* 28, 8354–8360. doi: 10.1523/JNEUROSCI.0616-08.2008

Holmes, C. (2013). Review: systemic inflammation and Alzheimer's disease. *Neuropathol. Appl. Neurobiol.* 39, 51–68. doi: 10.1111/j.1365-2990.2012.01307.x

Holmes, C., and Butchart, J. (2011). Systemic inflammation and Alzheimer's disease. *Biochem. Soc. Trans.* 39, 898–901. doi: 10.1042/BST0390898

Holtzman, D. M., Bales, K. R., Tenkova, T., Fagan, A. M., Parsadanian, M., Sartorius, L. J., et al. (2000). Apolipoprotein E isoform-dependent amyloid deposition and neuritic degeneration in a mouse model of Alzheimer's disease. *Proc. Natl. Acad. Sci. U S A* 97, 2892–2897. doi: 10.1073/pnas.050004797

Hooijmans, C. R., Rutters, F., Dederen, P. J., Gambarota, G., Veltien, A., van Groen, T., et al. (2007). Changes in cerebral blood volume and amyloid pathology in aged Alzheimer APP/PS1 mice on a docosahexaenoic acid (DHA) diet or cholesterol enriched Typical Western Diet (TWD). *Neurobiol. Dis.* 28, 16–29. doi: 10.1016/j.nbd.2007.06.007

Hughes, T. M., Kuller, L. H., Lopez, O. L., Becker, J. T., Evans, R. W., Sutton-Tyrrell, K., et al. (2012). Markers of cholesterol metabolism in the brain show stronger association with cerebrovascular disease than Alzheimer's disease. *J. Alzheimers Dis.* 30, 53–61. doi: 10.3233/JAD-2012-111460

Hughes, T. M., Lopez, O. L., Evans, R. W., Kamboh, M. I., Williamson, J. D., Klunk, W. E., et al. (2014). Markers of cholesterol transport are associated with amyloid deposition in the brain. *Neurobiol. Aging* 35, 802–807. doi: 10.1016/j.neurobiolaging.2013.09.040

Hughes, T. M., Rosano, C., Evans, R. W., and Kuller, L. H. (2013). Brain cholesterol metabolism, oxysterols and dementia. *J. Alzheimers Dis.* 33, 891–911. doi: 10.3233/JAD-2012-121585

Iadecola, C. (2004). Neurovascular regulation in the normal brain and in Alzheimer's disease. *Nat. Rev. Neurosci.* 5, 347–360. doi: 10.1038/nrn1387

Iuliano, L. (2011). Pathways of cholesterol oxidation via non-enzymatic mechanisms. *Chem. Phys. Lipids* 164, 457–458. doi: 10.1016/j.chemphyslip.2011.06.006

Iuliano, L., Crick, P. J., Zerbinati, C., Tritapepe, L., Abdel-Khalik, J., Poirot, M., et al. (2015). Cholesterol metabolites exported from human brai. *Steroids* doi: 10.1016/j.steroids.2015.01.026 [Epub ahead of print]

Iuliano, L., Monticolo, R., Straface, G., Spoletini, I., Gianni, W., Caltagirone, C., et al. (2010). Vitamin E and enzymatic/oxidative stress-driven oxysterols in amnestic mild cognitive impairment subtypes and Alzheimer's disease. *J. Alzheimers Dis.* 21, 1383–1392. doi: 10.3233/JAD-2010-100780

Jacob, K. D., Noren Hooten, N., Trzeciak, A. R., and Evans, M. K. (2013). Markers of oxidant stress that are clinically relevant in aging and age-related disease. *Mech. Ageing Dev.* 134, 139–157. doi: 10.1016/j.mad.2013.02.008

Jang, E. R., and Lee, C. S. (2011). 7-ketocholesterol induces apoptosis in differentiated PC12 cells via reactive oxygen species-dependent activation of NF-κB and Akt pathways. *Neurochem. Int.* 58, 52–59. doi: 10.1016/j.neuint.2010.10.012

Jaya Prasanthi, R. P., Schommer, E., Thomasson, S., Thompson, A., Feist, G., and Ghribi, O. (2008). Regulation of beta-amyloid levels in the brain of cholesterol-fed rabbit, a model system for sporadic Alzheimer's disease. *Mech. Ageing Dev.* 129, 649–655. doi: 10.1016/j.mad.2008.09.002

Jeitner, T. M., Voloshyna, I., and Reiss, A. B. (2011). Oxysterol derivatives of cholesterol in neurodegenerative disorders. *Curr. Med. Chem.* 18, 1515–1525. doi: 10.2174/092986711795328445

Jenner, A. M., Lim, W. L., Ng, M. P., Wenk, M. R., Shui, G., Sharman, M. J., et al. (2010). The effect of APOE genotype on brain levels of oxysterols in young and old human APOE epsilon2, epsilon3 and epsilon4 knock-in mice. *Neuroscience* 169, 109–115. doi: 10.1016/j.neuroscience.2010.04.026

Ji, Z. S., Miranda, R. D., Newhouse, Y. M., Weisgraber, K. H., Huang, Y., and Mahley, R. W. (2002). Apolipoprotein E4 potentiates amyloid beta peptide-induced lysosomal leakage and apoptosis in neuronal cells. *J. Biol. Chem.* 277, 21821–21828. doi: 10.1074/jbc.m112109200

Jiang, Q., Lee, C. Y., Mandrekar, S., Wilkinson, B., Cramer, P., Zelcer, N., et al. (2008). ApoE promotes the proteolytic degradation of Abeta. *Neuron* 58, 681–693. doi: 10.1016/j.neuron.2008.04.010

Jo, W. K., Law, A. C., and Chung, S. K. (2014). The neglected co-star in the dementia drama: the putative roles of astrocytes in the pathogeneses of major neurocognitive disorders. *Mol. Psychiatry* 19, 159–167. doi: 10.1038/mp.2013.171

Joshi, Y. B., and Praticò, D. (2015). The 5-lipoxygenase pathway: oxidative and inflammatory contributions to the Alzheimer's disease phenotype. *Front. Cell Neurosci.* 8:436. doi: 10.3389/fncel.2014.00436

Kakio, A., Nishimoto, S. I., Yanagisawa, K., Kozutsumi, Y., and Matsuzaki, K. (2001). Cholesterol-dependent formation of GM1 ganglioside-bound amyloid beta-protein, an endogenous seed for Alzheimer amyloid. *J. Biol. Chem.* 276, 24985–24990. doi: 10.1074/jbc.m100252200

Kakio, A., Nishimoto, S., Yanagisawa, K., Kozutsumi, Y., and Matsuzaki, K. (2002). Interactions of amyloid beta-protein with various gangliosides in raft-like membranes: importance of GM1 ganglioside-bound form as an endogenous seed for Alzheimer amyloid. *Biochemistry* 41, 7385–7390. doi: 10.1021/bi0255874

Keene, C. D., Cudaback, E., Li, X., Montine, K. S., and Montine, T. J. (2011). Apolipoprotein E isoforms and regulation of the innate immune response in brain of patients with Alzheimer's disease. *Curr. Opin. Neurobiol.* 21, 920–928. doi: 10.1016/j.conb.2011.08.002

Khandelwal, P. J., Herman, A. M., and Moussa, C. E. (2011). Inflammation in the early stages of neurodegenerative pathology. *J. Neuroimmunol.* 238, 1–11. doi: 10.1016/j.jneuroim.2011.07.002

Kierdorf, K., Wang, Y., and Neumann, H. (2010). . Immune-mediated CNS damage. *Results Probl. Cell Differ.* 51, 173–196. doi: 10.1007/400_2008_15

Kim, D. H., and Frangos, J. A. (2008). Effects of amyloid beta-peptides on the lysis tension of lipid bilayer vesicles containing oxysterols. *Biophys. J.* 95, 620–628. doi: 10.1529/biophysj.107.114983

Kim, H. A., Miller, A. A., Drummond, G. R., Thrift, A. G., Arumugam, T. V., Phan, T. G., et al. (2012). Vascular cognitive impairment and Alzheimer's disease: role of cerebral hypoperfusion and oxidative stress. *Naunyn Schmiedebergs Arch. Pharmacol.* 385, 953–959. doi: 10.1007/s00210-012-0790-7

Kim, J. H., Jittiwat, J., Ong, W. Y., Farooqui, A. A., and Jenner, A. M. (2010). Changes in cholesterol biosynthetic and transport pathways after excitotoxicity. *J. Neurochem.* 112, 34–41. doi: 10.1111/j.1471-4159.2009.06449.x

Kim, J., Basak, J. M., and Holtzman, D. M. (2009a). The role of apolipoprotein E in Alzheimer's disease. *Neuron* 63, 287–303. doi: 10.1016/j.neuron.2009.06.026

Kim, W. S., Chan, S. L., Hill, A. F., Guillemin, G. J., and Garner, B. (2009b). Impact of 27-hydroxycholesterol on amyloid-beta peptide production and ATP-binding cassette transporter expression in primary human neurons. *J. Alzheimers Dis.* 16, 121–131. doi: 10.3233/JAD-2009-0944

Kim, W. S., Hill, A. F., Fitzgerald, M. L., Freeman, M. W., Evin, G., and Garner, B. (2011). Wild type and tangier disease ABCA1 mutants modulate cellular amyloid-A production independent of cholesterol efflux activity. *J. Alzheimers Dis.* 27, 441–452. doi: 10.3233/JAD-2011-110521

Kim, Y. J., and Lee, C. S. (2010). Tyrosine kinase inhibitor AG126 reduces 7-ketocholesterol-induced cell death by suppressing mitochondria-mediated apoptotic process. *Neurochem. Res.* 35, 603–612. doi: 10.1007/s11064-009-0105-7

Kim, Y. J., Han, J. H., Han, E. S., and Lee, C. S. (2006). 7-Ketocholesterol enhances 1-methyl-4-phenylpyridinium-induced mitochondrial dysfunction and cell death in PC12 cells. *J. Neural Transm.* 113, 1877–1885. doi: 10.1007/s00702-006-0486-6

Koldamova, R. P., Lefterov, I. M., Ikonomovic, M. D., Skoko, J., Lefterov, P. I., Isanski, B. A., et al. (2003). 22R-hydroxycholesterol and 9-cis-retinoic acid induce ATP-binding cassette transporter A1 expression and cholesterol efflux in brain cells and decrease amyloid beta secretion. *J. Biol. Chem.* 278, 13244–13256. doi: 10.1074/jbc.m300044200

Koldamova, R., Fitz, N. F., and Lefterov, I. (2010). The role of ATP-binding cassette transporter A1 in Alzheimer's disease and neurodegeneration. *Biochim. Biophys. Acta* 1801, 824–830. doi: 10.1016/j.bbalip.2010.02.010

Koudinov, A. R., and Koudinova, N. V. (2005). Cholesterol homeostasis failure as a unifying cause of synaptic degeneration. *J. Neurol. Sci.* 229–230, 233–240. doi: 10.1016/j.jns.2004.11.036

Krabbe, G., Halle, A., Matyash, V., Rinnenthal, J. L., Eom, G. D., Bernhardt, U., et al. (2013). Functional impairment of microglia coincides with Beta-amyloid deposition in mice with Alzheimer-like pathology. *PLoS One* 8:e60921. doi: 10.1371/journal.pone.0060921

Kölsch, H., Heun, R., Kerksiek, A., Bergmann, K. V., Maier, W., and Lütjohann, D. (2004). Altered levels of plasma 24S- and 27-hydroxycholesterol in demented patients. *Neurosci. Lett.* 368, 303–308. doi: 10.1016/j.neulet.2004.07.031

Kölsch, H., Ludwig, M., Lütjohann, D., Prange, W., and Rao, M. L. (2000). 7alpha-Hydroperoxycholesterol causes CNS neuronal cell death. *Neurochem. Int.* 36, 507–512. doi: 10.1016/s0197-0186(99)00157-6

Kölsch, H., Ludwig, M., Lütjohann, D., and Rao, M. L. (2001). Neurotoxicity of 24-hydroxycholesterol, an important cholesterol elimination product of the brain, may be prevented by vitamin E and estradiol-17beta. *J. Neural. Transm.* 108, 475–488. doi: 10.1007/s007020170068

Lane-Donovan, C., Philips, G. T., and Herz, J. (2014). More than cholesterol transporters: lipoprotein receptors in CNS function and neurodegeneration. *Neuron* 83, 771–787. doi: 10.1016/j.neuron.2014.08.005

Latta, C. H., Brothers, H. M., and Wilcock, D. M. (2014). Neuroinflammation in Alzheimer's disease; A source of heterogeneity and target for personalized therapy. *Neuroscience* doi: 10.1007/978-1-4615-5405-9_3 [Epub ahead of print]

Lee, C. Y., Tse, W., Smith, J. D., and Landreth, G. E. (2011). ApoE promotes AA trafficking and degradation by modulating microglial cholesterol levels. *J. Biol. Chem.* 287, 2032–2044. doi: 10.1074/jbc.M111.295451

Leoni, V., and Caccia, C. (2011). Oxysterols as biomarkers in neurodegenerative diseases. *Chem .Phys. Lipids* 164, 515–524. doi: 10.1016/j.chemphyslip.2011.04.002

Leoni, V., Masterman, T., Mousavi, F. S., Wretlind, B., Wahlund, L. O., Diczfalusy, U., et al. (2004). Diagnostic use of cerebral and extracerebral oxysterols. *Clin. Chem. Lab. Med.* 42, 186–191. doi: 10.1515/cclm.2004.034

Leoni, V., Masterman, T., Patel, P., Meaney, S., Diczfalusy, U., and Björkhem, I. (2003). Side chain oxidized oxysterols in cerebrospinal fluid and the integrity of blood-brain and blood-cerebrospinal fluid barriers. *J. Lipid Res.* 44, 793–799. doi: 10.1194/jlr.m200434-jlr200

Lewis, J., Dickson, D. W., Lin, W. L., Chisholm, L., Corral, A., Jones, G., et al. (2001). Enhanced neurofibrillary degeneration in transgenic mice expressing mutant tau and APP. *Science* 293, 1487–1491. doi: 10.1126/science.1058189

Liu, B., and Hong, J. S. (2003). Role of microglia in inflammation-mediated neurodegenerative diseases: mechanisms and strategies for therapeutic intervention. *J. Pharmacol. Exp. Ther.* 304, 1–7. doi: 10.1124/jpet.102.035048

Liu, Q., Zerbinatti, C. V., Zhang, J., Hoe, H. S., Wang, B., Cole, S. L., et al. (2007). Amyloid precursor protein regulates brain apolipoprotein E and cholesterol metabolism through lipoprotein receptor LRP1. *Neuron* 56, 66–78. doi: 10.1016/j.neuron.2007.08.008

Luchsinger, J. A., and Mayeux, R. (2004). Dietary factors and Alzheimer's disease. *Lancet. Neurol.* 3, 579–587. doi: 10.1016/S1474-4422(04)00878-6

Luckhoff, H. K., Brand, T., van Velden, D. P., Kidd, M., Fisher, L. R., van Rensburg, S. J., et al. (2015). Clinical relevance of apolipoprotein e genotyping based on a family history of Alzheimer's disease. *Curr. Alzheimer Res.* 12, 210–217. doi: 10.2174/1567205012666150302154354

Luque-Contreras, D., Carvajal, K., Toral-Rios, D., Franco-Bocanegra, D., and Campos-Peña, V. (2014). Oxidative stress and metabolic syndrome: cause or consequence of Alzheimer's disease? *Oxid. Med. Cell. Longev.* 2014:497802. doi: 10.1155/2014/497802

Lyman, M., Lloyd, D. G., Ji, X., Vizcaychipi, M. P., and Ma, D. (2014). Neuroinflammation: the role and consequences. *Neurosci. Res.* 79, 1–12. doi: 10.1016/j.neures.2013.10.004

Lütjohann, D., Papassotiropoulos, A., Björkhem, I., Locatelli, S., Bagli, M., Oehring, R. D., et al. (2000). Plasma 24S-hydroxycholesterol (cerebrosterol) is increased in Alzheimer and vascular demented patients. *J. Lipid Res.* 41, 195–198.

Ma, M. T., Zhang, J., Farooqui, A. A., Chen, P., and Ong, W. Y. (2010). Effects of cholesterol oxidation products on exocytosis. *Neurosci. Lett.* 476, 36–41. doi: 10.1016/j.neulet.2010.03.078

Ma, W. W., Li, C. Q., Yu, H. L., Zhang, D. D., Xi, Y. D., Han, J., et al. (2015). The oxysterol 27-hydroxycholesterol increases oxidative stress and regulate nrf2 signaling pathway in astrocyte cells. *Neurochem. Res.* 40, 758–766. doi: 10.1007/s11064-015-1524-2

Maezawa, I., Maeda, N., Montine, T. J., and Montine, K. S. (2006a). Apolipoprotein E-specific innate immune response in astrocytes from targeted replacement mice. *J. Neuroinflammation* 7, 3–10. doi: 10.1186/1742-2094-3-10

Maezawa, I., Nivison, M., Montine, K. S., Maeda, N., and Montine, T. J. (2006b). Neurotoxicity from innate immune response is greatest with targeted replacement of E4 allele of apolipoprotein E gene and is mediated by microglial p38MAPK. *FASEB J.* 20, 797–799. doi: 10.1096/fj.05-5423fje

Maezawa, I., Zaja-Milatovic, S., Milatovic, D., Stephen, C., Sokal, I., Maeda, N., et al. (2006c). Apolipoprotein E isoform-dependent dendritic recovery of hippocampal neurons following activation of innate immunity. *J. Neuroinflammation* 25, 3–21. doi: 10.1186/1742-2094-3-21

Malaplate-Armand, C., Florent-Béchard, S., Youssef, I., Koziel, V., Sponne, I., Kriem, B., et al. (2006). Soluble oligomers of amyloid-beta peptide induce neuronal apoptosis by activating a cPLA2-dependent sphingomyelinase-ceramide pathway. *Neurobiol. Dis.* 23, 178–189. doi: 10.1016/j.nbd.2006.02.010

Manczak, M., Anekonda, T. S., Henson, E., Park, B. S., Quinn, J., and Reddy, P. H. (2006). Mitochondria are a direct site of Aβ accumulation in Alzheimer's disease neurons: implications for free radical generation and oxidative damage in disease progression. *Hum. Mol. Genet.* 15, 1437–1449. doi: 10.1093/hmg/ddl066

Mariani, E., Polidori, M. C., Cherubini, A., and Mecocci, P. (2005). Oxidative stress in brain aging, neurodegenerative and vascular diseases: an overview. *J. Chromatogr. B Analyt. Technol. Biomed. Life Sci.* 827, 65–75. doi: 10.1016/j.jchromb.2005.04.023

Martin, I., and Grotewiel, M. S. (2006). Oxidative damage and age-related functional declines. *Mech. Ageing Dev.* 127, 411–423. doi: 10.1016/j.mad.2006.01.008

Martins, I. J., Berger, T., Sharman, M. J., Verdile, G., Fuller, S. J., and Martins, R. N. (2009). Cholesterol metabolism and transport in the pathogenesis of Alzheimer's disease. *J. Neurochem.* 111, 1275–1308. doi: 10.1111/j.1471-4159.2009.06408.x

Marwarha, G., Dasari, B., Prasanthi, J. R., Schommer, J., and Ghribi, O. (2010). Leptin reduces the accumulation of Abeta and phosphorylated tau induced by 27-hydroxycholesterol in rabbit organotypic slices. *J. Alzheimers Dis.* 19, 1007–1019. doi: 10.3233/JAD-2010-1298

Marwarha, G., and Ghribi, O. (2014). Does the oxysterol 27-hydroxycholesterol underlie Alzheimer's disease-Parkinson's disease overlap? *Exp. Gerontol.* doi: 10.1016/j.exger.2014.09.013 [Epub ahead of print]

Marwarha, G., Raza, S., Prasanthi, J. R., and Ghribi, O. (2013). Gadd153 and NF-κB crosstalk regulates 27-hydroxycholesterol-induced increase in BACE1 and β-amyloid production in human neuroblastoma SH-SY5Y cells. *PLoS One* 8:e70773. doi: 10.1371/journal.pone.0070773

Marzolo, M. P., and Bu, G. (2009). Lipoprotein receptors and cholesterol in APP trafficking and proteolytic processing, implications for Alzheimer's disease. *Semin. Cell Dev. Biol.* 20, 191–200. doi: 10.1016/j.semcdb.2008.10.005

Mateos, L., Ismail, M. A., Gil-Bea, F. J., Leoni, V., Winblad, B., Björkhem, I., et al. (2011). Upregulation of brain renin angiotensin system by 27-hydroxycholesterol in Alzheimer's disease. *J. Alzheimers Dis.* 24, 669–679. doi: 10.3233/JAD-2011-101512

Mattson, M. P. (2004). Pathways towards and away from Alzheimer's disease. *Nature* 430, 631–639. doi: 10.1038/nature02621

Mayeux, R. (2003). Epidemiology of neurodegeneration. *Annu. Rev. Neurosci.* 26, 81–104. doi: 10.1146/annurev.neuro.26.043002.094919

Mazzetti, A. P., Fiorile, M. C., Primavera, A., and Lo Bello, M. (2015). Glutathione transferases and neurodegenerative diseases. *Neurochem. Int.* 82, 10–18. doi: 10.1016/j.neuint.2015.01.008

McGeer, E. G., and McGeer, P. L. (2010). Neuroinflammation in Alzheimer's disease and mild cognitive impairment: a field in its infancy. *J. Alzheimers Dis.* 19, 355–361. doi: 10.3233/JAD-2010-1219

McLellan, M. E., Kajdasz, S. T., Hyman, B. T., and Bacskai, B. J. (2003). In vivo imaging of reactive oxygen species specifically associated with thioflavine S-positive amyloid plaques by multiphoton microscopy. *J. Neurosci.* 23, 2212–2217.

Meaney, S., Heverin, M., Panzenboeck, U., Ekström, L., Axelsson, M., Andersson, U., et al. (2007). Novel route for elimination of brain oxysterols across the blood-brain barrier: conversion into 7alpha-hydroxy-3-oxo-4-cholestenoic acid. *J. Lipid Res.* 48, 944–951. doi: 10.1194/jlr.m600529-jlr200

Melov, S., Adlard, P. A., Morten, K., Johnson, F., Golden, T. R., Hinerfeld, D., et al. (2007). Mitochondrial oxidative stress causes hyperphosphorylation of tau. *PLoS One* 2:e536. doi: 10.1371/journal.pone.0000536

Michelucci, A., Heurtaux, T., Grandbarbe, L., Morga, E., and Heuschling, P. (2009). Characterization of the microglial phenotype under specific pro-inflammatory and anti-inflammatory conditions: Effects of oligomeric and fibrillar amyloid-beta. *J. Neuroimmunol.* 210, 3–12. doi: 10.1016/j.jneuroim.2009.02.003

Michikawa, M., Gong, J. S., Fan, Q. W., Sawamura, N., and Yanagisawa, K. (2001). A novel action of alzheimer's amyloid beta-protein (Abeta): oligomeric Abeta promotes lipid release. *J. Neurosci.* 21, 7226–7235.

Misonou, H., Morishima-Kawashima, M., and Ihara, Y. (2000). Oxidative stress induces intracellular accumulation of amyloid beta-protein (Abeta) in human neuroblastoma cells. *Biochemistry* 39, 6951–6959. doi: 10.1021/bi000169p

Mitomo, H., Chen, W. H., and Regen, S. L. (2009). Oxysterol-induced rearrangement of the liquid-ordered phase: a possible link to Alzheimer's disease? *J. Am. Chem. Soc.* 131, 12354–12357. doi: 10.1021/ja904308y

Morales, I., Guzmán-Martínez, L., Cerda-Troncoso, C., Farías, G. A., and Maccioni, R. B. (2014). Neuroinflammation in the pathogenesis of Alzheimer's disease. A rational framework for the search of novel therapeutic approaches. *Front. Cell Neurosci.* 8:112. doi: 10.3389/fncel.2014.00112

Morales, I., Jiménez, J. M., Mancilla, M., and Maccioni, R. B. (2013). Tau oligomers and fibrils induce activation of microglial cells. *J. Alzheimers Dis.* 37, 849–856. doi: 10.3233/JAD-131843

Mori, T., Paris, D., Town, T., Rojiani, A. M., Sparks, D. L., Delledonne, A., et al. (2001). Cholesterol accumulates in senile plaques of Alzheimer disease patients and in transgenic APP(SW) mice. *J. Neuropathol. Exp. Neurol.* 60, 778–785.

Mrak, R. E. (2012). Microglia in Alzheimer brain: a neuropathological perspective. *Int. J. Alzheimers Dis.* 2012:165021. doi: 10.1155/2012/165021

Mrak, R. E., and Griffin, W. S. (2005). Glia and their cytokines in progression of neurodegeneration. *Neurobiol. Aging* 26, 349–354. doi: 10.1016/j.neurobiolaging.2004.05.010

Mungarro-Menchaca, X., Ferrera, P., Morán, J., and Arias, C. (2002). beta-Amyloid peptide induces ultrastructural changes in synaptosomes and potentiates mitochondrial dysfunction in the presence of ryanodine. *J. Neurosci. Res.* 68, 89–96. doi: 10.1002/jnr.10193

Murphy, P. G., Borthwick, L. S., Johnston, R. S., Kuchel, G., and Richardson, P. M. (1999). Nature of the retrograde signal from injured nerves that induces interleukin-6 mRNA in neurons. *J. Neurosci.* 19, 3791–3800.

Naylor, R., Hill, A. F., and Barnham, K. J. (2008). Neurotoxicity in Alzheimer's disease: is covalently crosslinked A beta responsible? *Eur. Biophys. J.* 37, 265–268. doi: 10.1007/s00249-007-0243-2

Nelson, T. J., and Alkon, D. L. (2005). Oxidation of cholesterol by amyloid precursor protein and beta-amyloid peptide. *J. Biol. Chem.* 280, 7377–7387. doi: 10.1074/jbc.m409071200

Nieweg, K., Schaller, H., and Pfrieger, F. W. (2009). Marked differences in cholesterol synthesis between neurons and glial cells from postnatal rats. *J. Neurochem.* 109, 125–134. doi: 10.1111/j.1471-4159.2009.05917.x

Noguchi, N., Saito, Y., and Urano, Y. (2014). Diverse functions of 24(S)-hydroxycholesterol in the brain. *Biochem. Biophys. Res. Commun.* 446, 692–696. doi: 10.1016/j.bbrc.2014.02.010

Nunomura, A., Perry, G., Aliev, G., Hirai, K., Takeda, A., Balraj, E. K., et al. (2001). Oxidative damage is the earliest event in Alzheimer disease. *J. Neuropathol. Exp. Neurol.* 60, 759–767.

Nury, T., Samadi, M., Zarrouk, A., Riedinger, J. M., and Lizard, G. (2013). Improved synthesis and in vitro evaluation of the cytotoxic profile of oxysterols oxidized at C4 (4α- and 4β-hydroxycholesterol) and C7 (7-ketocholesterol, 7α- and 7β-hydroxycholesterol) on cells of the central nervous system. *Eur. J. Med. Chem.* 70, 558–567. doi: 10.1016/j.ejmech.2013.09.028

Oddo, S., Caccamo, A., Shepherd, J. D., Murphy, M. P., Golde, T. E., Kayed, R., et al. (2003). Triple-transgenic model of Alzheimer's disease with plaques and tangles: intracellular Abeta and synaptic dysfunction. *Neuron* 39, 409–421. doi: 10.1016/s0896-6273(03)00434-3

Okabe, A., Urano, Y., Itoh, S., Suda, N., Kotani, R., Nishimura, Y., et al. (2013). Adaptive responses induced by 24S-hydroxycholesterol through liver X receptor pathway reduce 7-ketocholesterol-caused neuronal cell death. *Redox Biol.* 2, 28–35. doi: 10.1016/j.redox.2013.11.007

Panza, F., D'Introno, A., Colacicco, A. M., Capurso, C., Pichichero, G., Capurso, S. A., et al. (2006). Lipid metabolism in cognitive decline and dementia. *Brain Res. Rev.* 51, 275–292. doi: 10.1016/j.brainresrev.2005.11.007

Papassotiropoulos, A., Lambert, J. C., Wavrant-De Vrièze, F., Wollmer, M. A., von der Kammer, H., Streffer, J. R., et al. (2005). Cholesterol 25-hydroxylase on chromosome 10q is a susceptibility gene for sporadic Alzheimer's disease. *Neurodegener. Dis.* 2, 233–241. doi: 10.1159/000090362

Papassotiropoulos, A., Lütjohann, D., Bagli, M., Locatelli, S., Jessen, F., Buschfort, R., et al. (2002). 24S-hydroxycholesterol in cerebrospinal fluid is elevated in early stages of dementia. *J. Psychiatr. Res.* 36, 27–32. doi: 10.1016/s0022-3956(01)00050-4

Park, L., Zhou, P., Pitstick, R., Capone, C., Anrather, J., Norris, E. H., et al. (2008). Nox2-derived radicals contribute to neurovascular and behavioral dysfunction in mice overexpressing the amyloid precursor protein. *Proc. Natl. Acad. Sci. U S A* 105, 1347–1352. doi: 10.1073/pnas.0711568105

Perry, V. H., Nicoll, J. A., and Holmes, C. (2010). Microglia in neurodegenerative disease. *Nat. Rev. Neurol.* 6, 193–201. doi: 10.1038/nrneurol.2010.17

Pfrieger, F. W. (2003). Outsourcing in the brain: do neurons depend on cholesterol delivery by astrocytes? *Bioessays* 25, 72–78. doi: 10.1002/bies.10195

Phan, H. T., Hata, T., Morita, M., Yoda, T., Hamada, T., Vestergaard, M. C., et al. (2013). The effect of oxysterols on the interaction of Alzheimer's amyloid beta with model membranes. *Biochim. Biophys. Acta* 1828, 2487–2495. doi: 10.1016/j.bbamem.2013.06.021

Popescu, B. O., Toescu, E. C., Popescu, L. M., Bajenaru, O., Muresanu, D. F., Schultzberg, M., et al. (2009). Blood-brain barrier alterations in ageing and dementia. *J. Neurol. Sci.* 283, 99–106. doi: 10.1016/j.jns.2009.02.321

Prasanthi, J. R., Huls, A., Thomasson, S., Thompson, A., Schommer, E., and Ghribi, O. (2009). Differential effects of 24-hydroxycholesterol and 27-hydroxycholesterol on beta-amyloid precursor protein levels and processing in human neuroblastoma SH-SY5Y cells. *Mol. Neurodegener.* 4:1. doi: 10.1186/1750-1326-4-1

Praticò, D., Uryu, K., Leight, S., Trojanoswki, J. Q., and Lee, V. M. (2001). Increased lipid peroxidation precedes amyloid plaque formation in an animal model of Alzheimer amyloidosis. *J. Neurosci.* 21, 4183–4187.

Puglielli, L., Friedlich, A. L., Setchell, K. D., Nagano, S., Opazo, C., Cherny, R. A., et al. (2005). Alzheimer disease beta-amyloid activity mimics cholesterol oxidase. *J. Clin. Invest.* 115, 2556–2563. doi: 10.1172/JCI23610

Puglielli, L., Konopka, G., Pack-Chung, E., Ingano, L. A., Berezovska, O., Hyman, B. T., et al. (2001). Acyl-coenzyme A: cholesterol acyltransferase modulates the generation of the amyloid beta-peptide. *Nat. Cell Biol.* 3, 905–912. doi: 10.1038/ncb1001-905

Puglielli, L., Tanzi, R. E., and Kovacs, D. M. (2003). Alzheimer's disease: the cholesterol connection. *Nat. Neurosci.* 6, 345–351. doi: 10.1038/nn0403-345

Qiu, L., Buie, C., Reay, A., Vaughn, M. W., and Cheng, K. H. (2011). Molecular dynamics simulations reveal the protective role of cholesterol in β-amyloid protein-induced membrane disruptions in neuronal membrane mimics. *J. Phys. Chem. B.* 115, 9795–9812. doi: 10.1021/jp2012842

Querfurth, H. W., and LaFerla, F. M. (2010). Alzheimer's disease. *N. Engl. J. Med.* 362, 329–344. doi: 10.1056/NEJMra0909142

Quintanilla, R. A., Orellana, J. A., and von Bernhardi, R. (2012). Understanding risk factors for Alzheimer's disease: interplay of neuroinflammation, connexin-based communication and oxidative stress. *Arch. Med. Res.* 43, 632–644. doi: 10.1016/j.arcmed.2012.10.016

Raber, J., Huang, Y., and Ashfordm, J. W. (2004). ApoE genotype accounts for the vast majority of AD risk and AD pathology. *Neurobiol. Aging* 25, 641–650. doi: 10.1016/j.neurobiolaging.2003.12.023

Račková, L. (2013). Cholesterol load of microglia: contribution of membrane architecture changes to neurotoxic power? *Arch Biochem Biophys.* 537, 91–103. doi: 10.1016/j.abb.2013.06.015

Ramesh, G., MacLean, A. G., and Philipp, M. T. (2013). Cytokines and chemokines at the crossroads of neuroinflammation, neurodegeneration and neuropathic pain. *Mediators Inflamm.* 2013:480739. doi: 10.1155/2013/480739

Reddy, P. H. (2011). Abnormal tau, mitochondrial dysfunction, impaired axonal transport of mitochondria and synaptic deprivation in Alzheimer's disease. *Brain Res.* 1415, 136–148. doi: 10.1016/j.brainres.2011.07.052

Reddy, P. H., and Beal, M. F. (2005). Are mitochondria critical in the pathogenesis of Alzheimer's disease? *Brain Res. Brain Res. Rev.* 49, 618–632. doi: 10.1016/j.brainresrev.2005.03.004

Reddy, P. H., and Beal, M. F. (2008). Amyloid beta, mitochondrial dysfunction and synaptic damage: implications for cognitive decline in aging and Alzheimer's disease. *Trends Mol. Med.* 14, 45–53. doi: 10.1016/j.molmed.2007.12.002

Reddy, P. H., McWeeney, S., Park, B. S., Manczak, M., Gutala, R. V., Partovi, D., et al. (2004). Gene expression profiles of transcripts in amyloid precursor protein transgenic mice: up-regulation of mitochondrial metabolism and apoptotic genes is an early cellular change in Alzheimer's disease. *Hum. Mol. Genet.* 13, 1225–1240. doi: 10.1093/hmg/ddh140

Reed, T. T. (2011). Lipid peroxidation and neurodegenerative disease. *Free Radic. Biol. Med.* 51, 1302–1319. doi: 10.1016/j.freeradbiomed.2011.06.027

Refolo, L. M., Malester, B., LaFrancois, J., Bryant-Thomas, T., Wang, R., Tint, G. S., et al. (2000). Hypercholesterolemia accelerates the Alzheimer's amyloid pathology in a transgenic mouse model. *Neurobiol. Dis.* 4, 321–331. doi: 10.1006/nbdi.2000.0304

Reid, P. C., Urano, Y., Kodama, T., and Hamakubo, T. (2007). Alzheimer's disease: cholesterol, membrane rafts, isoprenoids and statins. *J. Cell Mol. Med.* 11, 383–392. doi: 10.1111/j.1582-4934.2007.00054.x

Resende, R., Moreira, P. I., Proença, T., Deshpande, A., Busciglio, J., Pereira, C., et al. (2008). Brain oxidative stress in a triple-transgenic mouse model of Alzheimer disease. *Free Radic. Biol. Med.* 44, 2051–2057. doi: 10.1016/j.freeradbiomed.2008.03.012

Reynolds, A., Laurie, C., Mosley, R. L., and Gendelman, H. E. (2007). Oxidative stress and the pathogenesis of neurodegenerative disorders. *Int Rev Neurobiol.* 82, 297–325. doi: 10.1016/s0074-7742(07)82016-2

Rezai-Zadeh, K., Gate, D., Gowing, G., and Town, T. (2011). How to get from here to there: macrophage recruitment in Alzheimer's disease. *Curr. Alzheimer Res.* 8, 156–163. doi: 10.2174/1567212113451662050

Rosales-Corral, S., Reiter, R. J., Tan, D. X., Ortiz, G. G., and Lopez-Armas, G. (2010). Functional aspects of redox control during neuroinflammation. *Antioxid Redox Signal.* 13, 193–247. doi: 10.1089/ars.2009.2629

Roßner, S., Lange-Dohna, C., Zeitschel, U., and Perez-Polo, J. R. (2005). Alzheimer's disease β-secretase BACE1 is not a neuron-specific enzyme. *J. Neurochem.* 92, 226–234. doi: 10.1111/j.1471-4159.2004.02857.x

Royer, M. C., Lemaire-Ewing, S., Desrumaux, C., Monier, S., Pais de Barros, J. P., Athias, A., et al. (2009). 7-ketocholesterol incorporation into sphingolipid/cholesterol-enriched (lipid raft) domains is impaired by vitamin E: a specific role for alpha-tocopherol with consequences on cell death. *J. Biol. Chem.* 284, 15826–15834. doi: 10.1074/jbc.m808641200

Rubio-Perez, J. M., and Morillas-Ruiz, J. M. (2012). A review: inflammatory process in Alzheimer's disease, role of cytokines. *ScientificWorldJournal.* 2012:756357. doi: 10.1100/2012/756357

Sagare, A., Deane, R., Bell, R. D., Johnson, B., Hamm, K., Pendu, R., et al. (2007). Clearance of amyloid-beta by circulating lipoprotein receptors. *Nat. Med.* 13, 1029–1031. doi: 10.1038/nm1635

Saint-Pol, J., Candela, P., Boucau, M. C., Fenart, L., and Gosselet, F. (2013). Oxysterols decrease apical-to-basolateral transport of Aß peptides via an ABCB1-mediated process in an in vitro Blood-brain barrier model constituted of bovine brain capillary endothelial cells. *Brain Res.* 1517, 1–15. doi: 10.1016/j.brainres.2013.04.008

Saint-Pol, J., Vandenhaute, E., Boucau, M. C., Candela, P., Dehouck, L., Cecchelli, R., et al. (2012). Brain pericytes ABCA1 expression mediates cholesterol efflux but not cellular amyloid-β peptide accumulation. *J. Alzheimers Dis.* 30, 489–503. doi: 10.3233/JAD-2012-112090

Schipper, H. M. (2011). Apolipoprotein E: implications for AD neurobiology, epidemiology and risk assessment. *Neurobiol. Aging* 32, 778–790. doi: 10.1016/j.neurobiolaging.2009.04.021

Schönknecht, P., Lütjohann, D., Pantel, J., Bardenheuer, H., Hartmann, T., von Bergmann, K., et al. (2002). Cerebrospinal fluid 24S-hydroxycholesterol is increased in patients with Alzheimer's disease compared to healthy controls. *Neurosci. Lett.* 324, 83–85. doi: 10.1016/s0304-3940(02)00164-7

Serrano-Pozo, A., Muzikansky, A., Gómez-Isla, T., Growdon, J. H., Betensky, R. A., Frosch, M. P., et al. (2013). Differential relationships of reactive astrocytes and microglia to fibrillar amyloid deposits in Alzheimer disease. *J. Neuropathol Exp Neurol.* 72, 462–471. doi: 10.1097/NEN.0b013e3182933788

Shafaati, M., Marutle, A., Pettersson, H., Lövgren-Sandblom, A., Olin, M., Pikuleva, I., et al. (2011). Marked accumulation of 27-hydroxycholesterol in the brains of Alzheimer's patients with the Swedish APP 670/671 mutation. *J. Lipid Res.* 52, 1004–1010. doi: 10.1194/jlr.m014548

Sharma, S., Prasanthi, R. P. J., Schommer, E., Feist, G., and Ghribi, O. (2008). Hypercholesterolemia-induced Abeta accumulation in rabbit brain is associated with alteration in IGF-1 signaling. *Neurobiol. Dis.* 32, 426–432. doi: 10.1016/j.nbd.2008.08.002

Shea, T. B., Rogers, E., Ashline, D., Ortiz, D., and Sheu, M. S. (2002). Apolipoprotein E deficiency promotes increased oxidative stress and compensatory increases in antioxidants in brain tissue. *Free Radic. Biol. Med.* 33, 1115–1120. doi: 10.1016/s0891-5849(02)01001-8

Sheng, J. G., Mrak, R. E., Bales, K. R., Cordell, B., Paul, S. M., and Jones, R. A. (2000). Overexpression of the neuritotrophic cytokine S100beta precedes the appearance of neuritic beta-amyloid plaques in APPV717F mice. *J. Neurochem.* 74, 295–301. doi: 10.1046/j.1471-4159.2000.0740295.x

Shih, A. Y., Johnson, D. A., Wong, G., Kraft, A. D., Jiang, L., Erb, H., et al. (2003). Coordinate regulation of glutathione biosynthesis and release by Nrf2-expressing glia potently protects neurons from oxidative stress. *J. Neurosci.* 23, 3394–3406.

Shobab, L. A., Hsiung, G. Y., and Feldman, H. H. (2005). Cholesterol in Alzheimer's disease. *Lancet Neurol.* 4, 841–852. doi: 10.1016/S1474-4422(05)70248-9

Simard, A. R., Soulet, D., Gowing, G., Julien, J. P., and Rivest, S. (2006). Bone marrow-derived microglia play a critical role in restricting senile plaque formation in Alzheimer's disease. *Neuron* 49, 489–502. doi: 10.1016/j.neuron.2006.01.022

Smith, M. A., Rottkamp, C. A., Nunomura, A., Raina, A. K., and Perry, G. (2000). Oxidative stress in Alzheimer's disease. *Biochim. Biophys. Acta* 1502, 139–144. doi: 10.1016/S0925-4439(00)00040-5

Smith, M. A., Zhu, X., Tabaton, M., Liu, G., McKeel, D. W. Jr., Cohen, M. L., et al. (2010). Increased iron and free radical generation in preclinical Alzheimer disease and mild cognitive impairment. *J. Alzheimers Dis.* 19, 363–372. doi: 10.3233/JAD-2010-1239

Sochocka, M., Koutsouraki, E. S., Gasiorowski, K., and Leszek, J. (2013). Vascular oxidative stress and mitochondrial failure in the pathobiology of Alzheimer's disease: a new approach to therapy. *CNS Neurol. Disord. Drug Targets* 12, 870–881. doi: 10.2174/18715273113129990072

Sodhi, R. K., and Singh, N. (2013). Liver X receptors: emerging therapeutic targets for Alzheimer's disease. *Pharmacol. Res.* 72, 45–51. doi: 10.1016/j.phrs.2013.03.008

Sottero, B., Gamba, P., Gargiulo, S., Leonarduzzi, G., and Poli, G. (2009). Cholesterol oxidation products and disease: an emerging topic of interest in medicinal chemistry. *Curr. Med. Chem.* 16, 685–705. doi: 10.2174/092986709787458353

Sparks, D. L., Kuo, Y. M., Roher, A., Martin, T., and Lukas, R. J. (2000). Alterations of Alzheimer's disease in the cholesterol-fed rabbit, including vascular inflammation. Preliminary observations. *Ann. N Y Acad. Sci.* 903, 335–344. doi: 10.1111/j.1749-6632.2000.tb06384.x

Steffensen, K. R., Jakobsson, T., and Gustafsson, J. Å. (2013). Targeting liver X receptors in inflammation. *Expert Opin. Ther. Targets* 17, 977–990. doi: 10.1517/14728222.2013.806490

Streit, W. J., Xue, Q. S., Braak, H., and del Tredici, K. (2014). Presence of severe neuroinflammation does not intensify neurofibrillary degeneration in human brain. *Glia* 62, 96–105. doi: 10.1002/glia.22589

Stuart, L. M., Bell, S. A., Stewart, C. R., Silver, J. M., Richard, J., Goss, J. L., et al. (2007). CD36 signals to the actin cytoskeleton and regulates microglial migration via a p130Cas complex. *J. Biol. Chem.* 282, 27392–27401. doi: 10.1074/jbc.m702887200

Su, B., Wang, X., Lee, H. G., Tabaton, M., Perry, G., Smith, M. A., et al. (2010). Chronic oxidative stress causes increased tau phosphorylation in M17 neuroblastoma cells. *Neurosci. Lett.* 468, 267–271. doi: 10.1016/j.neulet.2009.11.010

Suzuki, S., Tanaka, K., Nagata, E., Ito, D., Dembo, T., and Fukuuchi, Y. (1999). Cerebral neurons express interleukin-6 after transient forebrain ischemia in gerbils. *Neurosci. Lett.* 262, 117–120. doi: 10.1016/s0304-3940(99)00051-8

Tai, L. M., Ghura, S., Koster, K. P., Liakaite, V., Maienschein-Cline, M., Kanabar, P., et al. (2015). APOE-modulated Aβ-induced neuroinflammation in Alzheimer's disease: current landscape, novel data and future perspective. *J. Neurochem.* 133, 465–488. doi: 10.1111/jnc.13072

Takeda, S., Sato, N., and Morishita, R. (2014). Systemic inflammation, blood-brain barrier vulnerability and cognitive/non-cognitive symptoms in Alzheimer disease: relevance to pathogenesis and therapy. *Front. Aging Neurosci.* 6:171. doi: 10.3389/fnagi.2014.00171

Tamagno, E., Bardini, P., Guglielmotto, M., Danni, O., and Tabaton, M. (2006). The various aggregation states of beta-amyloid 1-42 mediate different effects on oxidative stress, neurodegeneration and BACE-1 expression. *Free Radic Biol. Med.* 41, 202–212. doi: 10.1016/j.freeradbiomed.2006.01.021

Tanzi, R. E., and Bertram, L. (2005). Twenty years of the Alzheimer's disease amyloid hypothesis: a genetic perspective. *Cell* 120, 545–555. doi: 10.1016/j.cell.2005.02.008

Tchelingerian, J. L., Vignais, L., and Jacque, C. (1994). TNF alpha gene expression is induced in neurones after a hippocampal lesion. *Neuroreport* 5, 585–588. doi: 10.1097/00001756-199401000-00013

Terwel, D., Steffensen, K. R., Verghese, P. B., Kummer, M. P., Gustafsson, J. Å., Holtzman, D. M., et al. (2011). Critical role of astroglial apolipoprotein E and liver X receptor-α expression for microglial Aβ phagocytosis. *J. Neurosci.* 31, 7049–7059. doi: 10.1523/JNEUROSCI.6546-10.2011

Testa, G., Gamba, P., Badilli, U., Gargiulo, S., Maina, M., Guina, T., et al. (2014). Loading into nanoparticles improves quercetin's efficacy in preventing neuroinflammation induced by oxysterols. *PLoS One* 9:e96795. doi: 10.1371/journal.pone.0096795

Testa, G., Gamba, P., Di Scipio, F., Sprio, A. E., Salamone, P., Gargiulo, S., et al. (2012). Potentiation of amyloid-β peptide neurotoxicity in human dental neuron-like cells by the membrane lipid peroxidation product 4-hydroxynonenal. *Free Radic. Biol. Med.* 53, 1708–1717. doi: 10.1016/j.freeradbiomed.2012.08.581

Town, T., Nikolic, V., and Tan, J. (2005). The microglial "activation" continuum: from innate to adaptive responses. *J. Neuroinflammation* 2:24. doi: 10.1186/1742-2094-2-24

Urano, Y., Ochiai, S., and Noguchi, N. (2013). Suppression of amyloid-β production by 24S-hydroxycholesterol via inhibition of intracellular amyloid precursor protein trafficking. *FASEB J.* 27, 4305–4315. doi: 10.1096/fj.13-231456

Usui, K., Hulleman, J. D., Paulsson, J. F., Siegel, S. J., Powers, E. T., and Kelly, J. W. (2009). Site-specific modification of Alzheimer's peptides by cholesterol oxidation products enhances aggregation energetics and neurotoxicity. *Proc. Natl. Acad. Sci. U S A* 106, 18563–18568. doi: 10.1073/pnas.0804758106

Vance, J. E., Hayashi, H., and Karten, B. (2005). Cholesterol homeostasis in neurons and glial cells. *Semin. Cell Dev. Biol.* 16, 193–212. doi: 10.1016/j.semcdb.2005.01.005

Vaya, J., and Schipper, H. M. (2007). Oxysterols, cholesterol homeostasis and Alzheimer disease. *J. Neurochem.* 102, 1727–1737. doi: 10.1111/j.1471-4159.2007.04689.x

Verdier, Y., Zarándi, M., and Penke, B. (2004). Amyloid beta-peptide interactions with neuronal and glial cell plasma membrane: binding sites and implications for Alzheimer's disease. *J. Pept. Sci.* 10, 229–248. doi: 10.1002/psc.573

Vetrivel, K. S., and Thinakaran, G. (2010). Membrane rafts in Alzheimer's disease beta-amyloid production. *Biochim. Biophys. Acta.* 1801, 860–867. doi: 10.1016/j.bbalip.2010.03.007

Voloshyna, I., and Reiss, A. B. (2011). The ABC transporters in lipid flux and atherosclerosis. *Prog. Lipid Res.* 50, 213–224. doi: 10.1016/j.plipres.2011.02.001

von Bernhardi, R., Tichauer, J. E., and Eugenín, J. (2010). Aging-dependent changes of microglial cells and their relevance for neurodegenerative disorders. *J. Neurochem.* 112, 1099–1114. doi: 10.1111/j.1471-4159.2009.06537.x

Vukic, V., Callaghan, D., Walker, D., Lue, L. F., Liu, Q. Y., Couraud, P. O., et al. (2009). Expression of inflammatory genes induced by beta-amyloid peptides in human brain endothelial cells and in Alzheimer's brain is mediated by the JNK-AP1 signaling pathway. *Neurobiol. Dis.* 34, 95–106. doi: 10.1016/j.nbd.2008.12.007

Wahrle, S., Das, P., Nyborg, A. C., McLendon, C., Shoji, M., Kawarabayashi, T., et al. (2002). Cholesterol-dependent gamma-secretase activity in buoyant cholesterol-rich membrane microdomains. *Neurobiol. Dis.* 9, 11–23. doi: 10.1006/nbdi.2001.0470

Wahrle, S. E., Jiang, H., Parsadanian, M., Kim, J., Li, A., Knoten, A., et al. (2008). Overexpression of ABCA1 reduces amyloid deposition in the PDAPP mouse model of Alzheimer disease. *J. Clin. Invest.* 118, 671–682. doi: 10.1172/jci33622

Wahrle, S. E., Jiang, H., Parsadanian, M., Legleiter, J., Han, X., Fryer, J. D., et al. (2004). ABCA1 is required for normal central nervous system APOE levels and for lipidation of astrocyte-secreted APOE. *J. Biol. Chem.* 279, 40987–40993. doi: 10.1074/jbc.m407963200

Walsh, D. M., and Selkoe, D. J. (2007). A beta oligomers - a decade of discovery. *J. Neurochem.* 101, 1172–1184. doi: 10.1111/j.1471-4159.2006.04426.x

Waltl, S., Patankar, J. V., Fauler, G., Nusshold, C., Ullen, A., Eibinger, G., et al. (2013). 25-Hydroxycholesterol regulates cholesterol homeostasis in the murine CATH.a neuronal cell line. *Neurosci. Lett.* 539, 16–21. doi: 10.1016/j.neulet.2013.01.014

Wang, L., Schuster, G. U., Hultenby, K., Zhang, Q., Andersson, S., and Gustafsson, J. A. (2002). Liver X receptors in the central nervous system: from lipid homeostasis to neuronal degeneration. *Proc. Natl. Acad. Sci. U S A* 99, 13878–13883. doi: 10.1073/pnas.172510899

Wang, N., Yvan-Charvet, L., Lütjohann, D., Mulder, M., Vanmierlo, T., Kim, T. W., et al. (2008). ATP-binding cassette transporters G1 and G4 mediate cholesterol and desmosterol efflux to HDL and regulate sterol accumulation in the brain. *FASEB J.* 22, 1073–1082. doi: 10.1096/fj.07-9944com

Wang, Y., Li, M., Tang, J., Song, M., Xu, X., Xiong, J., et al. (2011). Glucocorticoids facilitate astrocytic amyloid-β peptide deposition by increasing the expression of APP and BACE1 and decreasing the expression of amyloid-β-degrading proteases. *Endocrinology* 152, 2704–2715. doi: 10.1210/en.2011-0145

Wegiel, J., Imaki, H., Wang, K. C., Wegiel, J., and Rubenstein, R. (2004). Cells of monocyte/microglial lineage are involved in both microvessel amyloidosis and fibrillar plaque formation in APPsw tg mice. *Brain Res.* 1022, 19–29. doi: 10.1016/j.brainres.2004.06.058

Weitz, T. M., and Town, T. (2012). Microglia in Alzheimer's Disease: It's All About Context. *Int. J. Alzheimers Dis.* 2012:314185. doi: 10.1155/2012/314185

Wood, W. G., Li, L., Müller, W. E., and Eckert, G. P. (2014). Cholesterol as a causative factor in Alzheimer's disease: a debatable hypothesis. *J. Neurochem.* 129, 559–572. doi: 10.1111/jnc.12637

Xiong, H., Callaghan, D., Jones, A., Walker, D. G., Lue, L. F., Beach, T. G., et al. (2008). Cholesterol retention in Alzheimer's brain is responsible for high beta- and gamma-secretase activities and Abeta production. *Neurobiol. Dis.* 29, 422–437. doi: 10.1016/j.nbd.2007.10.005

Xu, Q., Bernardo, A., Walker, D., Kanegawa, T., Mahley, R. W., and Huang, Y. (2006). Profile and regulation of apolipoprotein E (ApoE) expression in the CNS in mice with targeting of green fluorescent protein gene to the ApoE locus. *J. Neurosci.* 26, 4985–4994. doi: 10.1523/jneurosci.5476-05.2006

Yamanaka, K., Saito, Y., Yamamori, T., Urano, Y., and Noguchi, N. (2011). 24(S)-hydroxycholesterol induces neuronal cell death through necroptosis, a form of programmed necrosis. *J. Biol. Chem.* 286, 24666–24673. doi: 10.1074/jbc.m111.236273

Yan, S. D., Yan, S. F., Chen, X., Fu, J., Chen, M., Kuppusamy, P., et al. (1995). Non-enzymatically glycated tau in Alzheimer's disease induces neuronal oxidant stress resulting in cytokine gene expression and release of amyloid beta-peptide. *Nat. Med.* 1, 693–699. doi: 10.1038/nm0795-693

Yanagisawa, K. (2005). Cholesterol and amyloid beta fibrillogenesis. *Subcell. Biochem.* 38, 179–202. doi: 10.1007/0-387-23226-5_9

Yao, J., Irwin, R. W., Zhao, L., Nilsen, J., Hamilton, R. T., and Brinton, R. D. (2009). Mitochondrial bioenergetic deficit precedes Alzheimer's pathology in female mouse model of Alzheimer's disease. *Proc. Natl. Acad. Sci. U S A* 106, 14670–14675. doi: 10.1073/pnas.0903563106

Yau, J. L., Rasmuson, S., Andrew, R., Graham, M., Noble, J., Olsson, T., et al. (2003). Dehydroepiandrosterone 7-hydroxylase CYP7B: predominant expression in primate hippocampus and reduced expression in Alzheimer's disease. *Neuroscience* 121, 307–314. doi: 10.1016/s0306-4522(03)00438-x

Ye, S., Huang, Y., Müllendorff, K., Dong, L., Giedt, G., Meng, E. C., et al. (2005). Apolipoprotein (apo) E4 enhances amyloid beta peptide production in cultured neuronal cells: apoE structure as a potential therapeutic target. *Proc. Natl. Acad. Sci. U S A* 102, 18700–18705. doi: 10.1073/pnas.0508693102

Yoshimoto, N., Tasaki, M., Shimanouchi, T., Umakoshi, H., and Kuboi, R. (2005). Oxidation of cholesterol catalyzed by amyloid beta-peptide (Abeta)-Cu complex on lipid membrane. *J. Biosci. Bioeng.* 100, 455–459. doi: 10.1263/jbb.100.455

Yu, Y., and Ye, R. D. (2015). Microglial Aβ receptors in Alzheimer's disease. *Cell Mol. Neurobiol.* 35, 71–83. doi: 10.1007/s10571-014-0101-6

Zelcer, N., Khanlou, N., Clare, R., Jiang, Q., Reed-Geaghan, E. G., Landreth, G. E., et al. (2007). Attenuation of neuroinflammation and Alzheimer's disease pathology by liver x receptors. *Proc. Natl. Acad. Sci. U S A* 104, 10601–10606. doi: 10.1073/pnas.0701096104

Zhu, X., Lee, H. G., Casadesus, G., Avila, J., Drew, K., Perry, G., et al. (2005). Oxidative imbalance in Alzheimer's disease. *Mol. Neurobiol.* 31, 205–217. doi: 10.1385/mn:31:1-3:205

Zhu, X., Su, B., Wang, X., Smith, M. A., and Perry, G. (2007). Causes of oxidative stress in Alzheimer disease. *Cell. Mol. Life Sci.* 64, 2202–2210. doi: 10.1007/s00018-007-7218-4

16

Age-Related Inter-Region EEG Coupling Changes During the Control of Bottom–Up and Top–Down Attention

Ling Li and Dandan Zhao*

Key Laboratory for NeuroInformation of Ministry of Education, School of Life Science and Technology, University of Electronic Science and Technology of China, Chengdu, China

Edited by:
Junfeng Sun, Shanghai Jiao Tong University, China

Reviewed by:
Yu (Aaron) Tang, The University of Texas Southwestern Medical Center, USA
Jesse Jon Bengson, Center for Mind and Brain, USA

***Correspondence:**
Ling Li
liling@uestc.edu.cn

We investigated age-related changes in electroencephalographic (EEG) coupling of theta-, alpha-, and beta-frequency bands during bottom–up and top–down attention. Arrays were presented with either automatic "pop-out" (bottom–up) or effortful "search" (top–down) behavior to younger and older participants. The phase-locking value was used to estimate coupling strength between scalp recordings. Behavioral performance decreased with age, with a greater age-related decline in accuracy for the search than for the pop-out condition. Aging was associated with a declined coupling strength of theta and alpha frequency bands, with a greater age-related decline in whole-brain coupling values for the search than for the pop-out condition. Specifically, prefronto-frontal coupling in theta- and alpha-bands, fronto-parietal and parieto-occipital couplings in beta-band for younger group showed a right hemispheric dominance, which was reduced with aging to compensate for the inhibitory dysfunction. While pop-out target detection was mainly associated with greater parieto-occipital beta-coupling strength compared to search condition regardless of aging. Furthermore, prefronto-frontal coupling in theta-, alpha-, and beta-bands, and parieto-occipital coupling in beta-band functioned as predictors of behavior for both groups. Taken together these findings provide evidence that prefronto-frontal coupling of theta-, alpha-, and beta-bands may serve as a possible basis of aging during visual attention, while parieto-occipital coupling in beta-band could serve for a bottom–up function and be vulnerable to top–down attention control for younger and older groups.

Keywords: aging, electroencephalographic (EEG), visual pop-out, visual search, control of attention, inter-region phase coupling, theta, alpha

INTRODUCTION

Normal aging is associated with decline in the performance of a variety of cognitive functions, including effects observed in the visual search (Plude and Doussard-Roosevelt, 1989) and in the tasks involving both bottom–up attention and top–down attention, with a more prominent decline in tasks emphasizing top–down attention control (Greenwood et al., 1997; Kok, 2000; Madden et al., 2005; Madden, 2007; Lien et al., 2011; Li et al., 2013). Normal aging is correlated with changes in neural structure, including decline in brain volume (Scahill et al., 2003; Fotenos et al., 2008) and gray and white matter volumes (Raz et al., 2005; Gordon et al., 2008). Age-related losses in gray and white matter in medial-temporal, parietal, and frontal areas were reported. Hypotheses of age-related brain functional changes mainly include Compensation Related Utilization of Neural Circuits Hypothesis (CRUNCH) (Reuter-Lorenz and Lustig, 2005; Grady, 2008; Reuter-Lorenz and Cappell, 2008) and dedifferentiation hypothesis (Madden et al., 2007).

A variety of functional imaging, neurophysiological and neuropsychological studies have provided compelling evidence that frontoparietal networks play important roles in both top–down cognitive and bottom–up sensory factors of attention control (Corbetta and Shulman, 2002; Giesbrecht et al., 2003; Bledowski et al., 2004a,b Buschman and Miller, 2007; Husain and Nachev, 2007; Knudsen, 2007; Li et al., 2010). An aging study of visual attention has reported that older adults showed increased magnitude and spread of activity in fronto-parietal regions compared with younger adults, suggesting a compensation for a decline in overall bottom–up sensory input (dedifferentiation; Madden et al., 2007; see reviews Reuter-Lorenz and Park, 2010). However, activity decreases with aging in frontal cortex (Anderson et al., 2000; Milham et al., 2002; Johnson et al., 2004) and occipital cortex (Madden et al., 2004) were also reported in attention studies, pointing to an age-related decline in allocation of attentional resources efficiency (Lorenzo-López et al., 2008) or reduction in inhibitory control functions in attention (Colcombe et al., 2003; Madden et al., 2004; Andrés et al., 2006; Hasher et al., 2008). Performance has been found associated with fronto-parietal activation for older adults and with occipital activation for younger adults in top–down attention (Madden et al., 2007), but with prefrontal activation for younger adults and with deep gray matter structures for older adults in visual target detection (Madden et al., 2004). Increased activities in frontal regions associated with improved performance (Grady et al., 2002; Madden et al., 2004; Lorenzo-López et al., 2008; Vallesi et al., 2010), or with decreased performance (Madden et al., 2005) in older adults have also been reported in certain tasks. The CRUNCH interprets these contradictory results at some degree, whereby older adults use more or new neural circuits to accomplish tasks compared to younger adults.

A functional imaging study shows that aging is associated with decreased connectivity between areas within the fronto-parietal control network and between areas within the somatomotor network in a selective attention task, but with increased connectivity between the fronto-parietal and somatomotor network (Geerligs et al., 2014). Functional connectivity decreases with aging within the fronto-parietal regions during cue processing under executive control was reported (Madden et al., 2010). There has been study showing both selective increases between visual attention regions and supplementary motor area and decreases between sensorimotor systems and supplementary motor area in resting-state functional connectivity with age (Roski et al., 2013). In summary, aging is associated with lower connectivity within task-relevant networks and greater connectivity between the task-relevant networks and outside networks by functional imaging studies (Madden et al., 2005, 2010; Dennis et al., 2008; St Jacques et al., 2009; Geerligs et al., 2014), supporting the CRUNCH that older adults use more or new neural circuits to compensate for age-related decline.

In electrocephalogram (EEG) studies, older adults show reduced frontal theta activity during sustained attentional processes, and reduced theta connectivity strength within frontal regions and between frontal midline and temporal cortices during working memory maintenance (Kardos et al., 2014). Decreased posterior alpha activation in an attention network test (Deiber et al., 2013) and reduced beta activation in a visual attentional task correlated to alertness and sustaining attentional processes (Gola et al., 2012, 2013) with aging were reported. Aging is associated with decreased modularity and clustering and increased connectedness of anterior nodes in beta-band network during resting condition, pointing to a compensation of the anterior atentional system (Knyazev et al., 2015). These findings provide evidence that aging modulates distinct neural circuits at different oscillatory frequencies during attention functions. There is, however, relatively little evidence directly investigating aging-related functional connectivity by EEG in bottom–up and top–down attention together.

We used a paradigm based on a study in non-human primates by Buschman and Miller (2007) to investigate age-related coupling of different frequency bands during top-down and bottom-up attention control. Arrays were presented with either automatic "pop-out" (bottom–up) or effortful "search" (top–down) behavior to younger and older participants. Buschman and Miller found that fronto-extrastriate coherences were greater in the search than in the pop-out condition at low gamma-band (22–34 Hz) and parietal–extrastriate coherences were greater in the pop-out than in the search condition at high gamma-band (35–55 Hz). In a human EEG study, a double dissociation was reported, with significantly increased power from 4 to 24 Hz in parietal areas for pop-out targets and increased power from 4 to 24 Hz in frontal regions for search targets (Li et al., 2010). Greater frontal-parietal synchrony at low gamma-band frequencies for inefficient than efficient visual search were reported (Phillips and Takeda, 2009). Based on above neuroimaging and electrophysiology literatures, as well as the results from our previous studies (Li et al., 2010, 2013), we expected the differential roles of fronto-parieto-occipital connectivity at different lower oscillatory frequencies under both types of attention for younger and older groups. The purpose of the present study was to examine the effects of aging on functional connectivity at different oscillatory frequencies during visual search and simultaneously compare the fronto-parieto-occipital connectivity during top–down and bottom–up attention. We hypothesized that (a) aging and search condition are associated with decreases in connectivity due to a slowing in performance, and (b) connectivity at different oscillatory frequencies plays a differential role contributing to group and attentional control.

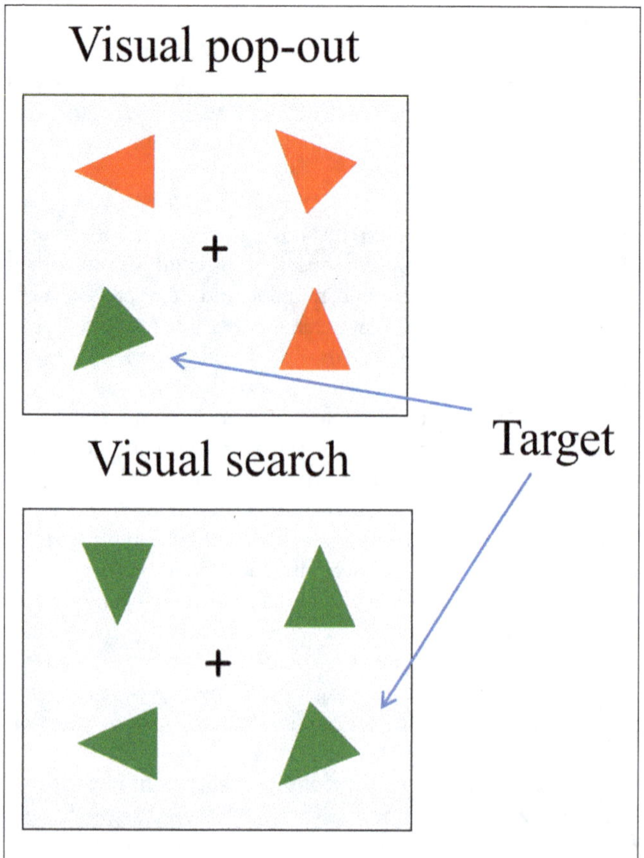

FIGURE 1 | An example of the stimulus array in the two experimental conditions. Each trial includes a target. In the **(up panel)**, the distractors differ from the target in both color and orientation, so that target detection is highly efficient and easy. In this pop-out condition, search is influenced primarily by the bottom–up attention. In the **(down panel)**, the distractors differ from the target only in orientation, so that target detection is less efficient and difficult. In this search condition, target detection is controlled mainly by top–down attention.

MATERIALS AND METHODS

Subjects

We utilized data reported in a previous study (Li et al., 2013) consisting of 13 younger subjects (6 females, mean age ± standard deviation = 23.9 ± 4.3 years, range from 18 to 35 years old) and 13 older subjects (6 females, mean age ± standard deviation = 63.1 ± 6.2 years, range from 52 to 75 years old). The mean numbers of years of education for the younger and older subjects were 15.9 ± 2.5 and 16.0 ± 2.2 years respectively. All the subjects were right-handed, had normal color vision, and had no history of neurological problems. None of the subjects were taking any psychotropic, neurological, or psychiatric medications at the time of testing. The experimental procedures were approved by the Committee for the Protection of Human Subjects for the University of California, Berkeley. Written Informed consent was obtained from all subjects prior to being tested.

Stimuli and Procedure

The stimuli were made up of 16 acute isosceles triangles, each with a particular color (red or green) and orientation [one of eight, (i-1) × 45°, $i = 1, 2, 3, 4, 5, 6, 7, 8$]. The triangles had two equal sides 6.5 cm in length and a third side 5.5 cm long, with an area of 16.20 cm × 16.20 cm. **Figure 1** illustrates an example of the stimulus sequence. After a 500 ms fixation cross, a target triangle (one of 16 triangles) appeared in the center of the screen for 1000 ms and was followed by a short 500 ms delay screen with a fixation cross. After the delay, a four stimulus array was presented, consisting of the target and three distracter triangles in the four quadrants of the screen. The target was randomly presented in one of these locations (upper-left, lower-left, upper-right, and lower-right). The center of each triangle was 6.2 cm vertical (either up or down) from the horizontal midline and 8.2 cm lateral (either right or left) from the vertical midline, resulting in stimuli at a visual angle of 5.34° from fixation. The array remained on the screen until a response and was followed by a 1000 ms fixation to show the end of the trial. Three distractor triangles were chosen to create the two main attention conditions in the experiment: "pop-out" and "search." The pop-out condition was created using distracters that differed from the target in both color and orientation (Treisman and Gelade, 1980), while the search condition was created by using distracters that differed from the target only in orientation. Half of the trials were in the pop-out condition and half were in the search condition. Half of the targets were presented in left visual field and half were in right visual field.

Subjects were asked to centrally fixate throughout the recording and to respond as quickly as possible whether the target was to the left or right of fixation. Participants used their right-hand for responding by pressing either button 1 for left or 2 for right from a computer key pad. Participants performed two practice blocks before starting the experiment and extra practice blocks were given as required until subjects were able to reach a mean accuracy of 80% in the task. After the practice, 12 experimental blocks comprising 32 trials each lasting about 2.5 min were run. There were 1–2 min breaks between blocks, with longer breaks every three blocks. E-prime (Psychology Software Tools, Pittsburgh, PA, USA) was used to present the stimuli and analyze the behavioral data.

Data Recording and Preprocessing

EEG was recorded by an ActiveTwo system (Biosemi, The Netherlands) with a 64 channel electrode cap. Right and left earlobes and four electrooculogram (EOG) were simultaneously recorded. EEG data were off-line referenced to the average of the right and left earlobes. EOG was measured from an electrode above and below the right eye to record vertical eye movements and electrodes on the outer canthus of each eye to measure horizontal eye movements. All channels were amplified with an analog bandpass filter of 0.06–208 Hz and were digitized at 1024 Hz.

Matlab was used for all data processing. Re-referenced EEG signals were filtered from 0.5 to 55 Hz with a two-way FIR bandpass filter (eegfilt.m from EEGLAB toolbox, Delorme and

Makeig, 2004) and segmented from 200 ms before the onset of the stimulus (visual array) to 1000 ms after the stimulus. Trials were rejected if they had an incorrect response or lacked a button press between 200 and 1500 ms (younger adults) or 200–2000 ms (older adults) after the onset of the stimulus array. Epochs with EOG artifacts were removed if there was a difference in amplitude between the two vertical EOG or between the two horizontal EOG of greater than 100 μV, or if there was more than 3 standard deviations (SDs) from the mean of the EOG difference wave. For each epoch, the linear drift was removed and the data was baseline corrected using the 200 ms pre-stimulus period. Finally, any epoch with a channel containing amplitudes of more than four standard deviations from the epoch mean was rejected. After above preprocessing, 537 trials remained for left pop-out targets, 480 trials remained for right pop-out targets, 479 trials remained for left visual search targets, and 424 trials remained for right search targets for the younger participants. 417 trials remained for left pop-out targets, 402 trials remained for right pop-out targets, 332 trials remained for left visual search targets, and 344 trials remained for right search targets for the older participants. These trials were used for ERP analysis (see in Li et al., 2010, 2013) and for the current EEG coupling analysis. At least 25 trials were included in the average for each condition.

EEG Cross-channel Coupling Analysis

To minimize the contribution of volume conduction and remove spurious coupling (Nunez et al., 1997; Lachaux et al., 1999), the following steps were applied to single trial of EEG data before the computation of the phase synchrony. Step 1: each single trial of 4 conditions (2 × 2, target condition and visual field) of every subject for both groups was filtered by the band-pass finite impulse response filters at 4 Hz intervals between 4 and 40 Hz. Totally signals of 9 frequency bands EEG were obtained. Step 2: we used a current source density (CSD) toolbox of MATLAB supplied by Kayser J. (http://psychophysiology.cpmc.columbia.edu/Software/CSDtoolbox/index.html) that implemented a spherical spline algorithm of Perrin et al. to estimate scalp current density (SCD) for EEG data (Perrin et al., 1989; Kayser and Tenke, 2006). The spline interpolation constant was set to 4.

After above SCD computation, the data from 200 ms before the onset of stimuli array to 1000 ms after the stimuli were used to estimate long-range neural phase synchrony in nine frequency bands by calculating phase-locking value (PLV). The PLV has been used to measure the bivariate phase synchronization in a number of EEG studies (Mormann et al., 2000; Quian Quiroga et al., 2002; Knyazev et al., 2015). The PLV between electrodes j and k, at each sample time t, across the N trials, were quantified as $PLV_{j,k,t}=\left|\frac{1}{N}\sum_{N} e^{i[\varphi_j(t)-\varphi_k(t)]}\right|$. Instantaneous phase $\varphi(t)$ of a signal was estimated by Hilbert transform.

The PLV takes on values between 0 and 1, but the PLV must first be normalized before it can be used as a metric of cross-electrode coupling strength. That is, we are interested in the properties of the distribution of phase difference between two electrodes. One way is to compare the actual mean PLV with a set of surrogate PLV created by offsetting phase of one signal by some large time lag. Two hundred surrogate PLV values for each frequency and time point were calculated, and the mean and standard deviation of surrogate PLV were estimated. Therefore, the normalized PLV [(real PLV – mean of surrogate PLV)/standard deviation of surrogate PLV] were defined as the modulation index used in this paper. For a given number of sample points, we can directly compare this normalized PLV for cross-electrode coupling strength across different pairs as well as different frequency bands which may have very different power levels. The normalized PLV index was computed for all pair-wise combinations of channels, generating 2016 (totally 64 channels) index values for each time point in 9 frequency bands in each condition for both groups. With $\alpha = 0.01$ and $N = 2016$ comparisons, an index value greater than 4.42 was required for significance by Bonferroni correction for multiple comparisons.

Statistical Analysis

Behavioral data were analyzed with a repeated measure ANOVA with condition (pop-out and search) and target visual field (left and right) as the within-subject factors and age (young and old) as the between-subject factor, followed by Bonferroni corrected t-tests if necessary with p-value <0.05 as a significant threshold.

Mean normalized PLV values and mean numbers of connection were calculated first by the mean of whole-brain significant coupling values in 0–600 ms time-window. Then mean normalized PLV multiplied by mean numbers of connection to obtain total coupling values. Finally, the total coupling values were analyzed with a repeated measure ANOVA with condition (pop-out and search) and target visual field (left and right) as the within-subject factors and age (young and old) as the between-subject factor for 9 frequency bands.

Eight regions of interest (ROIs) were selected including left prefrontal (Fp1, AF7, AF3, F5, F3, F1), right prefrontal (Fp2, AF8, AF4, F6, F4, F2), left central-frontal (FC5, FC3, FC1, C5, C3, C1), right central-frontal (FC6, FC4, FC2, C6, C4, C2), left central-parietal (CP5, CP3, CP1, P5, P3, P1), right central-parietal (CP6, CP4, CP2, P6, P4, P2), left parietal-occipital (PO7, PO3, O1), and right parieto-occipital (PO8, PO4, O2) regions (see **Figure 2**). Max normalized PLV values for all pair-wise combinations of eight regions of interest were calculated, generating 28 (totally 8 ROIs) index values for frequency bands of interest in four conditions for both groups. With $\alpha = 0.05$ and $N = 28$ comparisons, an index value greater than 2.91 was required for significance by Bonferroni correction for multiple comparisons. Each significant connectivity between ROIs were then analyzed with a repeated measure ANOVA with condition (pop-out and search) and target visual field (left and right) as the within-subject factors and age (young and old) as the between-subject factor for frequency bands of interest.

Linear relationship between above coupling values and behaviors were then tested by Pearson correlation coefficient for four conditions in both groups in each frequency band, respectively.

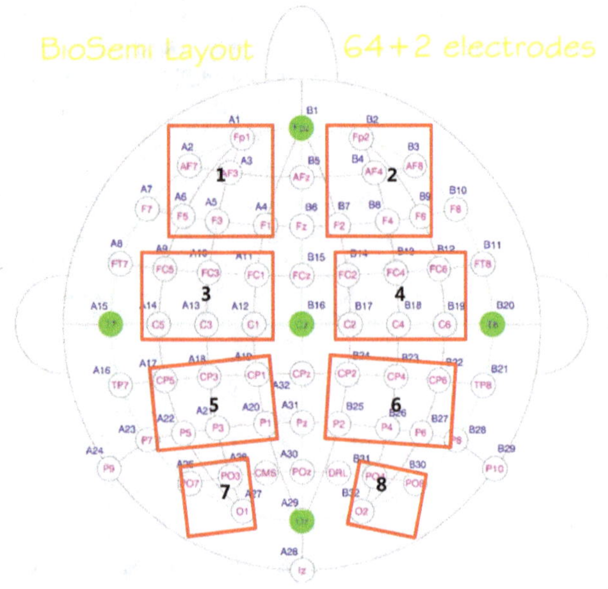

FIGURE 2 | Eight regions of interest (ROIs, marked by red rectangles) for inter-region analysis were selected including left prefrontal (Fp1, AF7, AF3, F5, F3, F1), right prefrontal (Fp2, AF8, AF4, F6, F4, F2), Left central-frontal (FC5, FC3, FC1, C5, C3, C1), right central-frontal (FC6, FC4, FC2, C6, C4, C2), Left central-parietal (CP5, CP3, CP1, P5, P3, P1), right central-parietal (CP6, CP4, CP2, P6, P4, P2), Left parietal-occipital (PO7, PO3, O1), and right parieto-occipital (PO8, PO4, O2) regions.

RESULTS

Behavioral Results

Mean reaction times (RTs) and accuracy rates are summarized in **Table 1** (mean ± standard deviation). There was a main effect of age (young and old), condition (pop-out and search), and target visual field (left and right) on mean RTs [age effect: $F(1,24) = 31.35$, $p < 0.001$; condition effect: $F(1,24) = 786.05$, $p < 0.001$; target visual field effect: $F(1,24) = 5.70$, $p = 0.025$, ANOVA], with slower RTs in the older subjects and in the search condition and in the left visual field target. However, there was no significant interaction in RTs among age, condition and target visual field. A main effect of age and condition was observed on accuracy rates [age effect: $F(1,24) = 19.75$, $p < 0.001$; condition effect: $F(1,24) = 88.55$, $p < 0.001$], with higher accuracy overall in the younger group and in the pop-out condition. There was a significant interaction in accuracy between age and condition [$F(1,24) = 14.28, p = 0.001$], showing an increased decline in accuracy for the older compared with the younger subjects in the search condition compared with the pop-out condition.

Reaction times and accuracy rates were assessed using a two-way repeated ANOVA with condition and target visual field for both groups, respectively. There was only a main effect of condition on mean RTs and accuracy rates for younger group [RTs: $F(1,12) = 449.51$, $p < 0.0001$; accuracy rates: $F(1,12) = 30.95$, $p < 0.001$], with quicker RTs and higher accuracy in the pop-out condition. For older group, there was a main effect of condition on mean RTs and accuracy rates [RTs: $F(1,12) = 355.06$, $p < 0.0001$; accuracy rates: $F(1,12) = 58.46$, $p < 0.001$], with quicker RTs and higher accuracy in the pop-out condition, and there was a main effect of target visual field only on RTs [$F(1,12) = 5.06, p = 0.044$], with slower RTs in the left visual field target.

EEG Coupling Results

Whole-brain Total Coupling Values

Supplementary Table S1 summarizes the statistical effects of three factors of age, condition, and target visual field and interaction on the total coupling values for 9 frequency bands. As can be seen in Supplementary Table S1, there was a main effect of age for total coupling values only in the theta and alpha bands [theta band: $F(1,24) = 9.28$, $p = 0.006$; alpha band: $F(1,24) = 5.89$, $p = 0.023$], and there was a main effect of condition in almost all frequency bands. Since there was not any effect of age or any interaction effect between age and other factors in the higher frequency bands (24–40 Hz), we did not report these results in the following analyses. In three beta bands (12–24 Hz) there was an interaction between age and target visual field, so that we averaged their coupling values as one beta band to analyze. Hence, the frequency bands of interest were theta (4–8 Hz), alpha (8–12 Hz), and beta (12–24 Hz) activities.

Table 2 presents the total coupling values of whole-brain in the theta, alpha, and beta frequency bands of two target visual fields for the pop-out and search conditions in younger

TABLE 1 | Behavioral results (mean ± SD).

Condition	Target visual field	RT (ms)		Accuracy (%)	
		Young	Old	Young	Old
Visual pop-out	Left	487.74 ± 106.82	704.91 ± 97.57	99.03 ± 1.16	97.75 ± 1.64
	Right	476.44 ± 94.39	678.11 ± 96.20	99.20 ± 0.87	98.16 ± 1.60
Visual search	Left	775.67 ± 129.86	1025.53 ± 74.26	92.74 ± 4.75	81.15 ± 9.35
	Right	768.45 ± 106.63	979.53 ± 148.64	93.13 ± 3.88	85.80 ± 7.64

Mean reaction times (RT, ms) and accurate rates (%) and their corresponding standard deviations as a function of condition and target visual field in younger and older subjects.

and older participants. For theta frequency band, there was a main effect of age (young and old) and target visual field (left and right), with bigger coupling values in the younger subjects only for search condition [independent t-tests, pop-out and left: $t_{(24)} = 2.39$, Bonferroni corrected $p > 0.05$; pop-out and right: $t_{(24)} = 2.23$, corrected $p > 0.05$; search and left: $t_{(24)} = 3.57$, corrected $p < 0.05$; search and right: $t_{(24)} = 2.79$, corrected $p < 0.05$]. There was an interaction between age and visual target field [$F(1,24) = 6.50$, $p = 0.018$], so that we tested two-way repeated measure ANOVA for the total coupling values with condition (pop-out and search) and target visual field (left and right) as the within-subject factors for both groups, respectively. There was only a main effect of target visual field for younger group [$F(1,24) = 9.26$, $p = 0.01$], with bigger coupling values in the left visual field target for pop-out condition [Paired t-tests, pop-out: $t_{(12)} = 2.74$, corrected $p < 0.05$; search: $t_{(12)} = 2.18$, corrected $p > 0.05$], but no such effect was present for the elderly group.

For alpha frequency band, there was a main effect of age and a marginal effect of condition on the total coupling values (Supplementary Table S1), and there was no significant interaction among age, condition and target visual field. The total coupling values were smaller for older compared to younger adults only in search condition [independent t-tests, pop-out and left: $t_{(24)} = 1.81$, corrected $p > 0.05$; pop-out and right: $t_{(24)} = 1.74$, corrected $p > 0.05$; search and left: $t_{(24)} = 3.52$, corrected $p < 0.05$; search and right: $t_{(24)} = 2.63$, corrected $p < 0.05$].

For beta frequency band, there was a main effect of condition [$F(1,24) = 7.10$, $p = 0.014$] and target visual field [$F(1,24) = 4.52$, $p = 0.044$], but no main effect was present in age. There was an interaction between age and visual target field [$F(1,24) = 6.40$, $p = 0.018$], so that we tested two-way repeated measure ANOVA for the total coupling values with condition (pop-out and search) and target visual field (left and right) as the within-subject factors for both groups, respectively. There was only a main effect of target visual field for younger group [$F(1,24) = 9.20$, $p = 0.01$], with bigger coupling values in the left visual field target for search condition [Paried t-tests, pop-out: $t_{(12)} = 2.23$, corrected $p > 0.05$; search: $t_{(12)} = 2.40$, corrected $p < 0.05$], but no such effect was present for the elderly group.

Supplementary Figure S1 illustrates the presence of significant positive linear relationship within the older adults between total coupling values and RTs in the pop-out condition with left visual field target in theta frequency band [Pearson correlation coefficient $(r) = 0.588$, $p = 0.035$]. A regression was used to test whether a quadratic relationship also contributed to the variance, but it was not significant [$r = 0.605$, $p = 0.103$]. All other correlation between total coupling values and RTs or accuracies was not significant ($p > 0.05$).

ROIs Coupling Value in Theta Frequency Band

Max normalized PLV values for all pair-wise combinations of eight regions of interest were calculated, generating 28 (totally 8 ROIs) index values for theta band (4–8 Hz) in four conditions for both groups. **Figure 3A** summarizes the main effect of age (blue line) and condition (red line) among eight regions of interest. As can be seen in **Figure 3A**, there was a main effect of age for coupling values on five long range connections, including the connections between left prefrontal and left central-frontal regions [1 and 3, $F(1,24) = 6.14$, $p = 0.02$], between right prefrontal and right central-frontal regions [2 and 4, $F(1,24) = 4.73$, $p = 0.04$], between right central-frontal and right central-parietal regions [4 and 6, $F(1,24) = 5.43$, $p = 0.03$], between left central-parietal and left parietal-occipital [5 and 7, $F(1,24) = 11.47$, $p = 0.002$], between right central-parietal and right parieto-occipital regions [6 and 8, $F(1,24) = 5.60$, $p = 0.04$], with smaller coupling values in older subjects. There was a main effect of condition for coupling values between left central-frontal and left central-parietal regions [3 and 5, $F(1,24) = 6.64$, $p = 0.017$], with smaller coupling values in the search condition.

For the connection between left prefrontal and central-frontal regions, there was an interaction between age and target visual field [$F(1,24) = 7.88$, $p < 0.001$], and there was no significant effect of condition. Hence we averaged the coupling values of the pop-out and search conditions, and applied repeated measure ANOVA with target visual field (left and right) as the within-subject factor and age (young and old) as the between-subject factor. **Figure 3B** shows the coupling values in both groups for both target fields. There was a main effect of age [$F(1,24) = 6.14$, $p = 0.02$] and an interaction between age and target field [$F(1,24) = 16.63$, $p < 0.001$], with bigger coupling values in left target than in right target for younger subjects [Paried t-tests, $t_{(12)} = 3.28$, $p = 0.007$] and bigger coupling values in right target than in left target for older subjects [Paried t-tests, $t_{(12)} = 2.43$, $p = 0.032$].

TABLE 2 | The total coupling values for all pair-wise combinations of electrodes in the theta, alpha, and beta frequency bands (mean ± SEM).

Condition	Target visual field	Theta band (4–8 Hz)		Alpha band (8–12 Hz)		Beta band (12–24 Hz)	
		Young	Old	Young	Old	Young	Old
Pop-out	Left	488.98 ± 64.69	270.28 ± 64.69	724.80 ± 130.16	391.14 ± 130.16	586.45 ± 81.01	433.29 ± 81.01
	Right	422.78 ± 55.43	248.36 ± 55.43	712.57 ± 137.41	375.45 ± 137.41	503.33 ± 74.08	410.13 ± 74.08
Search	Left	445.81 ± 52.71	179.77 ± 52.71	599.18 ± 70.38	249.36 ± 70.38	489.66 ± 56.17	277.76 ± 56.17
	Right	369.09 ± 43.39	198.13 ± 43.39	501.36 ± 60.03	278.36 ± 60.03	398.02 ± 54.24	316.03 ± 54.24

The total coupling values and their corresponding standard error of mean as a function of condition and target visual field in younger and older subjects.

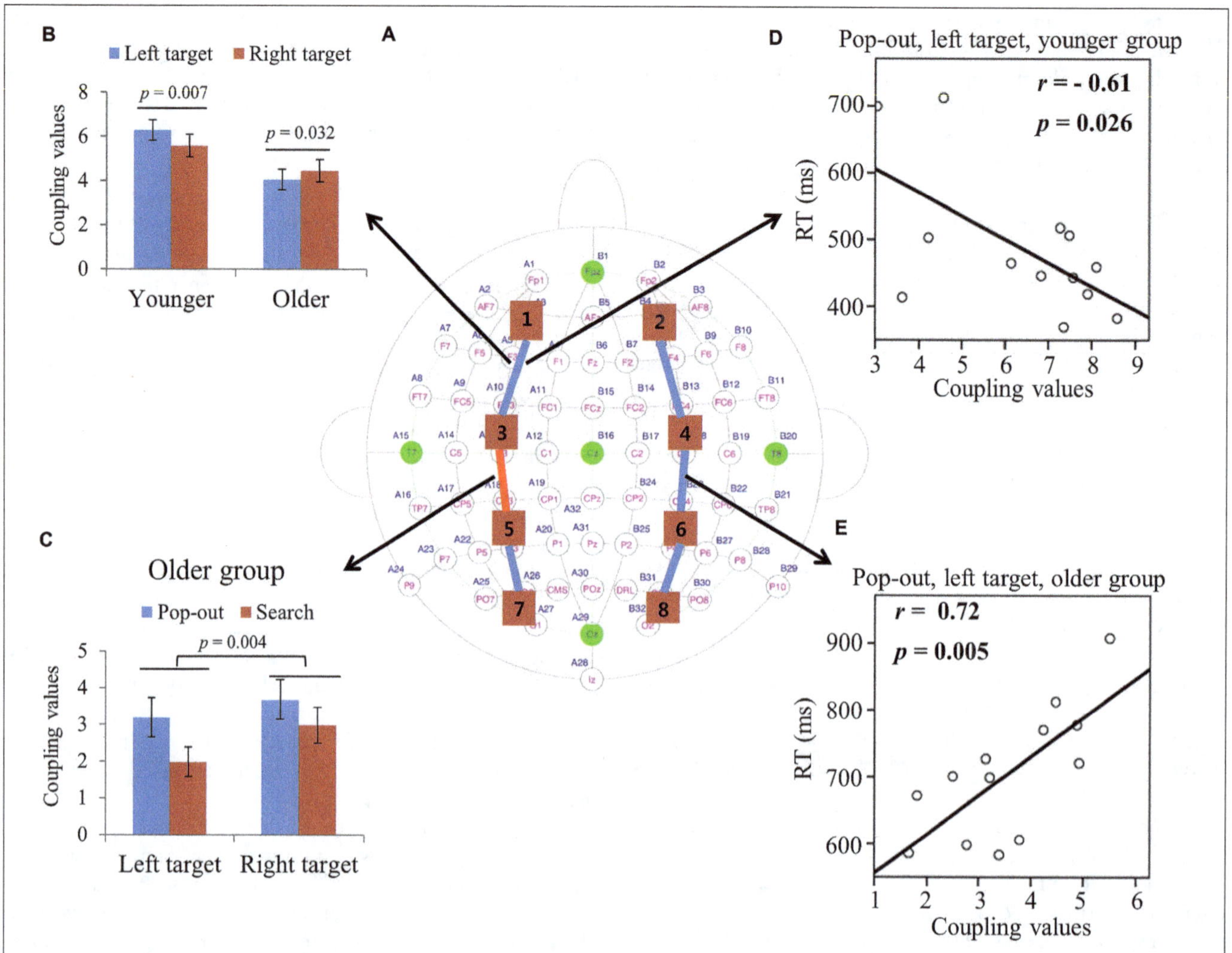

FIGURE 3 | (A) Inter-regions coupling in theta frequency band. Blue lines indicate main effect of age (younger > older) and red line indicates main effect of condition (pop-out > search). **(B)** Coupling values between left prefrontal and central-frontal regions as a function of target visual field in younger and older subjects, with greater coupling values in left target than in right target for younger subjects and greater coupling values in right target than in left target for old subjects. **(C)** Coupling values between left central-frontal and central-parietal regions as a function of target visual field in both conditions for older group, with greater values in pop-out condition and in right target, and no such effects for younger group. **(D)** Linear negative regression between mean RT and coupling value between left prefrontal and central-frontal regions for the pop-out condition with the left field target in the younger group. **(E)** Linear positive regression between mean RT and coupling value between right central-frontal and central-parietal regions for the pop-out condition with the left field target in the older group.

For the connection between left central-frontal and left central-parietal regions, there was an interaction between age and target visual field [$F(1,24) = 9.62$, $p = 0.005$]. Hence we divided the test into two repeated measure ANOVA with condition and target visual field as the within-subject factors for younger and older groups, respectively. There was a main effect of target field [$F(1,12) = 12.22$, $p = 0.004$] and condition [$F(1,12) = 5.69$, $p = 0.034$] for older group, with greater coupling values in the right field target and in the pop-out condition. There was no significant effect for the younger group. **Figure 3C** shows the coupling values in both conditions and target fields for older group. For the other four long range connections, there was no other significant effect.

Figure 3D illustrates the presence of significant negative linear relationship within the younger adults between coupling values of left prefrontal and central-frontal regions and RTs in the pop-out condition with left visual field target [$r = -0.61$, $p = 0.026$]. **Figure 3E** illustrates a significant positive linear relationship within the older adults between coupling values of right central-frontal and central-parietal and RTs in the pop-out condition with left visual field target [$r = 0.72$, $p = 0.005$]. All other correlation between coupling values and RTs or accuracies was not significant ($p > 0.05$).

ROIs Coupling Value in Alpha Frequency Band

Figure 4A summarizes the main effect of age (blue) and condition (red) among eight regions of interest. As can be seen in **Figure 4A**, there was a main effect of age for coupling values on two long range connections, including the connections between left prefrontal and left central-frontal regions [1 and

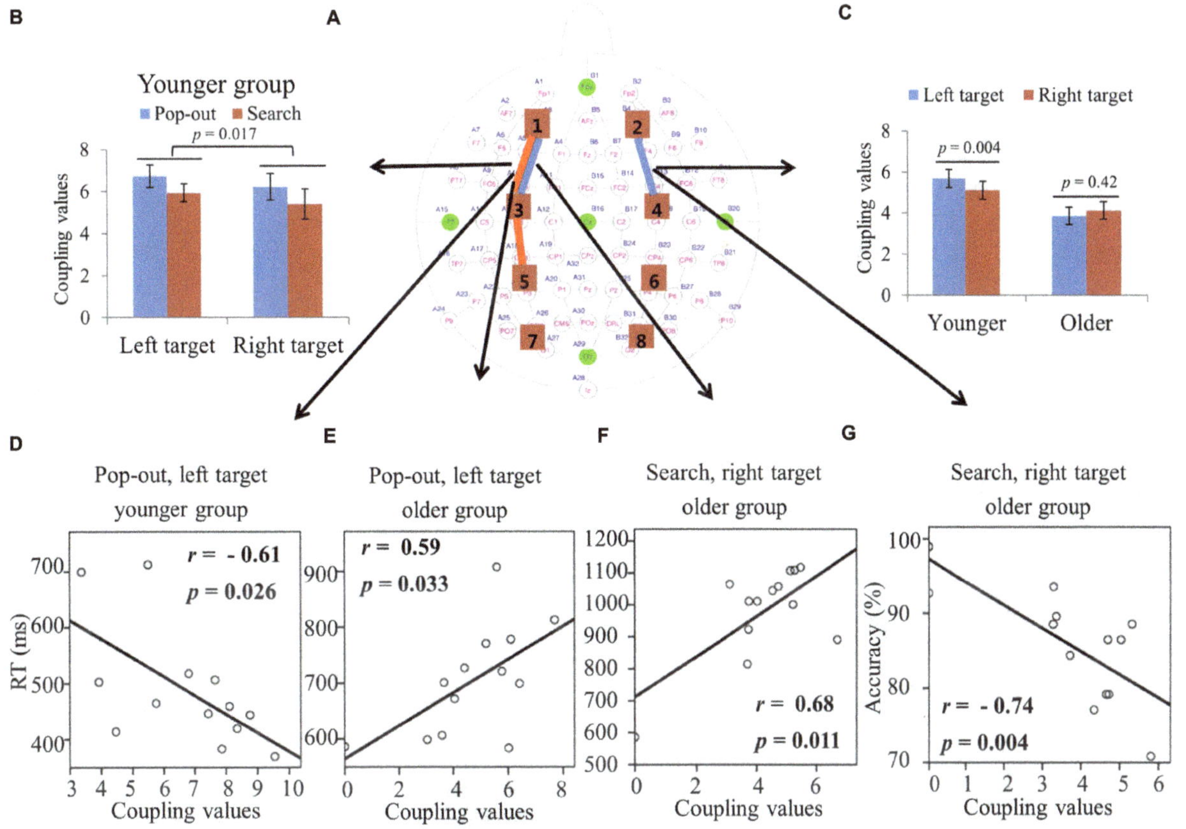

FIGURE 4 | (A) Inter-regions coupling in alpha frequency band. Blue lines indicate main effect of age (younger > older) and red line indicates main effect of condition (pop-out > search). **(B)** Coupling values between left prefrontal and central-frontal regions as a function of target field and condition in younger subjects, with greater coupling values in the left field target and in the pop-out condition. There was only a main effect of condition for the older group, with greater coupling values in the pop-out condition. **(C)** Coupling values between right prefrontal and central-frontal regions as a function of target field in younger and older subjects, with greater coupling values in left target than in right target for younger subjects and no difference between right and left targets for old subjects. **(D)** Linear negative regression between mean RT and coupling value between left prefrontal and central-frontal regions for the pop-out condition with the left field target in the younger group. Linear positive regression between mean RT and coupling value between left prefrontal and central-frontal regions for the pop-out condition with the left field target **(E)** and for the search condition with the right target **(F)** in the older group. **(G)** Linear negative regression between mean accuracy and coupling value between right prefrontal and central-frontal regions for the search condition with the right target in the older group.

3, $F(1,24) = 5.174$, $p = 0.03$], between right prefrontal and right central-frontal regions [2 and 4, $F(1,24) = 5.87$, $p = 0.02$], with smaller coupling values for older subjects. There was a main effect of condition for coupling values on connections between left prefrontal and left central-frontal regions [1 and 3, $F(1,24) = 14.03$, $p = 0.001$], between left central-frontal and left central-parietal regions [3 and 5, $F(1,24) = 5.87$, $p = 0.02$], with smaller coupling values in search condition.

For the connection between left prefrontal and central-frontal regions, there was an interaction between age and target visual field [$F(1,24) = 9.02$, $p = 0.006$]. Hence we divided the test into two repeated measure ANOVA with condition and target visual field as the within-subject factors for younger and older groups, respectively. There was a main effect of target field [$F(1,12) = 7.75$, $p = 0.017$] and condition [$F(1,12) = 5.09$, $p = 0.044$] for younger group, with greater coupling values in the left field target and in the pop-out condition. There was only a main effect of condition [$F(1,12) = 10.36$, $p = 0.007$] for the older group, with greater coupling values in the pop-out condition. **Figure 4B** shows the coupling values in both conditions and target fields for younger group.

For the connection between right prefrontal and central-frontal regions, there was an interaction between age and target visual field [$F(1,24) = 5.55$, $p = 0.03$], and there was no significant effect of condition. Hence we averaged the coupling values of the pop-out and search conditions, and applied repeated measure ANOVA with target visual field (left and right) as the within-subject factor and age (young and old) as the between-subject factor. **Figure 4C** shows the coupling values in both groups for both target fields. There was a main effect of age [$F(1,24) = 5.87$, $p = 0.02$] and an interaction between age and target field [$F(1,24) = 5.58$, $p = 0.03$], with bigger coupling values in left target than in right target for younger subjects [Paried t-tests, $t_{(12)} = 3.58$, $p = 0.004$]. Thus, greater bilateral prefronto-frontal coupling were shown in the left visual target for younger group.

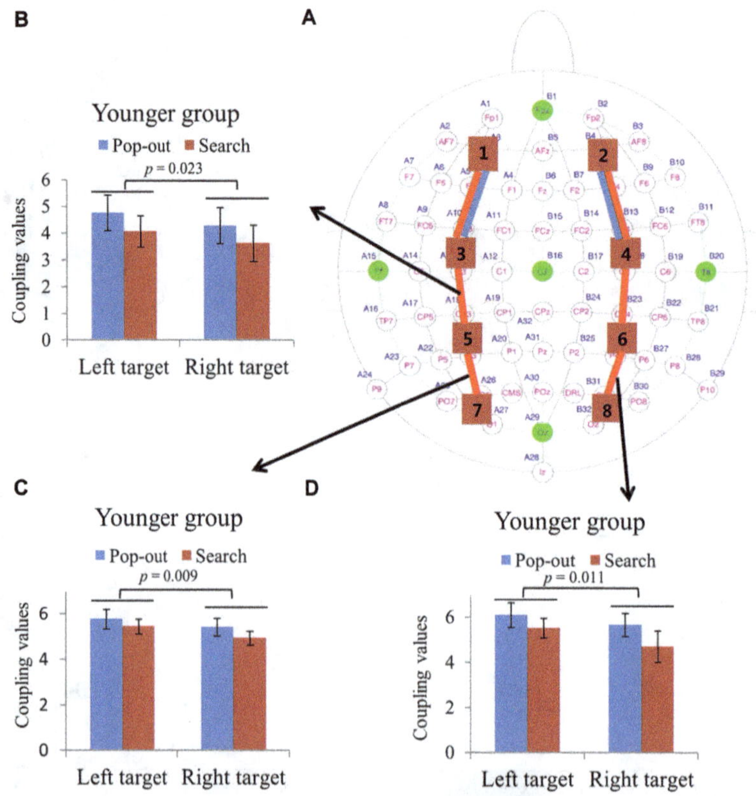

FIGURE 5 | (A) Inter-regions coupling in beta frequency band. Blue lines indicate main effect of age (younger > older) and red line indicates main effect of condition (pop-out > search). Coupling values between left central-frontal and central-parietal regions **(B)**, between left central-parietal and parietal-occipital regions **(C)**, and between right central-parietal and parietal-occipital regions **(D)** as a function of target field and condition in younger subjects, with bigger coupling values in left target than in right target, and no such effect was presented in the older group.

Figure 4D illustrates the presence of significant negative linear relationship within the younger adults between coupling values of left prefrontal and central-frontal regions and RTs in the pop-out condition with left visual field target [$r = -0.61$, $p = 0.026$]. **Figures 4E,F** illustrate the significant positive linear relationships within the older adults between coupling values of left prefrontal and central-frontal regions and RTs in the pop-out condition with left visual field target [$r = 0.59$, $p = 0.033$] and in the search condition with right visual field target [$r = 0.68$, $p = 0.011$], respectively. **Figure 4G** illustrates the significant negative linear relationship within the older adults between coupling values of right prefrontal and central-frontal regions and accuracies in the search condition with right visual field target [$r = -0.74$, $p = 0.004$]. All other correlation between coupling values and RTs or accuracies was not significant ($p > 0.05$).

ROIs Coupling Value in Beta Frequency Band

Figures 5A and **6A** summarizes the main effect of age and condition among eight regions of interest. As can be seen in **Figure 5A** with blue lines, there was a main effect of age for coupling values on two long range connections, including the connections between left prefrontal and left central-frontal regions [1 and 3, $F(1,24) = 5.49$, $p = 0.03$], between right prefrontal and right central-frontal regions [2 and 4, $F(1,24) = 5.03$, $p = 0.03$], with smaller coupling values for older subjects. In addition, there was a main effect of condition for those two frontal connections [1 and 3, $F(1,24) = 4.46$, $p = 0.045$; 2 and 4, $F(1,24) = 7.26$, $p = 0.01$] marked with red lines in **Figure 5A**, with smaller coupling values in search condition. There was a main effect of condition for coupling values between left central-frontal and left central-parietal regions [3 and 5, $F(1,24) = 4.87$, $p = 0.04$], between right central-frontal and right central-parietal regions [4 and 6, $F(1,24) = 5.96$, $p = 0.02$], between left central-parietal and left parietal-occipital [5 and 7, $F(1,24) = 5.81$, $p = 0.02$], between right central-parietal and right parieto-occipital regions [6 and 8, $F(1,24) = 7.75$, $p = 0.01$], with smaller coupling values in search condition (**Figure 5A**).

Due to the interaction between age and target visual field for these three connections [3 and 5, $F(1,24) = 4.29$, $p = 0.049$; 5 and 7, $F(1,24) = 7.54$, $p = 0.01$; 6 and 8, $F(1,24) = 4.38$, $p = 0.047$], we divided the test into two repeated measure ANOVA with condition and target field as the within-subject factors for both groups, respectively. There was only a main effect of target visual field [3 and 5, $F(1,12) = 6.73$, $p = 0.023$; 5 and 7, $F(1,12) = 9.69$, $p = 0.009$; 6 and 8, $F(1,12) = 8.93$, $p = 0.011$] for the younger group in these three connections, with bigger coupling values in left target than in right target, and no such effect was present for the older group. **Figures 5B–D** show the coupling values

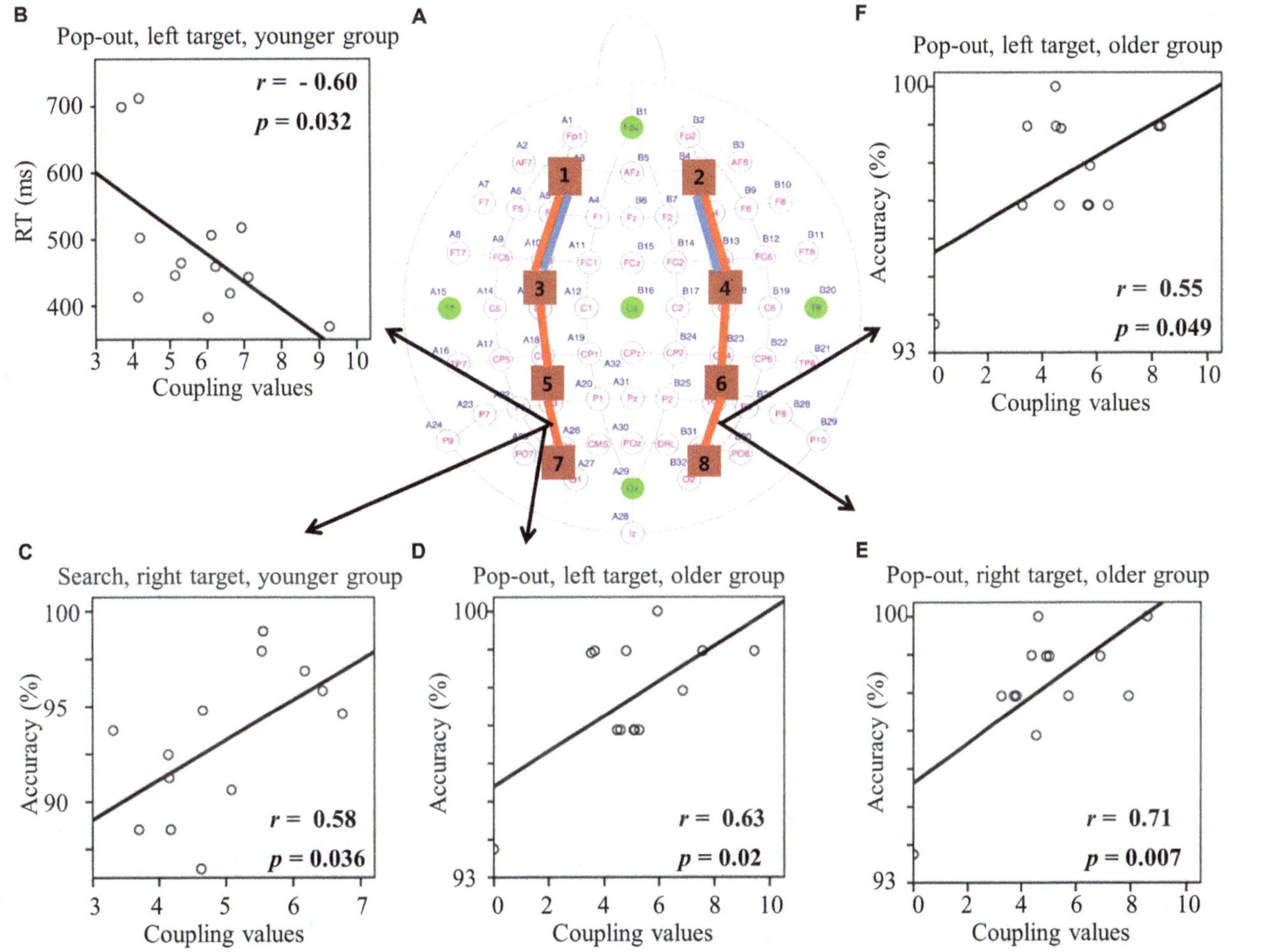

FIGURE 6 | (A) Inter-regions coupling in beta frequency band. Blue lines indicate main effect of age (younger > older) and red line indicates main effect of condition (pop-out > search). **(B)** Linear negative regression between mean RT and coupling value between left central-parietal and parietal-occipital regions for the pop-out condition with the left field target in the younger group. Linear positive regression between mean accuracy and coupling value between left central-parietal and parietal-occipital regions for the search condition with the right target in the younger group **(C)** and for the pop-out condition with the left target in the older group **(D)**. Linear positive regression between mean accuracy and coupling value between right central-parietal and parietal-occipital regions for the pop-out condition with the right target **(E)** and the left target **(F)** in the older group.

in both conditions and target fields for younger group at three connections.

For the coupling values between right prefrontal and central-frontal regions, there were significant positive linear relationships within the older subjects between values and RTs in all four conditions [pop-out and left: $r = 0.63$, $p = 0.02$; pop-out and right: $r = 0.61$, $p = 0.03$; search and left: $r = 0.58$, $p = 0.04$; search and left: $r = 0.58$, $p = 0.04$]. **Figures 6B,C** illustrate the significant positive linear relationships within the younger adults between coupling values of left central-parietal and parietal-occipital regions and performance in the pop-out condition with left target [RTs: $r = -0.60$, $p = 0.032$] and in the search condition with right visual field target [accuracy: $r = 0.58$, $p = 0.036$], respectively. **Figure 6D** illustrates the significant positive linear relationship within the older adults between coupling values of left central-parietal and parietal-occipital regions and accuracies in the pop-out condition with left target [$r = 0.63$, $p = 0.02$]. **Figures 6E,F** illustrate the significant positive linear relationships within the older adults between coupling values of right central-parietal and parietal-occipital regions and accuracies in the pop-out condition with left target [$r = 0.55$, $p = 0.049$] and right target [$r = 0.71$, $p = 0.007$], respectively. All other correlation between coupling values and RTs or accuracies was not significant ($p > 0.05$).

DISCUSSION

Aging Effects on Behavior and Inter-regions Coupling

Aging had prominent effects on both behavioral and EEG coupling strength under the control of top–down and bottom-up attention. Aging led to slowed RT and decreased accuracy (**Table 1**), indicating a slowing of cognitive performance with advancing age (Salthouse, 1996). Specifically, greater age-related reductions in accuracy in the search condition than in the pop-out condition were shown, suggesting additional attentional demands for older subjects with increased task complexity (Greenwood et al., 1997; Hommel et al., 2004; Madden et al., 2004, 2007).

Aging was associated with a declined whole-brain coupling strength of theta and alpha frequency bands, with a greater age-related decline in the search than in the pop-out condition (**Table 2**), in accord with their accuracy. Specifically, older adults showed a decreased lateral prefronto-frontal coupling in theta, alpha and beta frequency bands in both conditions (**Figures 3A**, **4A**, and **5A**), which confirmed the well-established age-related decline in allocation of attentional resources efficiency or reduction in inhibitory control functions in attention (Colcombe et al., 2003; Madden et al., 2004; Andrés et al., 2006; Hasher et al., 2008; Lorenzo-López et al., 2008; Gola et al., 2012; Deiber et al., 2013; Gola et al., 2013; Kardos et al., 2014).

Greater prefronto-frontal coupling (left lateral theta coupling, **Figure 3B**; and bilateral alpha coupling, **Figures 4B,C**), greater fronto-parietal coupling (left beta coupling, **Figure 5B**), and greater parieto-occipital coupling (bilateral beta coupling, **Figures 5C,D**) in the left target than in the right target for younger group were presented, suggesting a left visual field advantage (Holländer et al., 2005; Verleger and Smigasiewicz, 2015). This advantage might be related to the right hemispheric dominance in the ventral attentional network, which seems to particularly activate regions largely lateralized to the right hemisphere and involves right temporo-parietal and ventral frontal cortices in healthy subjects (Corbetta and Shulman, 2002; Shulman and Corbetta, 2012; Hong et al., 2015). Left visual field advantage was reduced with aging, supporting the Hemispheric Asymmetry Reduction in Older Adults (HAROLD) theory (Cabeza, 2002). Furthermore, older adults showed a greater left prefronto-frontal theta coupling (right two bars in **Figure 3B**) in the right visual target than in the left visual target, in accord with their quicker RTs, supporting the idea that older adults use bilateral neural circuits as compensation to accomplish visual search tasks (Reuter-Lorenz and Lustig, 2005; Grady, 2008; Reuter-Lorenz and Cappell, 2008). Interestingly, there was a greater left fronto-parietal theta coupling (**Figure 3C**) in the right visual target than in the left visual target for older group, whereas there was no difference for younger group. For younger group, left visual field advantage and the greater activity in the contralateral hemisphere (right visual target) for directing of attention may be counteracting, resulting in no difference between the right and left visual targets. For older group, the contribution of left visual field advantage is reduced, so that the activity in the contralateral hemisphere (right visual target) is in dominance, which is advantageous for task performance. These findings support the idea that right hemispheric dominance in the ventral attentional network is reduced to compensate for the inhibitory dysfunction with aging (Cabeza, 2002).

Attention Control Effects on Behavior and Inter-regions Coupling

The control of top–down and bottom–up attention had prominent effects on both behavioral and EEG coupling strength. Top–down control led to slowed RT and decreased accuracy for both groups (**Table 1**), indicating that the search task was sufficiently difficult to demand more cognitive effort (Treisman and Gelade, 1980). Top–down attentional control was associated with a declined whole-brain coupling strength of alpha and beta frequency bands, with a smaller coupling in the search than in the pop-out condition (**Table 2**). Specifically, search condition showed a decreased coupling of left fronto-parietal in theta and alpha frequency bands, of left prefronto-frontal in alpha-band, and of six inter-regions in beta-band compared to pop-out condition (**Figures 3A**, **4A**, and **5A**).

Pop-out target detection was mainly associated with greater parieto-occipital beta-coupling strength compared to search condition regardless of aging, in accord with their better performance, which confirmed previous findings that parietal power at beta-band (12–24 Hz) in human and parietal-extrastriate coherences at higher frequency band (35–55 Hz) in monkey were greater in the pop-out than in the search condition (Buschman and Miller, 2007; Li et al., 2010). This supports the idea that posterior parietal cortex is primarily responsible for the encoding of salient stimuli and automatic detection (Constantinidis and Steinmetz, 2005). Fronto-extrastriate coherences at intermediate frequency band (22–34 Hz) were greater in the search than in the pop-out condition (Buschman and Miller, 2007), but in the present study no significant difference in fronto-parietal theta-coupling strength between pop-out and search conditions for young subjects was observed (**Figure 3C**). This may be due to strict statistical method applied for significance in connections when constructing the network, as a result, weaker coupling may be ruled out. For example, if we use the normalized PLV values directly without threshold, a greater theta-coupling strength between left frontal and right occipital regions (regions 3 and 8) in the search than in the pop-out condition in left target for young subjects will be observed [3 and 8, paired t-test, $t_{(12)} = 3.59$, $p = 0.0037$]. We prefer to use strict statistical level to decrease the type I error. In summary, our results may indicate that the parieto-occipital coupling of beta-band could serve as a bottom-up function and be vulnerable to top–down attention control in both groups.

Relationships between Behavior and Inter-regions Coupling

The greater prefronto-frontal coupling showed better performance in theta and alpha bands for younger subjects (**Figures 3D** and **4D**), but worse performance in alpha and beta bands for older subjects (**Figures 4E–G**). These results provided additional information regarding the age-related change in the prefronto-frontal coupling in attentional control during the visual search task, suggesting that prefronto-frontal coupling for both groups may be generated by distinct brain cortices. An fMRI study has reported that younger individuals with higher levels of middle frontal gyrus activation exhibited better performance, and older individuals with higher levels of putamen activation showed worse performance during visual target detection (Madden et al., 2004). In present study, prefronto-frontal coupling results may most reflect connections within frontal gyrus for younger group, and most show connections within deep gray matter structures for older group in compensation for the age-related decline in visual search. Prefronto-frontal coupling was significant as a predictor of behavior for the younger and older groups, but in the opposite direction.

And the bigger parieto-occipital coupling in beta band led to better performance for both groups (**Figures 6B–F**), together with above results, indicating synchrony as a mechanism of attention (Miller and Buschman, 2013). Local synchrony between parieto-occipital cortices in beta-band and between prefronto-frontal cortices in theta, alpha and beta frequency bands may help the brain to improve its signal-to-noise ratio for better processing of bottom–up sensory input and top–down cognitive control, respectively. Parieto-occipital coupling in beta band was significant as a predictor of behavior for the younger and older groups in the same direction, and greater coupling may carry more bottom–up information.

In the current study, we found evidence for age-related changes in the differential roles of fronto-parieto-occipital connectivity at different oscillatory frequencies during the control of top–down and bottom–up attention. Together with evidence from past literature on the animal work on the networks contributing to top–down and bottom–up attention (Buschman and Miller, 2007; Miller and Buschman, 2013), these results suggest that bottom–up and top–down target lead to differential fronto-parieto-occipital connectivity at different oscillatory frequencies in younger and older adults. Greater prefronto-frontal coupling in theta and alpha-bands, fronto-parietal coupling in beta-band, and parieto-occipital coupling in beta-band in the left target than in the right target for younger group indicates a right hemispheric dominance in the ventral attentional network, which is reduced with aging to compensate for the inhibitory dysfunction. While pop-out target detection is mainly associated with greater parieto-occipital beta-coupling strength compared to search condition regardless of aging, in accord with their better performance. Prefronto-frontal coupling in theta, alpha, and beta bands and parieto-occipital coupling in beta band is a predictor of behavior for the both groups. Taken together these findings provide evidence that prefronto-frontal coupling of theta, alpha, and beta frequency bands may serve as a possible basis of aging during visual attention task, while parieto-occipital coupling in beta-band could serve for a bottom–up function and be vulnerable to top–down attention control for younger and older groups.

AUTHOR CONTRIBUTIONS

LL: Conceived, designed and performed the experiments. LL and DZ: Analyzed the data. LL: Wrote the paper.

ACKNOWLEDGMENTS

This research was supported by grants from the National Natural Science Foundation of China projects (NSFC, Nos. 61473062, 61203363, 91232725), 111 Project (B12027), and the Fundamental Research Funds for the Central Universities (ZYGX2014J077).

SUPPLEMENTARY MATERIAL

FIGURE S1 | Linear regression between mean reaction time (RT) and total coupling value for the pop-out condition with the left field target in the older group for theta frequency band. Each subject is marked as a circle, with 13 circles in total. Pearson correlation coefficient ($r = 0.588$) was significant ($p = 0.035$), indicating a positive linear correlation between RT and total coupling value in this condition.

REFERENCES

Anderson, N. D., Iidaka, T., Cabeza, R., Kapur, S., McIntosh, A. R., and Craik, F. I. M. (2000). The effects of divided attention on encoding- and retrieval-related brain activity: a PET study of younger and older adults. *J. Cogn. Neurosci.* 12, 775–792. doi: 10.1162/089892900562598

Andrés, P., Parmentier, F., and Escera, C. (2006). The effect of age on involuntary capture of attention by irrelevant sounds: a test of the frontal hypothesis of aging. *Neuropsychologia* 44, 2564–2568. doi: 10.1016/j.neuropsychologia.2006.05.005

Bledowski, C., Prvulovic, D., Goebel, R., Zanella, F. E., and Linden, D. E. (2004a). Attentional systems in target and distractor processing: a combined ERP and fMRI study. *Neuroimage* 22, 530–540. doi: 10.1016/j.neuroimage.2003.12.034

Bledowski, C., Prvulovic, D., Hoechstetter, K., Scherg, M., Wibral, M., Goebel, R., et al. (2004b). Localizing P300 generators in visual target and distractor processing: a combined event-related potential and functional magnetic resonance imaging study. *J. Neurosci.* 24, 9353–9360. doi: 10.1523/JNEUROSCI.1897-04.2004

Buschman, T. J., and Miller, E. K. (2007). Top-down versus bottom-up control of attention in the prefrontal and posterior parietal cortices. *Science* 315, 1860–1862. doi: 10.1126/science.1138071

Cabeza, R. (2002). Hemispheric asymmetry reduction in older adults: the HAROLD model. *Psychol. Aging* 17, 85–100. doi: 10.1037/0882-7974.17.1.85

Colcombe, A. M., Kramer, A. F., Irwin, D. E., Peterson, M. S., Colcombe, S., and Hahn, S. (2003). Age-related effects of attentional and oculomotor capture by onsets and color singletons as a function of experience. *Acta Psychol. (Amst.)* 113, 205–225. doi: 10.1016/S0001-6918(03)00019-2

Constantinidis, C., and Steinmetz, M. A. (2005). Posterior parietal cortex automatically encodes the location of salient stimuli. *J. Neurosci.* 25, 233–238. doi: 10.1523/JNEUROSCI.3379-04.2005

Corbetta, M., and Shulman, G. L. (2002). Control of goal-directed and stimulus-driven attention in the brain. *Nat. Rev. Neurosci.* 3, 201–215. doi: 10.1038/nrn755

Deiber, M. P., Ibanez, V., Missonnier, P., Rodriguez, C., and Giannakopoulos, P. (2013). Age-associated modulations of cerebral oscillatory patterns related to attention control. *Neuroimage* 82, 531–546. doi: 10.1016/j.neuroimage.2013.06.037

Delorme, A., and Makeig, S. (2004). EEGLAB: an open source toolbox for analysis of single-trial EEG dynamics including independent component analysis. *J. Neurosci. Meth.* 134, 9–21. doi: 10.1016/j.jneumeth.2003.10.009

Dennis, N. A., Hayes, S. M., Prince, S. E., Madden, D. J., Huettel, S. A., and Cabeza, R. (2008). Effects of aging on the neural correlates of successful item and source memory encoding. *J. Exp. Psychol. Learn. Mem. Cogn.* 34, 791–808. doi: 10.1037/0278-7393.34.4.791

Fotenos, A. F., Mintun, M. A., Snyder, A. Z., Morris, J. C., and Buckner, R. L. (2008). Brain volume decline in aging: evidence for a relation between socioeconomic status, preclinical Alzheimer disease, and reserve. *Arch. Neurol.* 65, 113–120. doi: 10.1001/archneurol.2007.27

Geerligs, L., Saliasi, E., Maurits, N. M., Renken, R. J., and Lorist, M. M. (2014). Brain mechanisms underlying the effects of aging on different aspects of selective attention. *Neuroimage* 91, 52–62. doi: 10.1016/j.neuroimage.2014.01.029

Giesbrecht, B., Woldorff, M. G., Song, A. W., and Mangun, G. R. (2003). Neural mechanisms of top-down control during spatial and feature attention. *Neuroimage* 19, 496–512. doi: 10.1016/S1053-8119(03)00162-9

Gola, M., Kaminski, J., Brzezicka, A., and Wrobel, A. (2012). Beta band oscillations as a correlate of alertness-changes in aging. *Int. J. Psychophysiol.* 85, 62–67. doi: 10.1016/j.ijpsycho.2011.09.001

Gola, M., Magnuski, M., Szumska, I., and Wrobel, A. (2013). EEG beta band activity is related to attention and attentional deficits in the visual performance of elderly subjects. *Int. J. Psychophysiol.* 89, 334–341. doi: 10.1016/j.ijpsycho.2013.05.007

Gordon, B. A., Rykhlevskaia, E. I., Brumback, C. R., Lee, Y., Elavsky, S., Konopack, J. F., et al. (2008). Neuroanatomical correlates of aging, cardiopulmonary fitness level, and education. *Psychophysiology* 45, 825–838. doi: 10.1111/j.1469-8986.2008.00676.x

Grady, C. L. (2008). Cognitive neuroscience of aging. *Year Cogn. Neurosci.* 1124, 127–144.

Grady, C. L., Bernstein, L. J., Beig, S., and Siegenthaler, A. L. (2002). The effects of encoding task on age-related differences in the functional neuroanatomy of face memory. *Psychol. Aging* 17, 7–23. doi: 10.1037/0882-7974.17.1.7

Greenwood, P. M., Parasuraman, R., and Alexander, G. E. (1997). Controlling the focus of spatial attention during visual search: effects of advanced aging and Alzheimer disease. *Neuropsychology* 11, 3–12. doi: 10.1037/0894-4105.11.1.3

Hasher, L., Lustig, C., and Zacks, R. (2008). "Inhibitory mechanisms and the control of attention," in *Variation in Working Memory*, eds A. R. A. Conway, C. Jarrold, M. J. Kane, A. Miyake, and J. N. Towse (New York, NY: Oxford University Press), 227–249.

Holländer, A., Corballis, M. C., and Hamm, J. P. (2005). Visual-field asymmetry in dual-stream RSVP. *Neuropsychologia* 43, 35–40. doi: 10.1016/j.neuropsychologia.2004.06.006

Hommel, B., Li, K. Z., and Li, S. C. (2004). Visual search across the life span. *Dev. Psychol.* 40, 545–558. doi: 10.1037/0012-1649.40.4.545

Hong, X., Sun, J., Bengson, J. J., Mangun, G. R., and Tong, S. (2015). Normal aging selectively diminishes alpha lateralization in visual spatial attention. *Neuroimage* 106, 353–363. doi: 10.1016/j.neuroimage.2014.11.019

Husain, M., and Nachev, P. (2007). Space and the parietal cortex. *Trends Cogn. Sci.* 11, 30–36. doi: 10.1016/j.tics.2006.10.011

Johnson, M. K., Mitchell, K. J., Raye, C. L., and Greene, E. J. (2004). An age-related deficit in prefrontal cortical function associated with refreshing information. *Psychol. Sci.* 15, 127–132. doi: 10.1111/j.0963-7214.2004.01502009.x

Kardos, Z., Toth, B., Boha, R., File, B., and Molnar, M. (2014). Age-related changes of frontal-midline theta is predictive of efficient memory maintenance. *Neuroscience* 273, 152–162. doi: 10.1016/j.neuroscience.2014.04.071

Kayser, J., and Tenke, C. E. (2006). Principal components analysis of Laplacian waveforms as a generic method for identifying ERP generator patterns: I. Evaluation with auditory oddball tasks. *Clin. Neurophysiol.* 117, 348–368. doi: 10.1016/j.clinph.2005.08.033

Knudsen, E. I. (2007). Fundamental components of attention. *Annu. Rev. Neurosci.* 30, 57–78. doi: 10.1146/annurev.neuro.30.051606.094256

Knyazev, G. G., Volf, N. V., and Belousova, L. V. (2015). Age-related differences in electroencephalogram connectivity and network topology. *Neurobiol. Aging* 36, 1849–1859. doi: 10.1016/j.neurobiolaging.2015.02.007

Kok, A. (2000). Age-related changes in involuntary and voluntary attention as reflected in components of the event-related potential (ERP). *Biol. Psychol.* 54, 107–143. doi: 10.1016/S0301-0511(00)00054-5

Lachaux, J. P., Rodriguez, E., Martinerie, J., and Varela, F. J. (1999). Measuring phase synchrony in brain signals. *Hum. Brain Mapp.* 8, 194–208.

Li, L., Gratton, C., Fabiani, M., and Knight, R. T. (2013). Age-related frontoparietal changes during the control of bottom-up and top-down attention: an ERP study. *Neurobiol. Aging* 34, 477–488. doi: 10.1016/j.neurobiolaging.2012.02.025

Li, L., Gratton, C., Yao, D., and Knight, R. T. (2010). Role of frontal and parietal cortices in the control of bottom-up and top-down attention in humans. *Brain Res.* 1344, 173–184. doi: 10.1016/j.brainres.2010.05.016

Lien, M. C., Gemperle, A., and Ruthruff, E. (2011). Aging and involuntary attention capture: electrophysiological evidence for preserved attentional control with advanced age. *Psychol. Aging* 26, 188–202. doi: 10.1037/a0021073

Lorenzo-López, L., Amenedo, E., Pascual-Marqui, R. D., and Cadaveira, F. (2008). Neural correlates of age-related visual search decline: a combined ERP and sLORETA study. *Neuroimage* 41, 511–524. doi: 10.1016/j.neuroimage.2008.02.041

Madden, D. J. (2007). Aging and visual attention. *Curr. Dir. Psychol. Sci.* 16, 70–74. doi: 10.1111/j.1467-8721.2007.00478.x

Madden, D. J., Costello, M. C., Dennis, N. A., Davis, S. W., Shepler, A. M., Spaniol, J., et al. (2010). Adult age differences in functional connectivity during executive control. *Neuroimage* 52, 643–657. doi: 10.1016/j.neuroimage.2010.04.249

Madden, D. J., Spaniol, J., Whiting, W. L., Bucur, B., Provenzale, J. M., Cabeza, R., et al. (2007). Adult age differences in the functional neuroanatomy of visual attention: a combined fMRI and DTI study. *Neurobiol. Aging* 28, 459–476. doi: 10.1016/j.neurobiolaging.2006.01.005

Madden, D. J., Whiting, W. L., and Huettel, S. A. (2005). "Age-related changes in neural activity during visual perception and attention," in *Cognitive Neuroscience of Aging: Linking Cognitive and Cerebral Aging*, eds R. Cabeza, L. Nyberg, and D. Park (New York, NY: Oxford University Press), 157–185.

Madden, D. J., Whiting, W. L., Provenzale, J. M., and Huettel, S. A. (2004). Age-related changes in neural activity during visual target detection measured by fMRI. *Cereb. Cortex* 14, 143–155. doi: 10.1093/cercor/bhg113

Milham, M. P., Erickson, K. I., Banich, M. T., Kramer, A. F., Webb, A., Wszalek, T., et al. (2002). Attentional control in the aging brain: insights from an fMRI study of the stroop task. *Brain Cogn.* 49, 277–296. doi: 10.1006/brcg.2001.1501

Miller, E. K., and Buschman, T. J. (2013). Cortical circuits for the control of attention. *Curr. Opin. Neurobiol.* 23, 216–222. doi: 10.1016/j.conb.2012.11.011

Mormann, F., Lehnertz, K., David, P., and Elger, C. E. (2000). Mean phase coherence as a measure for phase synchronization and its application to the EEG of epilepsy patients. *Physica D* 144, 358–369. doi: 10.1016/j.clinph.2013.09.047

Nunez, P. L., Srinivasan, R., Westdorp, A. F., Wijesinghe, R. S., Tucker, D. M., Silberstein, R. B., et al. (1997). EEG coherency. I: statistics, reference electrode, volume conduction, Laplacians, cortical imaging, and interpretation at multiple scales. *Electroencephalogr. Clin. Neurophysiol.* 103, 499–515. doi: 10.1016/S0013-4694(97)00066-7

Perrin, F., Pernier, J., Bertrand, O., and Echallier, J. F. (1989). Spherical splines for scalp potential and current density mapping. *Electroencephalogr. Clin. Neurophysiol.* 72, 184–187. doi: 10.1016/0013-4694(89)90180-6

Phillips, S., and Takeda, Y. (2009). Greater frontal-parietal synchrony at low gamma-band frequencies for inefficient than efficient visual search in human EEG. *Int. J. Psychophysiol.* 73, 350–354. doi: 10.1016/j.ijpsycho.2009.05.011

Plude, D. J., and Doussard-Roosevelt, J. A. (1989). Aging, selective attention, and feature integration. *Psychol. Aging* 4, 98–105. doi: 10.1037/0882-7974.4.1.98

Quian Quiroga, R., Kraskov, A., Kreuz, T., and Grassberger, P. (2002). Performance of different synchronization measures in real data: a case study on electroencephalographic signals. *Phys. Rev. E Stat. Nonlinear Soft Matter Phys.* 65:041903. doi: 10.1103/PhysRevE.65.041903

Raz, N., Lindenberger, U., Rodrigue, K. M., Kennedy, K. M., Head, D., Williamson, A., et al. (2005). Regional brain changes in aging healthy adults: general trends, individual differences and modifiers. *Cereb. Cortex* 15, 1676–1689. doi: 10.1093/cercor/bhi044

Reuter-Lorenz, P. A., and Cappell, K. A. (2008). Neurocognitive aging and the compensation hypothesis. *Curr. Dir. Psychol. Sci.* 17, 177–182. doi: 10.1111/j.1467-8721.2008.00570.x

Reuter-Lorenz, P. A., and Lustig, C. (2005). Brain aging: reorganizing discoveries about the aging mind. *Curr. Opin. Neurobiol.* 15, 245–251. doi: 10.1016/j.conb.2005.03.016

Reuter-Lorenz, P. A., and Park, D. C. (2010). Human neuroscience and the aging mind: a new look at old problems. *J. Gerontol. B Psychol. Sci. Soc. Sci.* 65, 405–415. doi: 10.1093/geronb/gbq035

Roski, C., Caspers, S., Langner, R., Laird, A. R., Fox, P. T., Zilles, K., et al. (2013). Adult age-dependent differences in resting-state connectivity within and between visual-attention and sensorimotor networks. *Front. Aging Neurosci.* 5:67. doi: 10.3389/fnagi.2013.00067

Salthouse, T. A. (1996). The processing-speed theory of adult age differences in cognition. *Psychol. Rev.* 103, 403–428. doi: 10.1037/0033-295X.103.3.403

Scahill, R. I., Frost, C., Jenkins, R., Whitwell, J. L., Rossor, M. N., and Fox, N. C. (2003). A longitudinal study of brain volume changes in normal aging using serial registered magnetic resonance imaging. *Arch. Neurol.* 60, 989–994. doi: 10.1001/archneur.60.7.989

Shulman, G. L., and Corbetta, M. (2012). "Two attentional networks. Identification and function within a larger cognitive architecture," in *Cognitive Neuroscience of Attention*, 2nd Edn, ed. M. I. Posner (New York, NY: Guilford Press), 113–128.

St Jacques, P. L., Dolcos, F., and Cabeza, R. (2009). Effects of aging on functional connectivity of the amygdala for subsequent memory of negative pictures: a network analysis of functional magnetic resonance imaging data. *Psychol. Sci.* 20, 74–84. doi: 10.1111/j.1467-9280.2008.02258.x

Treisman, A. M., and Gelade, G. (1980). A feature-integration theory of attention. *Cogn. Psychol.* 12, 97–136. doi: 10.1016/0010-0285(80)90005-5

Vallesi, A., Hasher, L., and Stuss, D. T. (2010). Age-related changes in transfer costs: evidence from go/nogo tasks. *Psychol. Aging* 25, 963–967. doi: 10.1037/a0020300

Verleger, R., and Smigasiewicz, K. (2015). Consciousness wanted, attention found: reasons for the advantage of the left visual field in identifying T2 among rapidly presented series. *Conscious. Cogn.* 35, 260–273. doi: 10.1016/j.concog.2015.02.013

17

The Lateralization of Intrinsic Networks in the Aging Brain Implicates the Effects of Cognitive Training

Cheng Luo [1], Xingxing Zhang [1], Xinyi Cao [2], Yulong Gan [1], Ting Li [3], Yan Cheng [2], Weifang Cao [1], Lijuan Jiang [2], Dezhong Yao [1] and Chunbo Li [2,4]**

[1] Key Laboratory for NeuroInformation of Ministry of Education, High-Field Magnetic Resonance Brain Imaging Key Laboratory of Sichuan Province, Center for Information in Medicine, School of Life Science and Technology, University of Electronic Science and Technology of China, Chengdu, China, [2] Shanghai Key Laboratory of Psychotic Disorders, Shanghai Mental Health Center, Shanghai Jiao Tong University School of Medicine, Shanghai, China, [3] Changning Mental Health Center, Shanghai, China, [4] Bio-X Institutes, Key Laboratory for the Genetics of Developmental and Neuropsychiatric Disorders, Ministry of Education, Shanghai Jiao Tong University, Shanghai, China

Edited by:
Michael Hornberger,
University of East Anglia, UK

Reviewed by:
Qing Jiao,
Taishan Medical University, China
Yuan Zhong,
Nanjing Normal University, China

***Correspondence:**
Dezhong Yao
dyao@uestc.edu.cn;
Chunbo Li
chunbo_li@163.com

Lateralization of function is an important organization of the human brain. The distribution of intrinsic networks in the resting brain is strongly related to cognitive function, gender and age. In this study, a longitudinal design with 1 year's duration was used to evaluate the cognitive training effects on the lateralization of intrinsic networks among healthy older adults. The subjects were divided into two groups randomly: one with multi-domain cognitive training over 3 months and the other as a wait-list control group. Resting state fMRI data were acquired before training and 1 year after training. We analyzed the functional lateralization in 10 common resting state fMRI networks. We observed statically significant training effects on the lateralization of two important RSNs related to high-level cognition: right- and left- frontoparietal networks (FPNs). The lateralization of the left-FPN was retained especially well in the training group but decreased in the control group. The increased lateralization with aging was observed in the cerebellum network (CereN), in which the lateralization was significantly increased in the control group, although the same change tendency was observed in the training group. These findings indicate that the lateralization of the high-level cognitive intrinsic networks is sensitive to multi-domain cognitive training. This study provides neuroimaging evidence to support the hypothesis that cognitive training should have an advantage in preventing cognitive decline in healthy older adults.

Keywords: aging, fMRI, lateralization, functional network, cognitive training

INTRODUCTION

The human brain is the most complex system in nature. The interhemispheric interaction is crucial to brain functions such as motor and cognitive processes. However, hemispheric specialization is also an obvious organizing principle for efficient information processing, such as leftward lateralization for speech and rightward lateralization for visuospatial attention (Corballis, 2014).

Postmortem and neuroimaging studies have displayed the asymmetries of the human brain (Goldberg et al., 2013). Recently, resting state functional magnetic resonance imaging (fMRI) has been widely used in the studies of the human brain in which it was organized into several intrinsic resting state networks (RSNs). More and more studies have provided the evidence to support the importance of these RSNs on the brain function, such as default mode and attention. In general, the spatial pattern of these RSNs is relatively stable across subjects. These RSNs demonstrate either spatial hemispheric symmetry, such as the default mode network (DMN) and sensorimotor network (SMN), or hemispheric asymmetry, such as the frontoparietal network (FPN) and attention network (Fox et al., 2006). Hemispheric symmetry, which is represented by the spatial lateralization of RSNs, may reflect the slight changes of RSNs in different states of the brain. For example, the lateralization is influenced by development (Kelly et al., 2009), gender (Agcaoglu et al., 2015) and diseases (Luo et al., 2014b). The lateralization of RSNs is also observed to be significantly altered in healthy older adults compared with younger adults (Agcaoglu et al., 2015; Seidler et al., 2015).

Neurodegeneration is associated with increasing age (Seidler et al., 2010), i.e., declining cognition and decreases in motor performance (Cheng et al., 2012; Brown et al., 2013). Physical activity and exercise have positive influences on neurodegeneration (Brown et al., 2013). It has been observed that directed cognitive training interventions will increase mental activity in older adults, helping them to resist age-related cognitive decline and even potentially reducing the risk of dementia (Gates and Valenzuela, 2010). In a previous behavioral study, we observed that cognitive training can improve multi-cognition in community-living older adults, including memory, attention and neuropsychological status (Cheng et al., 2012). However, the underlying brain mechanism allowing the training to enhance function has been unclear till now. Noninvasive neuroimaging techniques, especially fMRI, are used to investigate the association between the intervention and brain function. For example, musical training would enhance the functional connectivity in perceptual and motor systems (Luo et al., 2012a) and salience network (Luo et al., 2014a). Additionally, the motor-related exercise increased the integration of motor performance and imaging systems (Gong et al., 2015, 2016; Li et al., 2015a). MRI studies of aging adults have shown enlarged local cortex thickness and enhanced functional integration related to the expertise in cognitive and sensorimotor interventions (Boyke et al., 2008; Lustig et al., 2009; Cao et al., 2014; Li et al., 2014). Therefore, we hypothesized that the lateralization of RSNs found in resting state fMRI scanning might provide an approach to reflect the influence of cognitive training on healthy older adults.

In this study, to test our hypothesis, a longitudinal design with 1 year's duration was used to evaluate the cognitive training effects on the lateralization of intrinsic networks among healthy older adults. Healthy older adults with community-living were recruited and divided into two groups randomly: one received a multi-domain cognitive training over 3 months; the other was included in a wait-list control group. Resting state fMRI data were acquired before training and 1 year after training. The functional lateralization of 10 common resting state fMRI networks was evaluated between two groups using repeated measures analysis of variance (ANOVA).

MATERIALS AND METHODS

Participants

Forty healthy older adults were recruited from three community centers around Tongji Hospital in Shanghai via a dispatched notice/broadcasting by the local institute of community service from March 2008 to April 2008. All participants were admitted to the study after a personal interview according to the inclusion criteria as follows: normal functional capacity; independent living in the community; age (range: 65–75 years); educational level (more than 1 year); no abnormality in hearing, vision, or communication status; a score of 19 or above (the lower normal cut-off point of the MMSE score is due to the lower educational level in China than in the US; Li et al., 2006) using the Chinese version of the Mini-Mental State Examination (MMSE); and no physical disease or psychotic disorder. The subjects with obvious cognitive decline, a diagnosis of AD, a brain tumor, or serious neurological and/or psychiatric disorders such as major depressive disorder and schizophrenia were excluded in this study. All of participants underwent cognitive measurements and fMRI scanning at baseline and at 1 year after training. They were divided randomly into two groups, including the multi-domain training group (n = 23) and the control group (n = 17). One participant out of 23 in the multi-domain training group and one in the single-domain training group were excluded because of left-handedness, which would interrupt the study of the lateralization of brain (Mackey et al., 2013). This study was reviewed and approved by the Ethical Committee of the East China Normal University. This study was performed according to the recommendation of the Ethical Committee of the East China Normal University with written informed consent from all subjects. All subjects gave written informed consent in accordance with the Declaration of Helsinki.

Cognitive Interventions and Neuropsychological Tests

We conducted a randomized, controlled design to determine the effect of cognitive training on brain function and cognitive function (Cheng et al., 2012). The neuroimaging data and cognitive measurement were collected at baseline and at 1 year after training.

The multi-domain training group received 24 sessions (each session was 60 min) of cognitive training at a frequency of twice a week over a 12-week period, and the training procedure took place in a classroom in Tongji Hospital. The multi-domain cognitive training targeted memory, reasoning, problem-solving strategies, visual-spatial map reading skill developments, handcraft making, and health and physical exercise. A lecture about a common disease in aging people was presented during the first 15 min of each session. Then, the trainer taught the participants about a special cognitive strategy or technique via slide lecture during the second 30 min. The newly practiced skills were consolidated by dealing with some real-life problems during the last 15 min.

The wait-list control group served as a match for the social contact associated with cognitive training. The multi-domain training group and the control group attended a lecture about healthy living every 2 months (the training details are found in our previous study; Cheng et al., 2012).

To evaluate the effects of intervention on cognitive function, all measurements were administered at baseline and at 1 year after intervention, including the Repeatable Battery for the Assessment of Neuropsychological Status (RBANS, Form A), which has good validity and reliability in a Chinese community-living elderly sample (Lim et al., 2010; Cheng et al., 2011), the trail making test (TMT; Ashendorf et al., 2008), the visual reasoning test (Xiao et al., 2002) and the Color Word Stroop test (CWST; van Boxtel et al., 2001).

Data Acquisition

All participants were scanned using a Siemens 3T MRI Scanner (Erlangen, Germany) at baseline and at 1 year after training ending at East China Normal University, Shanghai, China. To minimize head motion, foam pads were used to fix the subjects' heads. High-resolution T1-weighted images were acquired using a magnetization-prepared rapid gradient-echo sequence, generating 160 slices (repetition time (TR) = 1900 ms, echo time (TE) = 3.43 ms, flip angle (FA) = 90 degrees, matrix size = 256 × 256, field of view (FOV) = 240 × 240 mm^2, slice thickness = 1 mm; no gap). Resting state functional images were acquired using a single-shot, gradient-recalled echo planar imaging sequence (TR = 2000 ms, TE = 25 ms and FA = 90 degrees, FOV = 240 × 240 mm^2, matrix = 64 × 64, slice thickness = 5 mm (no gap), 32 slices per volume). All subjects underwent a 310 s scanning to yield a total of 155 volumes. The subjects were instructed to rest with their eyes closed, not to think of anything in particular, and not to fall asleep.

Data Pre-process Analysis

Pre-processing of fMRI data were conducted using the SPM8 Software Package [statistical parametric mapping[1]]. The slice time correction, 3D motion detection and correction, spatial normalization and resample (3 mm × 3 mm × 3 mm), and spatial smoothing using an isotropic Gaussian kernel (6 mm full width at half maximum) were applied. The processing is identical to that used in prior studies (Chen et al., 2015; Jiang et al., 2016). Only the subjects with head motion less than 1.5 mm and 1.5° during fMRI acquisition were included in the following preprocessing. In addition, the translation and rotation of the subjects were assessed by frame wise displacement (FD),

$$FD_i = |\Delta d_{ix}| + |\Delta d_{iy}| + |\Delta d_{iz}| + |\Delta\alpha_i| + |\Delta\beta_i| + |\Delta\gamma_i|,$$

where i is the i-th time point, and $\Delta d_{ix} = d_{(i-1)x} - d_{ix}$ (similarly for the other head motion/rotation parameters; Power et al., 2012). No significant differences were found between groups in FD. Additional preprocessing in preparation included voxelwise nuisance correction by regressing out six motion signals.

[1]http://www.fil.ion.ucl.ac.uk/spm

ICA Decomposition

Similar to the approaches in our previous studies (Luo et al., 2012c; Li et al., 2015b), we first conducted spatial group ICA in which two times of data of all subjects were included in one group, using the GIFT Software, version 2.0a[2]. The time courses were temporally concatenated across subjects and reduced by means of principal component analysis in temporal domain, followed by an IC estimation using the FastICA algorithm. This algorithm was repeated 20 times in ICASSO[3], and the resulting components were clustered to estimate the reliability of the decomposition (Himberg et al., 2004). Dimension estimation on all subjects was performed using the minimum description length (MDL) criterion to determine the number of independent components (ICs). The ICs were back-constructed for each scans and each subject using the dual-regression approach (Zhang et al., 2010). Finally, we interrogated all components to identify RSNs. Ten RSNs were chosen based on the average power spectra and spatial map of the components such as in the previous studies (Luo et al., 2012c; Li et al., 2015b). Here, the power spectra of time course of ICs was analyzed, and the power spectra of the selected IC should show the frequency content was mainly concentrated below 0.1 Hz (Beckmann et al., 2005; Luo et al., 2012b).

Spatial Normalization to Symmetric Templates

To acquire the hemispheric symmetries' RSNs, the warping step was performed from the resulted RSNs to the symmetries' templates. First, the MNI template was warped to a symmetrized version of the MNI template because all subjects' functional images were normalized into the MNI template. Then, the MNI template was normalized to the symmetrized template. Finally, the warping parameters were applied to all components for the symmetrizing RSNs in all subjects.

Calculation of Voxelwise Homotopic Maps

The component values were initially normalized across voxels using z-score. The differences (B_v) between component values of both homotopic voxels on both sides of cerebral cortex were calculated using the following formula 1. As with our previous study (Agcaoglu et al., 2015), the difference was shown in a map with a positive difference ($R > L$) on the right side of the brain and negative difference ($L > R$) on the left side of the brain.

$$B_v = \begin{cases} (R_v - L_v)\ if\ R_v > L_v \\ (L_v - R_v)\ if\ L_v > R_v \\ 0 \quad otherwise \end{cases} \quad (1)$$

where R and L represents the right hemisphere and left hemisphere for each pairs of homotopic voxels v.

[2]http://icatb.sourceforge.net/
[3]http://research.ics.tkk.fi/ica/icasso

Hence, the voxelwise homotopic map was produced for each subject each RSN.

Laterality Cofactor

The laterality cofactor (LCF) was defined based on a voxelwise homotopic map, as in the previous study (Agcaoglu et al., 2015). The amount of laterality for a given RSN was calculated in the global laterality metric. The LCF was acquired by taking the differences between the sum of all intensities of laterality on the right and left hemispheres with respect to the sum of all intensities across the brain (Formula 2). The LCF was computed for the average models for each group. In addition, individual LCF was calculated to evaluate the alteration of LCFs related with training.

$$\mathrm{LCF} = \frac{S_l - S_r}{S_l + S_r} \tag{2}$$

Where S_l and S_r represents the sum of all intensities of laterality on the left and right hemispheres.

Statistical Test

For each of the components, one sample *t*-test was performed in voxelwise homotopic maps in three groups. Here, the pretraining fMRI data from all the subjects were included in one group; the second data were divided into training and control groups on the basis of receiving the training or not. For the three *t*-value maps, we then applied a mask to retain those voxels whose *t*-values exceed one standard deviation of the *t*-value across voxels. The thresholded *t*-maps were used to compute the LCFs of group level (Global LCF) according to the same formula to calculate the LCF (Formula 2).

According to the formula 2, the LCF value range was between −1 and 1. The Fisher-*z*-translation of individual LCF was performed for the distribution normality for each RSN. The individual LCF of each RSN was also evaluated used the ANOVA for repeated measurement data with *post hoc*, pair-wise Scheffe test in SPSS v20 (IBM Corp., Somer, NY, USA).

RESULTS

Demographic Information

At baseline, 23 subjects from the multi-domain training group and 17 subjects from the control group underwent cognitive measurements and fMRI scanning. Eighteen of the multi-domain training group and 14 of the control group finished the cognitive measurements and fMRI scanning at 1 year after the intervention. A total of eight participants withdrew, one due to death, two due to intestinal cancer, one due to her husband's death, one due to operation and three due to rejecting the scanning. No significant differences with regard to age, gender, education and MMSE score were found between the multi-domain training group and the control group (**Table 1**).

TABLE 1 | Demographic information of the subjects.

		Multi-domain training group	Control group	*p*
Age (year)	Baseline	70.61 ± 3.29	68.59 ± 3.24	0.838
	One-year Posttest	72.39 ± 3.43	70.85 ± 4.05	0.782
Gender (male)	Baseline	23 (16)	17 (9)	0.283
	One-year Posttest	18 (13)	14 (9)	0.631
Education (year)	Baseline	10.91 ± 3.65	10.64 ± 3.06	0.452
MMSE	Baseline	27.57 ± 2.57	28.17 ± 1.94	0.505
	One-year Posttest	27.72 ± 2.16	27.85 ± 2.31	0.900

Identification of RSN and Voxelwise Homotopic Maps

There were 45 components resulting from the group ICA. Ten components were selected as nonartifactual, relevant networks by visual inspection in accordance with published results (Luo et al., 2012c; Li et al., 2015b). The spatial maps of these RSNs were highly stable (reliability index >0.83) as determined by ICASSO. The 10 RSNs were shown in **Figure 1** and labeled as follows:

V1N: primary visual network. The visual cortex is often apparent in two separate components. This network showed spatial patterns consisting of primary visual area (Damoiseaux et al., 2006; Luo et al., 2012c).

V2N: the second visual network illustrated spatial patterns consisting of more lateral visual arear in the occipital lobe

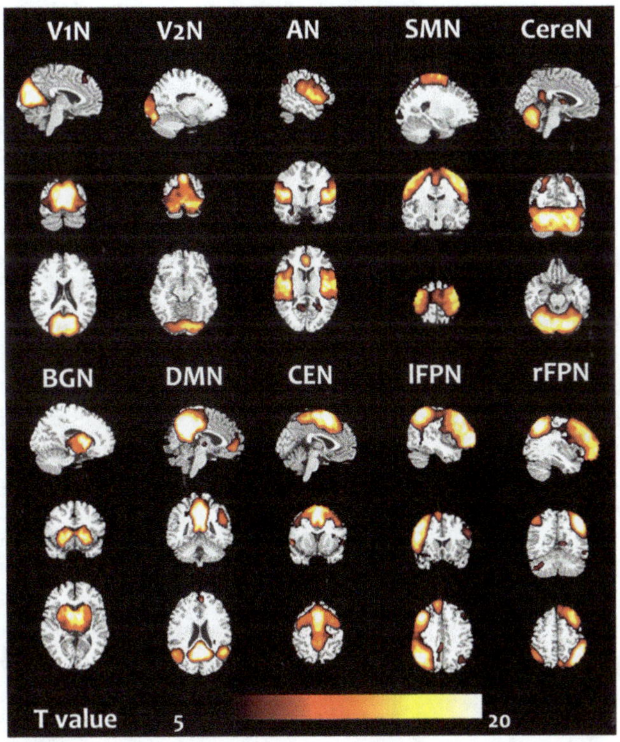

FIGURE 1 | Ten resting state networks (RSN) were chosen. The one sample *t*-test in the group included all subjects in the pre-training scans was performed.

which were previously known to be involved in visual processing (Damoiseaux et al., 2006; Luo et al., 2012c).

AN: auditory network (AN) primarily encompassed bilateral middle, superior temporal gyrus, temporal pole and insular, corresponded to the auditory system (Damoiseaux et al., 2006; Luo et al., 2012c).

SMN: sensorimotor network (SMN) was a network corresponding to sensory-motor function. This network includes pre- and postcentral gyrus, the primary sensorimotor cortices, and the supplementary motor area (Damoiseaux et al., 2006; Luo et al., 2012c).

CereN: cerebellum network included bilateral cerebellum hemispheres.

DMN: default mode network (DMN) mainly encompasses posterior cingulate cortex, medial prefrontal gyrus, bilateral superior frontal gyrus, and bilateral angular gyri (Raichle et al., 2001; Damoiseaux et al., 2006; Luo et al., 2012c).

lFPN: left lateral FPN (lFPN) along with right lateral FPN showed the similar spatial patterns with DAN consisting of regions previously known to be involved in goal-directed top-down processing (Damoiseaux et al., 2006; Luo et al., 2012c). This network primarily involved precuneus, inferior parietal lobule, middle frontal gyrus, superior parietal lobule.

rFPN: right lateral FPN (rFPN) including clusters lateralized to the right hemisphere putatively associated with DAN. lFPN and rFPN were the only maps to be strongly lateralized and were largely left–right mirrors of each other (Damoiseaux et al., 2006; Luo et al., 2012c).

CEN: central executive network showed spatial patterns consisting of the superior and middle prefrontal cortices, anterior cingulate and paracingulate gyri, and ventrolateral prefrontal cortex (Beckmann et al., 2005).

BGN: basal ganglia network, encompassed middle temporal gyrus, superior temporal gyrus, insular and temporal pole and corresponded to the auditory system (Luo et al., 2012b).

For 10 RSNs, their voxelwise homotopic maps were calculated for each group. Because the homotopic maps were similar to each other among groups, the group level maps resulted from the pre-training scans were illustrated in the **Figure 2**.

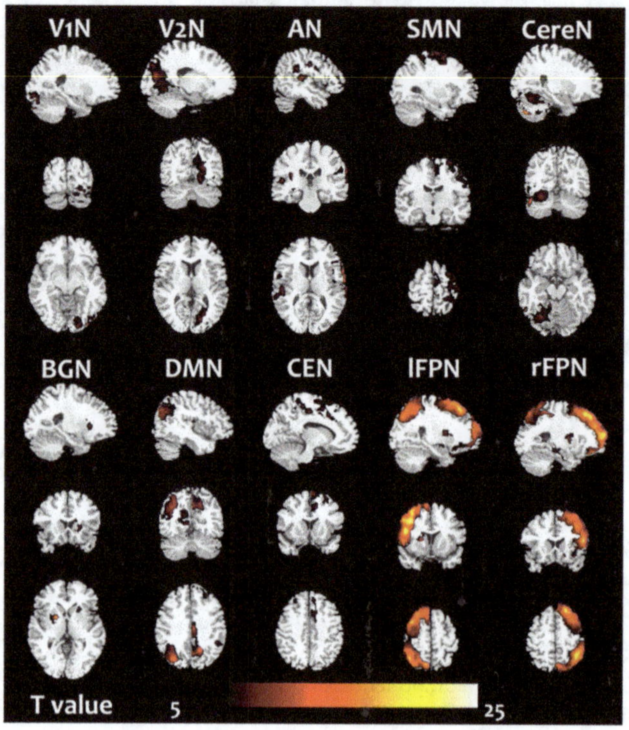

FIGURE 2 | The homotopic maps of the 10 RSN. The group level maps resulted from one sample t-test in the groups including the pre-training scans (before cognitive training) of all subjects.

Laterality Cofactors

In the three groups, the global LCF of each RSN were illustrated in **Figure 3**. According to the previous criteria (Agcaoglu et al., 2015), the LCFs are called highly lateralized when it has absolute value above 0.75 or has lateralized with absolute value above 0.2; the LCFs in rFPN and lFPN were highly lateralized in three groups. The remaining eight RSNs did not have marked lateralization, in which the LCFs have absolute value less than 0.2.

To investigate the influence of the multiple cognitive training on the laterality of RSN, the LCFs of each RSN and each subject were also evaluated (**Table 2**, **Figure 4**). After the Fisher r-to-z translation, a repeated measure ANOVA revealed that both groups improved their LCFs in CereN as indicated by a significant main effect of time ($F = 6.903$, $p = 0.015$). In addition, a significant training main effect on the LCF in rFPN ($F = 5.897$, $p = 0.021$) and lFPN ($F = 7.641$, $p = 0.01$), as well as interactions of LCF of lFPN ($F = 8.908$, $p = 0.006$), were observed. *Post hoc* analysis showed significantly increased LCF of lFPN in the training group compared with the control group at the second scan ($T = 3.48$, $p = 0.001$). Paired-sample t-tests revealed that the global LCF of CereN ($T = 2.30$, $p = 0.03$) was significantly increased after the training scan compared with the before-training scan in the control group but not in the training group. Similarly, compared with the before-training scan, the after-training scan showed the decreased LCF of lFPN ($T = 2.21$, $p = 0.04$) in the control group, whereas a marginal significant increase ($T = 2.02$, $p = 0.06$) was observed in the training group.

DISCUSSION

The lateralization of human brain function is an obvious sign reflecting functional specialization. Neurodegeneration would alter the functional specialization in aging. In this study, we used the LCF (Agcaoglu et al., 2015) of intrinsic networks resulting from the resting fMRI to investigate the effects of multi-domain cognitive training on healthy older adults. We observed statistically significant training effects on the lateralization of two important RSNs related to high-level cognition: right- and left- FPNs. In particular, the lateralization of lFPN were retained well in the training group but decreased in the control group. The increased lateralization with aging

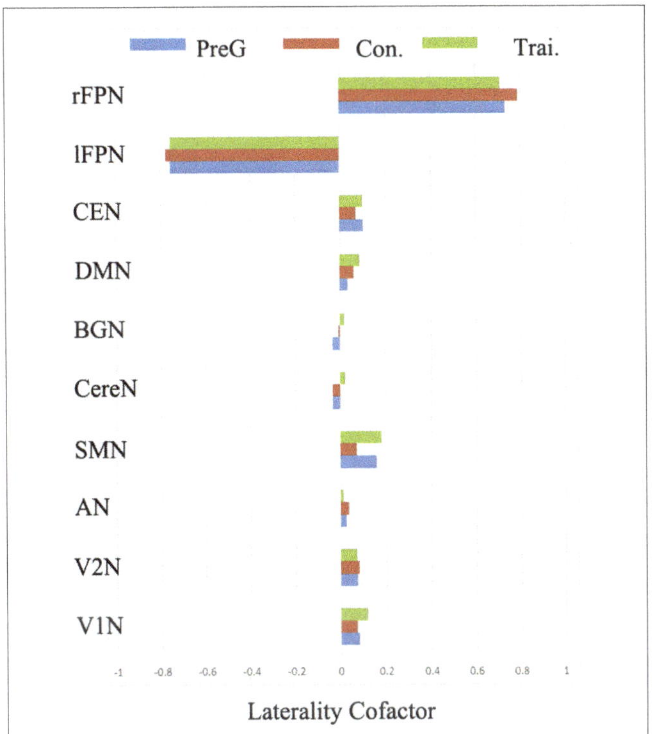

FIGURE 3 | The group level laterality cofactor (LCF) resulted from the three group *Bv* homotopic maps for each RSN. Three groups included the pre-training group including all subjects, the post-training group and the control group of the second scans.

was observed in the CereN, in which the lateralization was significantly increased in the control group, although the same change tendency was observed in the training group. These findings indicate that the lateralization of the high-level cognitive intrinsic networks is sensitive to multi-domain cognitive training. This study provides neuroimaging evidence to support the idea that cognitive training should have advantages in preventing the cognitive decline in healthy older adults.

Both human and animal studies indicates neural plasticity across the lifespan (Ball et al., 2002; Papp et al., 2009). A number of studies support the protective effects of late-life cognitive training on dementia (Ball et al., 2002; Wilson et al., 2002; Snowball et al., 2013). Our previous study has illustrated positive effects of multi-domain cognitive training interventions in healthy older adults. Here, the findings from neuroimaging were provided to uncover the potential brain changes to response the effects of interventions. The functional neuroimaging biomarkers can play an important role in detecting, assessing and diagnosing neurodegeneration (Horwitz and Rowe, 2011). In addition, there was altered intrinsic connectivity in the special targeted networks such as DMN and salience network to different neurodegenerative disorders (Seeley et al., 2009). Recently, the lateralization of RSNs was observed as an alteration accompanied by increased aging (Wilson et al., 2002). The hemispheric lateralization was also associated with enhanced cognitive ability (Gotts et al., 2013). Thus, the spatial pattern of intrinsic networks would be a candidate feature for the cognitive training intervention in older adults. Enhancement and maintenance of memory, visuospatial/construction and attention endured in healthy older adults with multi-domain cognitive interventions (Cheng et al., 2012). The changed lateralization of FPN and CereN which was observed in the cohort might be related to the brain mechanism of these behavior improvements.

The FPNs are associated with attention, cognitive performance and control processes. In the studies of resting state fMRI, the FPN is often identified using ICA. FPNs have marked asymmetry, which is involved in a multitude of cognitions; the right is more involved in monitoring processes whereas the left is putatively more involved in production processes (Cabeza et al., 2003). Combining lFPN and rFPN showed a similar spatial pattern, with a dorsal attention network consisting of regions previously known to be involved in goal-directed top-down processing (Damoiseaux et al., 2006; Luo et al., 2012c). Significant interactions of global LCF of lFPN were observed in this study. Global LCF of lFPN was significantly decreased in healthy controls whereas a marginal significant increase was observed in the training group. We presumed that the lateralization of lFPN would be an important predictor for maintenance of attention functioning and production processes. These findings implicated that the multi-domain cognitive training would contribute to the top-down attention function in the healthy older adults. Although the training main effects were also observed in the rFPN using repeated measure ANOVA, as indicated by the difference between the training group and control group, the training main effects might be stained by the initial distinction between groups (**Figure 4**). Thus the influence of training on the rFPN would not be evaluated directly in this study. In general, the FPN would be a target to multi-domain cognitive training.

Motor-related function decline is another physiological sign in old adults compared with younger adults. Accumulating evidence demonstrates decreased functional connectivity in the motor-related networks in aging, including the CereN and sensory-motor network (Tomasi and Volkow, 2012). Consistent with the previous studies, we found that the CereN is symmetrical at baseline (first scanning). However, improved lateralization of the CereN was observed in both group as indicated by a significant main effect of time in repeated measure ANOVA. The laterality significantly increased between two times of scans with interval of 1 year in healthy control groups whereas it did not in the training group. This finding reflected that the symmetry of the CereN was maintained in healthy older adults with multi-domain cognitive training. Recently, the functional connectivity studies indicate that the cerebellum participates in functional networks with motor control and cognitive processes (Habas et al., 2009; Krienen and Buckner, 2009). Thus, our findings might implicate that the multi-domain cognitive intervention contributed to the improvement of motor control in older adults. Actually, SMN would be directly related with motor performance (Zhang et al., 2015). Seidler et al. (2015) found greater network interactivity of SMN in older adults and suggested the protection

TABLE 2 | The results of the repeated measure ANOVA for the laterality cofactors of individual *Bv* maps in 10 RSNs.

		V1N	V2N	AN	SMN	CereN	BGN	DMN	CEN	lFPN	rFPN
Time main effects	*F* value	3.498	0.279	0.111	3.888	6.903	1.044	0.677	0.901	0.006	1.183
	P value	0.071	0.601	0.741	0.058	0.015*	0.315	0.417	0.35	0.939	0.285
Training main effects	*F* value	0.192	0.264	0.048	0.699	0.499	3.808	1.088	0.026	7.641	5.897
	P value	0.664	0.611	0.828	0.41	0.485	0.06	0.305	0.872	0.01*	0.021*
Interaction effects	*F* value	0.229	0.012	0.821	1.858	0.945	0.27	1.057	0.102	8.908	0.649
	P value	0.636	0.915	0.372	0.183	0.339	0.607	0.312	0.752	0.006*	0.427

*Note: *Represented the statistical significance $p < 0.05$.*

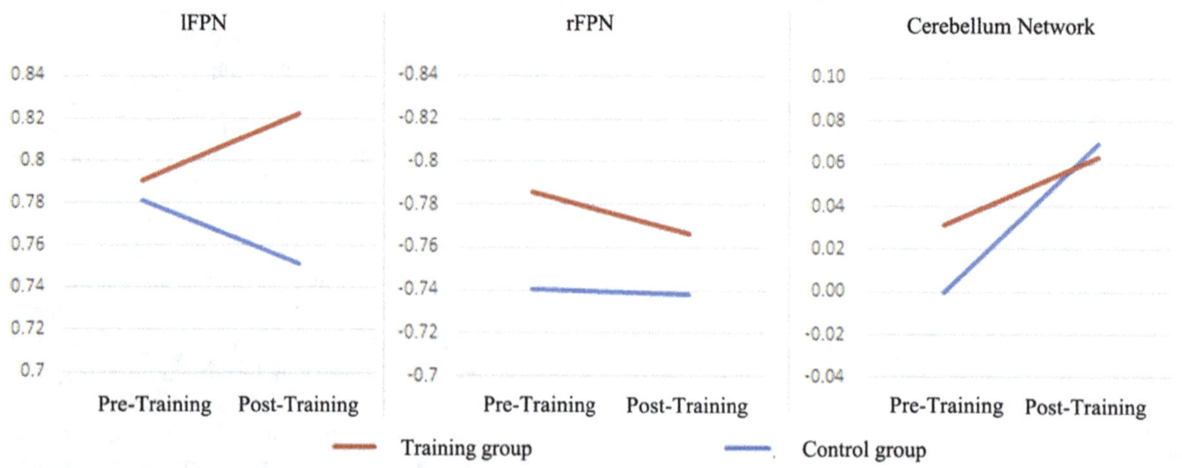

FIGURE 4 | The LCFs of individual *Bv* maps in the lFPN, rFPN and CereN. The repeated measure ANOVA were performed. The significance of statistical test was demonstrated in the **Table 2**.

against age declines in motor performance. However, no difference of the lateralization was found in the SMN in this study. It did not mean that the negative effects of cognitive training on the motor performance and motor prediction which are related with SMN are responsible. Future studies should focus on the various aspects of motor function associated with the cognitive intervention.

There are several limitations which should be mentioned here. First, the longitudinal design with 1-year duration was adopted in this study. The subjects were randomly grouped, and the behavior scores and genders were matched between groups. However, some connectivity features from the resting state fMRI might not match because their features could be calculated according to different methods. Thus, some features whose difference illustrated by repeated measure ANOVA might be stained by the mismatch in baseline (the first time) measures. Second, the relative small sample size would be another shortage of our study. In the future, more subjects should be recruited into the longitudinal study. Finally, the Group ICA was used to investigate the symmetry of the spatial pattern of RSNs. However, the number of ICs might be an underlying confounding factor. Till now, there has been no validated way to identify the number of ICs in ICA analysis. In this work, the MDL criteria implanted in GIFT software was used to determine the number of ICs.

In conclusion, lateralization of function is an important organization of the human brain. The distribution of intrinsic networks in the resting brain and their association with the multi-domain cognitive training is analyzed in this study. The lateralization of bilateral FPN and CereN was related to both aging and the multi-domain cognitive training in healthy older adults. These findings provide a neuroimaging evidence to support the positive effects of the cognitive training on enhancement and maintenance cognitive and motor function in healthy older adults.

AUTHOR CONTRIBUTIONS

Conceived and designed the work: CLi, CLuo and DY; Acquired the data: XC, TL, YC and LJ; Analyzed the data: WC, XZ, CLuo, YG, XC and YC; Wrote the article: CLuo, CLi and DY. All authors revised the work for important intellectual content. All of the authors have read and approved the manuscript.

ACKNOWLEDGMENTS

This study was funded by grants from the National Nature Science Foundation of China (81330032, 81371505, 81271547, 81471638), the Science and Technology Commission of Shanghai Municipality (134119a2501, 13dz2260500), the "111" project (B12027), SHSMU-ION Research Center for Brain Disorders.

REFERENCES

Agcaoglu, O., Miller, R., Mayer, A. R., Hugdahl, K., and Calhoun, V. D. (2015). Lateralization of resting state networks and relationship to age and gender. *Neuroimage* 104, 310–325. doi: 10.1016/j.neuroimage.2014.09.001

Ashendorf, L., Jefferson, A. L., O'Conno, M. K., Chaisson, C., Green, R. C., and Stern, R. A. (2008). Trail making test errors in normal aging, mild cognitive impairment and dementia. *Arch. Clin. Neuropsychol.* 23, 129–137. doi: 10.1016/j.acn.2007.11.005

Ball, K., Berch, D. B., Helmers, K. F., Jobe, J. B., Leveck, M. D., Marsiske, M., et al. (2002). Effects of cognitive training interventions with older adults: a randomized controlled trial. *JAMA* 288, 2271–2281. doi: 10.1001/jama.288.18.2271

Beckmann, C. F., Deluca, M., Devlin, J. T., and Smith, S. M. (2005). Investigations into resting-state connectivity using independent component analysis. *Philos. Trans. R. Soc. Lond. B Biol. Sci.* 360, 1001–1013. doi: 10.1098/rstb.2005.1634

Boyke, J., Driemeyer, J., Gaser, C., Buchel, C., and May, A. (2008). Training-induced brain structure changes in the elderly. *J. Neurosci.* 28, 7031–7035. doi: 10.1523/JNEUROSCI.0742-08.2008

Brown, B. M., Peiffer, J. J., and Martins, R. N. (2013). Multiple effects of physical activity on molecular and cognitive signs of brain aging: can exercise slow neurodegeneration and delay Alzheimer's disease? *Mol. Psychiatry* 18, 864–874. doi: 10.1038/mp.2012.162

Cabeza, R., Locantore, J. K., and Anderson, N. D. (2003). Lateralization of prefrontal activity during episodic memory retrieval: evidence for the production-monitoring hypothesis. *J. Cogn. Neurosci.* 15, 249–259. doi: 10.1162/089892903321208187

Cao, W., Luo, C., Zhu, B., Zhang, D., Dong, L., Gong, J., et al. (2014). Resting-state functional connectivity in anterior cingulate cortex in normal aging. *Front. Aging Neurosci.* 6:280. doi: 10.3389/fnagi.2014.00280

Chen, X., Duan, M., Xie, Q., Lai, Y., Dong, L., Cao, W., et al. (2015). Functional disconnection between the visual cortex and the sensorimotor cortex suggests a potential mechanism for self-disorder in schizophrenia. *Schizophr. Res.* 166, 151–157. doi: 10.1016/j.schres.2015.06.014

Cheng, Y., Wu, W., Feng, W., Wang, J., Chen, Y., Shen, Y., et al. (2012). The effects of multi-domain versus single-domain cognitive training in non-demented older people: a randomized controlled trial. *BMC Med.* 10:30. doi: 10.1186/1741-7015-10-30

Cheng, Y., Wu, W., Wang, J., Feng, W., Wu, X., and Li, C. (2011). Reliability and validity of the repeatable battery for the assessment of neuropsychological status in community-dwelling elderly. *Arch. Med. Sci.* 7, 850–857. doi: 10.5114/aoms.2011.25561

Corballis, M. C. (2014). Left brain, right brain: facts and fantasies. *PLoS Biol.* 12:e1001767. doi: 10.1371/journal.pbio.1001767

Damoiseaux, J. S., Rombouts, S. A., Barkhof, F., Scheltens, P., Stam, C. J., Smith, S. M., et al. (2006). Consistent resting-state networks across healthy subjects. *Proc. Natl. Acad. Sci. U S A* 103, 13848–13853. doi: 10.1073/pnas.0601417103

Fox, M. D., Corbetta, M., Snyder, A. Z., Vincent, J. L., and Raichle, M. E. (2006). Spontaneous neuronal activity distinguishes human dorsal and ventral attention systems. *Proc. Natl. Acad. Sci. U S A* 103, 10046–10051. doi: 10.1073/pnas.0604187103

Gates, N., and Valenzuela, M. (2010). Cognitive exercise and its role in cognitive function in older adults. *Curr. Psychiatry Rep.* 12, 20–27. doi: 10.1007/s11920-009-0085-y

Goldberg, E., Roediger, D., Kucukboyaci, N. E., Carlson, C., Devinsky, O., Kuzniecky, R., et al. (2013). Hemispheric asymmetries of cortical volume in the human brain. *Cortex* 49, 200–210. doi: 10.1016/j.cortex.2011.11.002

Gong, D., He, H., Liu, D., Ma, W., Dong, L., Luo, C., et al. (2015). Enhanced functional connectivity and increased gray matter volume of insula related to action video game playing. *Sci. Rep.* 5:9763. doi: 10.1038/srep09763

Gong, D., He, H., Ma, W., Liu, D., Huang, M., Dong, L., et al. (2016). Functional integration between salience and central executive networks: a role for action video game experience. *Neural Plast.* 2015, 2016:9803165. doi: 10.1155/2016/9803165

Gotts, S. J., Jo, H. J., Wallace, G. L., Saad, Z. S., Cox, R. W., and Martin, A. (2013). Two distinct forms of functional lateralization in the human brain. *Proc. Natl. Acad. Sci. U S A* 110, E3435–E3444. doi: 10.1073/pnas.1302581110

Habas, C., Kamdar, N., Nguyen, D., Prater, K., Beckmann, C. F., Menon, V., et al. (2009). Distinct cerebellar contributions to intrinsic connectivity networks. *J. Neurosci.* 29, 8586–8594. doi: 10.1523/JNEUROSCI.1868-09.2009

Himberg, J., Hyvärinen, A., and Esposito, F. (2004). Validating the independent components of neuroimaging time series via clustering and visualization. *Neuroimage* 22, 1214–1222. doi: 10.1016/j.neuroimage.2004.03.027

Horwitz, B., and Rowe, J. B. (2011). Functional biomarkers for neurodegenerative disorders based on the network paradigm. *Prog. Neurobiol.* 95, 505–509. doi: 10.1016/j.pneurobio.2011.07.005

Jiang, S., Luo, C., Liu, Z., Hou, C., Wang, P., Dong, L., et al. (2016). Altered local spontaneous brain activity in juvenile myoclonic epilepsy: a preliminary resting-state fMRI study. *Neural Plast.* 2016:3547203. doi: 10.1155/2016/3547203

Kelly, A. M., Di Martino, A., Uddin, L. Q., Shehzad, Z., Gee, D. G., Reiss, P. T., et al. (2009). Development of anterior cingulate functional connectivity from late childhood to early adulthood. *Cereb. Cortex* 19, 640–657. doi: 10.1093/cercor/bhn117

Krienen, F. M., and Buckner, R. L. (2009). Segregated fronto-cerebellar circuits revealed by intrinsic functional connectivity. *Cereb. Cortex* 19, 2485–2497. doi: 10.1093/cercor/bhp135

Li, G., He, H., Huang, M., Zhang, X., Lu, J., Lai, Y., et al. (2015a). Identifying enhanced cortico-basal ganglia loops associated with prolonged dance training. *Sci. Rep.* 5:10271. doi: 10.1038/srep10271

Li, Q., Cao, W., Liao, X., Chen, Z., Yang, T., Gong, Q., et al. (2015b). Altered resting state functional network connectivity in children absence epilepsy. *J. Neurol. Sci.* 354, 79–85. doi: 10.1016/j.jns.2015.04.054

Li, J., Luo, C., Peng, Y., Xie, Q., Gong, J., Dong, L., et al. (2014). Probabilistic diffusion tractography reveals improvement of structural network in musicians. *PLoS One* 9:e105508. doi: 10.1371/journal.pone.0105508

Li, C., Wu, W., Jin, H., Zhang, X., Xue, H., He, Y., et al. (2006). Successful aging in Shanghai, China: definition, distribution and related factors. *Int. Psychogeriatr.* 18, 551–563. doi: 10.1017/s1041610205002966

Lim, M. L., Collinson, S. L., Feng, L., and Ng, T. P. (2010). Cross-cultural application of the Repeatable Battery for the Assessment of Neuropsychological Status (RBANS): performances of elderly Chinese Singaporeans. *Clin. Neuropsychol.* 24, 811–826. doi: 10.1080/13854046.2010.490789

Luo, C., Guo, Z. W., Lai, Y. X., Liao, W., Liu, Q., Kendrick, K. M., et al. (2012a). Musical training induces functional plasticity in perceptual and motor networks: insights from resting-state FMRI. *PLoS One* 7:e36568. doi: 10.1371/journal.pone.0036568

Luo, C., Li, Q., Xia, Y., Lei, X., Xue, K., Yao, Z., et al. (2012b). Resting state basal ganglia network in idiopathic generalized epilepsy. *Hum. Brain Mapp.* 33, 1279–1294. doi: 10.1002/hbm.21286

Luo, C., Qiu, C., Guo, Z., Fang, J., Li, Q., Lei, X., et al. (2012c). Disrupted functional brain connectivity in partial epilepsy: a resting-state fMRI study. *PLoS One* 7:e28196. doi: 10.1371/journal.pone.0028196

Luo, C., Tu, S., Peng, Y., Gao, S., Li, J., Dong, L., et al. (2014a). Long-term effects of musical training and functional plasticity in salience system. *Neural Plast.* 2014:180138. doi: 10.1155/2014/180138

Luo, C., Yang, T., Tu, S., Deng, J., Liu, D., Li, Q., et al. (2014b). Altered intrinsic functional connectivity of the salience network in childhood absence epilepsy. *J. Neurol. Sci.* 339, 189–195. doi: 10.1016/j.jns.2014.02.016

Lustig, C., Shah, P., Seidler, R., and Reuter-Lorenz, P. A. (2009). Aging, training and the brain: a review and future directions. *Neuropsychol. Rev.* 19, 504–522. doi: 10.1007/s11065-009-9119-9

Mackey, A. P., Miller Singley, A. T., and Bunge, S. A. (2013). Intensive reasoning training alters patterns of brain connectivity at rest. *J. Neurosci.* 33, 4796–4803. doi: 10.1523/JNEUROSCI.4141-12.2013

Papp, K. V., Walsh, S. J., and Snyder, P. J. (2009). Immediate and delayed effects of cognitive interventions in healthy elderly: a review of current literature and future directions. *Alzheimers Dement.* 5, 50–60. doi: 10.1016/j.jalz.2008.10.008

Power, J. D., Barnes, K. A., Snyder, A. Z., Schlaggar, B. L., and Petersen, S. E. (2012). Spurious but systematic correlations in functional connectivity MRI networks arise from subject motion. *Neuroimage* 59, 2142–2154. doi: 10.1016/j.neuroimage.2011.10.018

Raichle, M. E., MacLeod, A. M., Snyder, A. Z., Powers, W. J., Gusnard, D. A., and Shulman, G. L. (2001). A default mode of brain function. *Proc. Natl. Acad. Sci. U S A* 98, 676–682. doi: 10.1073/pnas.98.2.676

Seeley, W. W., Crawford, R. K., Zhou, J., Miller, B. L., and Greicius, M. D. (2009). Neurodegenerative diseases target large-scale human brain networks. *Neuron* 62, 42–52. doi: 10.1016/j.neuron.2009.03.024

Seidler, R. D., Bernard, J. A., Burutolu, T. B., Fling, B. W., Gordon, M. T., Gwin, J. T., et al. (2010). Motor control and aging: links to age-related brain structural, functional and biochemical effects. *Neurosci. Biobehav. Rev.* 34, 721–733. doi: 10.1016/j.neubiorev.2009.10.005

Seidler, R., Erdeniz, B., Koppelmans, V., Hirsiger, S., Mérillat, S., and Jäncke, L. (2015). Associations between age, motor function and resting state sensorimotor network connectivity in healthy older adults. *Neuroimage* 108, 47–59. doi: 10.1016/j.neuroimage.2014.12.023

Snowball, A., Tachtsidis, I., Popescu, T., Thompson, J., Delazer, M., Zamarian, L., et al. (2013). Long-term enhancement of brain function and cognition using cognitive training and brain stimulation. *Curr. Biol.* 23, 987–992. doi: 10.1016/j.cub.2013.04.045

Tomasi, D., and Volkow, N. D. (2012). Aging and functional brain networks. *Mol. Psychiatry* 17, 471, 549–458. doi: 10.1038/mp.2011.81

van Boxtel, M. P., ten Tusscher, M. P., Metsemakers, J. F., Willems, B., and Jolles, J. (2001). Visual determinants of reduced performance on the stroop color-word test in normal aging individuals. *J. Clin. Exp. Neuropsychol.* 23, 620–627. doi: 10.1076/jcen.23.5.620.1245

Wilson, R. S., Mendes De Leon, C. F., Barnes, L. L., Schneider, J. A., Bienias, J. L., Evans, D. A., et al. (2002). Participation in cognitively stimulating activities and risk of incident Alzheimer disease. *JAMA* 287, 742–748. doi: 10.1001/jama.287.6.742

Xiao, S., Yao, P., Li, X., and Zhang, M. (2002). Neuropsychological testing profiles of patients with Alzheimer's disease and mild cognitive impairment: a case-control study. *Hong Kong J. Psychiatry* 12, 2–5.

Zhang, R., Yao, D., Valdés-Sosa, P. A., Li, F., Li, P., Zhang, T., et al. (2015). Efficient resting-state EEG network facilitates motor imagery performance. *J. Neural Eng.* 12:066024. doi: 10.1088/1741-2560/12/6/066024 [Epub ahead of print].

Zhang, H., Zuo, X. N., Ma, S. Y., Zang, Y. F., Milham, M. P., and Zhu, C. Z. (2010). Subject order-independent group ICA (SOI-GICA) for functional MRI data analysis. *Neuroimage* 51, 1414–1424. doi: 10.1016/j.neuroimage.2010.03.039

18

Brain Metabolic Stress and Neuroinflammation at the Basis of Cognitive Impairment in Alzheimer's Disease

*Fernanda G. De Felice * and Mychael V. Lourenco*

Institute of Medical Biochemistry Leopoldo de Meis, Federal University of Rio de Janeiro, Rio de Janeiro, RJ, Brazil

Edited by:
Fei Yin,
University of Southern California,
USA

Reviewed by:
Paula I. Moreira,
University of Coimbra,
Portugal
Enrique Cadenas,
University of Southern California,
USA

****Correspondence:***
Fernanda G. De Felice,
Institute of Medical Biochemistry
Leopoldo de Meis, Federal University
of Rio de Janeiro, Rio de Janeiro, RJ
21941-902, Brazil
felice@bioqmed.ufrj.br

Brain metabolic dysfunction is known to influence brain activity in several neurological disorders, including Alzheimer's disease (AD). In fact, deregulation of neuronal metabolism has been postulated to play a key role leading to the clinical outcomes observed in AD. Besides deficits in glucose utilization in AD patients, recent evidence has implicated neuroinflammation and endoplasmic reticulum (ER) stress as components of a novel form of brain metabolic stress that develop in AD and other neurological disorders. Here we review findings supporting this novel paradigm and further discuss how these mechanisms seem to participate in synapse and cognitive impairments that are germane to AD. These deleterious processes resemble pathways that act in peripheral tissues leading to insulin resistance and glucose intolerance, in an intriguing molecular connection linking AD to diabetes. The discovery of detailed mechanisms leading to neuronal metabolic stress may be a key step that will allow the understanding how cognitive impairment develops in AD, thereby offering new avenues for effective disease prevention and therapeutic targeting.

Keywords: Alzheimer's disease, amyloid-β oligomers, endoplasmic reticulum stress, inflammation, metabolic stress

Introduction

Incidence of Alzheimer's disease (AD) will greatly increase as world population ages (Prince et al., 2013) and changes in lifestyle observed in recent decades seem to be major contributors to such increased prevalence (Mattson, 2012; De Felice, 2013). Likewise, common diseases of modern adulthood, including obesity and diabetes mellitus, have been often regarded as AD risk factors (De Felice, 2013). Pioneering epidemiological studies connecting AD to diabetes initiated in the 1990s (Ott et al., 1996, 1999; Kalmijin et al., 1997) and were followed by several reports providing both clinical and experimental evidence into how these two disorders may course together (de la Monte, 2009; Matsuzaki et al., 2010; Crane et al., 2013; De Felice, 2013; De Felice et al., 2014).

Metabolic derangements, including inflammation, insulin resistance and endoplasmic reticulum (ER) stress, are known to underlie glucose intolerance and type 2 diabetes mellitus (T2DM) in peripheral tissues (Hotamisligil et al., 1995, 1996; Ozcan et al., 2004, 2006; Hotamisligil, 2006). A similar scenario has been recently described in the brains of patients that suffer from neurodegenerative disorders, such as AD. Neuropathology investigations have revealed that AD brains present several markers of insulin resistance, inflammation and ER stress (Hoozemans et al., 2005; Steen et al., 2005; Moloney et al., 2010; Bomfim et al., 2012; Talbot et al., 2012; O'Neill, 2013;

De Felice et al., 2014). In the following sections, we review current evidence indicating that a newly defined form of metabolic stress leads the path to cognitive decline in AD. The understanding of molecular mechanisms driving AD pathogenesis may shed new light on novel targets for drug development and offer strategies for disease prevention.

AD Pathogenesis

AD pathophysiology includes neuroinflammation, oxidative and ER stress, synapse loss and degeneration of specific neuronal populations (Selkoe, 2002; Ferreira and Klein, 2011; Mucke and Selkoe, 2012). Amyloid-β peptide (Aβ) is the main component of senile plaques that accumulate in AD brains (Masters et al., 1985), and substantial evidence indicates that Aβ is causally involved in AD (Mucke and Selkoe, 2012). Consolidated knowledge has established that soluble Aβ oligomers (AβOs; Lambert et al., 1998), and not necessarily the insoluble amyloid fibrils detected in senile plaques, promote direct damage to synapses, besides stimulating inflammatory response and cellular stress (Ferreira and Klein, 2011; Viola and Klein, 2015). These findings prompt AβOs, which are increased in AD brains (Gong et al., 2003; Xia et al., 2009), to be considered neurotoxins responsible for synapse and memory loss in AD early stages.

Very recent data has demonstrated that AβO actions stimulate pro-inflammatory mechanisms to impair neuronal insulin signaling and to trigger stress kinase activation, resulting in synapse and memory impairments in AD models (Bomfim et al., 2012; Lourenco et al., 2013; Ma et al., 2013). These events are quite similar to those acting in peripheral tissues to impair metabolism in diabetes and obesity (De Felice and Ferreira, 2014), in line with the idea that a form of metabolic stress develops in AD brains (Kapogiannis and Mattson, 2011; Yoon et al., 2012; De Felice and Ferreira, 2014). Such findings may impact translational research, as treating brain metabolic dysfunction might be a key strategy to fight neurological disorders.

Brain Metabolic Stress Mechanisms in AD

In peripheral tissues, prolonged inflammatory cascades lead to the activation of multiple cellular stress mechanisms that ultimately impair cell function and body metabolism (Hotamisligil, 2006; Gregor and Hotamisligil, 2011). In AD, evidence arising from *in vitro*, *in vivo* and neuropathology studies supports that such events occur throughout disease development and are linked to AβO neurotoxicity. Oligomers promote neuronal stress by instigating abnormal elevations in levels of tumor necrosis factor α (TNF-α) and reactive oxygen species (ROS), as well as activation in JNK/PKR signaling and increased eIF2α phosphorylation (eIF2α-P) levels in AD models (De Felice et al., 2007, 2014; Ma et al., 2009, 2013; Bomfim et al., 2012; Lourenco et al., 2013). In this context, pro-inflammatory signals appear to be directly responsible for defective insulin signaling and stress-mediated synapse loss caused by AβOs in neurons (Bomfim et al., 2012; Lourenco et al., 2013). This has led to a concept in which AβOs build up in pre-AD brains to cause inflammation (e.g., gliosis and cytokine production) and neuronal metabolic stress, ultimately leading to synaptic dysfunction and behavioral alterations. We next detail some of the mechanisms recently implicated in AD pathogenesis.

Unfolded Protein Response

Unfolded Protein Response (UPR) is defined as a collection of signaling pathways that respond to ER stress due to accumulation of misfolded proteins and/or impaired homeostasis. ER membrane sensors activate three signaling axes (ATF6α, IRE-1α/XBP-1s and PERK/eIF2α-P) to instigate transcriptional and translational alterations aimed at restoring cell homeostasis (Lai et al., 2007; Hetz et al., 2013). UPR signaling attenuates global translation and favors the synthesis of select transcription factors, such as ATF4, CHOP and Nrf2 (Buffington et al., 2014; Hetz and Mollereau, 2014). Under continued stress, however, these pathways may promote cell damage and death. This hormetic response pattern is thus critical to determine cell fate in such conditions (Mattson, 2008; Hetz, 2012).

Evidence for canonical UPR activation has been found in AD neurons (Hoozemans et al., 2005, 2009; Yoon et al., 2012) and in AD mouse models (Yoon et al., 2012; Ma et al., 2013). In accordance, AβOs trigger UPR in hippocampal neurons *in vitro* and *in vivo* (Chafekar et al., 2007; Casas-Tinto et al., 2011; Lourenco et al., 2013; Barbero-Camps et al., 2014), and experimental induction of ER stress leads to neuronal metabolic stress (Yoon et al., 2012), tau phosphorylation (Bose et al., 2011; van der Harg et al., 2014), stress kinase activation (Bose et al., 2011; Paquet et al., 2011) and cognitive impairment in mice (Lourenco et al., 2013). Further, alleviating ER stress with 4-phenylbutyrate, a chemical chaperone, promotes cognitive benefits in AD mouse models (Ricobaraza et al., 2009, 2010; Wiley et al., 2011; Lourenco et al., 2013).

Substantial recent evidence has proposed that UPR activation is a common feature of different neurodegenerative diseases, as deleterious impacts of UPR branches were reported in AD (Lourenco et al., 2013; Ma et al., 2013; Barbero-Camps et al., 2014; van der Harg et al., 2014), Parkinson's (Bellucci et al., 2011; Colla et al., 2012), Huntington (Lajole and Snapp, 2011), amyotrophic lateral sclerosis (ALS; Hetz et al., 2009; Kim et al., 2013) and prion diseases (Moreno et al., 2012). Correcting UPR activation further appears to be effective in preclinical models of prion infection (Moreno et al., 2012, 2013; Halliday et al., 2015) and ALS (Hetz et al., 2009; Kim et al., 2013), in addition to AD models (Ricobaraza et al., 2009, 2010; Lourenco et al., 2013; Ma et al., 2013). Therefore, it is likely that aberrant UPR signaling mediates brain dysfunction in a variety of neurological conditions (**Figure 1**).

eIF2α-P and Translational Repression

Under cellular stress, translational repression can be mediated by increased eIF2α phosphorylation (eIF2α-P), a regulatory factor essential for translation initiation in eukaryotes (Raven and Koromilas, 2008). PERK-mediated eIF2α-P is the main UPR branch leading to general protein synthesis repression and

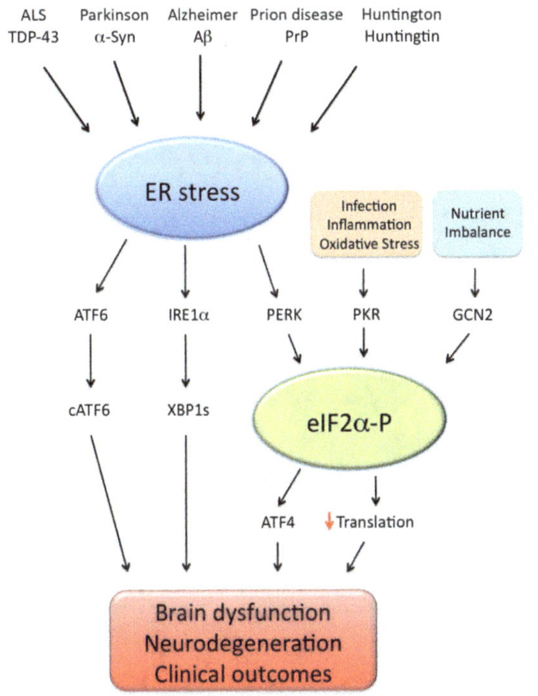

FIGURE 1 | Endoplasmic reticulum (ER) stress as a common denominator of neurodegenerative diseases. Brain ER stress is caused by several disease-associated stressors, including amyloid-β (Aβ; Alzheimer disease), α-synuclein (α-syn; Parkinson disease), prion protein (PrP; prion-related diseases), mutated huntingtin (Huntington and poly-Q diseases) and TAR DNA-binding protein of 43 kDa (TDP-43; amyotrophic lateral sclerosis, ALS). In such disorders, abnormal ER stress leads to the activation of three signaling pathways (ATF6; IRE1α/XBP1 s and PERK/eIF2α-P) collectively termed unfolded protein response (UPR). In parallel, events of infection, inflammation, nutrient deprivation and oxidative stress activate additional eIF2α kinases (namely PKR and GCN2), leading to abnormally high eIF2α-P levels, increased ATF4 production and impaired translation. Excessive UPR activity, eIF2α-P signaling and their downstream effectors impair cell function and may result in brain dysfunction and neurodegeneration, possibly explaining the clinical outcomes observed in neurodegenerative conditions.

facilitation of select mRNA translation (Buffington et al., 2014). Both PERK and eIF2α-P appear to be elevated in AD brains (Chang et al., 2002b; Yoon et al., 2012; Ma et al., 2013) and are induced by Aβ aggregates in neurons (Lee et al., 2010). Increased eIF2α-P has been further verified in other AD mouse models (Segev et al., 2012; Devi and Ohno, 2014).

Two other eIF2α kinases, namely the stress kinase PKR and the nutrient sensor GCN2, are enriched in the brain and have been reported to increase neuronal eIF2α-P (Costa-Mattioli et al., 2005; Lourenco et al., 2013; Roffé et al., 2013; Hetz and Mollereau, 2014), and thus emerge as candidates to explain increased eIF2α-P in AD.

Interestingly, deletion of either PERK or GCN2 in the brains of APP/PS1 mice decreases eIF2α-P levels, rescuing synapse plasticity and cognition (Ma et al., 2013). AβOs increase eIF2α-P through TNF-α-dependent PKR activation, thereby promoting synapse loss in hippocampal neurons and cognitive impairment in mice (Paquet et al., 2011; Lourenco et al., 2013). Providing clinical relevance to the findings observed in experimental models, PKR was found to be abnormally active in AD brains (Chang et al., 2002a; Paquet et al., 2011; Mouton-Liger et al., 2012b). Therefore, it is likely that PERK, GCN2, and PKR lead to increased eIF2α-P levels in AD.

Increased eIF2α-P levels also facilitate the translation of a small fraction of mRNAs (Buffington et al., 2014), among which is activating transcription factor 4 (ATF4), a protein linked to oxidative stress, enhanced γ-secretase activity and neuronal dysfunction when abnormally elevated (Mitsuda et al., 2007; Lange et al., 2008). ATF4 signaling further counteracts CREB1 pro-memory actions in mice (Costa-Mattioli et al., 2005; Rajasethupathy et al., 2012).

Recent findings demonstrated that ATF4 levels are increased in AD brains (Yoon et al., 2012; Baleriola et al., 2014) and in AD animal models (Ma et al., 2013; Devi and Ohno, 2014). Furthermore, soluble Aβ species appear to locally stimulate axonal ATF4 translation to propagate a neurodegenerative message in mice (Baleriola et al., 2014). Hence, eIF2α-P/ATF4 signaling has the potential to explain, at least in part, how disease progresses from defined brain regions in the beginning to a widespread forebrain dysfunction at later stages.

Translational repression instigated by eIF2α-P may be harmful to cognition, given that normal protein synthesis is required for memory (Flexner et al., 1964; Rossato et al., 2007). Accordingly, APP/PS1 mice present reduced brain protein synthesis in parallel to memory loss, and AβOs impair LTP-induced hippocampal protein synthesis (Ma et al., 2013). Nevertheless, the identity of memory-relevant translational products that are impacted in AD still remains to be determined.

Stress Kinase Activation

Cellular stress is also known to activate a family of protein kinases that mediate adaptive responses (Calay and Hotamisligil, 2013). These proteins are termed stress-sensitive kinases (or simply stress kinases) and include JNK, p38 MAPK, PKR, PERK and IKK, among other serine/threonine kinases (Vallerie and Hotamisligil, 2010; Hetz and Mollereau, 2014). Active stress kinases phosphorylate several protein targets to restore homeostasis. Nevertheless, their excessive or prolonged actions may trigger cell injury and, later, programmed cell death (Mattson, 2008; Vallerie and Hotamisligil, 2010; Hetz, 2012; De Felice et al., 2014).

Neuropathology studies have demonstrated abnormal activation of neuronal stress-sensitive kinases in AD brains. Indeed, abnormal phosphorylation of p38 MAPK (Hensley et al., 1999), JNK (Ma et al., 2009; Bomfim et al., 2012; Yoon et al., 2012), PERK (Hoozemans et al., 2005, 2009), PKR (Chang et al., 2002a; Paquet et al., 2011) and IKK (Talbot et al., 2012) have been reported in AD brains and might be core mediators of neuronal dysfunction. Accordingly, AβOs have been described to activate neuronal JNK and PKR to impair insulin signaling and synapse function (Ma et al., 2009; Bomfim et al., 2012; Lourenco et al., 2013), and transgenic animal models of AD exhibit similar alterations in JNK and PKR activity (Ma et al., 2009; Bomfim et al., 2012; Lourenco et al., 2013). Consistently, blocking either PKR or the brain-enriched JNK3 rescue cognitive impairments in AD mouse models (Yoon et al., 2012; Lourenco et al., 2013), suggesting that stress kinase activation lies upstream of synapse and memory impairment in AD.

An attractive possibility is that PKR further drives the activation of other MAPKs, such as p38MAPK and JNK, thus exacerbating neuronal damage. Very recent findings suggest that the interaction between PKR and the RNA-binding protein TRBP is essential to promote eIF2α-P and JNK activation under obesity-induced metabolic stress (Nakamura et al., 2015). A similar scenario might also develop in AD even independently of TNF-α, given that oxidative stress has been reported to activate neuronal PKR (Mouton-Liger et al., 2012a). Moreover, AβOs could activate PKR in glial cells to instigate MAPK-dependent actions, exacerbating neuroinflammatory responses in AD brains. These notions still demand further investigation.

Neuroinflammation

Elevated markers of inflammation are found in both AD animal models and human AD brains (Ferreira et al., 2014; Monson et al., 2014; Heneka et al., 2015). Consistently, evidence for gliosis and central infiltration of peripheral immune cells is often found in histopathological studies in AD mouse models (Yamanaka et al., 2012; Lourenco and Ledo, 2013; Yang et al., 2013; Baik et al., 2014; Ferreira et al., 2014; Monson et al., 2014).

Amyloid aggregates (ranging from oligomers to fibrils) induce a neuroinflammatory profile that may lead to synapse and neuronal damage (Combs, 2009; Pan et al., 2011; Lourenco et al., 2013; Medinas and Hetz, 2013; Parajuli et al., 2013; Heneka et al., 2015). Nevertheless, rather than deposited plaques, AβOs are thought to be core inducers of brain inflammation, given that they are potent microglial activators (Floden and Combs, 2006; Dhawan et al., 2012; Ledo et al., 2013) and diffuse throughout brain regions (Lambert et al., 1998; Forny-Germano et al., 2014; Viola and Klein, 2015). Accumulating evidence suggests that AβO-induced microglial activation releases TNF-α and other cytokines that, in turn, act on neurons to cause stress signaling and synapse injury (Floden and Combs, 2006; Sondag et al., 2009; Bomfim et al., 2012; Dhawan et al., 2012; Lourenco et al., 2013).

Therefore, neuroinflammation is considered to take place over the degenerative course of AD and to be linked to cognitive dysfunction. In fact, our recent results showed that AβO-triggered elevations in TNF-α levels orchestrate neuronal stress mechanisms to impair brain insulin signaling (Bomfim et al., 2012), synapses and cognition in animal models of AD (Lourenco et al., 2013; **Figure 2**). This cascade is mediated by stress kinases, including JNK and PKR, in the brains affected by AβOs (Lourenco et al., 2013). Since evidence suggests that reducing neuroinflammation can counteract memory deficits in AD mouse models (Medeiros et al., 2007; McAlpine et al., 2009; Kiyota et al., 2010; Bachstetter et al., 2012), a more complete understanding of how brain inflammation develops may lead to effective targeting of aberrant mechanisms underlying cognitive symptoms in AD.

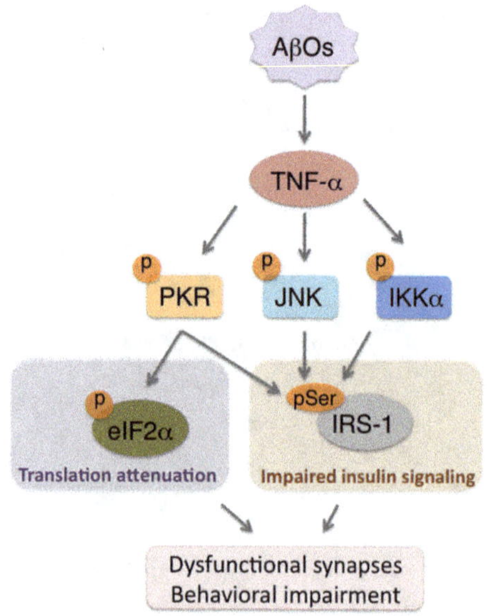

FIGURE 2 | AβOs trigger brain metabolic stress in Alzheimer's Disease (AD). Accumulation of AβOs in pre-AD brains instigates an inflammatory response that involves increased TNF-α production. TNF-α, in turn, acts on neurons to promote the activity of stress kinases (e.g., PKR, JNK, IKKα), which will serine phosphorylate both eIF2α-P to attenuate translation, and IRS-1 to impair insulin signaling. The combination of repressed protein synthesis and defective insulin signaling are components of a novel form of neuronal metabolic stress that may contribute to synapse deregulation and cognitive impairment in AD.

Metabolic Stress and Cognitive Function in AD

Experimental evidence has gathered inflammation, defective insulin signaling and cell stress to AD-linked neurotoxicity and neurodegeneration in a revised concept of metabolic stress (Paquet et al., 2011; Mouton-Liger et al., 2012a; Yoon et al., 2012; Ledo et al., 2013; Lourenco et al., 2013; Ma et al., 2013; Baleriola et al., 2014; De Felice et al., 2014). Although the classical alterations in glucose metabolism germane to metabolic impairments are observed in AD brains (Hoyer et al., 1988; Kapogiannis and Mattson, 2011; Chen and Zhong, 2013), the modern notion of metabolic stress also includes disturbances in proteostasis and activation of signaling pathways that mediate cellular stress.

In this context, the progressive build-up of AβOs in AD brains might trigger the activation of immune mechanisms, including glial cell reactivity and cytokine release that, in turn, lead to neuronal metabolic stress. A point of convergence of multiple stress pathways is found on elevated eIF2α-P levels. Accordingly, PKR, ER stress, eIF2α-P and ATF4 have been described as negative modulators of memory (Costa-Mattioli et al., 2007; Zhu et al., 2011; Rajasethupathy et al., 2012; Lourenco et al., 2013; Stern et al., 2013; Di Prisco et al., 2014; Ounallah-Saad et al., 2014). By acting together, such pathways might disrupt brain homeostasis and contribute to the cognitive decline observed in AD.

The precise mechanisms linking metabolic stress to synapse defects are still not fully understood, but the findings that increased eIF2α-P levels lead to LTP impairments (Ma et al., 2013) and synapse loss (Lourenco et al., 2013) in mice have provided initial clues on this causal relationship. Consistently, restoring normal brain eIF2α-P levels was shown to abrogate deficient levels of synaptic proteins and cognition (Lourenco et al., 2013; Ma et al., 2013), indicating a tight connection between eIF2α-P and synapse/memory integrity.

It is noteworthy that activation of PKR/eIF2α-P signaling (O'Connor et al., 2008; Devi and Ohno, 2010; Mouton-Liger et al., 2012a), as well as high-fat diet-induced metabolic stress (Wang et al., 2013) was shown to promote amyloidogenesis in a feed-forward cycle that might exacerbate amyloid pathology. It is thus tempting to speculate that accumulating injuries throughout life, including infections, diabetes and obesity, could instigate a brain metabolic stress scenario that includes ER stress and neuroinflammation to facilitate Aβ accumulation and sporadic AD onset at later stages of life (Herrup, 2010; Mattson, 2012; De Felice, 2013).

An unresolved question relates to whether brain insulin resistance could itself trigger AD-related phenomena, even in the absence of inflammation. In this regard, early studies using neuronal insulin receptor knockout (NIRKO) mice found that deficient brain insulin signaling causes abnormal tau phosphorylation without spatial memory impairment (Schubert et al., 2004). Recently, NIRKO mice were shown to develop anxiety and depressive-like behavior linked to altered dopamine metabolism (Kleinridders et al., 2015), and deletion of a single gene copy that encodes an insulin receptor subunit in the brain impairs synaptic plasticity and cognition (Nisticò et al., 2012). Nonetheless, it remains to be determined whether such mice develop brain metabolic stress in the presence or absence of neurotoxic stimuli. Future investigation may dissect the molecular steps that are required for metabolic stress-induced synapse impairments in an AD context.

Conclusions

Recent exciting evidence has connected AβO-induced neuronal stress to cognitive impairments in AD, in a mechanism that includes cytokine-induced activation of stress kinases and ultimately leads to neuronal and synapse dysfunction in AD experimental models (De Felice et al., 2007; Yoon et al., 2012; De Felice, 2013; Lourenco et al., 2013; Ma et al., 2013; Baleriola et al., 2014; De Felice and Ferreira, 2014; Ferreira et al., 2014). Hence, the combination of inflammation, neuronal insulin resistance, oxidative/ER stress and translational repression might generate a noxious scenario of brain metabolic stress to mediate and propagate synapse defects, resulting in cognitive deficits. In this context, ER stress and abnormal eIF2α-P levels emerged as key players in neuronal damage.

Sporadic AD is largely idiopathic, and it is noteworthy that Aβ-centric views of AD pathogenesis remain controversial (see Morris et al., 2014 for a critical review). Nonetheless, recent progress summarized here may have deep implications for disease prevention, as avoiding harmful events throughout life might reduce the risk of brain inflammation, metabolic stress and, consequently, of developing AD at later stages of life. Interrupting deleterious molecular pathways at prodromal stages will likely be the ideal strategy to delay AD progression. The identification of common AD drivers is imperative to establish effective therapeutics, and blocking neuronal metabolic stress at the earliest cognitive symptoms could offer a promising approach to minimize neuronal dysfunction and AD progression. Repurposing labeled anti-diabetic compounds could constitute an interesting option as they have been shown to attenuate AD-linked brain metabolic stress and memory dysfunction (Craft, 2012; De Felice et al., 2014). Future clinical trials may reveal whether these drugs, alone or in combination, are indeed effective in AD.

Acknowledgments

Work in De Felice lab has been supported by grants from Conselho Nacional de Desenvolvimento Científico e Tecnológico (CNPq), Fundação de Amparo à Pesquisa do Estado do Rio de Janeiro (FAPERJ) and Human Frontier Science Program (HFSP). MVL is supported by a CNPq predoctoral scholarship.

References

Bachstetter, A. D., Norris, C. M., Sompol, P., Wilcock, D. M., Goulding, D., Neltner, J. H., et al. (2012). Early stage drug treatment that normalizes proinflammatory cytokine production attenuates synaptic dysfunction in a mouse model that exhibits age-dependent progression of Alzheimer's disease-related pathology. *J. Neurosci.* 32, 10201–10210. doi: 10.1523/jneurosci.1496-12.2012

Baik, S. H., Cha, M. Y., Hyun, Y. M., Cho, H., Hamza, B., Kim, D. K., et al. (2014). Migration of neutrophils targeting amyloid plaques in Alzheimer's disease mouse model. *Neurobiol. Aging* 35, 1286–1292. doi: 10.1016/j.neurobiolaging.2014.01.003

Baleriola, J., Walker, C. A., Jean, Y. Y., Crary, J. F., Troy, C. M., Nagy, P. L., et al. (2014). Axonally synthesized ATF4 transmits a neurodegenerative signal across brain regions. *Cell* 158, 1159–1172. doi: 10.1016/j.cell.2014.07.001

Barbero-Camps, E., Fernández, A., Baulies, A., Martinez, L., Fernández-Checa, J. C., and Colell, A. (2014). Endoplasmic reticulum stress mediates amyloid beta neurotoxicity via mitochondrial cholesterol trafficking. *Am. J. Pathol.* 184, 2066–2081. doi: 10.1016/j.ajpath.2014.03.014

Bellucci, A., Navarria, L., Zaltieri, M., Falarti, E., Bodei, S., Sigala, S., et al. (2011). Induction of the unfolded protein response by alpha-synuclein in experimental models of Parkinson's disease. *J. Neurochem.* 116, 588–605. doi: 10.1111/j.1471-4159.2010.07143.x

Bomfim, T. R., Forny-Germano, L., Sathler, L. B., Brito-Moreira, J., Houzel, J. C., Decker, H., et al. (2012). An anti-diabetes agent protects the mouse brain from defective insulin signaling caused by Alzheimer's disease-associated Aβ oligomers. *J. Clin. Invest.* 122, 1339–1353. doi: 10.1172/jci57256

Bose, A., Mouton-Liger, F., Paquet, C., Mazot, P., Vigny, M., Gray, F., et al. (2011). Modulation of tau phosphorylation by the kinase PKR: implications in Alzheimer's disease. *Brain Pathol.* 21, 189–200. doi: 10.1111/j.1750-3639.2010.00437.x

Buffington, S. A., Huang, W., and Costa-Mattioli, M. (2014). Translational control in synaptic plasticity and cognitive dysfunction. *Annu. Rev. Neurosci.* 37, 17–38. doi: 10.1146/annurev-neuro-071013-014100

Calay, E. S., and Hotamisligil, G. S. (2013). Turning off the inflammatory, but not the metabolic, flames. *Nat. Med.* 19, 265–267. doi: 10.1038/nm.3114

Casas-Tinto, S., Zhang, Y., Sanchez-Garcia, J., Gomez-Velazquez, M., Rincon-Limas, D. E., and Fernandez-Funez, P. (2011). The ER stress factor XBP1s prevents amyloid- neurotoxicity. *Hum. Mol. Genet.* 20, 2144–2160. doi: 10.1093/hmg/ddr100

Chafekar, S. M., Hoozemans, J. J. M., Zwart, R., Baas, F., and Scheper, W. (2007). Aβ1–42induces mild endoplasmic reticulum stress in an aggregation State-dependent manner. *Antioxid. Redox Signal.* 9, 2245–2254. doi: 10.1089/ars.2007.1797

Chang, R., Suen, K.-C., Ma, C.-H., Elyaman, W., Ng, H.-K., and Hugon, J. (2002a). Involvement of double-stranded RNA-dependent protein kinase and phosphorylation of eukaryotic initiation factor-2alpha in neuronal degeneration. *J. Neurochem.* 83, 1215–1225. doi: 10.1046/j.1471-4159.2002.01237.x

Chang, R. C., Wong, A. K., Ng, H. K., and Hugon, J. (2002b). Phosphorylation of eukaryotic initiation factor 2 alpha (eIF2alpha) is associated with neuronal degeneration in Alzheimer's disease. *Neuroreport* 13, 2429–2432. doi: 10.1097/00001756-200212200-00011

Chen, Z., and Zhong, C. (2013). Decoding Alzheimer's disease from perturbed cerebral glucose metabolism: implications for diagnostic and therapeutic strategies. *Prog. Neurobiol.* 108, 21–43. doi: 10.1016/j.pneurobio.2013.06.004

Colla, E., Coune, P., Liu, Y., Pletnikova, O., Troncoso, J. C., Iwatsubo, T., et al. (2012). Endoplasmic reticulum stress is important for the manifestations of α-synucleinopathy *in vivo*. *J. Neurosci.* 32, 3306–3320. doi: 10.1523/jneurosci.5367-11.2012

Combs, C. K. (2009). Inflammation and microglia actions in Alzheimer's disease. *J. Neuroimmune Pharmacol.* 4, 380–388. doi: 10.1007/s11481-009-9165-3

Costa-Mattioli, M., Gobert, D., Harding, H., Herdy, B., Azzi, M., Bruno, M., et al. (2005). Translational control of hippocampal synaptic plasticity and memory by the eIF2alpha kinase GCN2. *Nature* 436, 1166–1173. doi: 10.1038/nature03897

Costa-Mattioli, M., Gobert, D., Stern, E., Gamache, K., Colina, R., Cuello, C., et al. (2007). eIF2α phosphorylation bidirectionally regulates the switch from short-to long-term synaptic plasticity and memory. *Cell* 129, 195–206. doi: 10.1016/j.cell.2007.01.050

Craft, S. (2012). Alzheimer disease: insulin resistance and AD—extending the translational path. *Nat. Rev. Neurol.* 8, 360–362. doi: 10.1038/nrneurol.2012.112

Crane, P. K., Walker, R., Hubbard, R. A., Li, G., Nathan, D. M., Zheng, H., et al. (2013). Glucose levels and risk of dementia. *N. Engl. J. Med.* 369, 540–548. doi: 10.1056/NEJMoa1215740

De Felice, F. G. (2013). Alzheimer's disease and insulin resistance: translating basic science into clinical applications. *J. Clin. Invest.* 123, 531–539. doi: 10.1172/JCI64595

De Felice, F. G., and Ferreira, S. T. (2014). Inflammation, defective insulin signaling and mitochondrial dysfunction as common molecular denominators connecting type 2 diabetes to Alzheimer disease. *Diabetes* 63, 2262–2272. doi: 10.2337/db13-1954

De Felice, F. G., Lourenco, M. V., and Ferreira, S. T. (2014). How does brain insulin resistance develop in Alzheimer's disease? *Alzheimers Dement.* 10, S26–S32. doi: 10.1016/j.jalz.2013.12.004

De Felice, F. G., Velasco, P. T., Lambert, M. P., Viola, K., Fernandez, S. J., Ferreira, S. T., et al. (2007). Aβ oligomers induce neuronal oxidative stress through an N-methyl-D-aspartate receptor-dependent mechanism that is blocked by the Alzheimer drug memantine. *J. Biol. Chem.* 282, 11590–11601. doi: 10.1074/jbc.m607483200

de la Monte, S. (2009). Insulin resistance and Alzheimer's disease. *BMB Rep.* 42, 475–481. doi: 10.5483/BMBRep.2009.42.8.475

Devi, L., and Ohno, M. (2010). Phospho-eIF2alpha level is important for determining abilities of BACE1 reduction to rescue cholinergic neurodegeneration and memory defects in 5XFAD mice. *PLoS One* 5:e12974. doi: 10.1371/journal.pone.0012974

Devi, L., and Ohno, M. (2014). PERK mediates eIF2alpha phosphorylation responsible for BACE1 elevation, CREB dysfunction and neurodegeneration in a mouse model of Alzheimer's disease. *Neurobiol. Aging* 35, 2272–2281. doi: 10.1016/j.neurobiolaging.2014.04.031

Dhawan, G., Floden, A. M., and Combs, C. K. (2012). Amyloid-β oligomers stimulate microglia through a tyrosine kinase mechanism. *Neurobiol. Aging* 33, 2247–2261. doi: 10.1016/j.neurobiolaging.2011.10.027

Di Prisco, G. V., Huang, W., Buffington, S. A., Hsu, C. C., Bonnen, P. E., Placzek, A. N., et al. (2014). Translational control of mGluR-dependent long-term depression and object-place learning by eIF2alpha. *Nat. Neurosci.* 17, 1073–1082. doi: 10.1038/nn.3754

Ferreira, S. T., Clarke, J. R., Bomfim, T. R., and De Felice, F. G. (2014). Inflammation, defective insulin signaling and neuronal dysfunction in Alzheimer's disease. *Alzheimers Dement.* 10(1 Suppl), S76–S83. doi: 10.1016/j.jalz.2013.12.010

Ferreira, S. T., and Klein, W. L. (2011). The Aβ oligomer hypothesis for synapse failure and memory loss in Alzheimer's disease. *Neurobiol. Learn. Mem.* 96, 529–543. doi: 10.1016/j.nlm.2011.08.003

Flexner, L. B., Flexner, J. B., Roberts, R. B., and De La Haba, G. (1964). Loss of recent memory in mice as related to regional inhibition of cerebral protein synthesis. *Proc. Natl. Acad. Sci. U S A* 52, 1165–1169. doi: 10.1073/pnas.52.5.1165

Floden, A. M., and Combs, C. K. (2006). Beta-amyloid stimulates murine postnatal and adult microglia cultures in a unique manner. *J. Neurosci.* 26, 4644–4648. doi: 10.1523/jneurosci.4822-05.2006

Forny-Germano, L., Lyra E Silva, N. M., Batista, A. F., Brito-Moreira, J., Gralle, M., Boehnke, S. E., et al. (2014). Alzheimer's disease-like pathology induced by amyloid-beta oligomers in nonhuman primates. *J. Neurosci.* 34, 13629–13643. doi: 10.1523/JNEUROSCI.1353-14.2014

Gong, Y., Chang, L., Viola, K. L., Lacor, P. N., Lambert, M. P., Finch, C. E., et al. (2003). Alzheimer's disease-affected brain: presence of oligomeric Aβ ligands (ADDLs) suggests a molecular basis for reversible memory loss. *Proc. Natl. Acad. Sci. U S A* 100, 10417–10422. doi: 10.1073/pnas.1834302100

Gregor, M. F., and Hotamisligil, G. S. (2011). Inflammatory mechanisms in obesity. *Annu. Rev. Immunol.* 29, 415–445. doi: 10.1146/annurev-immunol-031210-101322

Halliday, M., Radford, H., Sekine, Y., Moreno, J., Verity, N., Le Quesne, J., et al. (2015). Partial restoration of protein synthesis rates by the small molecule ISRIB prevents neurodegeneration without pancreatic toxicity. *Cell Death Dis.* 6:e1672. doi: 10.1038/cddis.2015.49

Heneka, M. T., Golenbock, D. T., and Latz, E. (2015). Innate immunity in Alzheimer's disease. *Nat. Immunol.* 16, 229–236. doi: 10.1038/ni.3102

Hensley, K., Floyd, R. A., Zheng, N.-Y., Nael, R., Robinson, K. A., Nguyen, X., et al. (1999). p38 kinase is activated in the Alzheimer's disease brain. *J. Neurochem.* 72, 2053–2058. doi: 10.1046/j.1471-4159.1999.0722053.x

Herrup, K. (2010). Reimagining Alzheimer's disease—an age-based hypothesis. *J. Neurosci.* 30, 16755–16762. doi: 10.1523/JNEUROSCI.4521-10.2010

Hetz, C. (2012). The unfolded protein response: controlling cell fate decisions under ER stress and beyond. *Nat. Rev. Mol. Cell Biol.* 13, 89–102. doi: 10.1038/nrm3270

Hetz, C., Chevet, E., and Harding, H. P. (2013). Targeting the unfolded protein response in disease. *Nat. Rev. Drug Discov.* 12, 703–719. doi: 10.1038/nrd3976

Hetz, C., and Mollereau, B. (2014). Disturbance of endoplasmic reticulum proteostasis in neurodegenerative diseases. *Nat. Rev. Neurosci.* 15, 233–249. doi: 10.1038/nrn3689

Hetz, C., Thielen, P., Matus, S., Nassif, M., Court, F., Kiffin, R., et al. (2009). XBP-1 deficiency in the nervous system protects against amyotrophic lateral sclerosis by increasing autophagy. *Genes Dev.* 23, 2294–2306. doi: 10.1101/gad.1830709

Hoozemans, J. J. M., Van Haastert, E. S., Nijholt, D. A. T., Rozemuller, A. J. M., Eikelenboom, P., and Scheper, W. (2009). The unfolded protein response is activated in pretangle neurons in Alzheimer's disease hippocampus. *Am. J. Pathol.* 174, 1241–1251. doi: 10.2353/ajpath.2009.080814

Hoozemans, J. J. M., Veerhuis, R., Haastert, E. S., Rozemuller, J. M., Baas, F., Eikelenboom, P., et al. (2005). The unfolded protein response is activated in Alzheimer's disease. *Acta Neuropathol.* 110, 165–172. doi: 10.1007/s00401-005-1038-0

Hotamisligil, G. S. (2006). Inflammation and metabolic disorders. *Nature* 444, 860–867. doi: 10.1038/nature05485

Hotamisligil, G. S., Arner, P., Caro, J. F., Atkinson, R. L., and Spiegelman, B. M. (1995). Increased adipose tissue expression of tumor necrosis factor-a in human obesity and insulin resistance. *J. Clin. Invest.* 95, 2409–2415. doi: 10.1172/jci117936

Hotamisligil, G. S., Peraldi, P., Budavari, A., Ellis, R., White, M. F., and Spiegelman, B. M. (1996). IRS-1-mediated inhibition of insulin receptor tyrosine kinase activity in TNF-α- and obesity-induced insulin resistance. *Science* 271, 665–668. doi: 10.1126/science.271.5249.665

Hoyer, S., Oesterreich, K., and Wagner, O. (1988). Glucose metabolism as the site of the primary abnormality in early-onset dementia of Alzheimer type? *J. Neurol.* 235, 143–148. doi: 10.1007/bf00314304

Kalmijin, S., Launer, L. J., Ott, A., Witteman, J. C., Hofman, A., and Breteler, M. M. (1997). Dietary fat intake and the risk of incident dementia in the Rotterdam study. *Ann. Neurol.* 42, 776–782. doi: 10.1002/ana.410420514

Kapogiannis, D., and Mattson, M. P. (2011). Disrupted energy metabolism and neuronal circuit dysfunction in cognitive impairment and Alzheimer's disease. *Lancet Neurol.* 10, 187–198. doi: 10.1016/S1474-4422(10)70277-5

Kim, H.-J., Raphael, A. R., Ladow, E. S., Mcgurk, L., Weber, R. A., Trojanowski, J. Q., et al. (2013). Therapeutic modulation of eIF2α phosphorylation rescues TDP-43 toxicity in amyotrophic lateral sclerosis disease models. *Nat. Genet.* 46, 152–160. doi: 10.1038/ng.2853

Kiyota, T., Okuyama, S., Swan, R. J., Jacobsen, M. T., Gendelman, H. E., and Ikezu, T. (2010). CNS expression of anti-inflammatory cytokine interleukin-4 attenuates Alzheimer's disease-like pathogenesis in APP+PS1 bigenic mice. *FASEB J.* 24, 3093–3102. doi: 10.1096/fj.10-155317

Kleinridders, A., Cai, W., Cappellucci, L., Ghazarian, A., Collins, W. R., Vienberg, S. G., et al. (2015). Insulin resistance in brain alters dopamine turnover and causes behavioral disorders. *Proc. Natl. Acad. Sci. U S A* 112, 3463–3468. doi: 10.1073/pnas.1500877112

Lai, E., Teodoro, T., and Volchuk, A. (2007). Endoplasmic reticulum stress: signaling the unfolded protein response. *Physiology (Bethesda)* 22, 193–201. doi: 10.1152/physiol.00050.2006

Lajole, P., and Snapp, E. L. (2011). Changes in BiP availability reveal hypersensitivity to acute endoplasmic reticulum stress in cells expressing mutant huntingtin. *J. Cell Sci.* 124, 3332–3343. doi: 10.1242/jcs.087510

Lambert, M. P., Barlow, A. K., Chromy, B. A., Edwards, C., Freed, R., Liosatos, M., et al. (1998). Diffusible, nonfibrillar ligands derived from Abeta1–42 are potent central nervous system neurotoxins. *Proc. Natl. Acad. Sci. U S A* 95, 6448–6453. doi: 10.1073/pnas.95.11.6448

Lange, P. S., Chavez, J. C., Pinto, J. T., Coppola, G., Sun, C. W., Townes, T. M., et al. (2008). ATF4 is an oxidative stress-inducible, prodeath transcription factor in neurons *in vitro* and *in vivo*. *J. Exp. Med.* 205, 1227–1242. doi: 10.1084/jem.20071460

Ledo, J. H., Azevedo, E. P., Clarke, J. R., Ribeiro, F. C., Figueiredo, C. P., Foguel, D., et al. (2013). Amyloid-β oligomers link depressive-like behavior and cognitive deficits in mice. *Mol. Psychiatry* 18, 1053–1054. doi: 10.1038/mp.2012.168

Lee, D. Y., Lee, K.-S., Lee, H. J., Kim, D. H., Noh, Y. H., Yu, K., et al. (2010). Activation of PERK signaling attenuates Abeta-mediated ER stress. *PloS One* 5:e10489. doi: 10.1371/journal.pone.0010489

Lourenco, M. V., Clarke, J. R., Frozza, R. L., Bomfim, T. R., Forny-Germano, L., Batista, A. F., et al. (2013). TNF-α mediates PKR-dependent memory impairment and brain IRS-1 inhibition induced by Alzheimer's β-amyloid oligomers in mice and monkeys. *Cell Metab.* 18, 831–843. doi: 10.1016/j.cmet.2013.11.002

Lourenco, M. V., and Ledo, J. H. (2013). Targeting Alzheimer's pathology through PPARγ signaling: modulation of microglial function. *J. Neurosci.* 33, 5083–5084. doi: 10.1523/JNEUROSCI.0172-13.2013

Ma, T., Trinh, M. A., Wexler, A. J., Bourbon, C., Gatti, E., Pierre, P., et al. (2013). Suppression of eIF2α kinases alleviates Alzheimer's disease–related plasticity and memory deficits. *Nat. Neurosci.* 16, 1299–1305. doi: 10.1038/nn.3486

Ma, Q. L., Yang, F., Rosario, E. R., Ubeda, O. J., Beech, W., Gant, D. J., et al. (2009). β-amyloid oligomers induce phosphorylation of tau and inactivation of insulin receptor substrate via c-Jun N-terminal kinase signaling: suppression by omega-3 fatty acids and curcumin. *J. Neurosci.* 29, 9078–9089. doi: 10.1523/JNEUROSCI.1071-09.2009

Masters, C. L., Simms, G., Weinman, N. A., Multhaup, G., Mcdonald, B. L., and Beyreuther, K. (1985). Amyloid plaque core protein in Alzheimer disease and down syndrome. *Proc. Natl. Acad. Sci. U S A* 82, 4245–4249. doi: 10.1073/pnas.82.12.4245

Matsuzaki, T., Sasaki, K., Tanizaki, Y., Hata, J., Fujimi, K., Matsui, Y., et al. (2010). Insulin resistance is associated with the pathology of Alzheimer disease: the Hisayama Study. *Neurology* 75, 764–770. doi: 10.1212/wnl.0b013e3181eee25f

Mattson, M. P. (2008). Hormesis defined. *Ageing Res. Rev.* 7, 1–7. doi: 10.1016/j.arr.2007.08.007

Mattson, M. P. (2012). Energy intake and exercise as determinants of brain health and vulnerability to injury and disease. *Cell Metab.* 16, 706–722. doi: 10.1016/j.cmet.2012.08.012

McAlpine, F. E., Lee, J., Harms, A. S., Ruhn, K. A., Blurton-Jones, M., Hong, J., et al. (2009). Inhibition of soluble TNF signaling in a mouse model of Alzheimer's disease prevents pre-plaque amyloid-associated neuropathology. *Neurobiol. Dis.* 34, 163–177. doi: 10.1016/j.nbd.2009.01.006

Medeiros, R., Prediger, R. D. S., Passos, G. F., Pandolfo, P., Duarte, F. S., Franco, J. L., et al. (2007). Connecting TNF-α signaling pathways to iNOS expression in a mouse model of Alzheimer's disease: relevance for the behavioral and synaptic deficits induced by amyloid-β protein. *J. Neurosci.* 27, 5394–5404. doi: 10.1523/jneurosci.5047-06.2007

Medinas, D. B., and Hetz, C. (2013). Proteostasis impairment: at the intersection between Alzheimer's disease and diabetes. *Cell Metab.* 18, 771–772. doi: 10.1016/j.cmet.2013.11.009

Mitsuda, T., Hayakawa, Y., Itoh, M., Ohta, K., and Nakagawa, T. (2007). ATF4 regulates gamma-secretase activity during amino acid imbalance. *Biochem. Biophys. Res. Commun.* 352, 722–727. doi: 10.1016/j.bbrc.2006.11.075

Moloney, A. M., Griffin, R. J., Timmons, S., O'connor, R., Ravid, R., and O'neill, C. (2010). Defects in IGF-1 receptor, insulin receptor and IRS-1/2 in Alzheimer's disease indicate possible resistance to IGF-1 and insulin signalling. *Neurobiol. Aging* 31, 224–243. doi: 10.1016/j.neurobiolaging.2008.04.002

Monson, N. L., Ireland, S. J., Ligocki, A. J., Chen, D., Rounds, W. H., Li, M., et al. (2014). Elevated CNS inflammation in patients with preclinical Alzheimer's disease. *J. Cereb. Blood Flow Metab.* 34, 30–33. doi: 10.1038/jcbfm.2013.183

Moreno, J. A., Halliday, M., Molloy, C., Radford, H., Verity, N., Axten, J. M., et al. (2013). Oral treatment targeting the unfolded protein response prevents neurodegeneration and clinical disease in prion-infected mice. *Sci. Transl. Med.* 5:206ra138. doi: 10.1126/scitranslmed.3006767

Moreno, J. A., Radford, H., Peretti, D., Steinert, J. R., Verity, N., Martin, M. G., et al. (2012). Sustained translational repression by eIF2α-P mediates prion neurodegeneration. *Nature* 485, 507–511. doi: 10.1038/nature11058

Morris, G. P., Clark, I. A., and Vissel, B. (2014). Inconsistencies and controversies surrounding the amyloid hypothesis of Alzheimer's disease. *Acta Neuropathol. Commun.* 2:135. doi: 10.1186/s40478-014-0135-5

Mouton-Liger, F., Paquet, C., Dumurgier, J., Bouras, C., Pradier, L., Gray, F., et al. (2012a). Oxidative stress increases BACE1 protein levels through activation of the PKR-eIF2α pathway. *Biochimica et Biophysica Acta (BBA) - Mol. Basis Dis.* 1822, 885–896. doi: 10.1016/j.bbadis.2012.01.009

Mouton-Liger, F., Paquet, C., Dumurgier, J., Lapalus, P., Gray, F., Laplanche, J.-L., et al. (2012b). Increased cerebrospinal fluid levels of double-stranded RNA-dependent protein kinase in Alzheimer's disease. *Biol. Psychiatry* 71, 829–835. doi: 10.1016/j.biopsych.2011.11.031

Mucke, L., and Selkoe, D. J. (2012). Neurotoxicity of amyloid-beta protein: synaptic and network dysfunction. *Cold Spring Harb. Perspect. Med.* 2:a006338. doi: 10.1101/cshperspect.a006338

Nakamura, T., Kunz, R. C., Zhang, C., Kimura, T., Yuan, C. L., Baccaro, B., et al. (2015). A critical role for PKR complexes with TRBP in immunometabolic regulation and eIF2alpha phosphorylation in obesity. *Cell Rep.* 11, 295–307. doi: 10.1016/j.celrep.2015.03.021

Nisticò, R., Cavallucci, V., Piccinin, S., Macrì, S., Pignatelli, M., Mehdawy, B., et al. (2012). Insulin receptor β-subunit haploinsufficiency impairs hippocampal late-phase LTP and recognition memory. *Neuromolecular Med.* 14, 262–269. doi: 10.1007/s12017-012-8184-z.

O'Connor, T., Sadleir, K. R., Maus, E., Velliquette, R. A., Zhao, J., Cole, S. L., et al. (2008). Phosphorylation of the translation initiation factor eIF2α increases BACE1 levels and promotes amyloidogenesis. *Neuron* 60, 988–1009. doi: 10.1016/j.neuron.2008.10.047

O'Neill, C. (2013). PI3-kinase/Akt/mTOR signaling: impaired on/off switches in aging, cognitive decline and Alzheimer's disease. *Exp. Gerontol.* 48, 647–653. doi: 10.1016/j.exger.2013.02.025

Ott, A., Stolk, R. P., Hofman, A., Van Harskamp, F., Grobbee, D. E., and Breteler, M. M. B. (1996). Association of diabetes mellitus and dementia: the rotterdam study. *Diabetologia* 39, 1392–1397. doi: 10.1007/s001250050588

Ott, A., Stolk, R. P., Van Harskamp, F., Pols, H. A. P., Hofman, A., and Breteler, M. M. B. (1999). Diabetes mellitus and the risk of dementia: the rotterdam study. *Neurology* 53, 1937–1937. doi: 10.1212/wnl.53.9.1937

Ounallah-Saad, H., Sharma, V., Edry, E., and Rosenblum, K. (2014). Genetic or pharmacological reduction of perk enhances cortical-dependent taste learning. *J. Neurosci.* 34, 14624–14632. doi: 10.1523/jneurosci.2117-14.2014

Ozcan, U., Cao, Q., Yilmaz, E., Lee, A. H., Iwakoshi, N. N., Ozdelen, E., et al. (2004). Endoplasmic reticulum stress links obesity, insulin action and type 2 diabetes. *Science* 306, 457–461. doi: 10.1126/science.1103160

Ozcan, U., Yilmaz, E., Ozcan, L., Furuhashi, M., Vaillancourt, E., Smith, R. O., et al. (2006). Chemical chaperones reduce ER stress and restore glucose homeostasis in a mouse model of type 2 diabetes. *Science* 313, 1137–1140. doi: 10.1126/science.1128294

Pan, X. D., Zhu, Y. G., Lin, N., Zhang, J., Ye, Q. Y., Huang, H. P., et al. (2011). Microglial phagocytosis induced by fibrillar beta-amyloid is attenuated by oligomeric beta-amyloid: implications for Alzheimer's disease. *Mol. Neurodegener.* 6:45. doi: 10.1186/1750-1326-6-45

Paquet, C., Mouton-Liger, F., Meurs, E. F., Mazot, P., Bouras, C., Pradier, L., et al. (2011). The PKR activator PACT is induced by Aβ: involvement in Alzheimer's disease. *Brain Pathol.* 22, 219–229. doi: 10.1111/j.1750-3639.2011.00520.x.

Parajuli, B., Sonobe, Y., Horiuchi, H., Takeuchi, H., Mizuno, T., and Suzumura, A. (2013). Oligomeric amyloid beta induces IL-1beta processing via production of ROS: implication in Alzheimer's disease. *Cell Death Dis.* 4:e975. doi: 10.1038/cddis.2013.503

Prince, M., Bryce, R., Albanese, E., Wimo, A., Ribeiro, W., and Ferri, C. P. (2013). The global prevalence of dementia: a systematic review and metaanalysis. *Alzheimers Dement.* 9, 63.e2–75.e2. doi: 10.1016/j.jalz.2012.11.007

Rajasethupathy, P., Antonov, I., Sheridan, R., Frey, S., Sander, C., Tuschl, T., et al. (2012). A role for neuronal pirnas in the epigenetic control of memory-related synaptic plasticity. *Cell* 149, 693–707. doi: 10.1016/j.cell.2012.02.057

Raven, J. F., and Koromilas, A. E. (2008). PERK and PKR: old kinases learn new tricks. *Cell Cycle* 7, 1146–1150. doi: 10.4161/cc.7.9.5811

Ricobaraza, A., Cuadrado-Tejedor, M., Marco, S., Pérez-Otaño, I., and García-Osta, A. (2010). Phenylbutyrate rescues dendritic spine loss associated with memory deficits in a mouse model of Alzheimer disease. *Hippocampus* 22, 1040–1050. doi: 10.1002/hipo.20883

Ricobaraza, A., Cuadrado-Tejedor, M., Perez-Mediavilla, A., Frechilla, D., Del Rio, J., and Garcia-Osta, A. (2009). Phenylbutyrate ameliorates cognitive deficit and reduces tau pathology in an Alzheimer's disease mouse model. *Neuropsychopharmacology* 34, 1721–1732. doi: 10.1038/npp.2008.229

Roffé, M., Hajj, G. N., Azevedo, H. F., Alves, V. S., and Castilho, B. A. (2013). IMPACT is a developmentally regulated protein in neurons that opposes the eukaryotic initiation factor 2alpha kinase GCN2 in the modulation of neurite outgrowth. *J. Biol. Chem.* 288, 10860–10869. doi: 10.1074/jbc.m113.461970

Rossato, J. I., Bevilaqua, L. R., Myskiw, J. C., Medina, J. H., Izquierdo, I., and Cammarota, M. (2007). On the role of hippocampal protein synthesis in the consolidation and reconsolidation of object recognition memory. *Learn. Mem.* 14, 36–46. doi: 10.1101/lm.422607

Schubert, M., Gautam, D., Surjo, D., Ueki, K., Baudler, S., Schubert, D., et al. (2004). Role for neuronal insulin resistance in neurodegenerative diseases. *Proc. Natl. Acad. Sci. U S A* 101, 3100–3105. doi: 10.1073/pnas.0308724101

Segev, Y., Michaelson, D. M., and Rosenblum, K. (2012). ApoE ϵ4 is associated with eIF2α phosphorylation and impaired learning in young mice. *Neurobiol. Aging* 34, 863–872. doi: 10.1016/j.neurobiolaging.2012.06.020

Selkoe, D. J. (2002). Alzheimer's disease is a synaptic failure. *Science* 298, 789–791. doi: 10.1126/science.1074069

Sondag, C. M., Dhawan, G., and Combs, C. K. (2009). Beta amyloid oligomers and fibrils stimulate differential activation of primary microglia. *Neuroinflammation* 6:1. doi: 10.1186/1742-2094-6-1

Steen, E., Terry, B. M., Rivera, E. J., Cannon, J. L., Neely, T. R., Tavares, R., et al. (2005). Impaired insulin and insulin-like growth factor expression and signaling mechanisms in Alzheimer's disease – is this type 3 diabetes? *J. Alzheimers Dis.* 7, 63–80.

Stern, E., Chinnakkaruppan, A., David, O., Sonenberg, N., and Rosenblum, K. (2013). Blocking the eIF2α kinase (PKR) enhances positive and negative forms of cortex-dependent taste memory. *J. Neurosci.* 33, 2517–2525. doi: 10.1523/JNEUROSCI.2322-12.2013

Talbot, K., Wang, H., Kazi, H., Han, L., Bakshi, K. P., Stucky, A., et al. (2012). Demonstrated brain insulin resistance in Alzheimer's disease patients is associated with IGF-1 resistance, IRS-1 dysregulation and cognitive decline. *J. Clin. Invest.* 122, 1316–1338. doi: 10.1172/JCI59903

Vallerie, S. N., and Hotamisligil, G. S. (2010). The role of JNK proteins in metabolism. *Sci. Transl. Med.* 2:60rv65. doi: 10.1126/scitranslmed.3001007

van der Harg, J. M., Nölle, A., Zwart, R., Boerema, A. S., Van Haastert, E. S., Strijkstra, A. M., et al. (2014). The unfolded protein response mediates reversible tau phosphorylation induced by metabolic stress. *Cell Death Dis.* 5:e1393. doi: 10.1038/cddis.2014.354

Viola, K. L., and Klein, W. L. (2015). Amyloid beta oligomers in Alzheimer's disease pathogenesis, treatment and diagnosis. *Acta Neuropathol.* 129, 183–206. doi: 10.1016/j.bpj.2014.11.1128

Wang, R., Li, J. J., Diao, S., Kwak, Y. D., Liu, L., Zhi, L., et al. (2013). Metabolic stress modulates Alzheimer's beta-secretase gene transcription via SIRT1-PPARgamma-PGC-1 in neurons. *Cell Metab.* 17, 685–694. doi: 10.1016/j.cmet.2013.03.016

Wiley, J. C., Pettan-Brewer, C., and Ladiges, W. C. (2011). Phenylbutyric acid reduces amyloid plaques and rescues cognitive behavior in AD transgenic mice. *Aging Cell* 10, 418–428. doi: 10.1111/j.1474-9726.2011.00680.x

Xia, W., Yang, T., Shankar, G. M., Smith, I. M., Shen, Y., Walsh, D., et al. (2009). A specific enzyme-linked immunosorbent assay for measuring β-amyloid protein oligomers in human plasma and brain tissue of patients with Alzheimer disease. *Arch. Neurol.* 66, 190–199. doi: 10.1001/archneurol.2008.565

Yamanaka, M., Ishikawa, T., Griep, A., Axt, D., Kummer, M. P., and Heneka, M. T. (2012). PPARγ/RXRα-induced and CD36-mediated microglial amyloid-β phagocytosis results in cognitive improvement in amyloid precursor protein/presenilin 1 mice. *J. Neurosci.* 32, 17321–17331. doi: 10.1523/JNEUROSCI.1569-12.2012

Yang, Y. M., Shang, D. S., Zhao, W. D., Fang, W. G., and Chen, Y. H. (2013). Microglial TNF-alpha-dependent elevation of MHC class I expression on brain endothelium induced by amyloid-beta promotes T cell transendothelial migration. *Neurochem. Res.* 38, 2295–2304. doi: 10.1007/s11064-013-1138-5

Yoon, S. O., Park, D. J., Ryu, J. C., Ozer, H. G., Tep, C., Shin, Y. J., et al. (2012). JNK3 perpetuates metabolic stress induced by Aβ peptides. *Neuron* 75, 824–837. doi: 10.3410/f.717965605.793466623

Zhu, P. J., Huang, W., Kalikulov, D., Yoo, J. W., Placzek, A. N., Stoica, L., et al. (2011). Suppression of PKR promotes network excitability and enhanced cognition by interferon-γ-mediated disinhibition. *Cell* 147, 1384–1396. doi: 10.1016/j.cell.2011.11.029

J.

19

C-reactive Protein, Advanced Glycation End Products, and their Receptor in Type 2 Diabetic, Elderly Patients with Mild Cognitive Impairment

Malgorzata Gorska-Ciebiada[1], Malgorzata Saryusz-Wolska[1], Anna Borkowska[1], Maciej Ciebiada[2] and Jerzy Loba[1]*

[1] *Department of Internal Medicine and Diabetology, Medical University of Lodz, Lodz, Poland,* [2] *Department of General and Oncological Pneumology, Medical University of Lodz, Lodz, Poland*

Edited by:
Jia Yao,
University of Southern California, USA

Reviewed by:
Paula I. Moreira,
University of Coimbra, Portugal
Chongren Tang,
University of Washington, USA

***Correspondence:**
Malgorzata Gorska-Ciebiada
magoca@poczta.onet.pl

Objective: The aim of the study was to evaluate serum levels of advanced glycation end products (AGEs), receptor for advanced glycation end products (RAGE), and C-reactive protein (CRP) in elderly patients with type 2 diabetes mellitus with and without mild cognitive impairment (MCI) and to determine the predictors (including AGEs, RAGE, and CRP levels) of having MCI in elderly patients with type 2 diabetes.

Methods: Two hundred seventy-six diabetics elders were screened for MCI (using the Montreal Cognitive Assessment: MoCA score). Data of biochemical parameters and biomarkers were collected.

Results: Serum AGEs, RAGE, and CRP levels were significantly increased in MCI patients compared to controls. In group of patients with MCI, serum RAGE level was positively correlated with AGEs level and with CRP level. RAGE, AGEs, and CRP concentrations were positively correlated with HbA1c levels and negatively correlated with MoCA score. The univariate logistic regression models revealed that variables, which increased the likelihood of diagnosis of MCI in elderly patients with type 2 diabetes were higher levels of HbA1c, RAGE, AGEs, CRP, TG, lower level of HDL cholesterol, previous CVD, HA, or use of HA drugs, hyperlipidemia, retinopathy, nephropathy, increased number of co-morbidities, older age, and less years of formal education. HA or use of HA drugs, previous CVD, higher level of RAGE and CRP, older age and less years of formal education are the factors increasing the likelihood of having MCI in elderly patients with type 2 diabetes in multivariable model.

Conclusion: In summary, serum AGEs, RAGE, and CRP are increased in the circulation of MCI elderly diabetic patients compared to controls. A larger population-based pro spective study needs to be performed to further confirm the relationship between AGEs, RAGE, and the cognitive decline or progress to dementia.

Keywords: AGEs, cognitive impairment, diabetes, elderly, RAGE

INTRODUCTION

Diabetes mellitus is one of the important chronic diseases worldwide.

The prevalence of type 2 diabetes mellitus (T2DM) raised rapidly in the last few decades (Wild et al., 2004). Complications include small and large vessels, eyes, kidneys, cranial, and peripheral nerves. Recent studies suggested that diabetes is a risk factor for cognitive decline and dementia in the elderly (Cukierman et al., 2005; Gorska-Ciebiada et al., 2009, 2014). T2DM has a highly complicated pathogenesis, so the etiology of cognitive impairment in diabetes is probably associated with many factors (Strachan et al., 1997). One of the recent hypotheses suggests that low-grade chronic inflammation is associated with mild cognitive impairment (MCI) or with cognitive decline (Yaffe et al., 2003; Schuitemaker et al., 2008). MCI is a transitional stage between normal cognitive aging and dementia. One large study has proven that some inflammatory parameters, such as C-reactive protein, TNF-α, and IL-6, are connected with cognitive dysfunction and decline (Yaffe et al., 2003). There are evidences from other population-based study that there are significant associations between CRP and MCI and with the attention and executive function domain score (Roberts et al., 2009). Another potential marker of cognitive dysfunction is a receptor for advanced glycation end products (RAGE). RAGE is a transmembrane receptor that belongs to the immunoglobulin super family of cell surface receptors. It interacts with its ligands and causes persistent inflammatory responses at vascular wall and vascular injuries, a major complication of diabetes (Neeper et al., 1992; Hori et al., 1996; Schmidt et al., 2000a; Kumano-Kuramochi et al., 2009). The major RAGE ligands in diabetes are advanced glycation end products (AGEs). They are derivatives of proteins, lipids, and ribonucleic acids. Serum AGEs levels increases with age and with diabetes or hyperglycemic states (Ulrich and Cerami, 2001). RAGE-mediated mechanisms play a crucial role in diabetes complications because they induce reactive oxygen species-mediated inflammation in vascular wall (Win et al., 2012). RAGE is also an important cell-signaling receptor involved in cognitive impairment. Recent studies report the association between RAGE levels and cognitive impairment in Alzheimer's disease (Deane and Zlokovic, 2007). Increased expression of RAGE was found in neurons and microglia in the hippocampus (Lue et al., 2001). Some authors have suggested that RAGE and other receptors could be involved in the injury of the brain in Alzheimer's disease and diabetes by microglial activation and oxygen-mediated neuroinflammation (Lue et al., 2012).

Data concerning serum AGEs and RAGE levels in MCI subjects with diabetes are lacking; therefore, the aim of the study was to (1) evaluate serum levels of AGEs, RAGE, and CRP in elderly patients with T2DM with and without MCI and (2) determine the predictors (including AGEs, RAGE, and CRP levels) of having MCI in elderly patients with T2DM.

MATERIALS AND METHODS

Study Population

A survey was conducted among unselected 276 elders who attended to outpatient clinic belonged to the Department of Internal Medicine and Diabetology, University Hospital no 1 in Lodz, Poland. A brief screening for recruitment was conducted by the investigators to identify potential participants. We included patients aged 65 and over with diabetes type 2 diagnosed minimum 1 year earlier, subjects who had been able to understand and cooperate with study procedures. The exclusion criteria were diagnosed depression or dementia, use of possible or known cognition-impairing drugs in the previous 3-month, presence of neoplasm, constant alcohol or substance abuse, severe visual, mobility, or motor coordination impairment, history of head trauma, inflammatory or infectious brain disease, severe neurological or psychiatric illness (**Table 1**).

Written informed consent was obtained from the participants at the beginning of the study. The first part of visit included a morning blood draw after a 10- to 12-h overnight fast, blood pressure measurements, height and weight assessment, and complete physical examination. Then, patients had eaten a breakfast followed by capillary glucose level measuring to ensure that participants were not hypoglycemic at the time of cognitive testing. The second part of visit took place in a private area in the clinic. Subjects completed a questionnaire describing baseline demographics and underwent cognitive testing.

Participant Characteristics, Clinical Evaluation, and Risk Factor Assessment

Demographic variables and possible risk factors were recorded in a standardized interview. Weight and height were measured to calculate body mass index [BMI = weight/height^2 (kg/m^2)]. The systolic and diastolic blood pressures (millimeter of mercury) were measured with the patient in sitting position after 5 min of rest. The detailed medical history of diabetes type 2 was taken and includes diabetes duration, currant treatment for diabetes and complications if present, family history of diabetes, co-morbid diseases of the patient [hyperlipidemia, hypertension, cardiovascular disease (CVD), lung disease, cancer, gastrointestinal tract diseases] and their treatment. Educational level was recorded in years of education. Smoking was classified as current, past, or never. Physical activity was recorded if any present. Diabetic vascular complications were assessed based on the existence of nephropathy, retinopathy, neuropathy, CVD, and stroke. Hypertension was defined as

TABLE 1 | The inclusion and exclusion criteria of the study.

The inclusion criteria
Age ≥65 years
Diabetes type 2 diagnosed minimum 1 year earlier
Full ability to understand and cooperate with study procedures
The exclusion criteria
Diagnosed depression or dementia
Use of possible or known cognition-impairing drugs in the previous 3-month
Presence of neoplasm
Constant alcohol or substance abuse
Severe visual, mobility, or motor coordination impairment
History of head trauma
Inflammatory or infectious brain disease
Severe neurological or psychiatric illness

either a history of hypertension or use of any antihypertensive agents, Hyperlipidemia defined as use of any lipid lowering agent or an untreated serum LDL cholesterol level 2.6 mmol/l or/and triglycerides 1.7 mmol/l.

Blood Biochemistry

After overnight fasting, blood samples were taken by venipuncture to assess serum levels of glycosylated hemoglobin (HbA1c), total cholesterol, triglycerides, low-density lipoprotein cholesterol (LDL-C), and high-density lipoprotein cholesterol (HDL-C). All the parameters were measured in a centralized laboratory.

Determination of Serum AGEs, RAGE, and CRP

The serum levels of AGEs, RAGE were assessed using ELISA kit (EIAab, Wuhan, China), and CRP was determined by Quantikine Human Immunoassay ELISA kit (R&D System, Minneapolis, MN, USA) according to the instructions of the manufacturer. Minimum detectable concentrations were 0.78 ng/ml for AGEs and 4.12 pg/ml for RAGE, 1×10^{-5} mg/l for CRP.

Neuropsychological Evaluations

All participants underwent the following tests: the Montreal Cognitive Assessment (MoCA) (Nasreddine et al., 2005) to evaluate the cognitive impairment, long version of the geriatric depression scale (GDS-30) (Yesavage et al., 1982–1983) to assessed the depressive mood, Katz Basic Activities of Daily living (BADL) and Lawton instrumental activities of daily living (IADL) questionnaires to collect information on daily activities (Lawton and Brody, 1969; Katz et al., 1970). The MoCA tests 8 cognitive domains, visual–spatial ability, attention, executive function, immediate memory, delayed memory, language, abstraction, calculation, and orientation, for a maximum total score of 30. The normal MoCA score is ≥26, with one point added if the subject has fewer than 12 years of formal education. The MoCA is better than other tools to detect MCI in the elderly patients with type 2 diabetes (Alagiakrishnan et al., 2013). MCI was diagnosed based on criteria established by the 2006 European Alzheimer's Disease Consortium, which are currently available standard test (Petersen, 2004; Portet et al., 2006). These criteria included absence of dementia. The cut-off points for MoCA scores (19/30) are recommended for the diagnosis of "dementia" in epidemiological studies. Patients with score 19 and below were excluded from the study as dementia and sent to psychiatrist for further care. The criteria mentioned above included also absence of major repercussions on daily life (in our study, measured by Katz BADL and Lawton IADL).

This interview was followed by GDS for mood assessment (Yesavage et al., 1982–1983). GDS consists of 30 items. Scores ranging from 0 to 9 were considered as normal, and 10 to 19 were considered to have depressive symptoms. Score 20 and above was excluded from the study as severe depressive symptomatology and sent to psychiatrist for further diagnosis.

According to criteria mentioned above 276 older subjects with diabetes type 2 were selected into groups: patients with MCI and controls (patients without MCI).

Ethics

The study was operated in accordance with the World Medical Association's Declaration of Helsinki. Each participant was assigned a number by which he/she was identified to keep his or her privacy. The approval was obtained from the independent local ethics committee of Medical University of Lodz No RNN/420/13/KB. The purpose, nature, and potential risks of the experiments were fully explained to the subjects, and all subjects gave written informed consent at the beginning of the study. The subjects had the full capacity to consent because they maintained general cognitive function and daily activities. We included only patients who had been fully able to understand and cooperate with study procedures. We excluded subjects with diagnosed depression or dementia. There was not any surrogate consent procedure (e.g., whereby next of kin or legally authorized representative) consented on the behalf of participants.

Statistical Analysis

All data are presented as means ± SD. Normality of distributions was assessed using the Shapiro–Wilk tests. The descriptive statistics the continuous variables using the Student's *t*-test or the Mann–Whitney *U* test whenever applicable and non-continuous variables using χ^2 test. Pearson correlation analysis for normally distributed variables and Spearman rank correlation for non-normally distributed variables were used to assess relationships. Simple logistic regression model was done in order to select the so-called independent factors that increase the selection risk of MCI in elderly patients with type 2 diabetes. Then, multivariable regression model was done in order to select the "strongest" factor from independent risk factors. To "optimize" the multivariable model, a stepwise approach was used (backward elimination with Wald criteria). Odds ratios (OR) were computed and presented with the 95% interval of confidence (CI). A p-value of <0.05 was considered statistically significant. Statistica 10.0 (StatSoft, Poland, Krakow) was used for analysis.

RESULTS

General Description of MCI Subjects and Controls

Table 2 describes the baseline characteristics of the study group. Compared with controls patients with MCI were significantly older, less educated, had a longer duration of diabetes, more were diagnosed with CVD, hypertension, hyperlipidemia, retinopathy, nephropathy, and other co-morbidities. MoCA score was significantly lower in subjects with cognitive impairment. The mean level of HbA1c and triglycerides was significantly higher, and level of HDL was lower in patients with MCI compared to controls. Furthermore, CRP was found to be increased in MCI patients compared to control group ($p < 0.001$). Lastly, there were no significant differences between the groups in sex, BMI, history of smoking, stroke, presence of neuropathy, depressive syndrome, type of the treatment, systolic and diastolic blood pressure, the plasma levels of fasting glucose, and total and LDL cholesterol ($p > 0.05$).

TABLE 2 | Demographic and clinical characteristics of type 2 diabetic elderly patients.

	All subjects	MCI	Controls	χ^2/Z	*p*-value
Number of patients	276	87	189		
Age (years)*	73.6 ± 4.8	75.7 ± 4.6	72.6 ± 4.6	−4.96	<0.001
Gender (female/male)	149/127	53/34	96/93	2.46	0.12
Education-years*	11.3 ± 2.4	9.7 ± 1.8	12.0 ± 2.2	7.97	<0.001
Smoked tobacco regularly	93 (33.7%)	26 (29.8%)	67 (35.4%)	0.83	0.36
Duration of T2DM (years)*	8.69 ± 6.23	11.25 ± 6.3	7.51 ± 5.85	−5.96	<0.001
Microvascular complications Retinopathy (%)*	121 (43.8%)	61 (70.1%)	60 (31.7%)	35.6	<0.001
Nephropathy (%)*	97 (35.1%)	43 (49.4%)	54 (28.5%)	11.37	0.007
Neuropathy (%)	56 (20.2%)	20 (22.9%)	36 (19.04%)	0.57	0.45
Macrovascular complications Previous CVD (%)*	109 (39.5%)	71 (81.6%)	38 (20.1%)	94.3	<0.001
Stroke (%)	14 (5.07%)	7 (8.04%)	7 (3.7%)	2.33	0.13
Previous HA/use of HA drugs (%)*	213 (77.2%)	80 (91.95%)	138 (73.01%)	18.3	<0.001
Hyperlipidemia (%)*	218 (78.9%)	81 (93.1%)	132 (69.8%)	12.87	<0.001
Co-morbidity (*n*)*	4.66 ± 3.11	7.07 ± 3.22	3.55 ± 2.33	−8.15	<0.001
Depressive syndrome (%)	82 (29.7%)	25 (28.7%)	57 (30.2%)	0.06	0.81
Treatment Insulin (%)	130 (47.1%)	42 (48.2%)	88 (46.5%)	0.07	0.79
OAD (%)	222 (80.4%)	71 (81.6%)	151 (79.8%)	0.11	0.74
MoCA score*	25.6 ± 3.07	21.6 ± 1.5	27.4 ± 1.3	13.34	<0.001
BMI (kg/m^2)	29.9 ± 3.67	30.4 ± 3.59	29.6 ± 3.68	−1.92	0.054
Systolic blood pressure (mmHg)	136.2 ± 15.9	136.5 ± 16.4	136.05 ± 15.8	−0.25	0.79
Diastolic blood pressure (mmHg)	75 ± 7.9	75.1 ± 8.0	74.9 ± 7.8	−0.09	0.92
Fasting plasma glucose (mmol/l)	129.3 ± 26.1	129.8 ± 27.2	129.1 ± 25.6	−0.14	0.88
HbA1c (%)*	7.24 ± 0.68	7.73 ± 0.71	7.01 ± 0.54	−7.5	<0.001
Serum cholesterol (mmol/l)	10.3 ± 2.18	10.31 ± 2.2	10.29 ± 1.71	−0.5	0.61
Serum LDL-C (mmol/l)	6.06 ± 1.67	6.01 ± 1.64	6.08 ± 1.73	−0.2	0.86
Serum triglycerides (mmol/l)*	9.65 ± 2.23	10.59 ± 2.68	9.22 ± 1.84	−6.6	<0.001
Serum HDL-C (mmol/l)*	2.5 ± 0.51	2.3 ± 0.6	2.67 ± 0.42	6.34	<0.001
CRP (mg/L)*	5.08 ± 2.8	7.6 ± 2.7	3.9 ± 2.0	−9.79	<0.001
AGEs (ng/ml)*	1.4 ± 1.06	2.19 ± 1.12	1.04 ± 0.82	−8.1	<0.001
RAGE (ng/ml)*	2.67 ± 1.68	4.24 ± 1.89	1.94 ± 0.91	−9.7	<0.001

**Significance, $p < 0.05$; comparing patients with MCI and those without MCI (controls).*
T2DM, diabetes type 2; OAD, oral anti-diabetic drug; CVD, cardiovascular disease; HA, hypertension; BMI, body mass index; CHOL, total cholesterol; CRP, C-reactive protein; AGEs, advanced glycation end products; RAGE, receptor for advanced glycation end products; HbA1c, glycosylated hemoglobin; HDL-C, high-density lipoprotein cholesterol; LDL-C, low-density lipoprotein cholesterol; MoCA, Montreal Cognitive Assessment,
Data are mean – SD values. Mann–Whitney U test (Z), or χ^2 test was used to test for significant differences.

Serum RAGE, AGEs, and CRP in MCI and Controls

Serum RAGE and AGEs levels were significantly increased in MCI patients compared to controls ($p < 0.001$). As expected, in group of diabetic elderly patients with MCI serum RAGE level was positively correlated with AGEs level ($r = 0.85$, $p < 0.001$) and with CRP level ($r = 0.54$, $p < 0.001$) (**Figures 1A–C**). Furthermore, RAGE, AGEs, and CRP concentrations were highly correlated with HbA1c levels (**Figures 2A–C**). We found also positive but weak correlation between these parameters and triglycerides levels and negative correlation with HDL levels. The results indicated that MoCA score was negatively correlated with RAGE, AGEs, and CRP levels (**Figures 3A–C**). Data are presented in **Table 3**.

Logistic Regression Models

Because many factors can influence the results we constructed the univariate logistic regression models and finally multivariable regression model to determine the predictors of having MCI in elderly patients with type 2 diabetes. The independent variables entered in the model at step one were demographic variables (age, gender, education), duration of diabetes, glycemic control (HbA1c level), CVDs (MI, angina, stroke), cardiovascular risk factors (BMI, smoking status, hyperlipidemia, previous HA or use of HA drugs), microvascular complications, presence of depressive syndrome, number of co-morbid conditions, levels of total, LDL, HDL cholesterol, triglycerides, AGEs, RAGE, and CRP. The univariate logistic regression models revealed that variables which increased the likelihood of having been diagnosed with MCI in elderly patients with type 2 diabetes were higher levels of HbA1c, RAGE, AGEs, CRP, TG, lower level of HDL cholesterol, previous CVD, HA or use of HA drugs, hyperlipidemia, retinopathy, nephropathy, increased number of co-morbidities, older age, and less years of formal education (**Table 4**).

Table 5 shows the results of modeling the risk of having MCI by multivariable regression. All variables presented in **Table 3** were introduced to this model. The multivariable model was optimized by the stepwise approach. HA or use of HA drugs, previous CVD, higher level of RAGE and CRP, older age and less years of formal education are the factors increasing the likelihood of having MCI in elderly patients with type 2 diabetes.

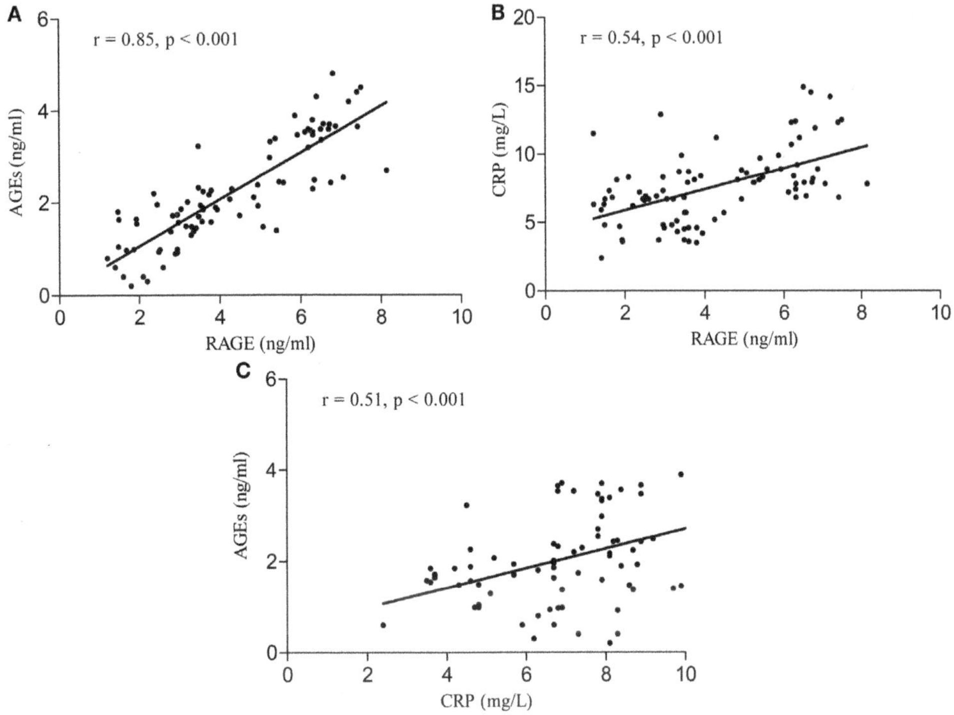

FIGURE 1 | (A) Correlation of RAGE with AGEs in group of diabetic elderly patients with MCI. **(B)** Correlation of RAGE with CRP in group of diabetic elderly patients with MCI. **(C)** Correlation of AGEs with CRP in group of diabetic elderly patients with MCI.

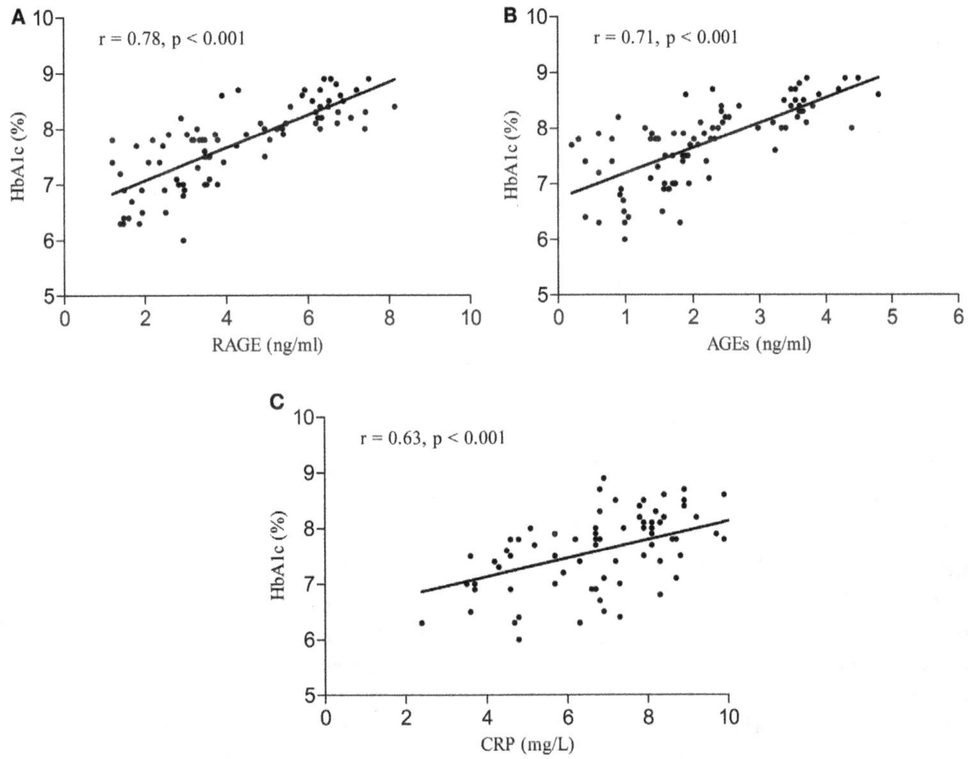

FIGURE 2 | (A) Correlation of HbA1c with RAGE in group of diabetic elderly patients with MCI. **(B)** Correlation of HbA1c with AGEs in group of diabetic elderly patients with MCI. **(C)** Correlation of HbA1c with CRP in group of diabetic elderly patients with MCI.

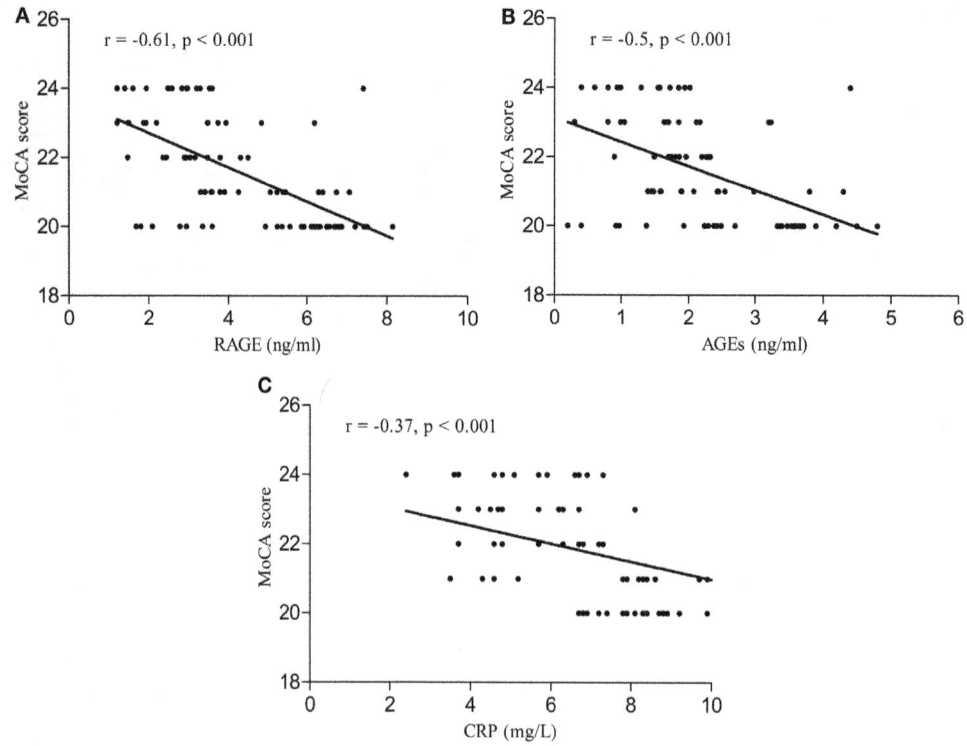

FIGURE 3 | (A) Correlation of MoCA score with RAGE in group of diabetic elderly patients with MCI. **(B)** Correlation of MoCA score with AGEs in group of diabetic elderly patients with MCI. **(C)** Correlation of MoCA score with CRP in group of diabetic elderly patients with MCI.

TABLE 3 | Relationship of serum levels of AGEs, RAGE, and CRP with other clinical indicators in group of diabetic elderly patients with MCI.

	AGEs	*p*	RAGE	*p*	CRP	*p*
	r		*r*		*r*	
MoCA score	−0.5	$p < 0.001$	−0.61	$p < 0.001$	−0.37	$p < 0.001$
HbA1c (%)	0.71	$p < 0.001$	0.78	$p < 0.001$	0.63	$p < 0.001$
Serum cholesterol (mmol/l)	0.1	0.33	0.12	0.25	0.35	0.001
Serum LDL-C (mmol/l)	0.06	0.6	0.08	0.43	0.27	0.01
Serum triglycerides (mmol/l)	0.26	0.014	0.37	$p < 0.001$	0.28	0.007
Serum HDL-C (mmol/l)	−0.2	0.056	−0.33	0.002	−0.19	0.06
AGEs (ng/ml)	1		0.85	$p < 0.001$	0.51	$p < 0.001$
RAGE (ng/ml)			1		0.54	$p < 0.001$
CRP (mg/l)					1	

**Significance, $p < 0.05$; r, correlation coefficient.*

BMI, body mass index; CHOL, total cholesterol; CRP, C-reactive protein; AGEs, advanced glycation end products; RAGE, receptor for advanced glycation end products; HbA1c, glycosylated hemoglobin; HDL-C, high-density lipoprotein cholesterol; LDL-C, low-density lipoprotein cholesterol; MoCA, Montreal Cognitive Assessment.

DISCUSSION

Our results show that patients with MCI had significantly higher CRP levels than controls. The increased CRP level is a predictor of cognitive impairment in elderly patients with type 2 diabetes. This result is consistent with recent reports. CRP – an acute-phase protein – is commonly used marker, which participates in low-grade inflammation in diabetes. It is mainly associated with the risk of DM complications. Other researchers had found serum levels of CRP were associated with cognition impairment and inversely correlated with MMSE and MoCA scores (Ge et al., 2013). In other studies, low-grade inflammation as reflected by serum CRP concentrations was found in subjects with cognitive dysfunction without dementia and in patients with non-amnestic MCI (Haan et al., 2008; Roberts et al., 2009). CRP is also associated with increased risk of CVD (Ridker et al., 1998). In our study, CRP as well as CVD is independent predictors of MCI in diabetic patients. Thus, the mechanism of the involvement of low-grade inflammation in cognitive impairment is not explained entirely by the presence of CVD in diabetic patients. CRP could initiate

TABLE 4 | Assessment results of the risk of having MCI in a simple logistic regression model in elderly patients with type 2 diabetes.

Variables analyzed	β	SE of β	*p*-value	OR	95% CI
Age (years)*	0.137	0.03	$p < 0.001$	1.15	1.08–1.22
Gender: female	0.2	0.1	0.12	1.2	0.49–1.59
Education (years)*	−0.639	0.09	$p < 0.001$	0.53	0.44–0.63
Smoked tobacco regularly	0.12	0.1	0.36	0.8	0.6–1.16
Duration of T2DM (years)*	0.097	0.02	$p < 0.001$	1.1	1.05–1.15
Previous stroke	0.41	0.27	0.14	1.5	0.87–2.58
Previous CVD*	1.43	0.16	$p < 0.001$	4.19	3.03–5.81
Previous HA or use of HA drugs*	0.88	0.22	$p < 0.001$	2.41	1.55–3.76
Hyperlipidemia*	0.72	0.21	0.001	2.01	1.35–3.12
Retinopathy*	0.8	0.14	$p < 0.001$	2.24	1.7–2.96
Nephropathy*	0.44	0.13	0.001	1.56	1.2–2.03
Neuropathy	0.11	0.01	0.45	1.12	0.82–1.53
Co-morbidity (*n*)*	0.426	0.05	$p < 0.001$	1.53	1.37–1.71
Depressive syndrome	0.03	0.01	0.8	0.96	0.73–1.27
BMI (kg/m^2)	0.058	0.03	0.1	1.06	0.98–1.13
HbA1c (%)*	1.69	0.23	$p < 0.001$	5.47	3.45–8.67
Serum cholesterol (mmol/l)	0.01	0.003	0.95	1.01	0.99–1.01
Serum LDL-C (mmol/l)	0.01	0.004	0.74	1.01	0.99–1.01
Serum triglycerides (mmol/l)*	0.02	0.004	$p < 0.001$	1.02	1.01–1.02
Serum HDL-C (mmol/l)*	−0.09	0.018	$p < 0.001$	0.91	0.87–0.94
CRP (mg/L)*	0.64	0.08	$p < 0.001$	1.9	1.62–2.22
AGEs (ng/ml)*	1.15	0.16	$p < 0.001$	3.17	2.31–4.34
RAGE (ng/ml)*	1.19	0.16	$p < 0.001$	3.28	2.42–4.45

**Significance, $p < 0.05$.*
β, regression coefficient; CI, confidence interval for odds ratio; OR, odds ratio; SE, standard error; T2DM, diabetes type 2; CVD, cardiovascular disease; HA, hypertension; BMI, body mass index; CHOL, total cholesterol; CRP, C-reactive protein; AGEs, advanced glycation end products; RAGE, receptor for advanced glycation end products; HbA1c, glycosylated hemoglobin; HDL-C, high-density lipoprotein cholesterol; LDL-C, low-density lipoprotein cholesterol.

TABLE 5 | Assessment results of the risk of having MCI in a multivariable logistic regression model in elderly patients with type 2 diabetes.

Variables analyzed	β	SE of β	*p*-value	OR	95% CI
Age (years)*	0.11	0.05	0.039	1.11	1.0–1.23
Education (years)*	−0.45	0.12	$p < 0.001$	0.64	0.5–0.82
Previous CVD*	1.2	0.24	$p < 0.001$	3.34	2.06–5.41
Previous HA or use of HA drugs*	1.24	0.41	0.002	3.48	1.56–7.76
CRP (mg/l)*	0.44	0.13	0.001	1.55	1.21–1.99
RAGE (ng/ml)*	0.67	0.23	0.004	1.95	1.24–3.06

**Significance, $p < 0.05$.*
β, regression coefficient; CI, confidence interval for odds ratio; OR, odds ratio; SE, standard error; CVD, cardiovascular disease; HA, hypertension; CRP, C-reactive protein; RAGE, receptor for advanced glycation end products.

immune cascade reactions leading to neurodegeneration via activating the complement system (Eagan et al., 2012).

Like CRP, AGEs–RAGE system stimulated by hyperglycemia could be responsible for the deterioration of cognition through an immune inflammatory pathway. AGEs – the products of non-enzymatic glycation on lysine and arginine residues accumulate in diabetic tissues – plays the important role in pathogenesis of diabetic complications. AGEs binds their receptor – RAGE and modulates cellular properties. Stimulation of RAGE results in activation of NADPH oxidase and generation of oxidation stress. Reactive oxygen species activate also formation of AGEs. In that way, the vicious circle is created – hyperglycemia induce AGEs generation, then after binding to RAGE increase oxidation stress and further production of AGEs (Kislinger et al., 1999; Wautier et al., 2001). Expression of RAGE is increased in CVD and in diabetes.

The frequency of cardiac events is higher and the progression of atherosclerosis is bigger in patients with diabetes compared to age-matched healthy controls. A lot of studies showed elevation of RAGE in diabetes and its association with diabetic complications and severity of the disease (Matsunaga-Irie et al., 2004; Yan et al., 2009). There are also data about increasing levels of AGEs with age and it is further enhancement by hyperglycemic state (Ulrich and Cerami, 2001). The interaction between AGEs and RAGE could result in higher inflammation in vascular wall via stimulation of oxidative stress. Activation of endothelial, smooth muscle cells and mononuclear phagocytes is highly associated with diabetic complications, such as nephropathy, retinopathy, and atherosclerosis (Schmidt et al., 2000b; Win et al., 2012).

Stimulation of RAGE play crucial role in the pathogenesis of T2DM and its complications, but RAGE is also an important cell-signaling receptor involved cognitive impairment. RAGE expression was found in different structures of the brain, in microglia, and astrocytes. In Alzheimer disease, RAGE expression was increased in inferior frontal cortex and hippocampus. The stimulation of RAGE in neurons can lead to increased inflammation through activation of the transcription faction NF-κB. In diabetes neuroinflammation, vascular injury and also activation of microglia could be driven by RAGE and the cascade of chemokines and cytokines (Lue et al., 2012).

In our study, AGEs and RAGE levels were significantly elevated in MCI subjects. The results are consistent with one study, which reported also higher level of AGEs in MCI subject with T2DM (Chen et al., 2011). The authors proposed possible the mechanism by which AGEs induce MCI in patients with type 2 diabetes. It is possible that AGEs stimulate endothelial dysfunction and followed the increased permeability of blood vessels. Thus, AGEs can accumulates in vascular wall and cause its injury. Other explanation could be higher inflammation and neural damage via inducing oxidative stress mediated by AGEs–RAGE interactions. AGEs could also activate microglia and destroy microtubular structure resulting in dysfunction of neurons (Chen et al., 2011).

In opposite to this result recent study was evaluated whether plasma levels of RAGE are altered in MCI and Alzheimer's disease. The authors did not found higher levels of RAGE in MCI but the study was performed among only 24 patients without vascular disease (only 16% of them had diabetes) (Marksteiner et al., 2014).

Expectedly, we found significant relationships between AGEs, RAGE, CRP, and glycosylated hemoglobin. Subjects with MCI had also more micro complications. Sustained hyperglycemia and development of diabetes complications can induce chronic low-grade inflammation and cell activation via AGEs–RAGE interaction. In agreement with our results, other studies reported that persistent hyperglycemia, indicated by elevated HbA1c, is an independent risk factor for the cognitive dysfunction (Ryan and Geckle, 2000).

In our previous work, we found that the presence of depressive syndrome is associated with higher levels of inflammatory markers in elderly patients with diabetes (Gorska-Ciebiada et al., 2015). Therefore, we put this parameter into logistic regression models; however, we revealed that the presence of depressive syndrome have no influence on the results.

Limitations

This study provides important insights into AGEs–RAGE system disturbances and low-grade inflammation pathologies underlying cognitive impairment in older diabetic patients; however, it is not without limitations. First, because our study population was relatively small, our results should be interpreted with caution. Second, the study was not designed as longitudinal prospective investigation. There have been few studies in which the cognitive declines in elderly diabetics were prospectively observed. However, the precise mechanisms underlying T2DM-related cognitive dysfunction or the development of dementia have not yet been elucidated. Furthermore, this investigation was limited to patients with diabetes, and therefore, an association between AGEs, RAGE, and CRP with other parameters in subjects without diabetes should also be assessed.

CONCLUSION

In summary, serum AGEs, RAGE, and CRP are increased in the circulation of MCI elderly diabetic patients compared to controls. Higher level of RAGE and CRP, HA or use of HA drugs, previous CVD, older age and less years of formal education are the factors increasing the likelihood of having MCI in elderly patients with type 2 diabetes. The precise mechanisms responsible for this finding are not entirely clear. A larger population-based prospective study needs to be performed to further confirm the relationship between AGEs, RAGE, and the cognitive decline or progress to dementia. As an option, targeting the AGEs–RAGE system in diabetes especially with cognitive impairments through specific pharmacologic interventions might result in a clinical benefit for these patients.

ACKNOWLEDGMENTS

The study was supported by non-profit grant of Medical University of Lodz no 502-03/8-072-03/502-64-052.

REFERENCES

Alagiakrishnan, K., Zhao, N., Mereu, L., Senior, P., and Senthilselvan, A. (2013). Montreal Cognitive Assessment is superior to standardized mini-mental status exam in detecting mild cognitive impairment in the middle-aged and elderly patients with type 2 diabetes mellitus. *Biomed Res. Int.* 11, 186106. doi:10.1155/2013/186106

Chen, G., Cai, L., Chen, B., Liang, J., Lin, F., Li, L., et al. (2011). Serum level of endogenous secretory receptor for advanced glycation end products and other factors in type 2 diabetic patients with mild cognitive impairment. *Diabetes Care* 34, 2586–2590. doi:10.2337/dc11-0958

Cukierman, T., Gerstein, H. C., and Williamson, J. D. (2005). Cognitive decline and dementia in diabetes – systematic overview of prospective observational studies. *Diabetologia* 48, 2460–2469. doi:10.1007/s00125-005-0023-4

Deane, R., and Zlokovic, B. V. (2007). Role of the blood-brain barrier in the pathogenesis of Alzheimer's disease. *Curr. Alzheimer Res.* 4, 191–197. doi:10.2174/156720507780362245

Eagan, D. E., Gonzales, M. M., Tarumi, T., Tanaka, H., Stautberg, S., and Haley, A. P. (2012). Elevated serum C-reactive protein relates to increased cerebral myoinositol levels in middle-aged adults. *Cardiovasc Psychiatry Neurol* 2012, 120540. doi:10.1155/2012/120540

Ge, X., Xu, X. Y., Feng, C. H., Wang, Y., Li, Y. L., and Feng, B. (2013). Relationships among serum C-reactive protein, receptor for advanced glycation products, metabolic dysfunction, and cognitive impairments. *BMC Neurol.* 13:110. doi:10.1186/1471-2377-13-110

Gorska-Ciebiada, M., Ciebiada, M., Barylski, M., and Loba, J. (2009). Diabetes mellitus in elderly according to new recommendations of Polish Diabetes Association. *Geriatria* 3, 147–150.

Gorska-Ciebiada, M., Saryusz-Wolska, M., Borkowska, A., Ciebiada, M., and Loba, J. (2015). Serum levels of inflammatory markers in depressed elderly patients with diabetes and mild cognitive impairment. *PLoS ONE* 10:e0120433. doi:10.1371/journal.pone.0120433

Gorska-Ciebiada, M., Saryusz-Wolska, M., Ciebiada, M., and Loba, J. (2014). Mild cognitive impairment and depressive symptoms in elderly patients with diabetes-prevalence, risk factors and co-morbidity. *J Diabetes Res* 2014, 179648. doi:10.1155/2014/179648

Haan, M. A., Aiello, A. E., West, N. A., and Jagust, W. J. (2008). C-reactive protein and rate of dementia in carriers and non carriers of apolipoprotein APOE4 genotype. *Neurobiol. Aging* 29, 1774–1782. doi:10.1016/j.neurobiolaging.2007.04.020

Hori, O., Yan, S. D., Ogawa, S., Kuwabara, K., Matsumoto, M., Stern, D., et al. (1996). The receptor for advanced glycation end-products has a central role in mediating the effects of advanced glycation end-products on the development of vascular disease in diabetes mellitus. *Nephrol. Dial. Transplant.* 11, 13–16. doi:10.1093/ndt/11.supp5.13

Katz, S., Downs, T. D., Cash, H. R., and Grotz, R. C. (1970). Progress in development of the index of ADL. *Gerontologist* 10, 20–30. doi:10.1093/geront/10.1_Part_1.20

Kislinger, T., Fu, C., Huber, B., Qu, W., Taguchi, A., Du Yan, S., et al. (1999). N(epsilon)-(carboxymethyl) lysine modifications of proteins are ligands for RAGE that activate cell signalling pathways and modulate gene expression. *J. Biol. Chem.* 274, 31740–31749. doi:10.1074/jbc.274.44.31740

Kumano-Kuramochi, M., Ohnishi-Kameyama, M., Xie, Q., Niimi, S., Kubota, F., Komba, S., et al. (2009). Minimum stable structure of the receptor for advanced glycation end product possesses multi ligand binding ability. *Biochem. Biophys. Res. Commun.* 386, 130–134. doi:10.1016/j.bbrc.2009.05.142

Lawton, M. P., and Brody, E. M. (1969). Assessment of older people: self-maintaining and instrumental activities of daily living. *Gerontologist* 9, 179–186. doi:10.1093/geront/9.3_Part_1.179

Lue, L. F., Andrade, C., Sabbagh, M., and Walker, D. (2012). Is there inflammatory synergy in type II diabetes mellitus and Alzheimer's disease? *Int. J. Alzheimers Dis.* 2012, 918680. doi:10.1155/2012/918680

Lue, L. F., Walker, D. G., Brachova, L., Beach, T. G., Rogers, J., Schmidt, A. M., et al. (2001). Involvement of microglial receptor for advanced glycation endproducts (RAGE) in Alzheimer's disease: identification of a cellular activation mechanism. *Exp. Neurol.* 171, 29–45. doi:10.1006/exnr.2001.7732

Marksteiner, J., Imarhiagbe, D., Defrancesco, M., Deisenhammer, E. A., Kemmler, G., and Humpel, C. (2014). Analysis of 27 vascular-related proteins reveals that NT-proBNP is a potential biomarker for Alzheimer's disease and mild cognitive impairment: a pilot-study. *Exp. Gerontol.* 50, 114–121. doi:10.1016/j.exger.2013.12.001

Matsunaga-Irie, S., Maruyama, T., Yamamoto, Y., Motohashi, Y., Hirose, H., Shimada, A., et al. (2004). Relation between development of nephropathy and the p22phox C242T and receptor for advanced glycation end product G1704T gene polymorphisms in type 2 diabetic patients. *Diabetes Care* 27, 303–307. doi:10.2337/diacare.27.2.303

Nasreddine, Z. S., Phillips, N. A., Bédirian, V., Charbonneau, S., Whitehead, V., Collin, I., et al. (2005). The Montreal Cognitive Assessment, MoCA: a brief screening tool for mild cognitive impairment. *J. Am. Geriatr. Soc.* 53, 695–699. doi:10.1111/j.1532-5415.2005.53221.x

Neeper, M., Schmidt, A. M., Brett, J., Yan, S. D., Wang, F., Pan, Y. C., et al. (1992). Cloning and expression of a cell surface receptor for advanced glycosylation end products of proteins. *J. Biol. Chem.* 267, 14998–15004.

Petersen, R. C. (2004). Mild cognitive impairment as a diagnostic entity. *J. Intern. Med.* 256, 183–194. doi:10.1111/j.1365-2796.2004.01388.x

Portet, F., Ousset, P. J., Visser, P. J., Frisoni, G. B., Nobili, F., Scheltens, P., et al. (2006). Mild cognitive impairment (MCI) in medical practice: a critical review of the concept and new diagnostic procedure. Report of the MCI Working Group of the European Consortium on Alzheimer's Disease. *J Neurol Neurosurg Psychiatry* 77, 714–718. doi:10.1136/jnnp.2005.085332

Ridker, P. M., Cushman, M., Stampfer, M. J., Tracy, R. P., and Hennekens, C. H. (1998). Plasma concentration of C-reactive protein and risk of developing peripheral vascular disease. *Circulation* 97, 425–428. doi:10.1161/01.CIR.97.5.425

Roberts, R. O., Geda, Y. E., Knopman, D. S., Boeve, B. F., Christianson, T. J., Pankratz, V. S., et al. (2009). Association of C-reactive protein with mild cognitive impairment. *Alzheimers Dement.* 9, 398–405. doi:10.1016/j.jalz.2009.01.025

Ryan, C. M., and Geckle, M. (2000). Why is learning and memory dysfunction in type 2 diabetes limited to older adults? *Diabetes Metab. Res. Rev.* 16, 308–315. doi:10.1002/1520-7560(2000)9999:9999<::AID-DMRR141>3.0.CO;2-X

Schmidt, A. M., Yan, S. D., Yan, S. F., and Stern, D. M. (2000a). The biology of the receptor for advanced glycation end products and its ligands. *Biochim. Biophys. Acta* 20, 99–111. doi:10.1016/S0167-4889(00)00087-2

Schmidt, A. M., Hofmann, M., Taguchi, A., Yan, S. D., and Stern, D. M. (2000b). RAGE: a multiligand receptor contributing to the cellular response in diabetic vasculopathy and inflammation. *Semin. Thromb. Hemost.* 26, 485–493. doi:10.1055/s-2000-13204

Schuitemaker, A., Dik, M. G., Veerhuis, R., Scheltens, P., Schoonenboom, N. S., Hack, C. E., et al. (2008). Inflammatory markers in AD and MCI patients with different biomarker profiles. *Neurobiol. Aging* 30, 1885–1889. doi:10.1016/j.neurobiolaging.2008.01.014

Strachan, M. W. J., Deary, I. J., Ewing, F. M. E., and Frier, B. M. (1997). Is type II diabetes associated with a decline in cognitive function? A critical review of published studies. *Diabetes Care* 20, 438–445. doi:10.2337/diacare.20.3.438

Ulrich, P., and Cerami, A. (2001). Protein glycation, diabetes, and aging. *Recent Prog. Horm. Res.* 56, 1–21. doi:10.1210/rp.56.1.1

Wautier, M. P., Chappey, O., Corda, S., Stern, D. M., Schmidt, A. M., and Wautier, J. L. (2001). Activation of NADPH oxidase by AGEs links oxidant stress to altered gene expression via RAGE. *Am. J. Physiol. Endocrinol. Metab.* 280, E685–E694.

Wild, S., Roglic, G., Green, A., Sicree, R., and King, H. (2004). Global prevalence of diabetes. Estimates for the year 2000 and projections for 2030. *Diabetes Care* 27, 1047–1053.

Win, M. T., Yamamoto, Y., Munesue, S., Saito, H., Han, D., Motoyoshi, S., et al. (2012). Regulation of RAGE for attenuating progression of diabetic vascular complications. *Exp. Diabetes Res.* 2012, 894605. doi:10.1155/2012/894605

Yaffe, K., Lindquist, K., Penninx, B. W., Simonsick, E. M., Pahor, M., Kritchevsky, S., et al. (2003). Inflammatory markers and cognition in well-functioning African-American and white elders. *Neurology* 61, 76–80. doi:10.1212/01.WNL.0000073620.42047.D7

Yan, S. F., Ramasamy, R., and Schmidt, A. M. (2009). Receptor for AGE (RAGE) & its ligands – cast into leading roles in diabetes & the inflammatory response. *J Mol Med (Berl)* 87, 235–247. doi:10.1007/s00109-009-0439-2

Yesavage, J., Brink, T., Rose, T., Lum, O., Huang, V., Adev, M., et al. (1982-1983). Development and validation of a geriatric depression screening scale: a preliminary report. *J. Psychiatr. Res.* 17, 37–49. doi:10.1016/0022-3956(82)90033-4

Permissions

All chapters in this book were first published in TMIABAN & BNARMI, by Frontiers; hereby published with permission under the Creative Commons Attribution License or equivalent. Every chapter published in this book has been scrutinized by our experts. Their significance has been extensively debated. The topics covered herein carry significant findings which will fuel the growth of the discipline. They may even be implemented as practical applications or may be referred to as a beginning point for another development.

The contributors of this book come from diverse backgrounds, making this book a truly international effort. This book will bring forth new frontiers with its revolutionizing research information and detailed analysis of the nascent developments around the world.

We would like to thank all the contributing authors for lending their expertise to make the book truly unique. They have played a crucial role in the development of this book. Without their invaluable contributions this book wouldn't have been possible. They have made vital efforts to compile up to date information on the varied aspects of this subject to make this book a valuable addition to the collection of many professionals and students.

This book was conceptualized with the vision of imparting up-to-date information and advanced data in this field. To ensure the same, a matchless editorial board was set up. Every individual on the board went through rigorous rounds of assessment to prove their worth. After which they invested a large part of their time researching and compiling the most relevant data for our readers.

The editorial board has been involved in producing this book since its inception. They have spent rigorous hours researching and exploring the diverse topics which have resulted in the successful publishing of this book. They have passed on their knowledge of decades through this book. To expedite this challenging task, the publisher supported the team at every step. A small team of assistant editors was also appointed to further simplify the editing procedure and attain best results for the readers.

Apart from the editorial board, the designing team has also invested a significant amount of their time in understanding the subject and creating the most relevant covers. They scrutinized every image to scout for the most suitable representation of the subject and create an appropriate cover for the book.

The publishing team has been an ardent support to the editorial, designing and production team. Their endless efforts to recruit the best for this project, has resulted in the accomplishment of this book. They are a veteran in the field of academics and their pool of knowledge is as vast as their experience in printing. Their expertise and guidance has proved useful at every step. Their uncompromising quality standards have made this book an exceptional effort. Their encouragement from time to time has been an inspiration for everyone.

The publisher and the editorial board hope that this book will prove to be a valuable piece of knowledge for researchers, students, practitioners and scholars across the globe.

List of Contributors

Antonio Zorzano
Molecular Medicine Program, Institute of Research in Biomedicine (IRB Barcelona), Barcelona, Spain
Departament de Bioquímica i Biologia Molecular, Facultat de Biologia, Universitat de Barcelona, Barcelona, Spain
CIBER de Diabetes y Enfermedades Metabólicas Asociadas, Instituto de Salud Carlos III, Barcelona, Spain

Marc Claret
CIBER de Diabetes y Enfermedades Metabólicas Asociadas, Instituto de Salud Carlos III, Barcelona, Spain
Diabetes and Obesity Research Laboratory, Institut d'Investigacions Biomèdiques August Pi i Sunyer, Barcelona, Spain

Shulan Hsieh
Cognitive Electrophysiology Laboratory: Control, Aging, Sleep, and Emotion (CASE), Department of Psychology, National Cheng Kung University, Tainan, Taiwan
Institute of Allied Health Sciences, National Cheng Kung University, Tainan, Taiwan

Mengyao Wu
Cognitive Electrophysiology Laboratory: Control, Aging, Sleep, and Emotion (CASE), Department of Psychology, National Cheng Kung University, Tainan, Taiwan
Department of Occupational Therapy, Shu-Zen Junior College of Medicine and Management, Kaohsiung, Taiwan

Chien-Hui Tang
Cognitive Electrophysiology Laboratory: Control, Aging, Sleep, and Emotion (CASE), Department of Psychology, National Cheng Kung University, Tainan, Taiwan

Amy Christensen and Christian J. Pike
Davis School of Gerontology, University of Southern California, Los Angeles, CA, USA

Xiangfei Hong
Shanghai Key Laboratory of Psychotic Disorders, Shanghai Mental Health Center, Shanghai Jiao Tong University School of Medicine, Shanghai, China
School of Biomedical Engineering, Shanghai Jiao Tong University, Shanghai, China

Yuelu Liu
Center for Mind and Brain, University of California, Davis, CA, USA

Junfeng Sun and Shanbao Tong
School of Biomedical Engineering, Shanghai Jiao Tong University, Shanghai, China

David A. S. Kaufman
Department of Psychology, Saint Louis University, St. Louis, MO, USA

Christopher N. Sozda
Department of Clinical and Health Psychology, University of Florida, Gainesville, FL, USA
Malcom Randall Veterans Administration Medical Center, Gainesville, FL, USA

Vonetta M. Dotson
Department of Clinical and Health Psychology, University of Florida, Gainesville, FL, USA

William M. Perlstein
Department of Clinical and Health Psychology, University of Florida, Gainesville, FL, USA
Malcom Randall Veterans Administration Medical Center, Gainesville, FL, USA
McKnight Brain Institute, University of Florida, Gainesville, FL, USA
Departments of Psychiatry, Saint Louis University, St. Louis, MO, USA
VA RR&D Brain Rehabilitation Research Center of Excellence, Malcom Randall Veterans Administration Medical Center, Gainesville, FL, USA

Bin-Yin Li and Hui-Dong Tang
Department of Neurology and Collaborative Innovation Center for Brain Science, Rui Jin Hospital Affiliated to Shanghai Jiao Tong University School of Medicine, Shanghai, China

Sheng-Di Chen
Department of Neurology and Collaborative Innovation Center for Brain Science, Rui Jin Hospital Affiliated to Shanghai Jiao Tong University School of Medicine, Shanghai, China
Laboratory of Neurodegenerative Diseases and Key Laboratory of Stem Cell Biology, Institute of Health Science, Shanghai Institutes for Biological Sciences, Chinese Academy of Science and Shanghai Jiao Tong University School of Medicine, Shanghai, China

Rommy von Bernhardi and Laura Eugenín-von Bernhardi
Department of Neurology, Faculty of Medicine, Pontificia Universidad Católica de Chile, Santiago, Chile

Jaime Eugenín
Laboratory of Neural Systems, Department of Biology, Faculty of Chemistry and Biology, Universidad de Santiago de Chile (USACH), Santiago, Chile

Angela Tam
McGill University, Montreal, QC, Canada
Douglas Mental Health University Institute, Research Centre, Montreal, QC, Canada
Centre de Recherche de L'institut Universitaire de Gériatrie de Montréal, Montreal, QC, Canada

Pierre Orban
Douglas Mental Health University Institute, Research Centre, Montreal, QC, Canada
Centre de Recherche de L'institut Universitaire de Gériatrie de Montréal, Montreal, QC, Canada

Christian Dansereau, AmanPreet Badhwar, Sylvie Belleville and Pierre Bellec
Centre de Recherche de L'institut Universitaire de Gériatrie de Montréal, Montreal, QC, Canada
Université de Montréal, Montreal, QC, Canada

Howard Chertkow, Amir Shmuel and Alain Dagher
McGill University, Montreal, QC, Canada

Alexandru Hanganu
Centre de Recherche de L'institut Universitaire de Gériatrie de Montréal, Montreal, QC, Canada
University of Calgary, Calgary, AB, Canada
Hotchkiss Brain Institute, Calgary, AB, Canada

Oury Monchi
Université de Montréal, Montreal, QC, Canada
University of Calgary, Calgary, AB, Canada
Hotchkiss Brain Institute, Calgary, AB, Canada

Pedro Rosa-Neto, Seqian Wang and John Breitner
McGill University, Montreal, QC, Canada
Douglas Mental Health University Institute, Research Centre, Montreal, QC, Canada

Saswati Paul and Jung-Soo Han
Department of Biological Sciences, Konkuk University, Seoul, South Korea

Won Kyung Jeon
Herbal Medicine Research Division, Korea Institute of Oriental Medicine, Daejeon, South Korea

Jennifer L. Bizon
Department of Neuroscience, College of Medicine, Evelyn F. and William L. McKnight Brain Institute, University of Florida, Gainesville, FL, USA

HyoungKyu Kim, Kwangsun Yoo, Jaeseung Jeong and Yong Jeong
Department of Bio and Brain Engineering, Korea Advanced Institute of Science and Technology, Daejeon, South Korea

Duk L. Na and Sang Won Seo
Department of Neurology, Samsung Medical Center, Sungkyunkwan University School of Medicine, Seoul, South Korea
Neuroscience Center, Samsung Medical Center, Seoul, South Korea

Weifang Cao, Yan Cheng Luo, Dezhong Yao and Changyue Hou
Key Laboratory for NeuroInformation of Ministry of Education, Center for Information in Medicine, High-Field Magnetic Resonance Brain Imaging Key Laboratory of Sichuan Province, School of Life Science and Technology, University of Electronic Science and Technology of China, Chengdu, China

Xinyi Cao, Cheng Luo and Lijuan Jiang
Shanghai Key Laboratory of Psychotic Disorders, Shanghai Mental Health Center, Shanghai Jiao Tong University School of Medicine, Shanghai, China

Ting Li
Shanghai Changning Mental Health Center, Shanghai, China

Chunbo Li
Shanghai Key Laboratory of Psychotic Disorders, Shanghai Mental Health Center, Shanghai Jiao Tong University School of Medicine, Shanghai, China
Bio-X Institutes, Key Laboratory for the Genetics of Developmental and Neuropsychiatric Disorders, Ministry of Education, Shanghai Jiao Tong University, Shanghai, China
Brain Science and Technology Research Center, Shanghai Jiao Tong University, Shanghai, China

Cátia F. Lourenço Ana Ledo and Cândida Dias
Center for Neuroscience and Cell Biology, University of Coimbra, Coimbra, Portugal

Rui M. Barbosa and João Laranjinha
Center for Neuroscience and Cell Biology, University of Coimbra, Coimbra, Portugal
Faculty of Pharmacy, University of Coimbra, Coimbra, Portugal

Yiwei Wang
Department of Clinical Pharmacy, School of Pharmacy, University of Southern California, Los Angeles, CA, USA

Roberta D. Brinton
Department of Pharmacology and Pharmaceutical Sciences, School of Pharmacy, University of Southern California, Los Angeles, CA, USA

David A. S. Kaufman and Cierra M. Keith
Department of Psychology, Saint Louis University, St. Louis, MO, USA

William M. Perlstein
Department of Clinical and Health Psychology, University of Florida, Gainesville, FL, USA
Department of Psychiatry, University of Florida, Gainesville, FL, USA
VA RR&D Brain Rehabilitation Research Center of Excellence, Malcom Randall Veterans Administration Medical Center, Gainesville, FL, USA

Paola Gamba, Gabriella Testa, Simona Gargiulo, Erica Staurenghi, Giuseppe Poli and Gabriella Leonarduzzi
Department of Clinical and Biological Sciences, School of Medicine, University of Turin, Orbassano, Torino, Italy

Ling Li and Dandan Zhao
Key Laboratory for NeuroInformation of Ministry of Education, School of Life Science and Technology, University of Electronic Science and Technology of China, Chengdu, China

Fernanda G. De Felice and Mychael V. Lourenco
Institute of Medical Biochemistry Leopoldo de Meis, Federal University of Rio de Janeiro, Rio de Janeiro, RJ, Brazil

Cheng Luo, Xingxing Zhang, Yulong Gan, Weifang Cao and Dezhong Yao
Key Laboratory for NeuroInformation of Ministry of Education, High-Field Magnetic Resonance Brain Imaging Key Laboratory of Sichuan Province, Center for Information in Medicine, School of Life Science and Technology, University of Electronic Science and Technology of China, Chengdu, China

Xinyi Cao, Yan Cheng and Lijuan Jiang
Shanghai Key Laboratory of Psychotic Disorders, Shanghai Mental Health Center, Shanghai Jiao Tong University School of Medicine, Shanghai, China

Ting Li
Changning Mental Health Center, Shanghai, China

Chunbo Li
Shanghai Key Laboratory of Psychotic Disorders, Shanghai Mental Health Center, Shanghai Jiao Tong University School of Medicine, Shanghai, China
Bio-X Institutes, Key Laboratory for the Genetics of Developmental and Neuropsychiatric Disorders, Ministry of Education, Shanghai Jiao Tong University, Shanghai, China

Malgorzata Gorska-Ciebiada, Malgorzata Saryusz-Wolska, Anna Borkowska, and Jerzy Loba
Department of Internal Medicine and Diabetology, Medical University of Lodz, Lodz, Poland

Maciej Ciebiada
Department of General and Oncological Pneumology, Medical University of Lodz, Lodz, Poland

Index

O

P

R

S

T

U

V

W

www.ingramcontent.com/pod-product-compliance
Lightning Source LLC
LaVergne TN
LVHW080946210926
848485LV00004B/778
* 9 7 8 1 6 3 9 8 9 0 8 5 9 *